Handbook of Emergency Response

Despite pre-emptive preparations, disasters can and do occur and are a fact of life. Whether natural disasters, catastrophic accidents, or terrorist attacks, the risk cannot be completely eliminated. A carefully prepared response is your best defense. This fully updated second edition of the *Handbook of Emergency Response* presents practical advice and guidelines on how to plan the coordinated execution of emergency response.

This handbook incorporates human factors and a systems engineering approach to emergency response project management. It provides cutting-edge research in developing a systematic structure for communication, cooperation, and coordination. Managing a project in the wake of a tragedy is complicated and involves various emotional, sentimental, reactive, and chaotic responses. This is the time when a structured communication model is most needed. This second edition includes important lessons learned and developments since the first edition was published, as well as additional information devoted to systems thinking and industrial engineering in planning for responses to emergencies. The reader will develop a thorough understanding of how to handle an emergency response using a systems approach.

The handbook is an ideal purchase for any student or practitioner of human factors, safety, systems engineering, events management, local or federal governance, or those in the emergency services.

LeeAnn Racz is a Supervising Engineer at ToxStrategies LLC in Fort Walton Beach, FL. Prior to this initiative, she was President and Founder of ClearView Environmental Engineering and Consulting, and she served for 23 years as a bioenvironmental engineer and civil engineer in the US Air Force. Dr Racz is a licensed professional engineer, certified industrial hygienist, and board-certified environmental engineer. She earned a BS in Environmental Engineering from California Polytechnic State University, San Luis Obispo, an MS in Biological and Agricultural Engineering from the University of Idaho, and a PhD in Civil and Environmental Engineering from the University of Utah. She has authored dozens of refereed journal articles, conference proceedings, magazine articles, and presentations, and edited six handbooks. Dr Racz is a member of several professional organizations and honor societies and has received numerous prestigious teaching and research awards.

Adedeji B. Badiru is Dean Emeritus and a retired Professor of Systems Engineering at the Air Force Institute of Technology (AFIT). He is a registered professional engineer and a fellow of the Institute of Industrial Engineers, as well as a fellow of the Nigerian Academy of Engineering. He has a BS degree in Industrial Engineering, an MS in Mathematics and an MS in Industrial Engineering from Tennessee University, and a PhD in Industrial Engineering from the University of Central Florida. He is the author of several books and technical journal articles and has received several awards and recognitions for his accomplishments. His special skills, experience, and interests center on research mentoring of faculty and graduate students.

ENVIRONMENTAL AND OCCUPATIONAL HEALTH SERIES

Series Editors:

LeeAnn Racz
Supervising Engineer, ToxStrategies LLC, Fort Walton Beach, Florida

Adedeji B. Badiru
Dean Emeritus, Graduate School of Engineering and Management, AFIT, Ohio

Handbook of Respiratory Protection:
Safeguarding Against Current and Emerging Hazards
LeeAnn Racz, Robert M. Eninger, and Dirk Yamamoto

Perfluoroalkyl Substances in the Environment:
Theory, Practice, and Innovation
David M. Kempisty, Yun Xing, and LeeAnn Racz

Total Health Exposure:
An Introduction
Kirk A. Phillips, Dirk P. Yamamoto, and LeeAnn Racz

Forever Chemicals:
Environmental, Economic, and Social Equity Concerns with PFAS in the Environment
David M. Kempisty and LeeAnn Racz

Environmental Ergonomics: Principles, Methods and Applications
Ken Parsons

Handbook of Emergency Response:
A Human Factors and Systems Engineering Approach, Second Edition
LeeAnn Racz and Adedeji B. Badiru

More Books Forthcoming

More about this series can be found at: https://www.crcpress.com/Environmental-and-Occupational-Health-Series/book-series/CRCENVOCCHEASER

Handbook of Emergency Response

A Human Factors and Systems Engineering Approach

Second Edition

Edited by
LeeAnn Racz
and Adedeji B. Badiru

CRC Press
Taylor & Francis Group
Boca Raton London New York

CRC Press is an imprint of the
Taylor & Francis Group, an **informa** business

Designed cover image: Getty Images

Second edition published 2026

by CRC Press
2385 NW Executive Center Drive, Suite 320, Boca Raton FL 33431

and by CRC Press
4 Park Square, Milton Park, Abingdon, Oxon, OX14 4RN

CRC Press is an imprint of Taylor & Francis Group, LLC

First edition published by CRC Press 2013

ISBN: 978-1-041-07348-2 (hbk)
ISBN: 978-1-041-09043-4 (pbk)
ISBN: 978-1-003-64817-8 (ebk)

DOI: 10.1201/9781003648178

Typeset in Times
by Deanta Global Publishing Services, Chennai, India

Contents

About the Editors

Adedeji Badiru is Dean Emeritus, Graduate School of Engineering and Management at the US Air Force Institute of Technology (AFIT). While serving as Dean, he had oversight for planning, directing, and controlling operations related to granting doctoral and master's degrees for the US Air Force. He was previously Professor and Head of Systems Engineering and Management at AFIT, Professor and Department Head of Industrial Engineering at the University of Tennessee, and Professor of Industrial Engineering and Dean of the University College at the University of Oklahoma. He is a registered Professional Engineer (PE), a certified Project Management Professional (PMP), a Fellow of the Institute of Industrial & Systems Engineers (IISE), a Fellow of the Industrial Engineering and Operations Management Society (IEOM), a Fellow of the Institute for Operations Research and Management Science (IORMS), and a Fellow of the Nigerian Academy of Engineering (Nigeria NAE). He is also a Program Evaluator for ABET. He holds a leadership certificate from the University Tennessee Leadership Institute. He has a BS in Industrial Engineering, an MS in Mathematics and an MS in Industrial Engineering from Tennessee Technological University, and a PhD in Industrial Engineering from the University of Central Florida. His areas of interest include mathematical modeling, systems design and integration, project management and optimization, innovation management, and productivity improvement. He is a prolific author, with over 45 books, over 40 book chapters, over 200 journal and magazine articles, and over 220 conference presentations. He is a member of several professional associations and scholastic honor societies. Professor Badiru, a world-renowned educator, has won several awards for his teaching, research, administrative, and professional accomplishments. He is the 2020 recipient of the Lifetime Achievement Award from Taylor and Francis publishing group. He was also a member of the AFIT team that won the 2019/2020 US Air Force Organizational Excellence Award. Professor Badiru is also the recipient of the 2022 BEYA career achievement award in the Government category and the 2024 Donald G. Newnan National Engineering Economy Teaching Excellence Award from the American Society for Engineering Education (ASEE). He also received the 2024 Tau Beta Pi Distinguished Alumnus award. He holds a US Trademark for the DEJI Systems Model for Design, Evaluation, Justification, and Integration. Badiru is a member of the Fulbright Specialists Program.

LeeAnn Racz is a supervising engineer at ToxStrategies LLC, where she consults on worldwide issues concerning risk from environmental and occupational hazards and exposures, including disasters and other emergencies. She has also been the President and Founder of ClearView Environmental Engineering and Consulting LLC, providing environmental and occupational health services to clients around the globe. Prior to her work as a consultant, she served for 23 years as a bioenvironmental engineer and civil engineer in the US Air Force, where she led responses to a myriad of emergencies, developed plans for natural and man-made disasters, and designed and conducted training for hundreds of other response personnel. Some highlights of Dr Racz's military assignments include squadron commander, Chief of Consultative Services at the US Air Force School of Aerospace Medicine, and Director of the Graduate Environmental Engineering and Science Program at AFIT. Dr Racz is a licensed Professional Engineer (PE), Certified Industrial Hygienist (CIH), and Board-Certified Environmental Engineer (BCEE). She is also a Program Evaluator for ABET. Dr Racz earned a BS in Environmental Engineering from California Polytechnic State University, San Luis Obispo, an MS in Biological and Agricultural Engineering from the University of Idaho, and a PhD in Civil and Environmental Engineering from the University of Utah. She has authored dozens of refereed journal articles, conference proceedings, magazine articles, presentations, and edited seven handbooks. Dr Racz is a member of several professional organizations and honor societies and has received numerous prestigious teaching and research awards.

List of Contributors

Adedeji B. Badiru
AB International Consulting Services
Beavercreek, OH

Lyle Burgoon
Raptor Pharm & Tox, Ltd.
New Hill, NC

Natasha Byrd
Utah Valley University
Provo, UT

Robert K. Campbell
Alliance Solutions Group
Newport News, VA

Damirson A. Co
University of Santo Tomas
Manila, Philippines

Stephan A. Devaux
Analytic Project Management
Waban, MA

Vinayak Dixit
University of New South Wales
Sydney, Australia

Amy G. Eddington
Utah Valley University
Provo, UT

John M. Flach
Wright State University
Perspicacity LLC
Beavercreek, OH

Alan C. Hale
ToxStrategies LLC
Dunkirk, MD

Brenda Jacklitsch
National Institute for Occupational Safety and Health
Cincinnati, OH

Tay Johannes
Air Force Institute of Technology
Wright-Patterson Air Force Base, OH

Cara Kneeland
Naval Air Force U.S. Pacific Fleet, U.S. Navy
San Diego, CA

Michael K. Lindell
Texas A&M University
College Station, TX

Chandini Raina MacIntyre
University of New South Wales
Sydney, Australia

Ann Marie Major
Pennsylvania State University
University Park, PA

Charlie A. Marquez
University of Santo Tomas
Manila, Philippines

David A. McEntire
Utah Valley University
Provo, UT

Brandon A. Miller
Oak Ridge National Laboratory
Knoxville, TN

Ahmed Usman Naibi
DGNB Consultants
Nigeria

Khalilat Usman Naibi
Federal Ministry of Innovation, Science, and Technology
Nigeria

Olufemi A. Omitaomu
Oak Ridge National Laboratory
Knoxville, TN

LeeAnn Racz
ToxStrategies LLC
Fort Walton Beach, FL

Melanie Robison
Utah Valley University
Provo, UT

Brian D. Simpson
U.S. Air Force Research Laboratory
Wright-Patterson Air Force Base, OH

Nagendra Singh
Oak Ridge National Laboratory
Knoxville, TN

Aisha Tarfa
AB International Consulting Services
Brandenburg an der Havel, Germany

W. Jon Williams
National Institute for Occupational Safety and Health
Pittsburgh, PA

Brian Wolshon
Louisiana State University
Baton Rouge, LA

Preface

Disasters are a fact of life. Natural disasters, catastrophic accidents, and terrorist attacks have the potential to present risks to health, property, and life as we know it. Preparation is key to responding to such disasters. Rapid response, effective information flow, leveraging social media, and first-responder coordination are essential for providing critical medical services to victims, recovering key services and infrastructure, and restoring order to chaos.

This two-part handbook presents an integrative guide for emergency response project management following emergencies resulting from accidental, man-made, or natural disasters. The collection of chapters is an update to the first edition and provides a mix of human factors and systems engineering approaches. Part 1 includes chapters that present organizational and planning issues central to emergency response, as well as their solutions. Important concepts in Part 1 include organizational resiliency, creating effective response communications, risk communication, critical path drag, evacuation planning, damage assessment, biosecurity threats, responding to radiation incidents, and understanding the impacts of heat. Part 2 focuses on human factors and management considerations, including discussions on environmental considerations. In particular, Part 2 presents topics such as coordinated project management, systems models in emergency response, emergency response process improvement, learning curve implications, and environmental factors associated with emergencies.

Coordinated response plans are essential in emergencies. The interdependencies of factors make a modern systems approach imperative for a harmonized and effective emergency response. This handbook provides an important guide for organizations as they prepare for emergencies before crises occur.

Part I

Organizational and Planning Solutions

1 Resilient Organizations Overcome Challenges to Unified Response

Robert K. Campbell

1.1 INTRODUCTION

Emergency response continues to mature as our nation captures lessons learned, improves the National Frameworks, adopts the National Incident Management System, implements resource typing and the National Qualification System, and continuously improves capabilities through the National Preparedness System. However, response operations are locally executed, state-managed, and federally supported. While the federal government, through the Federal Emergency Management Agency (FEMA), has established robust doctrines for conducting preparedness activities and response, the emergency response operations and coordination begin locally. There are many obstacles to effective emergency response, such as lack of preparedness, resilience, resources, operational coordination, etc. However, arguably the most critical obstacle remains the lack of unified response operations among responders, which is driven by human factors. This chapter explores the internal and external challenges and influences that determine an organization's ability to achieve a unified response. Resilient organizations have the ability to overcome many of these challenges, and establishing resilience through several decisive actions during the pre-incident phase is essential. For this reason, this chapter will focus heavily on leadership responsibilities, pre-incident preparedness, and building resilience in addition to typical response mission area tactics.

Over the last 20 years, there have been a series of monumental incidents that have revealed challenges in responders' ability to successfully respond to an incident. Many of these have been uncovered in after-action reports, legislative changes, and updates to important emergency management doctrine.

- 9/11 revealed the lack of interoperable communication systems among different disciplines.
- Hurricane Katrina revealed the lack of integration and unity among all levels of government to swiftly respond.
- Hurricane Maria revealed competing political interests and inconsistent priorities between the local, territory, and federal governments.

DOI: 10.1201/9781003648178-2

- The Arkema Chemical disaster in the aftermath of Hurricane Harvey revealed the lack of operational coordination between the incident command (fire) and law enforcement (members were exposed to hazardous chemical combustion byproducts while driving through the isolation zone).
- Initial response to the West Fertilizer Company incident revealed that despite having been trained and certified in the incident command system (ICS), initial responders failed to establish incident command, coordinate priorities, and make timely decisions to evacuate the area.
- Local, state, and federal responses to the Ebola virus and COVID-19 demonstrated the confusing effects of inconsistent and contradictory risk communication to the public.
- The East Palestine train derailment highlighted the challenges facing rural and tribal community first responders when faced with an overwhelming incident that requires organizing, directing, and coordinating primarily external resources from surrounding counties, state, federal, and rail/private organizations.

This chapter begins with an overview of the types of incidents emergency responders face before introducing various challenges to unified response operations. It concludes with an examination of solutions for overcoming these challenges, such as crisis-ready leadership, building resilience, strategies, preparedness activities, and implementation.

1.2 SPECTRUM OF INCIDENTS

The escalating scale and scope of response operations require response core capabilities such as operational coordination and adherence to the National Incident Management System. There are 15 FEMA response core capabilities designed to address various threats and hazards. **Incidents** result from the fruition of threats or hazards. A **threat** is a "natural, technological, or human-caused occurrence, individual, entity, or action that has or indicates the potential to harm life, information, operations, the environment, and/or property" (FEMA 2006). A **hazard** is "something that is potentially dangerous or harmful, often the root cause of an unwanted outcome" (FEMA 2006). While hazards exist throughout our communities, they are often controlled or limited in a way that yields a benefit while outweighing the risk of an adverse outcome. Threats and hazards may be natural, technological, or human-caused. Our risk profile associated with threats and hazards continues to evolve. This evolution is driven by climate change, geopolitical circumstances, advances in technology, and an increase in vulnerabilities from aging infrastructure, population growth, changing demographics, and lack of adequate capacity for essential services and utilities. According to the 2023 National Preparedness Report, the greatest capability gaps are in Fire Management and Suppression; Logistics and Supply Chain Management; Public Health, Healthcare, and Emergency Medical Services (EMS); and Long-Term Vulnerability Reduction core capabilities (FEMA 2023b). In 2019, rural and tribal jurisdictions cited the greatest gaps in Operational Coordination,

Operational Communications, Planning, and Long-Term Vulnerability Reduction (Lang 2019).

The Operational Coordination core capability is described by FEMA as, "Establish and maintain a unified and coordinated operational structure and process that appropriately integrates all critical stakeholders and supports the execution of Core Capabilities."

The Long-Term Vulnerability core capability is described by FEMA as, "Build and sustain resilient systems, communities, and critical infrastructure and key resources lifelines so as to reduce their vulnerability to natural, technological, and human-caused threats and hazards by lessening the likelihood, severity, and duration of the adverse consequences."

The spectrum of incidents is a way of describing the scale of incidents that responders encounter. An **incident** is

> an occurrence, natural or human-caused, that requires a response to protect life or property. Incidents can, for example, include major disasters, emergencies, terrorist attacks, terrorist threats, civil unrest, wildland and urban fires, floods, hazardous materials spills, nuclear accidents, aircraft accidents, earthquakes, hurricanes, tornadoes, tropical storms, tsunamis, war-related disasters, public health and medical emergencies, and other occurrences requiring an emergency response.
>
> **(FEMA 2006)**

Therefore, threats and hazards can lead to incidents when the risk occurs. As an incident escalates in scale, so does the number and type of responders involved in the incident.

An abnormal event is an incident that can be handled internally by an organization. For example, a small spill of formaldehyde by a laboratory technician can be handled with a locally available spill kit and a trained technician with personal protective equipment (PPE). A small grease fire at a local restaurant may be extinguished by a trained cook with an ABC-rated fire extinguisher. However, once an incident escalates or presents a risk that cannot be managed internally, someone declares an emergency by dialing 9-1-1, calling upon responders, and seeking external resources.

An **emergency** is "any incident, whether natural, technological, or human-caused, that requires responsive action to protect life or property" (FEMA 2006). Small, defined emergencies may only require a single-discipline response, such as a fire department responding to a fire. But as the scale and scope of the emergency grows, it may require a multidisciplinary response. For example, a rail accident may involve fire, law enforcement, emergency medical services, hazardous material response, and rail response teams. For larger incidents, responders from outside of the local area may be called upon, or the incident might impact multiple jurisdictions, as may be the case with a flood or tornado. Multidiscipline, multiagency response operations can be complex and present numerous challenges to the incident commander, who must integrate responders into the ICS in accordance with the National Incident Management System (NIMS). While an incident commander may have authority over those from within his jurisdiction, there may be limits and constraints on how he may employ resources from other agencies and jurisdictions. This can be particularly challenging for small, rural jurisdictions as was the case in the West Texas and East Palestine incidents cited earlier. In both cases, incident commanders were highly dependent on external resources and responders that were not owned by their jurisdiction, but they had the authority (and liability) for incident management. An emergency can escalate into a crisis when reaching a decision or tipping point with rapidly increasing severity or destabilization.

Farazmand (2001) defines a **crisis** as follows:

> Crises involve events and processes that carry severe threat, uncertainty, an unknown outcome, and urgency. … Most crises have trigger points so critical as to leave historical marks on nations, groups, and individual lives. Crises are historical points of reference, distinguishing between the past and the present. … Crises come in a variety of forms, such as terrorism (New York World Trade Center and Oklahoma bombings), natural disasters (Hurricanes Hugo and Andrew in Florida, the Holland and Bangladesh flood disasters), nuclear plant accidents (Three-Mile Island and Chernobyl), riots (Los Angeles riot and the Paris riot of 1968, or periodic prison riots), business crises, and organizational crises facing life-or-death situations in a time of rapid environmental change. … Crises consist of a 'short chain of events that destroy or drastically weaken' a condition of equilibrium and the effectiveness of a system or regime within a period of days, weeks, or hours rather than years. … Surprises characterize the dynamics of crisis situations. … Some crises are processes of events leading to a level of criticality or degree of intensity generally out of control. Crises often have past origins and diagnosing their original sources can help to understand and manage a particular crisis or lead it to alternative state of condition.

The key characteristics of a crisis are uncertainty, technical complexity, high severity, potential for large-scale engagement, multifaceted, secondary effects, and urgency. An escalating emergency that encounters a crisis that is not resolved or contained can lead to a disaster.

A **disaster** is "an occurrence of a natural catastrophe, technological accident, or human-caused event that has resulted in severe property damage, deaths, and/or multiple injuries" (FEMA 2006). Disasters require the mobilization of national and international resources to respond and recover, and often take extended time periods to fully recover and restore communities to their pre-incident status. Disasters are particularly deleterious to impoverished populations as they usually live in vulnerable locations, lack the financial and social resources to sustain themselves outside of their homes, and require outside assistance for basic needs. Additionally, there are several other socially vulnerable populations that require further consideration when building a culture of preparedness throughout the community. Factors to consider include: non-English speakers, literacy, age (i.e., elderly and children), accessibility to transportation, and physical and mental disabilities, among many others (Campbell 2023). FEMA has identified 21 factors that comprise the community resilience challenges index based on researching multiple similar indices and considering their impact on outcomes.

Before moving on to the next section, it is worth mentioning the five mission areas of emergency management and how they correspond to the phases of an incident. The five mission areas are: prevention, protection, mitigation, response, and recovery. These are often thought to be stove-piped because they are different "areas" and have their own "framework" under the National Frameworks. Nevertheless, it is important to highlight that these mission areas have considerable overlap and interdependencies. Despite this chapter's focus on "unified response," emergency managers and responders need to be engaged across all mission areas. For example, building prevention and mitigation capabilities can reduce the capacity needed during response operations. Under the National Recovery Framework, recovery begins pre-incident by establishing recovery outcomes and coordination between concurrent response and recovery operations; they are not distinct, sequential phases of the incident. Overcoming challenges to unified response begins pre-incident with planning, operational coordination and communication, and preempting incident impacts through prevention, protection, and mitigation. Building resilience in a community and its infrastructure can also reduce the need for response. Minimizing the need for response and quickly navigating from response to recovery reduces the adverse impact on lives, property, the environment, and the economy. But if a response is not unified due to a lack of pre-incident foundation, response operations may be prolonged.

1.3 CHALLENGES TO UNIFIED RESPONSE OPERATIONS

There are numerous challenges to unified response operations. Over many years of consulting, planning, training, and exercising with diverse businesses of all sizes, local, state, and federal governments, military, and international clients, we have compiled thousands of observations that form the basis of the challenges listed below. While comprehensive, there are certainly more challenges than can reasonably be covered in this chapter; this chapter focuses on the most salient challenges that need attention. This section will explore these challenges in no particular order. The purpose of this section is to highlight the challenges in order to frame the discussion and solutions needed.

1.3.1 Size

As outlined in the above section, the size, scope, and scale of the incident drives the need for multidiscipline, multijurisdiction response operations. The ICS provides an organizational framework for responders. The Emergency Operations Center (EOC) provides a coordination center for various emergency support functions (ESFs). Both structures are important to operational coordination and communication. In addition to the ICS organizational structure, larger responses will also require communication systems such as common operating pictures, audio/video communication systems, joint information centers, and public alerting/warning systems. Span of control can become a significant challenge as the size of the operation grows. Proactive and regular communication becomes more important to ensure command and control of the situation.

In the aftermath of the West Fertilizer incident, Frank Patterson established an incident command to handle the destruction of part of the community from the fertilizer-grade ammonium nitrate explosion and subsequent fire at the West Fertilizer Company. During his tenure as incident commander, many volunteers and state and federal agencies appeared on scene, offering both assistance and attempting to take control of the incident. His frequent communications and updates to everyone involved helped maintain control as other mobile command posts appeared despite their lack of authority or involvement in the actual response. Frequent communication from the incident commander to update the responders on the situation ensured that he maintained command and control of the response operation (Campbell 2023).

1.3.2 Staffing

Another challenge to response operations is the number and type of staff available to support response operations and coordination. In many rural communities, it is not uncommon for emergency managers and responders to delay establishing an EOC due to a lack of staffing. When an EOC is established, the staff in the EOC performs multiple roles, filling more than one ESF. Responders on scene focus on operations with less emphasis on logistics and planning, as the priority is controlling and containing the incident. Staff bandwidth constrains what activities responders can undertake and how quickly they can execute the mission. Additionally, many rural communities are served by volunteer responders who often have jobs in industry, agriculture, or mining. While these volunteers are just as dedicated as their career counterparts, they often lack the ability to take extra time off work from their primary jobs to complete the extensive training that their career, full-time counterparts are afforded. This often results in a lower level of training and competency (e.g., Hazmat Awareness vs Hazmat Operations), which limits their ability to respond offensively to more complex, severe incidents. These situations require the deployment of external teams to support offensive response operations required to contain and control an incident.

1.3.3 Resource Limitations

All communities face resource limitations based on available funding, equipment, staffing, facilities, and external parties such as debris removal teams, contractors, utility responders, and state resources. Community leaders operate their jurisdictions on a fixed budget and must make risk-based budgetary decisions to best serve their community. This requires risk acceptance as it is impossible to fund measures to prevent and mitigate against every risk. Small jurisdictions inherently operate on small budgets yet face many of the same threats and hazards that larger jurisdictions face. This challenge drives the need for wise prioritization of limited resources.

1.3.4 Equipment Compatibility and Interoperability

As technology advances, responders use and interface with an increasing variety of technologies and tools within the teams and among supporting response elements. Some of these technologies include communication systems (e.g., common operating systems, cursor-on-target, radio networks to include encryption, GPS, computer networks for information sharing, emergency alerting and notification systems, etc.); unmanned systems such as ground-based robots, boats and submersibles, and aircraft; hazardous materials sensors; personal protective equipment; heavy equipment for debris removal. Each technology performs a unique function. Within each type of equipment or technology, there are many vendors, models, and designs, which may not be compatible with competitor products or the communications infrastructure used by responders. For example, unmanned aircraft systems (UAS) use a variety of radio frequencies to operate and send data back to the ground station. Deconflicting the radio frequencies used by various technologies and communication devices can present several challenges, especially when external teams arrive on the scene to assist with operations. While these technologies have come a long way in exporting data in common formats and protocols so that it can be shared and imported into common operating pictures, a classic example of incompatibility was an early attempt to use a UAS in response and recovery to a hazmat derailment.

Case Study: In 2012, a shipment of hazardous materials derailed in Jefferson County, Kentucky. The derailment occurred on the side of a mountain in an area that was difficult to reach or view. While responders and contractors deployed to clean up the spill, the incident commander needed a way to observe and monitor the activities. When a fire ignited after contractors attempted to move a car containing butadiene, a flammable substance, the incident commander authorized the use of a UAS to provide enhanced situational awareness as the fire threatened an adjacent car containing hydrogen fluoride. He employed an Aerion Datron Scout UAS operated by a contractor. While this was one of the first-known UAS applications in a hazmat incident, there were several lessons learned related to interoperability. First, the UAS could not stream video to unsupported ground stations. Second, video data was stored on an SD card that was onboard the UAS. After returning from its mission, the video file would be downloaded from the SD card and then shared. Third, the video format was not compatible with video viewers in use by the jurisdiction, so the file format had to be converted. The UAS industry has come a long way since these lessons were learned. Most UAS are capable of streaming video in compatible formats to ground stations for further export and sharing. However, some issues remain, such as ownership of the data, export of the video and flight data to servers in foreign countries, proprietary navigation systems and software, compatibility among UAS when used together, and regulatory restrictions and waivers for use in public safety operations. Some states have banned the use of certain foreign-manufactured UAS over data security concerns, which continues to raise challenges for users.

Other equipment compatibility and interoperability concerns stem from long-standing communication systems, such as radios, encryption, access, and interoperability among responders to monitor and communicate with each other. With different manufacturers and technologies in use among response teams, the lack of operational communication can frustrate the unity of effort and teamwork in response operations.

An analysis of environmental, health, and safety risks during the 9/11 response highlighted problems with worker exposure to asbestos, heavy metals, silica, and other inhalation hazards from smoke, dust, and debris operations. Few workers wore respiratory protection. Those responders that did wear respirators found replacement cartridges in short supply, and those that were available were often incompatible with the specific respirators in use. Today, response organizations are standardizing equipment and PPE to realize savings and maximize interoperability within their communities. However, not all PPE and respiratory protection devices are compatible as they are certified as a complete system by the manufacturer.

Detection systems used in hazmat response operations are also manufacturer-specific, and consumable supplies are often restricted to use with the manufacturer's equipment for good reasons. Product-specific limitations, cross-sensitivities, and procedures make it challenging for responders to employ multiple detection devices with consistency and compatibility during response operations. Generic sensors such as photo-ionization detectors, flame ionization detectors, and Geiger-Müller detectors provide responders with quantified hazard response concentrations or dose, respectively, but without proper calibration or identification of the specific chemical or isotope, the quantified output could be misleading. Responders employing similar products from different manufacturers may receive widely varying results, which appear in conflict. For example, the Rae Systems MultiRae® gas detector utilizes electrochemical sensors similar to the Industrial Scientific SafeCore® multigas detector. However, differences in software and sensitivity can yield different results. The MultiRae software had a tendency to over-respond to a hazard before settling down to the actual concentration over time, whereas the SafeCore software is tuned for more accurate responses but may experience an apparent delay in response as the output concentration approaches the actual concentration. Likewise, the SafeCore software may be slower to recover after the sensor is exposed to hazards. This phenomenon was reported during 60 trials and comparative analysis at Dugway Proving Ground, Utah, during Technology Experimentation and Characterization Field Trials (TECFT) 2020 when testing and evaluating Alliance Solutions Group, Inc.'s ArgusElite® Hazmat UAS (Campbell 2020). These phenomena are not wrong, but rather, they illustrate differences in how the product was designed to serve its customers. This example highlights the need to understand the capabilities, limitations, compatibility of hardware and software, and differences in equipment outputs used in operational decision-making.

Standardization of equipment across responders may seem like the solution, as FEMA-driven resource typing strives to ensure standardized capabilities. A US Air Force project solicited recommendations for standardization of all detection equipment located at all installations. This effort entailed reviewing 15,000 line items of equipment at 80+ installations and making recommendations for selecting and achieving a standardized equipment set for each installation to procure. There are many benefits to this approach (e.g., standardized logistics, power needs during deployments, training, and lifecycle management). However, there are also some pitfalls to be avoided. Each community faces different hazards. In this example, there are various industries in each community that use different chemicals that could pose a threat, requiring detection, identification, quantification, and risk-based decision-making. Allowing some flexibility within the standardization process to ensure localization of capabilities to address localized risks should be considered as it was during this project.

1.3.5 Personnel Qualifications and Credentialing

As mentioned earlier in the context of differing levels of hazmat training and certification between volunteer and career firefighters, teams may adopt different standards for competency, training, and certification. One common difference is the certification body for hazmat response training. While all hazmat responders are required to comply with Occupational Safety and Health Administration (OSHA) HAZWOPER regulations, public safety responders tend to gravitate towards International Fire Service Accreditation Congress (IFSAC) certification, while private sector responders tend to adopt the Pro-Board certification. The challenge arises when integrating private and public sector hazmat teams in a response and recognizing that there may be some differences in the competency of these teams based on their training and certifications. This issue also extends into emergency medical technician training and certification. The challenge for the incident commander lies in understanding how he can employ different resources during response operations without compromising public and responder safety.

Furthermore, the issue of different certifications complicates the credentialing process. As teams arrive on scene and they are vetted for competence, some organizations may have a discipline-centric view on the issue of acceptable certifications and could inadvertently dismiss some credentialed responders because of the lack of alignment with their certification. Credentialing is an important part of the integration process because it assures responders that their team members are competent and trained to perform their assigned tasks.

1.3.6 Politics, Power, and Pride

Political interests of different organizations play a factor in the lack of integrated response operations. Competing interests unfortunately take precedence over providing swift aid to those in need. While most government organizations have accountability systems in place, some developing nations rely heavily on nongovernmental organizations (NGOs) such as the UN, Red Cross, Red Crescent, and others. While there are many reputable NGOs capable and interested in providing relief and aid, some are biased or have alternative interests that inhibit an integrated response operation.

In Eastern Afghanistan, after the April 2009 earthquake, it took the provincial government about 30 days to respond with assistance to affected communities. Additionally, some NGOs were reluctant to share their capabilities and resources with the government to protect their autonomy and ability to respond in a way that advanced their mission. For example, the Afghan Red Crescent touts its neutrality as an organization that cannot be seen as siding with militants, the government, or foreign militaries. Therefore, they choose efficacious and opportune situations to respond and provide support based on their capabilities and resources. NGOs also derive their funding and resources based on the publication of their accomplishments during a response. This independence precludes them from effectively coordinating with the government in a way that optimizes the overall response operations. Therefore, the government often does not know where NGO resources are providing aid to disaster victims. Each organization vies for recognition by being able to meet the needs of disaster victims without coordination or sharing of information and resources. This makes it extremely difficult for the government to know the real-time needs of disaster victims and stage a coordinated response operation that employs the most appropriate organization in the right place based on proximity and capability. Finally, in some cases, disaster response resources are misappropriated by local leaders, precluding effective distribution to those in need. This results in a false sense of accomplishment for those leaders who provided the resources to a certain district or village. Deployment of aid in developing countries like Afghanistan continues to be a major organizational challenge due to political factors.

The more recent example related to Hurricane Maria illustrates how power, politics, and media may thwart efforts to establish a unified response. In the aftermath of Hurricane Maria, the governor of Puerto Rico used the media to disparage the federal response effort, claiming that they lacked food and water. Meanwhile, adequate food and water supplies existed on the island, but the lack of distribution and management of these supplies exacerbated the situation as pallets of water sat in warehouses. The island had a more pressing issue. Power and communications systems had been disabled during the disaster, making coordination nearly impossible. Lack of power also contributed to an inability to resume cell tower operations, refrigerate medicines, and provide air conditioning for residents exposed to heat. While FEMA marshaled a response to Puerto Rico's requests for assistance, power politics affected how they prioritized and delivered aid. Instead of delivering teams of utility experts to resurrect the disabled power grid and communications systems, they delivered more water at the behest of the local government and building media pressure. This example not only highlights the importance of unity of effort but also underscores the importance of local preparedness, plans, and organic capabilities in stabilizing disrupted services that are essential to normal operations within a community.

The Community Lifelines toolkit was established by FEMA after this hurricane season to provide a process for evaluating and communicating the status of disrupted lifelines to senior leaders in an effort to prioritize resource allocation. FEMA created Community Lifelines to reframe incident information, understand and communicate incident impacts using plain language, and promote unity of effort across the whole community to prioritize efforts to stabilize the lifelines during incident response (FEMA 2023a).

Organizational pride can also stymie unified response operations. Teams that train together, build trusting relationships among team members, and develop a sense of organizational pride are often resistant to sharing information, allowing outsiders into their team, and providing resources where they become dependent on integration with other teams. This example is clearly illustrated by Gen. (ret.) Stanley McChrystal in his book *Team of Teams*, where he explains how he overcame insular attitudes among many of the coalition's most elite yet stove-piped organizations in the fight against Al-Qaeda in Iraq (McChrystal 2015). This challenge is real at all levels of government and in the business community. As teams progress through storming, norming, and forming, team identity and pride become a challenge to integrating with other teams in a way that ensures successful leveraging of resources. This is usually apparent to me when we run exercises for our clients.

As multiple disciplines and agencies come together to participate in an exercise, we commonly observe a propensity for decision-makers to resist the integration of external resources into the ICS and their operations. There may be some good reasons for this reluctance as explained above in the section on credentialing. Usually, this conflict becomes apparent when we get to the point in a hazmat exercise where the responsible party has been conducting initial response operations, and the first responding fire department arrives on scene and begins forming the ICS without including the responsible party's team of responders. This usually leads to a discussion on credentialing, training, standards, and unified command. Next, we often observe law enforcement participation occurring in a stove-pipe, and not as part of the ICS. When specialized teams such as regional hazmat teams or rail incident responders arrive on the scene, either the incident commander wants to hand off incident command or struggles to integrate these teams where they traditionally belong (in the Hazmat Group under the Operations Section).

Unified response operations are not easy to implement. Trust plays an important factor, but organizational pride creates some artificial boundaries that prevent sharing information, collaborating, and responding in unison to the situation. While these examples highlight special forces and fire departments, other organizations struggle with this challenge. It may manifest itself in the form of a "turf battle" where organizations contradict each other, disagree over how to integrate and work together, or respond on their own without coordination. The Freedom Industries incident in West Virginia captures this issue across multiple organizations. Instead of participating in a Joint Information Center, local, state, and federal agencies publicly contradicted each other over the safety of the drinking water system after Freedom Industries discharged 10,000 gallons of Methylcychohexanemethanol (MCHM) and glycol into the Elk River, overloading the water treatment plant, and contaminating the drinking water system (CSB 2017). The Centers for Disease Control and Prevention (CDC), which was not involved in the initial response, provided uncoordinated information to the public. An elected official drank the water during a press briefing and declared it "safe" while no data existed to establish a "safe" level of the contaminants. Unlike a traditional hazmat spill where the fire department and hazmat teams lead the response, this became a public health emergency much like the Ebola virus and COVID-19, so the ICS structure and participants varied from traditional response operations. While regulatory oversight and responsibilities for incidents like this are comprised of multiple shared lanes, integration into the ICS and unified response presents multiple challenges and turf battles, which ultimately lead to a confused and frightened public.

These examples illustrate how the challenges associated with politics, power, and pride can influence emergency response operations. Emergency responders and leaders cannot ignore these human factors when conducting response operations.

1.3.7 Training and Exercises

Some obstacles to unified response are rooted in training and exercise disparities among different organizations. FEMA defines training as "to make proficient with specialized instruction and practice." In contrast, an exercise is an evaluated event that may be discussion- or operations-based. Both training and exercises are part of the preparedness cycle. The outcome of an exercise includes an after-action report/improvement plan, which leads to continuous improvement of capabilities. There is certainly a place for unit-specific training and exercises to ensure that the unit has the competence to perform its responsibilities proficiently. However, it may be a rare circumstance where a solo unit responds to an emergency. By definition, there will likely be at least two parties involved: the party that declared the emergency and the response team. Therefore, it is important for both entities (and any others that may become involved) to train and exercise together so that they are able to integrate, communicate, coordinate, control, and recover from the incident.

At the unit responder level, organizations define their training requirements based on standards (American National Standards Institute, National Fire Protection Association (NFPA), mission essential tasks, and regulatory [OSHA, the Environmental Protection Agency (EPA), etc.]), qualifications, and/or required competencies. Unit responders train to their respective standards, but these may not apply to all organizations. For example, law enforcement may not adopt NFPA standards, while fire departments commonly adopt NFPA standards. This can create a barrier to sharing common terminology, accepted level of proficiency, and integration into a unified command structure. Another example is the numerous standards set by different organizations for sampling procedures (i.e., Department of Justice, HHS, DHS, ASTM, Department of Defense, etc.). While different training curricula and standards may bring multifaceted approaches and perspectives, thereby adding value, the different training curricula and standards also can create conflict and uncertainty over who is actually trained to the appropriate standard for the response situation. It is important for responders who are going to work together to define, adopt, and implement consistent standards where applicable. In many cases, there will be multiple standards that apply due to the various regulatory bodies overseeing response operations (i.e., OSHA, EPA, DOT, etc.) and various standards which are often based on a profession or activity. After 9/11, the Department of Homeland Security established the NIMS to improve operational coordination, communication, and response. The NIMS is comprised of several key components: resource management, information sharing, and command and control. These components have led to the standardization of terminology, incident command system, resource typing, national qualification system, and methods of sharing information. While implementation of the NIMS is required for federal grant recipients, it is not required but encouraged for those in the private sector. Training to different standards among response organizations without coordination has led to numerous challenges and even deadly consequences.

Attempting to execute someone else's responsibilities or performing at a higher level can lead to deadly consequences. On April 17, 2013, the West Fire Department responded to a fire at the West Fertilizer Company in West, Texas. The team was trained and certified to the Hazmat Awareness level and had completed independent study courses through FEMA's Emergency Management Institute on ICS, NIMS, and the National Response Framework (CSB 2016). As volunteer firefighters, they had completed a basic fire training course. Some responders were trained to a higher level. However, while these courses provided knowledge-level training on incident command and how to identify and report a hazardous material incident, 12 responders attempted to extinguish a fire that was beyond their training and available resources. According to OSHA regulations and NFPA standards for hazmat training, offensive actions in a hazmat incident require Hazmat Technician-level training and certification. Sadly, this incident escalated and resulted in a deadly explosion. The Chemical Safety Board investigation identified the lack of appropriate training for this situation and that responders did not implement an incident command system or establish incident objectives. This is an example of a training gap that was later addressed by FEMA through establishing courses that went beyond the knowledge level and incorporated application, synthesis, and judgment to ensure that responders more clearly understood their capabilities and limitations and possessed the ability to make good decisions during a crisis.

Exercises can comprise a wide range of scale, scope, and participation. Discussion-based exercises such as seminars and tabletop exercises can test knowledge of plans, procedures, and understanding of responsibilities. Operations-based exercises such as drills, functional exercises, and full-scale exercises can test the performance of responders in executing plans, procedures, and responsibilities. An exercise series consists of an escalating series of exercises whereby participation and execution grow with each exercise. Exercises with ambiguous objectives, scenarios, scope, or evaluation criteria can lead to frustration and personality-driven outcomes rather than objective and constructive feedback on improving capabilities. While many organizations are comfortable conducting internal exercises, failure to include external response organizations preempts the ability to learn from challenges that may be encountered when working with different resources and capabilities such as communication devices, organizational structures and liaisons, equipment, and differing competencies.

1.3.8 Funding

There are several challenges related to funding and unified response: insufficient funding, limitations on grant funding allowable use, unfunded mandates, discipline-specific funding, lack of community-wide coordination and approval process, and competing interests. In general, communities are not able to prepare for all threats and hazards due to limited resources. This requires prioritization at the organization or community level based on risk, as the jurisdiction's budget is not able to eliminate or mitigate all risks.

Most federal grants define allowable expenses and prohibit certain types of expenses depending on the type of grant. For example, some grants allow for staff augmentation while prohibiting the purchase of equipment, whereas other grants are specifically designed for equipment purchases but prohibit staff augmentation. The challenge for those involved in response operations is to piece the grant funding together like a puzzle where different grants and disciplines bring unique pieces of the puzzle in the form of grant funding for specific resources in such a way that the community completes the puzzle and ultimately builds capabilities. The risk is that each discipline pursues grant funds for its own department instead of contributing and aligning its grant funding with the priorities of the community.

Another challenge is unfunded mandates from the federal government. A classic example is the Emergency Planning Community Right to Know Act (EPCRA), which requires governors of each state to establish planning districts (i.e., Local Emergency Planning Committees [LEPC]) and requires the development of an emergency response plan that is reviewed and updated annually. The EPA, which promulgates and enforces this regulation, does not provide funding or grants to the community to assist with implementation of these requirements. However, the Department of Transportation Pipeline and Hazardous Materials Safety Administration collects fees from transporters to fund the Hazardous Materials Emergency Preparedness grant, which is commonly used by LEPCs to fund planning and training activities (but there must be a transportation component). So, organizations and communities must collaborate on how they are going to fund the capabilities needed and comply with regulations such as EPCRA.

1.3.9 Leadership

The leadership challenges to unified response are growing in complexity for several reasons: growing interdependence across sectors impacted by the disaster, inability to identify leaders based on the type of disaster and form unified command structures accordingly, uninformed decision-making, and a culture of reaction instead of proactive investments prior to a disaster.

As we have seen with COVID-19, there is a high degree of interdependence across sectors, supply chains, and even among government departments. While COVID-19 was a public health emergency, the cascading effects of decisions made at the state and federal level adversely impacted mental health, education outcomes, and the economy. In the wake of the 2017 Hurricane and Wildfire season, FEMA established

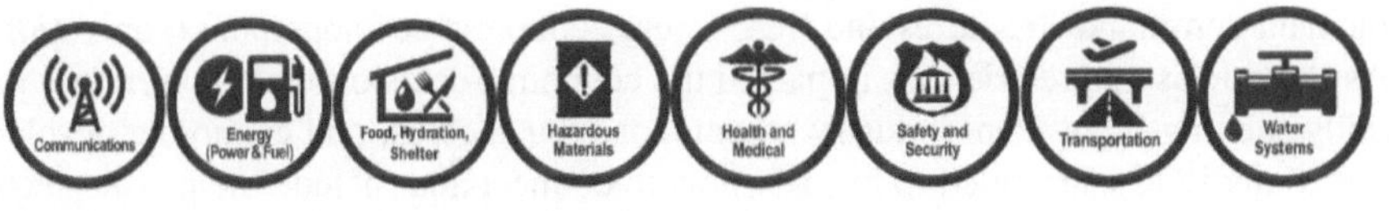

FIGURE 1.1 Community lifelines

the Community Lifelines toolkit to help states prioritize impacts to essential services that are needed for a community to function (i.e., lifelines) and communicate the status of lifelines along with requests for Lines of Effort from federal agencies to stabilize the lifelines. There are eight lifelines with components and subcomponents, as shown in Figure 1.1. These lifelines are also interdependent. For example, communications are not possible without power, and safety and security require transportation. Even across industries, we are seeing a high degree of interdependence between utilities and businesses, suppliers and manufacturers, transporters and retailers, and raw materials industries such as timber and construction.

When one sector of the economy is impacted by a disaster, there is a cascading effect on other sectors and industries. When the Colonial Pipeline computer system was hacked, the company was not able to track and bill for fuel issued to transporters. As a precaution to prevent further damages, the company shut down the pipeline and disbursement of fuel to transporters. This resulted in regional fuel shortages at gas stations and airports along the East Coast, impacting transporters, retailers, and consumers. While the company contacted the FBI and a private information technology (IT) consultant to resolve the cyber-attack, the widespread nature of impacts across multiple sectors and areas beckoned for a unified response.

Several of these examples also highlight the difficulty in identifying the incident commander or those who should be part of a unified command. During many hazmat exercises, a consistent observation is the hesitation or reluctance of public safety responders to form a unified command with the responsible party. While not always the case, many see sharing command with the responsible party as a conflict of interest, but often, the responsible party has the ability to bring the right resources to bear during the response operations. Nowhere is this more clearly illustrated than with the oil/gas and rail industries. Both industries experience significant economic impact when operations are disrupted, so they are committed to containing any spills, cleaning up the environment, and restoring operations as quickly as possible. These priorities may pose competing interests to public safety; therefore, it is essential for a unified command that includes public safety representation.

At the outset of COVID-19, the Department of Health and Human Services was poised to lead any federal response to a pandemic, but at the last minute, FEMA was directed to lead the response. Similar situations played out across the country as public health departments established an incident command system, but due to the scale of the crisis, many departments and leaders were overwhelmed by the complexity and far-reaching impacts. Some departments worked with their state to request an incident management team to help manage the ICS until the response stabilized. Others needed to increase their bandwidth. Noticeably absent from many incident command structures and EOCs were economic development organizations. As shutdowns and restrictions impacted the economy, decision-makers were not initially seeking input from industry associations, businesses, and economic developers. Many EOCs struggled to identify how to connect and include the private sector in the EOC. Identifying the right leaders and inviting them into the decision-making structure is essential; otherwise, impact and risk are simply shifted from one domain (public health) to another (economy, education, and mental health). In the case of COVID-19, some have argued that the cure was worse than the disease. This underscores the importance of leadership and decision-making.

In order to make the best decisions, leaders need high-quality information in a timely manner. But this is not always possible, as was the case with a novel coronavirus, a tropical storm that intensifies to a Category 5 hurricane overnight, or an unexpected militant attack. Leaders have increased their sense of situational awareness through purchasing new technologies such as common operating pictures, GIS services, and warning systems. While these technologies are helpful, situational awareness is increased with the ability to collect and share relevant information and project how the risk profile will change in the future. This enables leaders to make informed decisions. Stove-pipes of information, unwillingness to share intelligence, and inability to get the right information to the right decision-makers impede effective leadership during a crisis. While there has been much progress with the formation of fusion centers and information-sharing systems, more expertise and discipline are needed to gather the right information and make meaningful projections into the future. This was evident during the COVID-19 crisis as health departments, the CDC, and the Department of Defense established sets of criteria (e.g., percent vaccinated, percent positivity on PCR tests, fatality rate, etc.) that drove specific mitigation practices (e.g., distancing, masking, restrictions on gathering, etc.). While many leaders acted out of an abundance of caution for public health, there was a tradeoff in prioritizing public health outcomes over social, economic, and educational outcomes. The selection of metrics reflected lagging instead of leading indicators, and mitigation measures reflected traditional pandemic plan countermeasures, which assumed large droplet spread. While some leaders focused on the past, other leaders used predictive models and updated their approach to prevention and mitigation measures once learning that COVID-19 spread through bioaerosols, which required a shift in mitigation measures.

As the global climate and geopolitical threats continue to change, leaders not only need to be informed about the current threats and hazards, but they need to shift their risk management approach from reliance on historical data to future-based risk analysis. Many leaders focus on historical data to make future decisions without regard to changing demographics, climate, transnational and national threats, migration, and social attitudes because the past is objective, easy to measure, and somewhat manageable. Future threats and hazards are harder to predict and sometimes tainted with biases based on the source of information. Leaders must look past political and social agendas and seek out credible information in the age of disinformation. Unfortunately, many leaders are rewarded for short-term success but not long-term investments that may yield long-term success. Our communities need leaders with the moral courage and vision to make long-term investment decisions that outweigh short-term wins.

While this is not an exhaustive discussion of all of the challenges facing unified response, these summary categories and examples illustrate that there are many barriers to overcoming unified response. The rest of this section is dedicated to finding solutions to overcome these challenges. As indicated in the last paragraph on leadership, one of the key solutions is shifting one's thinking from response to resilience and preparedness. Response is reactive. Resilience and preparedness are proactive. On a timeline of an incident, response occurs after the incident while building resilience and enhancing preparedness occur well before the incident occurs. Thus, in this book on emergency response, we must shift the focus to pre-incident actions that include prevention, protection, mitigation, preparedness, recovery outcomes, and resilience. What we do pre-incident to shape the battlefield and set the conditions for swift and successful response will do more to improve response operations than focusing solely on response operations. Overcoming the challenges to a unified response is truly a human factors challenge, not a tactical response challenge.

1.4 OVERCOMING THE CHALLENGES

In *Crisis-Ready Leadership: Building Resilient Organizations and Communities* (Campbell 2023), the book elaborates on how to develop a crisis-ready leader through various tools, methods, case studies, and profiles of exemplary crisis leaders. This section references several key points from that book as it applies to this chapter on how resilient organizations overcome challenges to unified response and introduce new material related to achieving a unified response.

1.4.1 Crisis-Ready Leadership

Crisis-ready leadership begins pre-incident. To be prepared for response operations, responders must plan, train, and exercise in realistic and challenging environments. All preparation begins pre-incident. The decisions related to a community's risk profile, risk management investments, planning, equipment purchases, mutual aid agreements, training, and exercises are made by leaders. An inherent risk for all organizations and communities is that a crisis could occur. Therefore, all leaders must be crisis-ready. A crisis-ready leader is marked by several attributes, as shown in Table 1.1 (Campbell, 2023). Developing these attributes includes study, training, practice, openness to feedback, and a commitment to personal and professional improvement. Additionally, crisis-ready leaders must be ready for a crisis at any moment. They must be able to overcome the stress associated with a crisis and make good judgments, leading response operations into stabilization and swift recovery.

Crisis-ready leaders acquire a long-term vision that is rooted in an understanding of future risks, the rate of changing risk profiles, a commitment to building resilience, and a stable, thriving community. An effective leader envisions the future with all its threats and opportunities, then plots a course to navigate the organization through the challenges into the future. Notice that effective leaders do not wait

TABLE 1.1
Attributes of a Crisis-Ready Leader

Character Traits	Knowledge	Skills and Abilities
• Humility • Integrity • People smarts • Moral courage	• Self-awareness • Know the plan • Situational awareness with leading indicators • Multidisciplinary knowledge	• Communication • Complex problem-solving and design thinking • Trust building • Decisiveness
Additional Advice • Surround yourself with competent leaders and advisors • Control the operations tempo • Maintain objectivity		

for bad things to happen and simply respond. Effective leaders see the future and make decisions and investments and set priorities to make the envisioned future a reality and set the conditions under which they will lead the response. Good leaders represent a force for driving the changes needed to get there. Great leaders influence others to be on their team and participate fully in making these changes a reality. Empowering others not only builds the team but also builds sustaining commitment to the long-term vision beyond the leader's tenure.

Building resilient organizations and communities that overcome challenges in emergency response, especially unified operations, begins with leadership. Without effective leadership, the remaining solutions will not come to fruition.

1.4.2 Building Resilience

Building resilience is an integral part of overcoming challenges to unified response because resilience sets the conditions for success by creating an operating environment that can withstand stressors and rebound, thereby creating momentum in the right direction, i.e., towards recovery. The hard work of baking resilience into systems, organizations, communities, and teams happens before an incident, not during or after the incident (although the recovery process affords opportunities to develop recovery outcomes that build resilience). This requires leaders who understand the potential risks and cast a long-term vision for success, as many resilience-building initiatives require long-term investments.

1.4.2.1 Defining Resilience

The Merriam-Webster Dictionary defines "**resilience**" as:

1. the capability of a strained body to recover its size and shape after deformation caused especially by compressive stress
2. an ability to recover from or adjust easily to misfortune or change

"**Community Resilience**" is defined by the National Institute of Standards and Technology (NIST) as "the ability of a community to prepare for anticipated natural hazards, adapt to changing conditions, and withstand and recover rapidly from disruptions" (National Institute of Standards and Technology, 2020).

1.4.2.2 Types of Resilience

When discussing resilience, it is important to define the type of resilience and boundaries around the entity of concern so that appropriate measures can be taken. In an interdependent world, this can be challenging as excluding a major component of your system can result in a shift of risk from one component to the other in the name of resilience. Using a capitals approach to determining the components of the system provides a comprehensive framework for both communities and organizations.

FEMA incorporated the University of South Carolina Hazards & Vulnerability Research Institute's Baseline Resilience Indicators for Communities (BRIC) into the National Risk Index (University of South Carolina 2022). While there are multiple resilience indicators and models, this model works well for the community context. The BRIC index utilizes 49 variables across six broad capitals. These capitals and some sample variables include:

Human Well-Being/Cultural/Social: physical attributes of populations, values, and belief systems (educational attainment equality, pre-retirement age, personal transportation access, communication capacity, English language competency, non-special needs populations, health insurance, mental health support, food security, access to physicians)

Economic/Financial: economic assets and livelihoods (homeownership, employment rate, racial/ethnic income inequality, non-dependence on primary/tourism sector employment, gender income inequality, business size, large retail with regional/national distribution, federal employment).

Infrastructure/Built Environment/Housing: buildings and infrastructure (sturdier housing types, temporary housing availability, medical care capacity, evacuation routes, housing stock construction quality, temporary shelter availability, school restoration potential, industrial re-supply potential, high-speed internet infrastructure).

Institutional/Governance: access to resources and the power to influence their distribution (mitigation spending, flood insurance coverage, governance performance regimes, jurisdictional fragmentation, disaster aid experience, local disaster training, population stability, nuclear accident planning, crop insurance coverage).

Community Capacity: social networks and connectivity among individuals and groups (volunteerism, religious affiliation, attachment to place, political engagement, citizen disaster training, civic organizations).

Environmental/Natural: natural resource base and environmental conditions (local food supplies, natural flood buffers, energy use, perviousness, water stress).

A similar approach can be implemented in the organizational resilience context. The leader's role is to create a culture of resilience by understanding their risks, risk tolerance, and rate that the risk profile is changing. This drives leaders to evaluate their capabilities compared with their vulnerabilities and then design resilience into their systems. Taking a capitals approach to determining resilience indicators for an organization leads to the following:

Human Capital: employees, vendors, access to qualified labor; recruiting, hiring, onboarding systems, feedback/evaluation systems; indicators may include utilization, turnover, productivity, customer satisfaction, and compensation equity.

Infrastructure: facility, equipment, supplies, internet, transportation, cyber-infrastructure; indicators may include adequacy of built environment for hazards, internet bandwidth, supply chain capacity and redundancy, power reliability.

Financial Capital: cash reserves, customer diversification, backlog, liquidity, assets, insurance; indicators may include cash reserve/current liabilities, percentage of revenue from largest customer, backlog/annual revenue, current assets/current liabilities, insurance coverage/assets.

Intellectual Capital: intellectual property, knowledge management and preservation, information systems.

Governance/Systems: management systems that include policies, procedures, assignment of responsibilities, and associated plans such as continuity of operations.

Hazards will present unique stressors and subsequently impact the system in different ways. This process overlaps and parallels with the preparedness cycle. One way to think of the relationship between preparedness and resilience is that resilience can be an aspiring goal within the preparedness cycle. The preparedness cycle builds capabilities through identifying and assessing risks, developing plans, building resources, training, exercises, and improvement. An organization can be prepared without achieving resilience, so the resilience goal entails considering how each step of preparedness builds resilience. Another way to think of the relationship is that a culture of preparedness integrates resilience to reduce the consequences and risk of the hazard. Resilience reduces risk through prevention and mitigation investments that reduce the frequency and/or severity of the hazard on a system (i.e., community or organization). Preparedness builds capabilities to respond to and recover from risks. Both are necessary and work together. The following framework for building resilience follows a systematic pathway (Campbell 2023).

1. Define the system (e.g., community, business, school, economy, market, etc.).
2. Identify local, relevant hazards and assess the risk. These are the stressors that will be applied to your system.
3. Identify the components of the system that are impacted by the hazards.

4. Identify interdependent components and the extent of impact.
5. Aggregate the impact on all components based on the risk of each hazard.
6. Determine vulnerabilities within the system.
7. Develop strategies to strengthen components to enhance resilience.
8. Evaluate and prioritize resilience measures that increase system-wide resilience.
9. Implement actions to increase resilience.

1.4.2.3 Six R's of Resilience

While there are multiple indices for measuring resilience, most of these systems are rooted in utilizing some variable (e.g., unemployment, households without a vehicle) or a weighting method. These systems may be biased to the indices selected or weighted and may not accurately reflect a holistic measure of resilience for a community or organization. For example, FEMA's Community Resilience Challenges Index identifies 22 social demographic indicators from the American Community Survey, but does not address the adequacy of local government systems, continuity of government, preparedness, capabilities, or continuity of operations. Similarly, the CDC's Social Vulnerability Index is based on social demographic data but not public health and healthcare system capacity and capabilities. Therefore, the "Six R's of Resilience" provide a more comprehensive measure for the resilience of a system.

The Six R's of Resilience outlines several attributes of resilient systems that can be used to formulate resilience measures or evaluate the extent of a system's resilience. While there are some overlaps and interdependencies, this model approaches resilience measures from multiple perspectives that are descriptive of a resilient system. The Six R's are described below:

Ready: How well is the system prepared for the hazards and threats outlined in its risk profile? How prepared is the organization to take advantage of opportunities in a timely manner?

Redundant: Are redundancies built into essential components of the system (e.g., redundant sources of supply, methods for product/service delivery, key staffing, financing and banking, revenue/customer diversification, etc.)?

Repairable: How easily and quickly can an essential component of the system be repaired if it is damaged? Are the supplies, resources, and procedures in place to return the damaged component to an operable state within the required timeframe?

Resistant: How resistant to damage are the essential components of the system (e.g., are structures built to a standard that can resist or prevent damage from hazards such as flooding, wind, hail, blasts, etc.)?

Robust: How strong and persistent are the system and its components when facing disruptions? Is the system mature, defined, managed, scalable, and replicable?

Reserves: Have leaders adequately established and maintained reserves such as sufficient cash to maintain operations during cash flow interruptions, liquid assets that can be converted to cash, excess personnel capacity to deal with staffing shortages, adequate inventory reserves, or additional space to accommodate physical distancing or take advantage of process modifications?

1.4.3 Develop Strategies

The third part of overcoming challenges to unified response requires the development of strategies. Just as building resilience requires leadership, vision, and investment, so does developing strategies. The following section outlines some key elements to developing strategies for overcoming the various challenges of unified emergency response. It should not be a surprise that organizational alignment is a key starting point.

1.4.3.1 Organizational SWOT Analysis

Each organization needs situational awareness in order to know its current status of preparedness. Preparedness for what? Do we have the right capabilities and capacities? How are we monitoring our capabilities to ensure we can confidently claim readiness? This begins with conducting an analysis of strengths, weaknesses, opportunities, and threats (SWOT) (Table 1.2).

In order to complete a SWOT analysis, the organization needs to understand its operating environment. There are several tools for doing this, but it often begins with key stakeholders identifying the various conditions in which they are operating, as these conditions could affect the organization. An analysis of political, economic, social, technological, environmental, and legal (PESTEL) factors is a useful tool for this exercise. For example:

- How are politics and political priorities affecting preparedness initiatives?
- What economic trends could impact purchasing power, employment, tax revenues, etc.?
- What social trends in our community could result in greater needs, vulnerabilities, or strengths?
- What changes in technology could enhance the way response operations are conducted or put those operations at greater risk?
- How are environmental regulations impacting emergency response operations?
- What are the legal changes or trends that could impact response operations?

TABLE 1.2
SWOT Analysis

	Positive Impacts	**Negative Impacts**
Internal Forces	Strengths	Weaknesses
External Forces	Opportunities	Threats

These are just example questions to help responders and community leaders explore and identify operating conditions, challenges, and trends that could affect response operations.

Once these factors are identified, stakeholders should conduct a SWOT analysis, first identifying organizational strengths and weaknesses in light of the PESTEL analysis. For example, a fire department might identify the following strengths and weaknesses:

Strength: All firefighters are trained to Fire Fighter level 2 and Hazmat Operations.
Weakness: The departments are staffed at 75%, which puts a strain on department personnel and presents a risk to the community.

These internal strengths and weaknesses provide situational awareness across the organization.

Next, stakeholders examine external opportunities and threats that could positively or negatively impact their organization or community in light of the PESTEL analysis, as outlined in the examples below.

Opportunities: an increase in grant funding availability for certain initiatives.
Threats: cyber-attacks, an increase in civil unrest/dissatisfaction with government, and climate change.

The resulting SWOT analysis captures input from stakeholders and helps to identify some trends, but more importantly, the analysis can be used to formulate some goals and direction for the organization. Organizations should identify steps that leverage their strengths to shore up weaknesses, take advantage of opportunities, and defend against threats. New initiatives may emerge from this exercise. The next step in developing a strategy is to identify where your organization is currently at and where it needs to go, at least the direction and some initial objectives in that direction. A PESTEL and SWOT analysis can help you do that. Objectives should be supported by goals, action items, and accountability by defining who is responsible for each action, when it will be completed, the resources needed, and how you will monitor and measure progress. An additional benefit of this group exercise is that it creates buy-in and alignment within the organization. This overcomes some of the internal obstacles to a unified response.

1.4.3.2 Networking, Relationships, and Resource Inventory

Few communities and organizations have the full capacity and capabilities to respond to every type and scale of incident. While all disasters are local (so the saying goes), the locality often requires external support in the form of unique resources or additional capacity to respond to the incident. These resources are traditionally sourced through the EOC under the NIMS framework. However, as we discussed earlier regarding obstacles to a unified response, merging external resources with local resources presents several challenges. Therefore, networking, building relationships, and identifying resources needed prior to the incident can help overcome the challenges of unified response operations.

Networking involves getting to know those in your community, outside your community at the regional, state, and federal levels of government, private sector partners and liaisons such as economic development organizations, and non-profit organizations such as community-based, faith-based, and national-level resources. Networking has been hampered some due to COVID-19, but state, regional, and national-level conferences are rebounding and offering opportunities to get to know other potential partners and resources.

Relationships are built on trust, not simply an exchange of business cards, although that could be the beginning of a relationship. Relationships take time to forge along shared experiences. Certainly, a major disaster can forge relationships for a lifetime, but we would prefer to forge those relationships before the incident so that we know who we can call and trust to support us. Trust is like an account, such as the Trust Account illustrated in Figure 1.2. Trust is built by three types of deposits: integrity, competence, and respect.

Integrity is doing what you say you are going to do and being honest and forthcoming. **Competence** is demonstrating that you can correctly deliver the expected product, result, or service. **Respect** is treating others with dignity, deference, and as you would want to be treated.

Each time a person demonstrates integrity, competence, or respect, they make a deposit into the Trust Account, and the balance increases. However, when a person fails to do what they said they were going to do, delivers shoddy results, or prioritizes others' needs as secondary, that person makes a withdrawal from the Trust Account. Sometimes, these withdrawals are unintentional, without malice, but the end result is the same. The level of trust ultimately determines the strength of the relationship. It may be time to reassess our relationships and make some investments for the long term. This can be difficult on a day-to-day basis, but here are a few practical ways to make "deposits" in Trust Accounts that result in "investments" in relationships:

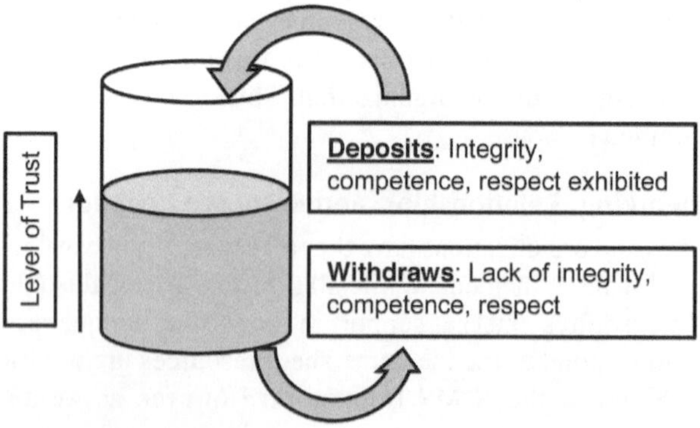

FIGURE 1.2 Trust account illustrated

- Invite your network into the planning process when you update your local and regional plans.
- Invite your network to a training that you host (e.g., host a FEMA course and make it a regional initiative; most of these courses are delivered in your community for free).
- Invite your network to participate in an exercise. The demands for more exercises are increasing beyond many organizations' capacity to plan and conduct these exercises. We are pulled in many directions. But there are increasing opportunities to observe or participate without committing the entire organization's staff and resources. Look for these opportunities to create shared experiences and learn more about other organizations' resources.
- Team with others in your network on grant proposals, projects, and initiatives.
- Team with other jurisdictions to share the cost of a consultant's services and make it a regional effort instead of a local effort.

Resources are also scarce, but one of the Six R's of Resilience is Reserves. It is important to build adequate reserves, but this is not always possible, practical, or wise stewardship of funds. Identifying other organizations that have the resources that you might need and establishing mutual aid agreements to leverage those resources can help build capacity. One pitfall of this strategy is that many other organizations may be doing the same thing with the same resource owner, so it is important to understand what other mutual aid agreements are in place and their method for prioritizing and allocating resources when there are competing interests. With an abundance of resource typing and the national qualification system, it is becoming easier to identify and request standardized resources through the federal system. But in some cases, your community might need unique resources that are not accessible through this system.

1.4.4 Public-Private Partnerships

Eighty-five percent of the community's critical resources are controlled by the private sector (e.g., telecommunications, internet service providers, banking systems, railroads, power generation, the electric grid, fuel stations, airlines, etc.). For many communities, public-private partnerships begin and end with the utility companies. While this is certainly a good start, utilities comprise just some of the essential services in a community. During COVID-19, we realized the importance of employment and the wider array of services provided by the private sector (e.g., grocery stores, meatpacking facilities, farms, government contractors, road maintenance contractors, educators, healthcare workers, construction workers, and the list goes on). COVID-19 redefined essential workers and highlighted the interdependence and fragility of our economy based on supply chains. Emergency response operations are rarely a "public sector-only" event. Most large-scale disasters will require a whole community effort to respond. Severe weather events require power restoration and debris removal.

Train derailments require cooperation and collaboration among the rail operator, first responders, and environmental restoration contractors. Cyber-attacks require IT professionals, law enforcement, and the entity that has been victimized by the attack (which could be a utility, government, or pipeline operator). Because emergency response operations will likely involve more private sector involvement than working with a utility company, include the private sector in your network, relationships, and resources. Invite them into the community planning, training, and exercises. Forge partnerships that are win-win; many public-private partnerships make the mistake of only defining what the private sector can do for the public sector. A more balanced discussion is needed to build reserves, capacity, and flexibility and ensure a strong economy during and after an incident. Here are a few examples:

- Identify environmental restoration contractors in response plans and establish Indefinite Delivery-Indefinite Quantity contracts with these vendors to ensure agreements are in place before the disaster. This protects against price gouging and ensures the vendor is compensated fairly.
- Work with hotels to establish agreements to house responders or displaced persons during a disaster. This averts lost revenue from a lack of visitors to the hotels during an incident while providing necessary housing for those impacted.
- Establish a retainer with private IT forensic consultants to assist with response to a cyber-attack.
- Exercise flexibility with retail and dining establishments to ensure continuity of operations during incidents. Many jurisdictions closed streets or granted variances to enable outdoor dining during COVID-19.
- Use grant funds to invest in redundant fiber communications systems within the community; move telecommunications and power lines underground where above-ground lines are at risk from weather-related disruptions.
- Make infrastructure investments that are beneficial for the business community, mitigating hazards to their establishments.

1.4.5 Organizational Development

There are two aspects to organizational development strategies to overcoming challenges to emergency response: internal organizational development and external organizational development. Internal organizational development consists of systems and capabilities-driven strategies. External organizational development entails filling the gaps in desired or target capabilities with external partners through mutual aid agreements and public-private partnerships, as discussed in the previous section.

Internal organizational development begins with adopting a management system along with a standard to which the system is established. There are several relevant emergency management and response related-standards, such as the Emergency Management Standard (ANSI/EMAP 5-2019), Standard on Continuity, Emergency, and Crisis Management (NFPA Std 1600), and Security and Resilience Emergency Management Guidelines for Incident Management (ISO 22320:2018). While these standards cover broader emergency management programs, there are emergency response elements to each. Implementation of these standards requires the development and implementation of a system comprised of risk assessments, plans, procedures, resources, communications, and other elements. Adopting an independent standard establishes a commitment to the adoption of industry best practices and continuous improvement, which leads to organizational maturity. Regardless of whether the standard requires third-party audits, this practice can identify blind spots, provide new perspectives, and enhance accountability. The commitment to continuous improvement prevents stagnation and propels development.

1.4.6 Strategic Planning, Development, and Communications

Comprehensive Preparedness Guide (CPG) 201, *Threat and Hazard Identification and Risk Assessment and Stakeholder Preparedness Review*, and the National Preparedness System provide communities with methods for building capabilities (FEMA 2018). These align well with strategic planning and decision-making. The following steps are established in CPG 201 and the National Preparedness System.

Comprehensive Preparedness Guide 201

Step 1: Identify the Threats and Hazards of Concern
Step 2: Give the Threats and Hazards Context
Step 3: Establish Capability Targets
Step 4: Assess Capabilities
Step 5: Identify and Address Capability Gaps
Step 6: Describe Impact of Funding Sources

National Preparedness System

Part 1: Identify and Assess Risks
Part 2: Estimate Capability Requirements
Part 3: Build and Sustain Capabilities
Part 4: Plan to Deliver Capabilities
Part 5: Validate Capabilities
Part 6: Review and Update

1.4.6.1 Identify Capability Requirements

Identifying capability requirements begins with a risk assessment to understand the context of the risks facing a community. While many risk assessments rely heavily on historical data such as the National Oceanic and Atmospheric Administration (NOAA) databases of weather events, active shooter data from law enforcement databases, and hazardous material incidents from the National Response Center database, it is important to consider trends in order to predict the future risk profile for the community. Changing climate, aging infrastructure, advancing technologies, and increased nation-state threats should be accounted for during this exercise. The

TABLE 1.3
Response Core Capabilities

Planning	Fatality Management Services	Operational Communications
Public Information and Warning	Fire Management and Suppression	Public Health, Healthcare, and Emergency Medical Services
Operational Coordination	Logistics and Supply Chain Management	Situational Assessment
Infrastructure Systems	Mass Care Services	On-Scene Security, Protection, and Law Enforcement
Critical Transportation	Mass Search and Rescue Operations	Environmental Response/ Health and Safety

future risk profile could be expressed in a contextualized scenario-based summary that highlights expected impacts or a quantitative representation. Whichever the method, planners will need to establish target capabilities and estimate their capability requirements. Then, planners should conduct a capability gap analysis based on current capabilities and those needed to respond effectively to the future risk profile for the community. These gaps become the basis for strategic planning.

1.4.6.1.1 Preparedness System

FEMA has identified 32 core capabilities that span the five mission areas of emergency management. Fifteen of these capabilities support the response mission area. These core capabilities are shown in Table 1.3.

Building these capabilities entails planning, resource procurement, organization, training, and exercises to validate the capabilities. Each capability includes targets based on risk and/or desired capabilities. Preparedness can be measured for each capability based on the set targets and how well entities can achieve those targets based on exercise performance. Capability status is relayed through the Stakeholder Preparedness Review and is often compiled at the state emergency management organization. Capability gaps should be communicated to local and state decision-makers to ensure that they are aware of any gaps so that they can either accept the risk, invest in capabilities, or request assistance (usually in the form of state and federal grants but sometimes through local leadership).

1.4.6.1.2 Implementation

Finally, these strategies need to be implemented. After prioritizing capability gaps and initiatives, there are several actions that will enhance capabilities: planning, organizational development, equipping, training, and exercises.

1.4.6.2 Planning, Organizing, and Equipping

Collaborative planning is essential to building unified emergency response capabilities. Stove-piped plans fail to engage cross-discipline organizations and ensure effective interfaces and assumptions are in place. Team-based planning ensures shared assumptions, goals, and seamless interfaces among different departments and disciplines. Following a process such as the six-step Comprehensive Preparedness Guide 101 ensures a standardized approach to planning and minimizes hidden agendas. Collaborative planning ensures that plans are interoperable with other plans. Without stakeholder involvement in the planning process, planners are unaware of other capabilities, plans, and resources. Seek to understand the positions, interests, and capabilities within other organizations to address these needs. Include lessons learned from recent real-world events and exercises. Vet the plan adequately to ensure stakeholders have an opportunity to review and provide input on the plan; this creates buy-in, especially when their input is included. Apply best practices and lessons learned from previous incidents.

While there is much value in the planning process, the goal should be to arrive at a useful, actionable plan that aids in response decision-making. Many plans provide generic information but fail to establish action levels that drive decision-making. Having developed several hundred pandemic/infectious disease plans, we found that establishing action levels based on the situation, severity, and impact, despite having imperfect and incomplete information, enabled decision-makers to manage the incident rather than react to the situation with merely standard operating procedures. Decision points are critical points in a scenario where decision-makers have an opportunity to make a decision that controls, contains, or deescalates the incident. Plans should provide sufficient information within the context of a situation to ensure incident management across multiple organizations.

There are several tenets that guide developing response plans. These include minimizing duplication from other plans by establishing cross-references, as this reduces the possibility of differences during plan revision. Second, accurate information enhances situational awareness and thereby accelerates the decision cycle. In many incidents, it takes time to gather information, but if known information can be compiled and provided in advance, then incident commanders can make faster, better decisions. For example, in hazardous material emergency response plans, we typically include hazmat facility profiles containing contact information, plume model outputs, a list of vulnerable facilities, and the hazmat facility's capabilities. This type of information leads to a pre-incident action plan and enables swift decision-making, as public protective actions will take considerable time to implement. Third, clarify roles and responsibilities so that responders know which organization is responsible for the various tasks involved in response operations. This minimizes any confusion during the incident. Finally, ensure the plan and associated procedures are comprehensive (i.e., there are no gaps) and interoperable (i.e., the fire department actions align with law enforcement actions).

After developing the plan, train on and test it. After completing a new plan or revision, it is essential to test the plan through seminars and tabletop exercises. This is a key step in creating buy-in for different organizations to integrate into a seamless response team. The seminar gives all parties an opportunity to read and learn about the threat, the responder's capabilities (which should be outlined in the plan), the response structure, key decisions, response actions, and tools. A tabletop exercise gets responders working together, making decisions (sometimes decisions that could not be made during the planning workshops), and hopefully agreeing on how they will respond. If there are shortcomings or inaccuracies in the plan, then those can be addressed after the tabletop exercise.

Exercise design and planning also can offer opportunities to build collaborations. During the course of several large functional and full-scale exercises, reviewing the plans in advance of the exercise design enables the engagement of stakeholders on inconsistencies, inadequate procedures, poor assumptions, and bad procedures that would not work. Due to the expense of the exercises, it is important to resolve these issues as much as possible with the stakeholders before designing and running the exercise. If you can predict the major observations and items that will be on the improvement plan before you design the exercise, then it is not worth running the exercise. In addition, many response teams identify additional problems with their plans during the course of conducting training in preparation for exercises.

At one US military installation's medical group, it was clear that the mass casualty incident plan was not going to work while conducting refresher training involving medical teams, which included a few mock casualties. The teams were tripping over each other, did not have all of the necessary supplies, such as IV stands (this was a large clinic with ancillary services, not an inpatient hospital), and the patient flow through the clinic was not logical. This occurred even after several improvements to the plan were made in the two months leading up to the exercise. At the end of the training, the medical group commander asked the participants for ideas and feedback. This meeting quickly turned into a white-board session that lasted two hours, with the best ideas coming from the lowest-ranking personnel. By the next morning, in preparation for the exercise, they had modified team positions and the facility (they improvised with the resources on hand). After the 100-person mass casualty incident (MCI) exercise, the hot wash was electric with cheers, and the large clinic was ready to handle an MCI. The key to bringing together many on-base response teams and off-base responders was collaborative planning; team-based response training in concepts of operation, equipment, and procedures; collaborative-based functional exercises; more planning; and a full-scale MCI exercise.

1.4.6.2.1 Community-based Capabilities

Having done an extensive analysis of response capabilities based on current publications, instructions, and observations during 2,100+ exercises, it is clear that the siloed approach to capability development does not work well. This has led to multiple disciplines claiming responsibility for the same task, multiple equipment sets with different users and different procedures, similar equipment items with different capabilities yielding different measurements (which appear to provide the operators with conflicting data and ultimately lead to lost confidence in these units by the incident commander), and unknown capabilities among first response disciplines that should be integrating during a response. One solution to this issue is to take a community-based approach to building capabilities.

Collaborating across disciplines ensures that grant funding aligns with capability development and reduces overlap with other organizations. Integration and interoperability of new equipment, standardization of training, and procedure development can be streamlined with collaborative planning and resourcing. Community emergency planners should identify which disciplines will be funded to build and maintain the capabilities. This might include several disciplines working together to procure equipment, train together, and create the right team capability.

Enterprise-wide planning for large companies, healthcare organizations, regional response teams, and military teams should define and standardize resource procurements to ensure they align with the risk and need rather than each organization and department making purchasing decisions in a vacuum. As many have learned, the sustainment cost is usually more than the initial purchase, so developing a sustainment plan prior to procurement could lead to more collaboration.

An effective community-based plan ensures that the capabilities are built based on the location-specific risks. This enables the locality to tailor their capabilities and capacities accordingly. It also helps consolidate resources and integrate responders while eliminating unnecessary redundancies. When integration occurs, responders become more familiar with their counterpart's resources, knowledge, and equipment so that they can train together effectively and standardize their procedures. Ultimately, the community becomes better prepared for response because they are ready to respond together as a knowledgeable, integrated response team.

1.4.6.2.2 Whole Community Engagement

This section has focused on a few technical response aspects of effective planning. Let us close on the concept of whole community planning because this affects unified response operations. The whole community is diverse and consists of the public, community-based organizations, businesses, schools, industries, public sector, agriculture, and non-profit organizations. But within these categories, there are still more diverse and unique situations that must be considered, especially among the public. Within each community, people experience inequities during disasters due to a variety of access and functional needs, historic inequities, and situations that create a disadvantage. These inequities result in greater impacts on some populations and the preponderance of resources being utilized to save lives, protect health, and address the economic impacts on those who are most affected. These adverse impacts then result in cascading effects such as job loss, lower employment, default on credit cards and loans, lost tax revenue, loss of social and cultural resources and knowledge, and migration. To achieve more equitable outcomes during the response to incidents, planners must do a better job accounting for the whole population and its various needs. According to a national survey of over 300 emergency managers, local emergency plans do not adequately identify and address the needs of underserved populations: the homeless (only 22% of plans), public transit-dependent (only 24% of plans), and non-English speaking (only 41% of plans) populations (National Association of Counties 2019). Inequities like this result in disparate outcomes to incidents and often demand significant response resources, further threatening a unified response operation. It is incumbent on planners to apply an equity lens in the planning process by utilizing available information and collaborating with community-based organizations, non-profit organizations, and faith-based organizations.

1.4.6.3 Training

Utilizing and training in NIMS-based response operations helps improve interoperability and aligns response operations. It is important to ensure responders are properly trained to fulfill their responsibilities during an incident. This begins by clearly defining the expected competencies (i.e., knowledge, skills, abilities, and attitudes needed to perform the task) and level of proficiency (i.e., the level of competence needed) required. For training to be effective, participants must complete training with learning objectives that adequately align with the required competencies and level of proficiency. For example, if incident commanders need to be able to apply principles of NIMS and the ICS by completing an incident action plan, then the course needs to deliver this level of training along with verification that the learning objectives associated with application have been achieved. Unfortunately, we often settle for training with a multiple-choice test at the awareness or knowledge level, not the application or judgment level.

In 2020, AIHA published a list of competencies for using direct reading instruments in industry and response operations due to the numerous deadly incidents related to misinterpretation of these instruments by users who lacked the appropriate level of training (AIHA 2020). In 2022, NFPA published standard 470 to define the various competencies associated with different levels of hazmat response (NFPA 2022). These consensus organizations are leading the way in establishing best practices that are industry-wide and not specific to any single discipline. Responders should seek out applicable standards and then identify training plans that align with responder responsibilities.

Over the last couple of decades, we have achieved success at various levels of government by clearly identifying the competencies needed and delivering realistic training that delivers appropriate learning objectives. In 2005, a new training program for the US Air Forces in Europe, dubbed the CBRN Challenge™, identified the knowledge, skills, and abilities needed by military response teams to successfully survive and operate through a chemical, biological, radiological, and nuclear (CBRN) attack. This week-long training program brought together three different disciplines involved in response operations and provided knowledge of CBRN agents and their physiological effects on specific mission sets, as well as how to detect, identify, and quantify these agents. The different response organizations used different equipment, often had their own procedures, and performed different functions for different purposes. The training involved the skills needed to operate the detection equipment by engaging participants in following procedures and the ability to interpret the results, while familiarizing partner organizations with each others' capabilities. However, the training could not stop there, as their mission-essential tasks entailed risk management and risk communication in an ICS structure. Therefore, we engaged participants in realistic scenarios where they performed their response operations with the equipment, interfaced with the other organizations that participated in the training, and required them to analyze the information gathered (rather than report raw data results) and make risk-based recommendations to commanders who would engage in questions and need to balance operational risks, not just health-based risks. After all, it would be easy to recommend wearing PPE or evacuating the area to protect one's health, but if those were not possible due to mission requirements, then alternatives would need to be formulated to optimize operations and the overall mission. The CBRN Challenge™ achieved higher-level learning objectives where participants were required to synthesize information from other response teams about operational mission tasks and evaluate all of the information to negotiate the best course of action. This training stressed participants with realism, time pressure, and required performance of exacting tasks (there were no injects when participants could not operate their equipment due to dead batteries or misinterpretation of the results). The training not only trained each discipline in how to respond, but it also built interoperable teams. Participants often commented about the relationships built with other organizations during the training. The CBRN Challenge™ set the stage for many other training venues.

After the US Chemical Safety Board (CSB) made recommendations to FEMA concerning deficiencies in national training in the wake of the West Fertilizer Company tragedy, a partnership was developed with Georgia Tech Research Institute to design, develop, and deliver similar courses to equip planners and incident commanders with the information, skills enhancement, and abilities needed to navigate complex crises involving hazardous materials.* Since the existing level of national training lacked attention to higher-level learning objectives, we carefully designed these courses to address the shortfalls identified by the CSB. These courses were extremely popular as they were requested in 40 localities in 25 states over a two-year period. These courses engaged the whole community of participants in planning and forging better-working relationships among organizations in the community. They stretched participants who filled different roles in the ICS than they normally filled. Ultimately, the training built relationships across organizations and sometimes jurisdictions, enhancing trust and improving operational coordination.

Regrettably, organizations sometimes state that they are reluctant to invite other organizations into their training because they are not ready; they want to be prepared before embarrassing themselves in front of another organization, or they do not want to let other organizations know about their capabilities, latest equipment, or special procedures. Unfortunately, these communities are not ready for a real incident where they will need to integrate with other organizations. Training together is a great way to build trust, share information, build relationships, and improve interoperability, operational coordination, and communication.

1.4.6.4 Exercises

Having conducted over 2,000 exercises, we have observed the greatest gain in capabilities and benefits from conducting the right type of training along with an exercise series. An exercise series is a series of exercises over a period of time that build on the previous exercises, such as a tabletop exercise that is followed up a year later in a functional exercise that is similar in scenario. A strong emphasis on training at the

* MGT-457 On-scene Crisis Leadership and Decision Making for Hazmat Incidents and MGT-458 Building Whole Community Engagement for LEPCs.

same scale and scope is necessary to gradually build the capabilities that will lead to success during evaluated exercises. Over the course of several hundred week-long combined training and exercise events, we have found significant capability gains by combining training with exercises using a systematic building block approach. This ensures a successful exercise based on proper training, rehearsals, and integration of first-response disciplines interfacing at the right pace to ultimately yield the most value while focusing on more critical issues during a full-scale exercise.

Exercise purists may argue for completely separating training and exercises with a focus on using exercises to measure capabilities on any given day. However, exercises are expensive, time-consuming, and contribute to organizational learning (even though they are not defined as training, this is a benefit). Thus, we advocate for ensuring the right type of training, building up to a full-scale exercise while ensuring that participants are ready and improving throughout the series by addressing areas for improvement before moving on to the next exercise. Conducting a full-scale exercise when participants are not adequately trained and prepared does not serve the responders or community well. If the goal is to improve preparedness and capabilities, then careful timing and sequencing of the right type of training and exercises can ensure that organizations are on pace to reach their goals while receiving the feedback associated with an evaluated exercise. The exercise is not the goal; rather, building capabilities and preparing the organization for anticipated risk aligns best with the national preparedness goal.

A properly designed and scoped exercise starts with clear objectives that can lead to evaluation criteria. While an exercise may not be funded or scoped to encompass every participant and detail, controllers and evaluators play an important role in ensuring the exercise achieves the objectives through the presented scenario and that participant performance is measured against established criteria. Deviating from either will likely lead to frustration and disengagement. For these reasons, we have found much success with employing experts in the controller and evaluator roles so that they have sufficient knowledge to engage participants where appropriate and make informed observations during the evaluation process. We also prefer to utilize evaluators representing multiple disciplines, as this adds value and external insight into the response process and reduces bias from one single discipline. Controller interaction should be minimal. Injects should flow from a natural communication system through the right channel or organization. This begins with a diverse exercise planning team representing the various stakeholders that will participate in the exercise. Including external perspectives can also lead to more realism and insights that will improve interoperability among response organizations. After-action reports can become politicized or biased if external evaluators are not invited to participate on the evaluation team.

1.5 SUMMARY

There are multiple challenges and obstacles to unified response operations that inhibit different disciplines and jurisdictions from effectively executing the response and swiftly transitioning into recovery and restoration (Table 1.4). These challenges

TABLE 1.4
Summary of Challenges and Solutions to Unified Response

Challenges and Obstacles to Unified Response	Solutions for Achieving Unified Response
Incident Size	Develop Crisis-Ready Leaders
Limited Staffing	Build Resilience into the Organization
Resource Limitations	Develop Organizational Strategies
Equipment Compatibility and Interoperability	Enhance Preparedness
Personnel Qualifications and Credentialing	
Politics, Power, and Pride	
Inadequate Training	
Insufficient Funding	
Leadership	

and obstacles are often rooted in the organization prior to the response and therefore should be addressed pre-incident. The table above summarizes the challenges and the solutions to overcoming them. Implementing these solutions requires organizational leadership that understands how the future risks will require a multiagency, multijurisdiction response and how to take steps to resolve obstacles to a unified response. As we have covered in this chapter, resilient organizations are best apt to overcome these challenges because they have the characteristics needed to resolve challenges to integration, interoperability, communication, organizational maturity, and preparedness. Resilient organizations possess six key characteristics that enable this: they are ready, robust, repairable, and resistant; they also have adequate reserves and built-in redundancies. These characteristics are enabled by relationships with other organizations.

REFERENCES

AIHA (2020). *Technical Framework: Guidance on Use of Direct Reading Instruments. https://www.aiha.org/education/frameworks/technical-framework-guidance-on-use-of-direct-reading-instruments* .

Campbell, B. (2020). *Technology Experimentation & Characterization Field Trials 2020: ArgusElite® Analysis Report*, Alliance Solutions Group, Inc., Newport News, VA.

Campbell, B. (2023). *Crisis-ready Leadership: Building Resilient Organizations and Communities*, Wiley, Hoboken, NJ.

Chemical Safety Board (2017). *Investigative Report Chemical Spill Contaminates Public Water Supply in Charleston, West Virginia.* https://www.csb.gov/west-fertilizer-explosion-and-fire-/

Farazmand, A. (2001). "Introduction – Crisis and Emergency Management." Chapter 1 in *Handbook of Crisis and Emergency Management*, (ed. Farazmand, A.), Marcel Dekker, Inc., New York and Basel.

FEMA (2006). *Hazards, Disasters and U.S. Emergency Management: An Introduction*, https://training.fema.gov/hiedu/docs/hazdem/appendix%20-%20select%20em-related%20terms%20and%20definitions.doc#:~:text=Crisis%3A%20%E2%80%9C%E2%80%A6,and%20property%20of%20its%20members%E2%80%A6 (accessed October 2, 2021).

FEMA (2018). *Threat and Hazard Identification and Risk Assessment (THIRA) and Stakeholder Preparedness Review (SPR) Guide, Comprehensive Preparedness Guide (CPG) 201*, 3rd edition, https://www.fema.gov/emergency-managers/risk-management/risk-capability-assessment (accessed August 29, 2023).

FEMA (2023a). Community lifelines, https://www.fema.gov/emergency-managers/practitioners/lifelines (accessed December 26, 2023).

FEMA (2023b). *National Preparedness Report.*Available at: *https://www.fema.gov/sites/default/files/documents/fema_2023-npr.pdf (accessed June 17, 2025)..*

FEMA (n.d.). Glossary, https://www.fema.gov/about/glossary (accessed December 24, 2023).

Lang, K., et al. (2019). *National Tribal & Rural Training Needs Assessment, Rural Domestic Preparedness Consortium.* https://ruraltraining.org/wp-content/uploads/2020/04/2019_National_Tribal__Rural_Training_Needs_Assessment-Finalv1.pdf.

McChrystal, G. S. A., Silverman, D., Collins, T., et al. (2015). *Team of Teams*, Portfolio Penguin, London.

National Institute of Standards and Technology (NIST) (2020). *Community Resilience*, https://www.nist.gov/topics/community-resilience. (accessed January 8, 2022).

National Association of Counties (2019). *Managing Disasters at the County Level: A National Survey.*https://www.naco.org/sites/default/files/documents/Emergency%20Management%20in%20County%20Government_03.25.19.pdf

National Association of Fire Protection (2022). *Hazardous Materials/Weapons of Mass Destruction (WMD) Standard for Responders. https://www.nfpa.org/product/nfpa-470-standard/p0470code/nfpa-470-hazardous-materials-weapons-of-mass-destruction-wmd-standard-for-responders-2022/47022.*

University of South Carolina (2022). *Hazards and Vulnerability Research Institute,* https://artsandsciences.sc.edu/geog/hvri/bric (accessed January 9, 2022).

2 A Multi-layered Dynamic Systems Model of Disaster Response

John Flach, Brian Simpson, and Cara Kneeland

2.1 INTRODUCTION

This chapter presents a dynamic systems model of emergency response that is informed by recent insights into military command and control, embodied cognition, economics, and more generally into the nature of complex natural systems. We begin by considering some antiquated assumptions often embedded in conventional approaches to the performance of humans and organizations. Next, we present an alternative framework for thinking about emergency response as a complex, multi-layered dynamic system. The functioning of this model is illustrated using examples from interviews with emergency response personnel and published after-action reviews of emergency response events. Additionally, we suggest attributes of organizations that will enhance their overall resilience and ability to cope with the uncertainties that are endemic to emergency situations.

The model presented here can be thought of as a model of organizational decision-making or sensemaking. As such, it reflects three means of coordination suggested by Thompson (1967). It is intended to provide a useful context for thinking about organizational sensemaking as described by Weick (1995) and the challenges associated with managing teams of teams as described by McChrystal (2015). Further, there are obvious parallels with models of individual cognition and sensemaking. For example, the three layers are somewhat analogous to Rasmussen's (1986) three levels of information processing: knowledge-, rule-, and skill-based. The idea of multiple, coupled dynamic loops is consistent with Rasmussen's (1986) decision ladder, which shows how the coupling of perception and action varies across the different levels of information processing. The need to frame problems and to evaluate and change frames to keep pace with changing situational demands is consistent with the Klein et al. (2006) Data Frame Theory of sensemaking. Finally, this model provides plausible explanations for the qualitative distinctions observed in decisionmaking (e.g., intuitive/System 1 vs. analytical/System 2) in terms of emergent properties, rather than as distinct cognitive mechanisms (e.g., Kahneman, 2011).

DOI: 10.1201/9781003648178-3

2.1.1 A Straw Man: Conventional Wisdom

Conventionally, organizational and human behaviors have been modeled using linear models that tend to emphasize a causal sequence of information-processing stages that begin with current knowledge (e.g., in the head of a human leader or formalized in doctrine), which sets up procedures for formulating plans and making proper decisions (e.g., taking into account the intended outcomes, available resources, opportunities, and threats), which are then implemented as a sequence of actions. Generally, the models include feedback as an error signal indicating when the intended consequences are not being realized. This leads to a repeat of the same causal sequence – update knowledge, revise plan, and act to implement the new plan.

Figure 2.1 shows four examples that illustrate the implicit linear assumptions that have shaped how we think about the performance of humans and organizations. The first example (A) is in the context of military command and control. The Marine Corps manual on command and control (MCDP 6; 1996) describes this conventional view:

> The traditional view of command and control sees "command" and "control" as operating in the same direction: from the top of the organization toward the bottom. Commanders impose control on those under their command; commanders are "in control" of their subordinates, and subordinates are "under the control" of their commanders.
>
> **(p. 39–40)**

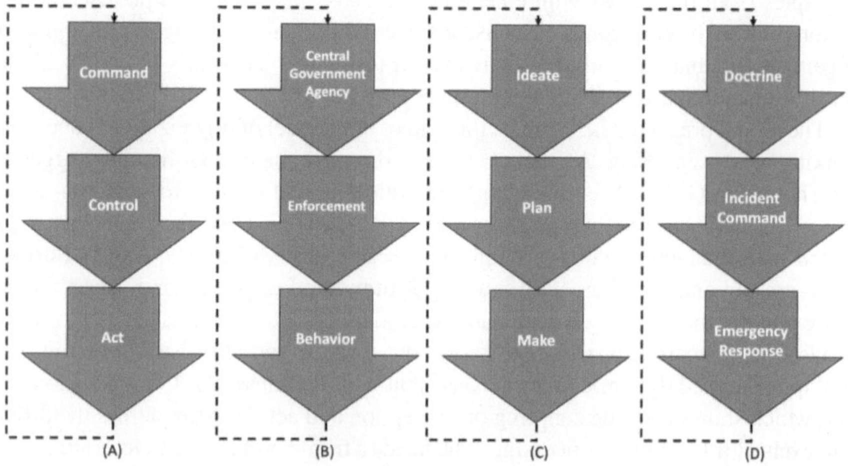

FIGURE 2.1 Conventional frameworks for thinking about the performance of individuals and organizations in multiple contexts.

The second context (B) reflects conventional assumptions about managing common pool resources like water irrigation systems, fisheries, or forests. As Elinor Ostrom (2010) describes, the conventional assumption was that without the imposition of regulations by a central government agency, people would compete to maximize their own local (selfish) interests, and this would inevitably lead to the *tragedy of the commons*, exhausting the resource and having tragic consequences for all who depend on that resource.

The third context (C) reflects conventional assumptions about human creativity. Kerr and Frasca (2021) refer to this model of creativity as a "God model" because it models creativity as if the creator acts like a "God of creation" who can "think things into being." They write:

> With most of our current models of creativity, we can see that they have unconsciously carried forward the classical linear model (ideate, plan, make) that never had to actually address the question of how novelty is possible because it was taken for granted that God alone created.
>
> **(p. 41)**

The fourth context (D) reflects our own observations based on after-action analyses of emergency response events and the explanations for unsatisfying outcomes. As in the other examples, there is an assumption of an a priori plan or doctrine that is enforced by an authority and determines the action. When outcomes are unsatisfying, there is a strong tendency to attribute the unsatisfying results to failures to follow established doctrine or to implement plans properly. While this attribution may sometimes be warranted, there is often an implicit assumption that the situation being evaluated conforms to the past experiences that led to the dogma or inspired the plans. This tends to underestimate the complexity and uniqueness of each disaster. Often, these after-action reviews are too quick to terminate analysis and attribute failures to "human error" when deviations from established doctrine and plans are discovered. However, with deeper analysis, it will often be discovered that these deviations reflect failed experiments where people were applying sound judgment to cope with novelty and surprise.

2.1.2 Common Misconceptions

When we look across the different conventional models illustrated in Figure 2.1, we see three common misconceptions: 1) underestimating the complexity and uncertainty of natural ecologies; 2) underestimating the dependence on feedback and the importance of the coupling of perception and action for adapting to the realities of complex ecologies; 3) underestimating the ability of people to leverage local structure (e.g., ecological rationality; heuristics) and social relations (e.g., trust) to successfully muddle through and cope with complexity.

2.1.2.1 Complexity

Disasters and emergency operations typically require coordination across many agents, distributed in space and time, who are dealing with multidimensional, dynamically evolving situations. Thus, no single agent (human or automated) has the capacity to have full awareness of all the relevant factors. Further, each disaster or emergency event is unique. There will inevitably be surprises that cannot be anticipated in the development of standard procedures or in the formulation of a plan. According to complexity science, the resulting uncertainty is not something that can be solved by gathering more data. Rather, due to the presence of nonlinear interactions and the potential for small changes to result in dramatically different outcomes, there is never enough data. This is typically illustrated by the butterfly effect – the idea that something as small as a butterfly flapping its wings can have a dramatic effect on future weather patterns (e.g., where a tornado forms). The point is that it is impossible to monitor all the butterflies – and other minor perturbations that ultimately contribute to the weather. The key here is to understand that there will always be potentially significant factors that cannot be known in advance. Thus, uncertainty is endemic.

The important implication of this is that no single agent (e.g., leader) can have accurate or complete situational awareness. Thus, building situational awareness will require collaboration and communication across multiple agents, each with a unique perspective on the event. However, even then, the awareness achieved will be limited in accuracy and scope. Surprise will be inevitable. Further, because of the uniqueness of each event, blind adherence to standard procedures or to a plan will rarely lead to satisfying outcomes. Thus, hypotheses and plans must always be considered tentative, and the organization must be prepared to adapt the standards and plans to accommodate uncertainty and surprise. With respect to the conventional models in Figure 2.1:

- **Military command and control** systems need to adopt a "mission command" style in which commanders provide command intent but do not try to micromanage field operations. They must trust the field level officers and give them the authority to adapt to the circumstances on the ground (MCDP 6; 1996).
- **Managing shared resources** is typically achieved through multi-level polycentric control that leverages the social intelligence of communities to self-organize processes for avoiding the tragedy of the commons (Ostrom, 2010).
- **Innovation** typically emerges from active engagement with situations; it involves smart muddling to explore diverse possibilities and to stimulate creativity and discovery (Kerr and Frasca, 2021).

2.1.2.2 Feedback

In order to cope with the uncertainty and complexity of natural events, it is necessary to "close the loop" – that is, to monitor the consequences of actions and use the information (i.e., feedback) to adjust actions, plans, and assumptions to achieve satisfactory outcomes. In essence, every action is a test of situational awareness, generating feedback that can be used to better tune the coupling of perception and action. When the consequence of an action is surprising (in either a negative or positive direction), this is an indication that situational awareness is lacking in some respect. For example, in taking a road trip, surprise could be due to situational factors (e.g., unexpected traffic), the wrong action (e.g., oversteering), a deficient plan (e.g., the wrong route), or incorrect assumptions (e.g., about the availability of fuel stations). Note that this is different from a simple servomechanism (e.g., a thermostat) where the "error" signal is simply a deviation from a goal or set point. In any complex situation, the source of the "error" or "surprise" can be somewhat ambiguous – and thus, it will take some sensemaking to determine whether the actions, the plan, the underlying assumptions, or all three ultimately need to be adjusted to achieve a satisfactory outcome.

A critical aspect of stability for feedback control is the temporal demands of the events. A key feature of the model to be presented will be an understanding of the natural time constants for different levels of control, relative to the temporal demands that determine temporal windows of opportunity.

2.1.2.3 Human Expertise

Unfortunately, humans are often regarded as the weakest link when it comes to complex work. A great deal of research has been conducted to catalog the limitations of humans as information processors (e.g., Wickens, 1984). Thus, it is not unusual for technologists to endeavor to design the human out of complex systems and replace them with more powerful autonomous systems (e.g., Artificial Intelligence). However, there is increasing evidence that the perceptual and logical puzzles that have been used to assess human capabilities in the laboratory are not representative of the demands of the natural world. These sterile environments typically do not account for the skills that allow people to cope with their everyday natural environments. Further, these laboratory observations do not fit with observations of human experts working in complex domains (e.g., Klein, 2023). In contrast to the conventional view, Ostrom (2010) summarizes a conclusion that is shared by many others who have observed the behavior of experts in their natural fields of endeavor:

> humans have a more complex motivational structure and more capability to solve social dilemmas than posited in earlier rational-choice theory. Designing institutions to force (or nudge) entirely self-interested individuals to achieve better outcomes has been the major goal posited by policy analysts for governments to accomplish for much of the past half century. Extensive empirical research leads me to argue that instead, a core goal of public policy should be to facilitate the development of institutions that bring out the best in humans. We need to ask how diverse polycentric institutions help or hinder the innovativeness, learning, adapting, trustworthiness, levels of cooperation of participants, and the achievement of more effective, equitable, and sustainable outcomes at multiple scales.
>
> **(Ostrom, 2010, pp. 664–665)**

Thus, the case can be made that when it comes to the type of sensemaking required to manage the uncertainty and ambiguities that are endemic to complex work domains like disaster response, humans are uniquely capable. The growing power of information technologies (including satellite communications, portable computing devices, machine learning, and artificial intelligence) is undeniable. However, we believe that these technologies belong in human-autonomous team environments and should be designed as tools to support human experts, compensating for limitations and enhancing capabilities, rather than as substitutes or replacements for those experts.

2.2 SOME OBSERVATIONS

Over the last four years, we have interviewed first responders and reviewed after-action evaluations of emergency events. This work was motivated by an interest in assessing the impact of new technologies (e.g., GPS, mobile communications, enhanced mapping, and tracking technologies) on coordination and control during distributed, complex operations. This chapter will focus on two aspects of these observations and the implications for modeling emergency response behaviors. Specifically, this involved 1) the importance of incident command, and 2) the impact of organizational culture.

2.2.1 Incident Command

The importance of incident command to the success of emergency operations was a recurrent theme in many of our interviews, and this was found to be particularly true in firefighting operations. We heard and read about both excellent (e.g., Washington Naval Yard) and poor (e.g., Uvalde) examples of incident command. One interview, in particular, illustrated the role and potential value of having a layer of control focused on incident command. The incident was a multi-vehicle accident involving multiple serious injuries in a rural area. A dump truck drove over the top of a car, critically injuring and trapping a woman in the car. The truck then went off the side of the road and hit two young girls who were rollerblading along the road – both of whom were critically injured. The dump truck then hit another pick-up truck, which subsequently hit a tree and resulted in moderate injuries to the occupants of that pick-up truck.

Three paramedics arrived at the scene:

> So, I'm pulling up and I'm like "Holy Cow!" I have two paramedics and me, I have to get two helicopters, I have to get three or four mutual aid medical units, I need another mutual aid rescue truck, and another mutual aid engine. This is the middle of a rural area. So, I know it's going to take a while for all that to get here. So, I took command. I started calling for all these resources and I'm sorting stuff. This lady comes running up saying she's a nurse. [I say,] "Here's my first aid kit, go help that girl." A police officer shows up, "what do you need?" "Go help that girl."
>
> I'm a paramedic and I'm not rendering treatment to these people. I don't know which one to go to first if I were, but I decided that I need to coordinate all this or else we're only going to save one, and my goal was to save them all. And that's what happened, they all lived.
>
> I didn't save any of those lives. I just got the resources that they needed as quick as possible, so we could handle it all…
>
> … getting the resources, getting the helicopters, getting them to the hospital within the golden hour, that's how I felt that I contributed to the whole incident.

It is unlikely that the seriously injured people would have gotten to trauma centers within the golden hour if all three paramedics had focused on directly treating the injured at the scene. Thus, the fact that one person took on the responsibility of incident command was critical to the ultimate success of this operation. In this instance, incident command provided an important perspective and additional layer of control over the direct work of the paramedics treating the injured, the volunteers who show up to the scene, and the additional support that includes the helicopter pilots and trauma center staff.

2.2.2 Organizational Culture

The person who described the accident above was a fire chief at the time of the interview. He was well versed in the standards for incident command as documented in the Department of Homeland Security's *National Incident Management System* (2008) report. This report evolved from the experiences of managing large forest fires and is now the national standard for fire and police departments with respect to incident command. However, in interviews with both police and fire personnel, we discovered that the two organizations are not equally enthusiastic about these guidelines. In fact, we heard multiple accounts of situations where police either bypassed the incident command or participated only reluctantly. This suggested to us that there was another layer in the dynamics of organizational response that reflected the cultures of the participating organizations. That is, organizations come to emergency operations with different experiences and expectations based on their work and training within their home organizations.

One obvious difference between police and fire is that police officers are often on patrol as individuals, but in contrast, firefighters typically come to events as teams. Thus, police departments place a high value on independence and personal initiative, and fire departments tend to place a high value on teamwork and coordination. Also, note that police are trained that in the case of active shooting incidents, engaging the shooter is the highest priority and establishing incident command is secondary. However, even in active shooter events, establishing incident command to coordinate the potentially large and diverse teams who respond to the emergency remains an important step. This is illustrated in the after-action review of an active shooter event at the Washington Naval Yard (2013). In this incident, an officer set up an incident command outside the building to coordinate the activities of multiple shooter teams attempting to track down the shooter. As the event evolved, this officer coordinated with the teams in the building and controlled when additional teams could enter the building. On the other hand, an after-action review of the 2022 mass shooting at a school in Uvalde, TX (Department of Justice 2024) found that the failure to establish incident command was a contributing factor that led to poor situational awareness and misinterpretation of the event as a barricaded shooter incident, rather than an active shooter incident.

The key inference from these observations is that in addition to an incident command layer, there is a third layer impacting the dynamics of emergency response that reflects the prior knowledge, standards, and expectations that organizations impose on their members. This layer shapes how incident command is implemented, as well as how basic skills and expectations are trained to enable mutual adjustment among individual first responders.

2.3. AN ALTERNATIVE MODEL

As noted earlier (see Figure 2.1), the idea of a command hierarchy with multiple levels is not novel. However, our observations and the research in other domains reviewed above suggest that the coupling between levels is much more intimate and dynamic than is assumed in the classical hierarchical models. Rather than visualizing the coupling between levels as the passing of information through a series of stages, we suggest that the coupling is better modeled as a nesting in which outer stages set up constraints on the processing in inner stages, as illustrated in Figure 2.2. The nesting creates an adaptive system in which changes in outer levels (e.g., dynamic re-planning) can impact the degrees of freedom or possibilities for action in the inner levels. In essence, this is a self-organizing system where the changes to outer loops are continually redesigning the possibilities for the inner loops.

Figure 2.3 shows a more detailed view of a polycentric control system with three nested levels that reflect: 1) the direct activity of first responders (mutual adjustment); 2) incident command (planning); and 3) the organizational culture (standardization). These three levels correspond roughly with Thompson's (1967) three means that organizations use to coordinate activity: standardization, planning, and mutual adjustment. A critical aspect of this model is that all three levels get feedback resulting from the consequences of actions during the disaster event. However, the time constant of the various loops is different, and the focus of attention will typically be different – reflecting different access to information and different spheres of action.

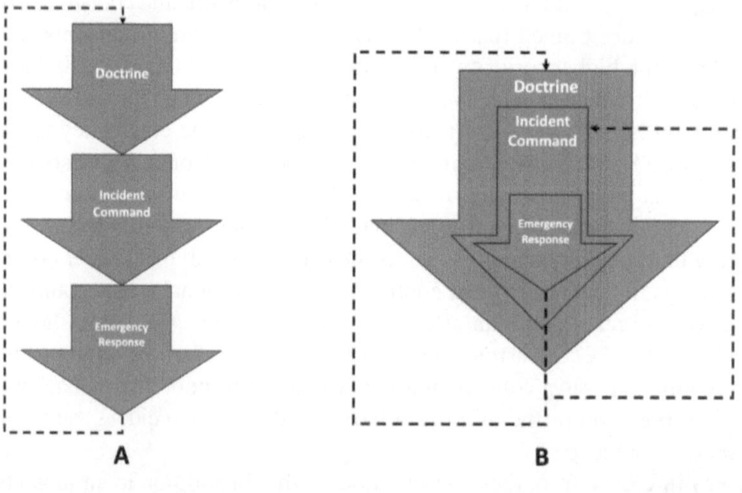

FIGURE 2.2 The classical hierarchical model (A) is contrasted with a model in which the layers are nested such that outer layers "design" or shape the possibilities of inner layers.

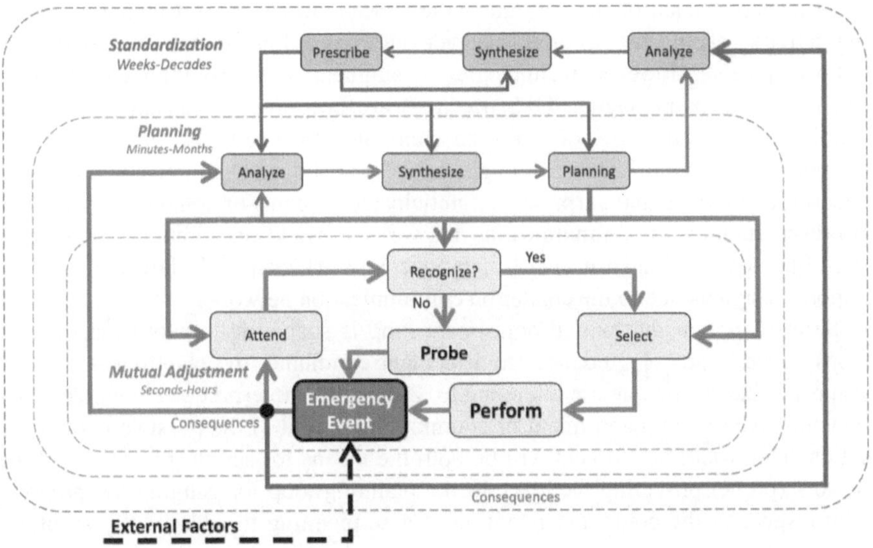

FIGURE 2.3 A more detailed model of a multi-layered, nested polycentric control system.

For example, in the multi-vehicle accident described above, two of the paramedics were attending to and treating specific patients. These paramedics were focused on the immediate needs of their specific patients and were not aware of the total number of people who were injured or the expected arrival time of the helicopters. The person who took over incident command had a better overview of the situation. He knew the total number of victims and was able to direct volunteers to specific patients. He was also in direct contact with the helicopters, helping them to identify an appropriate landing area. With respect to the organizational culture, the account of this accident will be used by the future fire chief to impress upon the people in his command the importance of incident command. In the interview, he mentioned the need to impress upon his officers the importance of ensuring one individual stays in their command vehicles to focus on incident command, resisting their natural urges to get directly involved in firefighting activities.

2.3.1 Mutual Adjustment Cycle

The mutual adjustment cycle is the innermost loop in the polycentric control system. It involves the emergency response personnel who are "on the ground," directly responding to the disaster. This might include firefighters, police, emergency healthcare workers, and local volunteers. These people are directly involved in moment-to-moment adaptations to the events on the ground. This loop has the shortest time constant and can respond immediately to adapt to rapid changes at the scene. These rapid responses typically require real-time coordination of activities among multiple people under dynamically changing situations, often involving high degrees of risk.

Until recently, much of the communication for coordinating and mutually adjusting activities would be via direct contact (i.e., voice, line of sight, and dedicated radio channels). However, technologies to augment direct communications (e.g., cell phones, text messaging, GPS tracking) are becoming increasingly available. The increased availability of real-time communication networks greatly expands the potential for coordinating through mutual adjustment to adaptively respond to uncertain situations and surprises not anticipated in plans or standard procedures. However, monitoring communication networks can add an additional burden on front-line workers, and we heard many accounts where people failed to pick up important signals due to the chatter on communication networks.

Performance in the mutual adjustment loop is shaped by inputs from the two loops above. Plans or guidance from incident command (the planning layer) will shape 1) what the people are attending to, 2) how they interpret or recognize situations relative to command intent or common goals, and 3) the possible options for action. The front-line workers will be both the means for action (perform) and the sensors (probe) providing feedback to the planning loop for gauging the progress with respect to the command intent and for re-planning to address any surprises encountered.

Performance in the mutual adjustment loop is also shaped by the standards and expectations that are created through training and experience reflected in the outermost loop (standardization layer). The training in the standardization layer shapes expectations and skills at the mutual adjustment level with potentially positive and negative consequences. For example, the benefit of standard practices is that they allow for automatic responses that reduce the cognitive load when responding to common or expected situations. However, a potential risk is that sometimes these practices can be applied mindlessly in situations that deviate from the norm in unexpected or unrecognized ways. Another benefit of standard practices is that the activities are predictable, thus facilitating coordination with others who know the standards. Note that Figure 2.3 shows only a single standardization layer; however, in practice, every organization participating in the disaster event will typically have unique standard practices and expectations reflecting the specific nature of that organization's long-time experiences and cultures. Thus, we have observed that the standard practices of different *teams* (e.g., police and fire) can be a source of friction and conflict. This can perhaps be mitigated by joint training exercises; however, such exercises are rare due to the expense and logistics required.

While the mutual adjustment layer has the shortest time constant allowing quick responses to events, the individuals are limited in their access to information and do not have the capacity to integrate information that is distributed in time and space to gain "top sight" on the situation. This opens the possibility that in responding quickly to local events, the people may ultimately be working at cross purposes with regards to achieving the overall objectives of the organization. Thus, the constraints imposed by the outer layers in terms of plans and standards can facilitate coordination at the mutual adjustment level. On the other hand, micromanagement that demands strict adherence to plans and requires authorization for any deviations can inhibit the ability of people to intelligently adapt to dynamic situations.

2.3.2 Planning Cycle

The planning cycle for regional disaster events would represent the people and activities in an incident command center. Ideally, all the organizations participating in the event would be represented here, and ideally, they would function as a joint command – sharing information and participating in setting goals/objectives, developing plans, and issuing commands and instructions to the people in the field. The goal is to achieve unity of command to provide clear, unambiguous guidance (e.g., common ground) for mutual adjustments by the front-line workers.

The planning layer receives updates about evolving situations on the ground from multiple sources within the mutual adjustment layer. This feedback is analyzed relative to past experiences and standards of operations (from the outer loop) and synthesized into new plans and guidance for the front-line operators. Typically, this involves a continuous re-planning or "flexecution" (Klein, 2007) process in which plans are constantly evaluated and adjusted relative to evolving situations on the ground. Because it takes time to integrate the information coming from multiple sources to achieve accurate situational awareness, the planning loop has a much longer time constant than the mutual adjustment loop. For example, slowed responses from incident command to the mutual adjustment level may result in instability as ground operators may be getting guidance from incident command that is based on outdated information. The appropriate time constant for the planning loop depends on the speed at which the environment or situation evolves. Thus, efforts to micromanage actions at the mutual adjustment level from a centralized incident command center will sometimes result in instability due to the inability to respond within short windows of opportunity. On the positive side, however, due to the broader access to information, the incident command center has the capacity to pick up patterns and trends that are not visible to the people directly engaged with the situation. This big-picture perspective can allow the planning cycle to frame the problem in a way that simplifies and/or increases the efficiency of the mutual adjustment efforts of the people on the ground. By providing a big-picture perspective, the planning layer can often help the people on the ground to anticipate and prepare for changes that can be forecasted based on the more global patterns and trends.

2.3.3 Standardization Cycle

The outermost loop reflects the process of organizational learning. This cycle takes the activities and consequences of an event or events as input to be analyzed (e.g., in after-action reviews or historical analyses). The products of these analyses are then implemented as new doctrine, principles, and standard procedures that are communicated through mentoring and training. These create what is often referred to as the culture of the organization, and this culture constrains how planning and mutual adjustment will be framed for future events. For example, the National Incident Management System includes principles and standard procedures that reflect experience from managing many prior disasters, mostly involving large forest fires. This is now recommended as a national standard for guiding responses to all regional disasters.

The standardization cycle has the longest time constant and is typically integrating information gleaned from a long history of experience covering multiple prior events. The contributions of this layer are difficult to observe in the operations of a single organization because this layer reflects the hidden assumptions and tacit knowledge that are typically shaping performance in the background. However, the impact of this layer becomes particularly salient in situations where people from different organizations (with different training and cultures) must cooperate to deal with a complex event like a regional disaster. The different learning and training processes across organizations can result in different *cultures* that can clash in the planning and mutual adjustment processes of an event where cooperation is required for efficient coordination and ultimate success. As noted above, clashes between fire and police cultures were a recurrent theme in our interviews with emergency responders. McChrystal's (2015) *Team of Teams* provides an interesting account of the challenges of achieving coordination when teams from different operational cultures must coordinate activities to get the job done. The military has recently begun to address the opportunities and challenges of achieving skilled coordination across diverse teams from different cultures in efforts to formalize doctrine for Joint All Domain Operations (JADO) (US Air Force, 2021). A key challenge in both disaster management and military operations is that joint exercises designed to train multiple teams together are logistically difficult and extremely expensive with respect to time and money.

Finally, while the organizational learning that occurs in the standardization cycle can significantly shape how people plan and how they respond to situations on the ground during an event, the influence of feedback in this loop will typically not be evident during the event. The learning will often benefit from after-action reviews and reflection. Thus, the impact of learning in the standardization loop will become more evident in subsequent events.

2.3.4 Resilience as an Emerging Property

The three components described above are being modeled as a system of three coupled, closed-loop-circuits. All three loops are provided with feedback in terms of consequences of actions on the ground. The inner loop focuses on utilizing feedback to react to rapidly evolving situations on the ground. The middle loop focuses on integrating information from distributed sources to detect trends and patterns that allow short- and long-term forecasting to anticipate and prepare for coming events on the ground. The outer loop reflects the integration of information across many events that contributes to organizational learning, skill development, and standardization. Note that there is also an embedded planning loop (coupling between standardization layer and planning layer) that allows plans to be "tested" relative to long-term experiences before implementing them in the mutual adjustment layer. Thus, it is possible to consider and reject a plan before acting on it.

The implication of the coupling across layers is that the dynamics within each component need to be considered in the context of the interactions with other components. Further, there are properties of the whole (e.g., organizational resilience) that emerge from these interactions and are difficult or impossible to infer from independent analyses of the components in isolation. Essentially, the resilience of an organization reflects the ability to adapt to surprises in order to achieve a satisfying outcome in a complex, uncertain world. Because of the nonlinearities associated with couplings where outer layers are dynamically constraining, designing, or shaping the processes of inner layers, there is no analytical way to optimize organizational resilience. However, numerous constructs have been suggested that can help organizations wrestle with the challenges of resilience. These include constructs such as *polycentric control* (Ostrom, 1999; Wilson, 2019; Woods & Branlat, 2010), *subsidiarity* (e.g., Sage & Cuppan, 2001), *command intent* (Klein, 1993, 1994; Shattuck, 2000), and *essential friction* (Rochlin, 1998).

The construct of *polycentric control* was identified by Ostrom (1999) in relation to her studies of how communities are able to avoid depleting a common pool of resources through mutual cooperation. The problem of managing a common resource is often referred to as the *tragedy of the commons* problem. As noted in the introduction, it has been assumed that without centralized control, communities will compete to maximize their own local interests, and this will inevitably lead to depletion of the common resource and tragic consequences for all who depend on that resource. Ostrom's work challenges this assumption. She noted that conventional approaches that rely heavily on a centralized authority often fail to solve this type of problem. However, under certain conditions, including collective choice arrangements, monitoring, and fast and fair conflict resolution, diverse communities are often able to avoid the tragedy of the commons. In terms of the model depicted in Figure 2.3, the conditions described by Ostrom reflect a dynamic coupling where stability is achieved through mutual adjustments across local autonomous communities (innermost loop), who operate within a set of collective agreements based on shared principles of fairness (outermost loop – standardization) that are enforced through conflict resolution at the planning level (middle loop).

The principle of *subsidiarity* has been discussed by Sage and Cuppan (2001) in relation to the distribution of authority within federations of systems. In classical hierarchical models such as those illustrated in Figure 2.1, the delegation of authority is presumed to be top-down, as if authority resides naturally with a central agency. However, the principle of subsidiarity suggests that authority should reside at the local level. The implication is that people or sub-organizations should have the authority to flexibly make decisions in response to their local situations with minimal constraint from a central authority who is not directly engaged in the situation. This recognizes that in highly dynamic situations, the people at the local levels have direct information that generally will enable stable adaptation through mutual adjustment. In federations of systems, centralized planning authority should only be used for problems that require information that is beyond the capacity of the local agencies. The main point is that people on the ground can be trusted to make smart decisions if they have adequate information.

The military construct of *command intent* is closely related to the principle of subsidiarity. The key point is that military commanders should avoid micromanaging the junior officers in the field of battle. Thus, in planning for military engagements, the plans should emphasize the overall purpose or goal of the operations and should trust field officers to adapt to local circumstances and events in ways that they judge will best satisfy the overall command intent. As with the principle of subsidiarity, the construct of command intent recognizes that local situational dynamics are happening at a pace that is too fast to allow stable adjustments to be made in the planning (or standardization) loops. When this is the case, stability of the whole depends heavily on the capacity for mutual adjustment in the innermost loop of the model in Figure 2.3. This capacity of military organizations to adapt through mutual adjustment is greatly enhanced by the availability of advanced information networks that allow direct, real-time communications between distributed units in the field, reducing dependence on a central command.

Rochlin's (1998) construct of *essential friction* reflects a balancing counterweight to extreme applications of the constructs of subsidiarity and command intent. In physical systems friction is often seen as wasted energy. However, at the same time, some degree of friction (or damping) is essential for stable control in most situations. In the organizational context, constraints from higher levels to lower levels, such as standards of practice and the need for local actors to get approval from authorities in an incident command center, can be seen as friction that slows down or hampers creative adaptation at the mutual adjustment level. However, as with physical systems, Rochlin points out that some degree of friction is essential for stability. Without these constraints, the system can become unstable due to impetuous mutual adjustments that may reflect limitations of local information and conflicting local values. Thus, the key point is that the propagation of constraints from outer to inner levels in our model can play an essential role in dampening local noise and increase overall stability of the organization.

The need for *friction* was observed in the after-action review of a mass shooting incident at the Washington Navy Yard (Washington, DC Metropolitan Police Department, 2013). At least 117 officers from eight different organizations entered the building during the initial search for the shooter. Upon establishing incident command outside the building, an officer restricted access to the building, so that self-responding officers were not allowed to enter the building without checking-in and getting permission. This allowed control over people entering the building and allowed people already in the building to be alerted when a new team was admitted to the building. While this check-in policy could be perceived as friction by officers eager to protect victims from an active shooter, it was necessary to avoid confusion and potential friendly-fire accidents. In this case, the incident commander also restricted non-uniformed officers from joining the search for the shooter, so that they would not be mistakenly identified as the shooter.

In our model, each of the above constructs can be framed as the need to balance constraints across a multi-layered, coupled control system to reflect differential access to information and differential time lags in making sense of the information. In essence, constraints from outer loops frame the degrees of freedom for adaptations in inner loops. A proper framing will generally simplify the control problems within the inner loops, while an improper framing may impede or complicate the inner loop control problems. Note that there is no single absolute best solution to this balancing problem. Rather, framing, stability, and resilience are always determined in relation to the situations that organizations must cope with to succeed. However, it is possible to generalize from control theory to claim that to succeed in highly dynamic environments, organizations will require a high capacity for mutual adjustment. In such environments, the planning and standardization loops are simply too slow to keep pace with the situated demands. However, the skills developed over experience with prior events (standards of practice) may facilitate quick adaptations at the local level. In more stable environments, the benefits of prior experience applied through standardization and planning will generally lead to more efficient and stable operations. In the case of disaster management, resilience may depend heavily on the capacity for fast mutual adjustments during the initial stages of a disaster, when things on the ground are changing rapidly. However, prior preparations and the recovery process following a disaster may benefit from more deliberate policy development (standardization) and planning.

2.4 SUMMARY AND CONCLUSIONS

In discussions of organizational dynamics, a distinction is often made between hierarchical/centralized vs. flat/networked forms of organizations, as if these are distinct types. However, the multi-layered model in Figure 2.3 suggests that this is actually a continuum in which organizations vary in the degree of coupling across three nested control loops. Organizations typically characterized as hierarchical tend to rely heavily on standardization and planning loops to constrain/coordinate actions at the mutual adjustment level. Organizations typically characterized as networked tend to allow more flexibility for decisionmaking and real-time coordination at the mutual adjustment level. Note that for large, distributed organizations, the capability for mutual adjustment will ultimately depend on real-time communication networks that allow people to be aware of each other's actions. However, Rochlin (1997) warns that these networks can also be misused as a means for micromanagement, in which a central authority uses the communication network to enforce compliance, thus limiting the capacity for mutual adjustment.

With our model, resilience reflects the degree to which the constraints across the three levels fit the demands of the situations with which the organizations must cope. Resilience in highly dynamic environments requires a high capacity for mutual adjustment and for dynamic re-planning or flexecution. However, standardization and planning constraints can lead to both greater efficiency and accuracy in less dynamic environments. Note also that environments are typically not stationary, so that a resilient organization will typically have to be constantly tuning the coupling across levels (i.e., learning from each event, dynamically reframing problems) to keep aligned with changing situational dynamics.

As previously noted, the model in Figure 2.3 is intended as a model of organizational decisionmaking or sensemaking. As such, it provides a useful context for thinking about the organizational sensemaking described by Weick (1995) and the challenges associated with managing teams of teams described by McChrystal (2015). Further, there are also obvious parallels with models of individual cognition and sensemaking. For example, the three layers are somewhat analogous to Rasmussen's (1986) three levels of information processing: knowledge-, rule- and skill-based. The idea of multiple, coupled dynamic loops is consistent with Rasmussen's (1986) decision ladder, which shows how the coupling of perception and action varies across the different levels of information processing. The need to frame problems and to evaluate and change frames to keep pace with changing situational demands is consistent with Klein, Moon, and Hoffman's (2006) Data Frame Theory of sensemaking. Finally, this model can explain the qualitative distinctions observed in decisionmaking (e.g., intuitive/System 1 vs. analytical/System 2) in terms of emergent properties, rather than as distinct cognitive mechanisms (e.g., Kahneman, 2011).

In summary, we hope our model provides a useful framework for generalizing some of the intuitions and principles of stability derived from quantitative analyses of closed-loop dynamic systems to better understand the dynamics and emerging properties of organizations in relation to resilience. In this respect, we hope that some of the qualitative performance shifts and emergent properties of organizational dynamics will be less mysterious, and the value of some of the constructs for assessing the resilience of organizations will be more obvious.

2.5 ACKNOWLEDGMENTS

Our recent work interviewing domain experts in the field of emergency operations was supported by funding from the Air Force Research Laboratories, Wright-Patterson, AFB. We want to thank Tim Shaw and Jim Gruenberg for sharing their experiences in emergency operations and for introducing us to other domain experts. They also allowed us to observe tabletop exercises using the Aware software, which has been designed to improve coordination during emergency operations. The views expressed are those of the authors and do not necessarily reflect the official policy or position of the Department of the Air Force, the Department of Defense, or the US government.

REFERENCES

Department of Homeland Security (2008). *National Incident Management System.* Washington, DC: U.S. Department of Homeland Security.

Department of Justice (2024). Critical Incident Review: Active Shooter at Robb Elementary School. Available at: https://portal.cops.usdoj.gov/resourcecenter/content.ashx/cops-r1141-pub.pdf (accessed June 13, 2025).

Kahneman, D. (2011). *Thinking, Fast and Slow.* New York: Farrar, Straus and Giroux.

Kerr, I. & Frasca, J. (2021) Innovating emergent futures: The innovation design approach for change and worldmaking. Monee, IL: Emergent Futures Lab Press.

Klein, G. A. (1993). *Characteristics of Commander's Intent Statements* (Tech. Rep., ContractsMDA903-90-C-0032 and MDA903-92-C-0098). Arlington, VA: U.S. Army Research Institute for the Behavioral and Social Sciences.

Klein, G. A. (1994). A script for the commander's intent statement. In A. H. Levis & I. S. Levis (Eds.), *Science of Command and Control: Part III. Coping with Change* (pp. 75–86). Fairfax, VA: AFCEA International Press.

Klein G, Jalaeian M, Hoffman RR and Mueller ST (2023) The plausibility transition model for sensemaking. Front. Psychol. 14:1160132.https://www.frontiersin.org/journals/psychology/articles/10.3389/fpsyg.2023.1160132/full

Klein, G., Moon, B., & Hoffman, R. R. (2006). Making sense of sensemaking 2: A macrocognitive model. *IEEE Intelligent Systems,* September/October, pp. 88–92.

Klein, G. A. (2007). Flexecution as a paradigm for replanning, part 1. *IEEE Intelligent Systems,* September/October, pp. 79–83.

McChrystal, S. (2015). *Team of Teams.* New York: Penguin Books.

Ostrom, E. (1999). Coping with tragedies of the commons. *Annual Review of Political Science, 2,* 493–535.

Ostrom, E. (2010). Beyond markets and states: Polycentric governance of complex systems. *American Economic Review, 100*(June), 641–672.

Sage, A. P., & Cuppan, C. D. (2001). On the systems engineering and management of systems of systems and federations of systems. *Information-Knowledge-Systems Management,* 2(4), 245–325.

Shattuck, L. (2000). Communicating intent and imparting presence. *Military Review, 80*(2), 66–72.

Thompson, J. (1967). *Organizations in Action.* New York: McGraw Hill.

Rasmussen, J. (1986). *Information Processing and Human-Machine Interaction.* New York: North Holland.

Rochlin, G. I. (1997). *Trapped in the Net.* Princeton, NJ: Princeton University Press

Rochlin, G. I. (1998). Essential friction: Error-control in organizational behavior. In N. Akerman (Ed.), *The Necessity of Friction.* Boulder, CO: Westview Press.

U.S. Air Force (2021). *The Department of the Air Force Role in Joint All-Domain Operations.* Air Force Doctrine Publication 2-99. https://www.doctrine.af.mil/Portals/61/documents/AFDP_3-99/AFDP%203-99%20DAF%20role%20in%20JADO.pdf.

U.S. Marine Corps (1996). *Command and Control* (MCDP 6). Washington, DC: Department of the Navy.

Washington, DC Metropolitan Police Department (2013). After action report Washington Navy Yard, September 16. www.mpdc.dc.gov.

Weick, K. (1995). *Sensemaking in Organizations.* Thousand Oaks, CA: Sage Publications.

Wickens, C. D. (1984). Processing resources in attention. In R. Parasuraman & R. Davies (Eds.), Varieties of attention (pp. 63–101). New York: Academic Press.

Wilson, D. S. (2019). The tragedy of the commons: How Elinor Ostrom solved one of life's greatest dilemmas. *Economics.* evonomics.com/tragedy-of-the-commons-elinor-ostrom/.

Woods, D. D., & Branlat, M. (2010). Hollnagel's test: Being 'in control' of highly interdependent multi-layered networked systems. Cogn Tech Work 12, 95–101.

3 Creating Effective Response Communications

Tay Johannes

3.1 INTRODUCTION

The ability to communicate accurately, comprehensively, and concisely in an emergency or crisis is not simply aspirational or a convenience; it is an absolutely critical need. Emergency communications play a key role in saving lives, facilitating a unity of effort, and enabling targeted resource employment regarding events that range from natural to man-made disasters and emergencies. With an increasingly dynamic world, the need for robust and resilient communication systems becomes increasingly apparent. This chapter delves into several crisis and emergency response communication considerations and offers general guidelines with methods and concepts for approaching response communications.

An emergency or crisis requires timely and accurate communication with first responders, government officials, the public, and the media. A wide range of emergencies or crises affect organizations from house fires to earthquakes or from vandalism to terrorism. Management and control of these incidents require a sound communications approach to ensure the best possible outcome. Success in response communications requires development, adaptation, and thorough planning. Without putting considerable effort into each of these, failure is almost guaranteed.

3.2 STRATEGIC ELEMENTS OF RESPONSE COMMUNICATIONS

Successful response communication strategy has four strategic elements as a foundation that include: stakeholders, organizational leadership, planning, and situational awareness. We will characterize each of these elements and start with a look at the stakeholders element.

3.2.1 Stakeholders in Response Communications

Response communications is a process of incoming and outgoing information to and from major stakeholders who are either producers or consumers of information or both. In an emergency response situation, the emergency communication

 DOI: 10.1201/9781003648178-4

activities of stakeholders vary based on their roles and responsibilities in the crisis. Stakeholders here will typically fall into one of the following broad categories that include:

- First responders: Fire, law enforcement, emergency medical, public works.
- Survivors: Those directly affected or impacted by a specific event.
- Public officials: Mayors, commissioners, councils, other elected officials.
- Volunteer groups: American Red Cross, Salvation Army, etc.
- Business community: Services (food or lodging), public works (not first response).
- Media: Various news services (the strongest link to the general public).
- General public: All others impacted by emergency events.

These roles will undoubtedly have a wide spectrum of information processes and flows depending on the emergency situation and how formal or informal the group structure is. Given these general roles for stakeholders in response communications, leaders and leadership emerge in varying degrees of influence within these stakeholder groups. Understanding how that leadership emerges within the group depends on a group dynamic often referred to as organizational leadership.

3.2.2 Organizational Leadership in Response Communications

Organizational leadership establishes the basis for both internal and external communication; how committed or engaged leaders are to their organizations will be a major determinant in the success of communication activities. The organizational leader provides vision, focus, and endorsement for establishing, expanding, and adjusting lines of communication with organization staff, partners, and the public. These various contributions by the organizational leader to emergency communication highlight several planning actions. Arguably, these planning actions may be the most critical parts of response communications.

3.2.3 Planning in Response Communications

Understanding the planning process requires a slightly philosophical mindset and may be the most important part of the leadership commitment to communications. The quote "Plans are worthless, but planning is everything" is often attributed to Dwight D. Eisenhower, who served as the 34th President of the United States from 1953 to 1961. Eisenhower was a five-star general in the United States Army during World War II and served as Supreme Commander of the Allied Expeditionary Forces in Europe. The essence of the quote highlights a philosophy that, while specific plans may not be strictly followed due to highly dynamic emergency responses, the process of planning itself is invaluable. The act of planning helps individuals and organizations anticipate challenges, understand the broader implications, and explore areas of flexibility with unforeseen events during emergency responses.

3.2.4 Situational Awareness in Response Communications

The National Response Framework (NRF) developed, published, and released by the Federal Emergency Management Agency highlights and emphasizes the need to gain and maintain situational awareness. Situational awareness has been defined in many different ways. First identified as a US Air Force concept for fighter pilots, courtesy of Colonel John Boyd's "observe-orient-decide-act loop" or OODA loop (as referenced in von Lubitz 2008, 562). Putting this in aviation community vernacular, "A pilot with good situational awareness flies ahead of the plane." It involves being aware of what is happening around you, understanding the significance of those events, and anticipating what might happen next. This action enables follow-on actions of activating and deploying key resources and capabilities, coordinating response actions, and then demobilizing. In a more general context, situational awareness, as discussed by Human Factors practitioners and researchers in the Enhanced Safety through Situational Awareness Integration (ESSAI), is defined as:

> the perception of the elements in the environment within a volume of time and space, the comprehension of their meaning, and the projection of their status in the near future.
>
> **(Endsley 1988, 98)**

A lessons-learned report by the White House on the national response to Hurricane Katrina made special mention of situational awareness in the findings. The White House committee found that inadequate situational awareness during the response resulted in decision-makers using incorrect and incomplete information (Townsend 2006, 97–98). This use of incorrect and incomplete information (with a corresponding loss of situational awareness) introduces a physical aspect of situational awareness that came as a result of communication infrastructure failures. The damaged infrastructure included:

- Communication facilities and backup power supply systems' destruction.
- Over three million phone lines down in Louisiana, Mississippi, and Alabama.
- Thirty-eight 911 call centers down.
- Over 2,000 wireless network cell sites offline.
- 37 of 41 radio stations off-the-air in New Orleans (Townsend 2006, 5–10).

Impaired response, command, control, and situational awareness were all cited as the results of the massive communication damage and the failure to adequately plan for alternatives (Townsend 2006, 3). The failures highlight a broader systemic situation in the physical realm for situational awareness and needed resiliency within the broader situational awareness processes.

Aside from the physical infrastructure priorities for achieving situational awareness, a need for stakeholders to communicate and share situational awareness establishes the concept of stakeholders having and working from a common operating picture. The common operating picture is a key concept and principle described in the National Incident Management System (NIMS) as an overview of an incident made through collecting and organizing various types of information from various responsible sources to support coordinated decision-making (FEMA 2017). This facilitates consistent information regarding the incident for on-scene responders and off-scene command and support personnel, including asset availability and location and status of requests. The development of a common operating picture and common situational awareness for first responders is considered a key issue by the National Academy of Sciences in addressing the issue of providing the most effective assistance to those affected by disasters (National Academy of Sciences 2007, 49–50). The common operating picture, listed first under NIMS concepts and principles, also emerges within the strategic concept within the NRF:

> In the event of an act of terrorism, natural disaster, or other emergency, the NOC [National Operations Center], as the principal operations center for DHS [Department of Homeland Security], coordinates and integrates information from the NOC components to provide situational awareness and a common operating picture for the entire Federal Government, as well as for local, state, tribal, territorial, and insular area governments, as appropriate, to ensure that accurate and critical terrorism and disaster-related information reaches government decision makers in a timely manner.
>
> **(DHS 2019, 24)**

A common operating picture is a shared perspective of various emergency support functions that allows the calibration of situational awareness at the support functions' level. The NRF identifies, defines, and elaborates on fifteen emergency support functions, each with a separate annex that includes purpose, capability, members, and operational concepts. A list of emergency support functions is shown in Table 3.1.

TABLE 3.1
Emergency Support Functions (ESFs) of the National Response Framework

ESF #1 Transportation	**ESF #2 Communications**	**ESF #3 Public works and engineering**	**ESF #4 Firefighting**
ESF #5 Emergency management	ESF #6 Mass care, emergency assistance, housing, and human services	ESF #7 Logistics management and resource support	ESF #8 Public health and medical services
ESF #9 Search and rescue	ESF #10 Oil and hazardous materials response	ESF #11 Agriculture and natural resources	ESF #12 Energy
ESF #13 Public safety and security	ESF #14 Cross-sector business and infrastructure	ESF #15 External affairs	

Incident management under the NIMS doctrine offers some general response-based questions such as: what resource and how much is needed; where and when is this resource needed; and who gets it. Upon closer inspection of the common operating picture, many different facets begin to appear. Information needs at the detailed level show some variability due to specific mission tasks, type of event, location, phase of response, demographics, time period, and so forth. Though the common operating picture serves the response system's overall unity of effort, variation in detail focus is apparent across various information users.

3.3 A SYSTEM CHARACTERIZATION OF RESPONSE COMMUNICATIONS

Successful emergency responses require communication systems that are adaptable to a wide variety of situations. These communication systems must convey messages that are timely and accurate, routed properly, and in a format that ensures clarity and efficient understanding. The most effective communication systems in response are characterized by seven basic elements:

1. Communications planning
2. Information coming in
3. Information going out
4. Messengers
5. Staffing
6. Training and exercises
7. Monitoring, updating, and adapting (Haddow et al. 2021, 194)

Balancing these elements requires a systems approach and substantial effort by a dedicated communications team.

The communications team is made up of select individuals oriented to higher organizational perspectives relative to the organization's vision and strategy. Ideally, the team members would include senior representatives vested with some decision authority. Where possible, the most senior personnel (along with their enabling authorities) would come from the following functions:

- Corporate communication leader (such as a chief information officer)
- Public affairs
- Operations
- Legal
- Security and/or safety
- Human resources
- Information technology (IT)

The team leader (typically the chief information officer) would assemble and orchestrate team activities and meetings and act as the conduit to overall organizational leadership. The communications team fulfills an important role in establishing an effective communications system and implementing its basic elements, which are addressed in the following sections. The first section, perhaps the most important element, is planning the emergency response communications.

3.3.1 Communications Planning

When considering the various hazards and threats to an organization, it is almost impossible to establish the range of events and predict how and when they will occur. Regardless, emergency communications planning must focus on delivering information to stakeholders and identifying the mechanisms of transfer. As the team executes planning, the organization's strategic objectives and vision play a leading role in establishing policy, identifying stakeholders, and characterizing desired outcomes. The communications planning process tracks the flow of information from sources to end users and how the information evolves, changes, and is transmitted. The communications team must maintain a current list of contacts that are sources of information and consumers of information, including the media and key personnel within the organization. The emergency communications team should keep this list readily available for emergency responses.

For effective planning, planners should address common communications issues in emergency response. These five common issues with communications are:

1. Loss of primary communications networks: direct and indirect (i.e., sometimes the network operation is impacted by loss of power, physical damage, etc.). Often, a communication system failure is due to overload or exceedance of system carrying capacity. To be addressed later, a response can improve with exercises and training that truly test the system limits.
2. Failure to plan for and enact alternatives for such outages. In a scenario where a disaster destroys a communication tower, it impacts not just a single system but rather multiple systems such as landline phones (microwave links), cell phones, and radios all at once. To reduce the cost of maintenance and other fees (but increasing the chances of risk), various communication systems tend to cluster (communication towers, duct banks, and other network nodes).
3. In organizations that use hand-held communication devices (i.e., radios) in emergency response, loss of communications discipline – open mikes, radio discipline, "walking" over other transmissions, proximity of transmitters causing interference, mike too close, yelling causing overdrive conditions, slurring, etc.
4. Ignorance of radio propagation (cannot be in a valley and expect low frequencies, which propagate through a ground wave, to get out), ignorance of distance/interference issues, etc.
5. Interoperability issues with external equipment resources (including things such as different encryption, different frequencies, etc.) (Phelps 2016), (United States Council of Mayors 2004).

3.3.2 Information Coming In

Established and mature lines of communication (information coming in) are critically important for the emergency communications team and must be credible and resilient. Because sources are not inherently consistent, the communications team will need to establish working relationships with each source before an emergency occurs. Familiarity with the sources not only improves awareness of their message content and abilities but also enables the team to anticipate potential variations and organizational dynamics of the information provided. The emergency communications team must establish some capacity to identify and integrate new sources of information that emerge during an emergency event.

With each line of communication (information source), the team must establish information procedures and formats that will expedite processing and acting on the information coming in. The team must work with each source to ensure a proper understanding of the type, content, and timing of information delivered. In situations where direct interaction might be limited or not available, the communication team should acknowledge these limitations and establish processes to either validate the messages through separate avenues or structure the information format so that it is perhaps self-validating. Obviously, in some situations, immediate interaction with the message is not required.

3.3.3 Information Going Out

In addition to planning efforts with sources (information coming in), the emergency communications team should plan efforts with information consumers (information going out). The scope of information leaving the organization should be reviewed by the team and assessed for consistency with organizational goals and objectives. Again, format, content, and timing planning factors similar to the evaluation of incoming information are key considerations for information going out. A comprehensive, in-depth analysis of stakeholder organizations (such as the general public, first responders, government officials, etc.) and their expectations for information going out will be needed to ensure the lines of communication are complete.

3.3.4 Messengers

A key consideration of both information flowing in and out of the organization is the credibility of the message. The quickest and simplest approach to credibility is the deliberate and intentional selection of the messenger. The messenger should be a recognizable leader within the organization and someone with a reputation of at least knowing and being involved with the activities communicated and at most being in direct control. Alternatively – especially on information going out to external stakeholders – the messenger will require some cultivation or development of this recognition. Currently, we see a lot of automation in communication, so the messenger may not always be a person. Even in dealing with a system-generated message, the need for recognition and credibility remains the same whether it is developed or in need of development.

3.3.5 Staffing

As time progresses, having a dedicated communication staff is becoming rarer in both larger and smaller organizations. Certainly, having a staff is more likely in larger organizations; however, even for those organizations, the trend is towards smaller staffs. Regardless of the organizational scale, overall trends are emerging towards distributed communication staffing (often pushed by the advancement of information technology). Communication planning must appropriately address the cases of dedicated communication staff as well as distributed staff that would include most or all of the organization. The communication team must align and adapt the planning efforts to various staff situations and constructs.

3.3.6 Training and Exercises

Effective response communications require well-trained personnel (messengers and staff) throughout the system in the processes that generate, transmit, and receive information and are tested through comprehensive exercises. Training and exercises, using various emergency-related scenarios, practically and effectively test emergency communication in a controlled environment and create opportunities to evaluate information flow processes for both incoming and outgoing communication. Training should support overall organizational objectives in emergency response communications in the following forms:

- Stakeholder engagement: Develop operational competence with specific lines of communication as they pertain to incoming or outgoing information, the character and content of that information, timing, and other situational contexts.
- Social media: Learn how to orchestrate the operations of various social media accounts, manage an online profile, and maintain linkages to stakeholders that reinforce existing lines of communication (more on this later in section 3.4 Social Networks and New Media).
- Outreach: Learn how to leverage communication resources in efforts to cultivate common interests with various stakeholders so that the organization can make progress towards emergency preparedness and hazard mitigation goals through pooling resources, reducing competing/conflicting efforts, and promoting mutual assistance.

Training and exercises are complementary processes – exercises test what the organization has incorporated into training. The communication system requires exercises to test the communications operations during emergency responses as a method of identifying strengths and weaknesses, identifying opportunities for improvement, and establishing some baseline experiences that are extremely valuable for real-world responses. Exercises are also a good way to test and challenge organizational assumptions that are made both deliberately and tacitly.

3.3.7 Monitoring, Updating, and Adapting

With the final element of communication capability being monitoring, updating, and adapting, a common theme and challenge in many emergencies and disasters is information overload. In general, information overload is due to the information age we live in and the ubiquitous bombardment of information available everywhere, all the time. The emergency communication team needs to analyze the organization's exposure to all this information to not only prioritize the lines of communication but also establish a filtering process for dealing with irrelevancy (noise), redundancy, and conditions of too much information. To establish a good filtering process, the emergency communications team should take action on the phases of emergency decision-making:

- Assessment: A quick initial assessment is critical in knowing the what, when, and where of an event. Collect basic facts such as whether the event is over, developing, or ongoing and its severity during initial emergency response actions.
- Identify key groups: In given situations, a hierarchy of response involvement emerges with various stakeholders. Distinguish information priorities and potentially conflicting needs.
- Course of action development: Determine warning and/or emergency notification content with respect to the mission and anticipated response. In addition to content, the communication team must also consider the implications for the organization, given its capabilities and constraints.
- Evaluation: Determine lessons learned from the decision-making processes. Retrospectively assess how well the communication system met the short-term and long-term needs within the organization and external to the organization. Consider feedback loops within the communication system that allowed it to adapt to dynamic conditions.

Monitoring, adapting, and updating elements also have physical considerations. Ideally, an emergency communications center should be close to the organization's emergency operations center. The center should be equipped to support internal and external information flow, including considerations for redundancy based on system priorities and the nature of the emergency event. As determined by the various threat scenarios, the center should have backups in terms of both physical infrastructure and information assets.

3.4 SOCIAL NETWORKS AND NEW MEDIA

New communication methods, specifically social media, have grown immensely popular and extraordinarily capable. Connectivity and versatility continue to increase the widespread adoption along with the revolutionary aspects of personal/private interaction brought on by social media. The public's reflexive response in emergencies now is to grab their smartphone and hit video record. Unlike the transportation system, the communication system, especially with smartphone technology, has increased "anywhere" access to information and communications. Due to today's higher expectations for nationwide connectivity, communication delays with stakeholders and those directly controlling or influencing the response operations are not tolerated for very long. Transparency and the official and unofficial releases of information coupled with the national level commitment to open government have led to an expectation of immediate and almost instantaneous release of good or bad information. Social media has influenced emergency response communications by competing with, and sometimes even eclipsing, public messaging access. This is an age of unprecedented access and the ability to inform in real time through the manipulation of new media capabilities.

3.4.1 Social Media Benefits

The organization Information Systems for Crisis Response and Management (ISCRAM) is a community of researchers, practitioners, and professionals who are interested in the development and application of information systems for managing crises and emergencies. They focus on leveraging technology and information systems to enhance the preparedness, response, recovery, and overall management of disasters and crises. During their 2021 workshop on social media for disaster response and resilience, they identified four areas where social media provided substantial value for crisis management:

- real-time and ongoing situational awareness;
- rapid insights in the immediate aftermath of disaster;
- integration with heterogeneous, multi-modal data; and
- flexible value across the crisis management cycle (Lorini et al. 2021).

Social media is the go-to source for immediate and in-depth information about general events; with crises, the demand for this kind of information spikes. The daily routine uses of social media give it the familiarity that human nature relies on during stressful events. As the scale of emergency events or disasters increases, the occurrence of crisis-related developments and cross-issues also rises. Social media offers potential insights on these tangential developments and some visibility on potential influences. To improve emergency management and the needed situational awareness for evolving crises and spin-off emergencies, the imperative to process, integrate, and make sense of information is critical. Social media offers what we need here, with something called multi-modal data, which can be defined as different modes of data such as text, images, and video. Integrating this social data with more authoritative data like geospatial analytics, graphic information systems (GIS), satellite imagery, and other sensor-type data may be the key to the next evolution of situational awareness development and creating common operating picture platforms.

Finally, the flexible value proposition highlights how social media potentially fulfills the emergency manager data needs across an event lifecycle, from the initial determining the extent, evaluating the efficacy of response efforts (like a feedback loop mechanism), and forecasting efforts required during future recovery efforts.

3.4.2 Social Media Barriers

The ISCRAM group also acknowledged during the same 2021 workshop four barriers to leveraging social media in emergency management in the following areas:

- Information overload and uncertainty in automated filtering.
- Misinformation and its consequences.
- Validation and verification.
- Formatting information (Lorini et al. 2021).

The highly familiar information overload has broadly become a common experiential issue for many emergency managers to varying degrees. It is easy to imagine an operation center being flooded with waves of information that include both critical data and, perhaps to a greater extent, irrelevant and incomplete data. Early efforts to create automated filters for the information tidal wave have left many critics skeptical. Researchers have worked on technologies to create some type of social media filters through the use of artificial intelligence (AI), machine learning, natural language processing, and other processing algorithms with some success (Lorini et al. 2021).

Various organizations process emergency information differently depending on the situation, timing, goals, and objectives, thus driving different uses of social media information. Regarding the filtering out of irrelevant information, dealing with misinformation is imperative. One project to deal with social media and misinformation worth considering is called "Project EPIC" (Empowering the Public with Information in Crisis). Project EPIC, started in September 2009, was funded by the National Science Foundation. A group of students and faculty from the Universities of Colorado, Boulder and the University of California, Irvine formed a "multi-disciplinary, multi-university, multi-lingual research effort to support the information needs of members of the public during times of mass emergency" (UC-Boulder 2023). In an age of social media, the project looked at "behavioral and technical knowledge of computer mediated communication to the world of crisis studies and emergency response… studying massive wide scale coordination across the internet, and conducting action research and employing participatory design oriented approaches." The study aimed to "look beyond today's state of the art and anticipate future socio-technical change" (UC-Boulder 2023). During the COVID-19 pandemic, Project EPIC transitioned to its latest form focused on information sciences research into disinformation (accidental) and misinformation (intentional).

The validation and verification of information are becoming concerns for credibility and communication message security due to questions about the imposed risks of information being inaccurate. Using social media as a data source for communication is somewhat risky, and emergency managers need resources to determine social media data trustworthiness prior to taking action. As seen in the Hurricane Sandy response, fake social media postings and photoshopped images were distractions from factual, relevant information (Phelps 2016, 40)

A final barrier to using social media lies in practical concerns about its information format. During an emergency event when time is severely limited, there is little tolerance for delay in reformatting social media information into a usable or compatible format. Formats need to be reconciled much earlier than during the response phase. A common format or format element would be geo-referencing, which is common with imagery. There are also various universal textual formats like text files and comma-separated values (CSV), as well as tabular forms. Finally, to close the discussion on information format, we must consider the notion of language format. Multilinguistic technology solutions may drive emergency communication formats to replicate messaging in other languages.

To address applying social media information resources, organizations are increasingly becoming more engaged with social media by integrating various social media tools into their websites and communications strategies. For over ten years, FEMA has incorporated social media into its communication plans to improve transparency in the response and recovery operations, along with opening channels for receiving unofficial data and information inputs (FEMA 2023)

3.4.3 Future of Social Media in Emergency Communications

Some researchers are looking for information technologies to capture more information and piece it all together to maximize situational awareness. In 2007, IBM developed an artificial intelligence machine, Watson, as a means to help the medical field assess patients' symptoms and search all available medical information to conclude the most likely cause. IBM Watson was a data analytics processor that used natural language processing, a technology that analyzes human speech for meaning and syntax. But in May 2018, IBM discontinued the development of Watson to expand into other areas of AI, with its most recent AI project called watsonx. Through secure means and collaborative workspace, this AI accesses organizational data resources and automates AI processes to deliver generative AI within organizational applications to train, tune, and distribute models (IBM 2023). As another example, Facebook's relevancy engines are recognizing common things that people are posting about, like locations, birthdays, holidays, news events, etc., and then are grouping them by topic for expedient review. This technology could be harnessed to focus on events such as disasters and feed information into an emergency response center. Other platforms, such as YouTube, Snapchat, TikTok, etc., offer shared access to photos, videos, texts, and drawings. Leveraging these platforms with their varying operating conditions and capabilities could support meeting information and data requirements during a response as well as offer various options for messaging the public during crisis and emergency events.

As social media grows in popularity and demand for resources, this new communication resource presents additional risks for responders – a dependency on information networks that may not reach all sections of society. Of particular concern are vulnerable and disadvantaged segments of the population who lack the means and abilities necessary to access social media. In the same way that past considerations have been made for, for example non-English speakers and the hearing impaired, new considerations arise with each new social media platform or process. As an example of an access issue, the homeless are not likely to be most effectively informed of critical emergency messages via social media interaction if they don't have regular access to a computer or mobile communication devices like smartphones.

3.5 CONCLUSIONS

Communication is a fundamental element of emergency response. Comprehensive communication planning is also fundamental and an essential ingredient for success in emergency response. Sharing and receiving the right information at the right time with the public, government officials, and the media is crucial in making sure emergency response and recovery efforts run smoothly. Emergency communication information captured during responses may also inform us about approaches to risk reduction and impact mitigations for future disasters. Clearly communicating policies, goals, and priorities to the organization and stakeholders enhances adoption and support, as well as promotes a more efficient response operation. Finally, leveraging traditional media and social media for information is a must for emergency planning and response, creating enhanced and robust situational awareness.

REFERENCES

Department of Homeland Security. 2019. *National Response Framework*. 4th ed. Washington, DC: Government Printing Office.

Endsley, M. R. 1988. Design and evaluations for Situational Awareness enhancement. In *Proceedings of the Human Factors Society 32nd Annual Meeting,* Human Factors Society, Santa Monica, CA. October 24-28.

Federal Emergency Management Agency. 2017. *National Incident Management System*. https://www.fema.gov/emergency-managers/nims (accessed on December 27, 2023).

Federal Emergency Management Agency. 2023. *Social Media Policies*. https://www.fema.gov/about/news-multimedia/social-media/policies (accessed on January 1, 2024).

Haddow, G. D., Bullock, J. A., & Coppola, D. P. 2021. *Introduction to Emergency Management*, 7th ed. Cambridge, MA: Elsevier Butterworth Heinemann.

IBM. 2023. *IBM Watson to Watsonx*. https://www.ibm.com/watson (accessed on December 29, 2023).

Lorini, V., Castillo, C., Peterson, S., Rufalo, P., Purohit, H., Pajarito, D., Porta de Albuquerque, J., & Buntain, C. 2021. Social media for emergency management: Opportunities and challenges at the intersection of research and practice. In *Proceedings of the 18th Annual ISCRAM Conference—Blacksburg, VA, USA, May 2021* (pp. 39–44). https://idl.iscram.org/files/valeriolorini/2021/2372_ValerioLorini_etal2021.pdf. (accessed on December 28, 2023).

von Lubitz, D. K. J. E. 2008. Medical readiness for operations other than war: Boyd's OODA loop and training using advanced distributed simulation technology. *International Journal of Risk Assessment and Management* 9(4): 409–432.

National Academy of Sciences. 2007. *Successful Response Starts with a Map: Improving Geospatial Support for Disaster Management.* Washington, DC: National Academies Press. http://www.nap.edu/catalog/11793.html (accessed on December 29, 2023).

Phelps, R. 2016. Lessons learned from Hurricane Sandy. *Risk and Resilience Hub*, January 25. https://www.riskandresiliencehub.com/2119/ (accessed on December 28, 2023).

Townsend, F. F. 2006. *The Federal Response to Hurricane Katrina: Lessons Learned.* Washington DC: Office of the Assistant to the President for Homeland Security and Counterterrorism. https://georgewbush-whitehouse.archives.gov/reports/katrina-lessons-learned/ (accessed on December 29, 2023).

University of Colorado-Boulder. 2023. *Project EPIC at the University of Colorado Boulder.* https://epic.colorado.edu/ (accessed on December 29, 2023).

United States Council of Mayors. 2004. Interoperability survey: A 192-city survey. In *Archive 72nd Annual Meeting.* https://www.usmayors.org/ (accessed on December 29, 2023).

4 Effectively Communicating Risk and Uncertainty to the Public in Crises

Lyle D. Burgoon

4.1 THE PRINCIPLES OF EFFECTIVE CRISIS COMMUNICATIONS

There are six principles that govern effective communications, regardless of the crisis and audience. These principles are:

- Trust: Build trust with your communities before the crisis (using these principles) so that your communities will trust your communications during the crisis.
- Honesty: Always tell the truth.
- Transparency: Explain what you know, explain what you don't know, and explain why and how you know what you know and don't know. If you do not know the answer, say so.
- Timeliness: Communicate at a time when your audience can take action; communicate when the situation changes and requires an update.
- Appropriateness: Use language that is appropriate and approachable for your audience.
- Ownership: Own any and all mistakes, and correct those mistakes as soon as possible.

These six principles, when used together, will help to ensure the success of present and future communications. These principles build trust between the community and the crisis communication agency and officers.

4.2 TRUST: HOW YOUR HISTORY WITH YOUR AUDIENCE WILL HELP OR HINDER YOU

The audience for crisis communications will have preconceived notions about the trustworthiness of your organization based on its prior interactions, observations,

 DOI: 10.1201/9781003648178-5

and the interactions and observations of trusted others. Under Reichart's theory of "expectational gaps," differences between how an organization has behaved and an audience member's construct of how an organization should behave (i.e., the expectational gap) will influence the perception one holds about the organization (Reichart, 2003).

If you or your organization have reputational issues with your audience, your audience will be less inclined to believe and trust you. It is generally recognized that trust is formed from many factors working together that we have a duty to expect from our institutions. These include ensuring communications, even before a crisis, are transparent (i.e., good and bad information is shared appropriately and in a timely manner without requiring coercion), that the institution is operating in an ethical manner (i.e., not causing intentional harm), and that institutions do and act in the ways they say they will (Badu et al., 2023). Unsurprisingly, once trust is lost, it may never be regained (Slovic, 1993).

Crisis communicators have a lot of pre-work that needs to be done before any given crisis occurs. In many ways, this pre-work is not any different from how most of us have been trained for team sports. The first lesson we teach is that we should treat others the way we want to be treated. All of us want to be treated with respect. Part of respect is being truthful to each other and avoiding deception. If we are all honest with each other, then we can begin to trust each other. Once we have trust, we can work together knowing that our teammates will execute their jobs properly and to the best of their abilities. As we practice together, we are, in effect, rehearsing for the real deal. Ultimately, our audience is part of the team as well. If they believe they can trust us, and they believe we can do our jobs right, then we will continue to grow that trust. But, as noted by Slovic (1993), once someone loses our trust, we may never regain it.

Thus, when we make mistakes, we must own them, and we must take that ownership as soon as possible (Willink and Babin, 2015). This is what transparency is all about. We need to be open. We need to give the good news and the bad news. And we need to give the bad news and own our mistakes (and mistakes are a type of bad news) openly, of our own accord, without being coerced. This is discussed more fully in section 4.4: Transparency.

4.3 HONESTY: ALWAYS TELL THE TRUTH

The building blocks for trust are honesty. Being honest is more than just avoiding being dishonest (Miller, 2021). Being honest includes being intellectually honest – saying that we do not know something when that is the case. Guessing or speculating without qualification is not necessarily lying to the public, but it is not being honest either.

The ethics around honesty are pretty clear – if you are honest, then there is generally little risk of harm. We will not consider those boundary cases and thought experiments that rarely occur in real life (e.g., Kant's example of a murderer at the door) and will focus on the ethics of communications. Specifically, we will consider a situation that happens often in public health communication – noble lies (Brown and de Barra, 2023).

Brown and de Barra (2023) view the purpose of noble lies as helping the state/government. Although that is one purpose, noble lies can have other purposes. That is why I define noble lies differently and state that they are generally lies told by those in power to effect some change that they deem positive. For instance, a parent telling their child that Santa Claus has a 24/7 worldwide surveillance system whereby he can keep score of when the child is behaving well or not is clearly a lie; however, it is told so that the parent gets something they deem positive – good behavior from their child.

The problem with noble lies is that they are lies – they are not the truth. And we cannot control how people will react to finding out that the noble lie is in fact a falsehood. Generally, though, once people understand that the noble lie was, in fact, a lie, they will no longer trust the source of the noble lie.

What this means is that lies, once discovered, regardless of their purpose, will decrease trust. In a democratic society, trust in those in power is especially important. Federal employees are often reminded that their jobs are a direct result of the public's trust, and that federal employees have an obligation to keep that trust.

What does this mean for emergency response communicators? It is simple – always be honest in your communications. Do not attempt to deceive people. Recognize that noble lies, once discovered, will destroy trust. In the case study, we will examine a case of a noble lie from the COVID-19 pandemic.

4.4 TRANSPARENCY: EXPLAINING WHAT YOU DO AND DO NOT KNOW

Being transparent and being honest tend to run hand-in-hand. To be fully honest, one needs to be transparent. I separate honesty from transparency when I write about communications because transparency is such a critical concept that it deserves to be discussed separately. However, one cannot be fully honest without being transparent.

A communicator who is transparent will explain what they know, explain what they don't know, and explain why and how they know what they know and don't know. Transparent communicators state that they do not know the answer when appropriate. These are all important aspects of being honest.

If a transparent communicator does these things, what do they not do? Transparent communicators avoid guessing or speculating. If they do need to guess, they will make it obvious that they are guessing. In addition, providing a rationale for the guess is important so that receivers (people who receive the message) can make their own judgments as to the quality of the guess. Providing the rationale also provides additional transparency about how the communicator came to their guess.

When might a communicator need to guess? Generally, guesses are made when we are making predictions about the future. For instance, "We do not know for sure, but we believe the bridge on Roberts' Road will flood during this rain event" is quite obviously a guess. The words "we do not know for sure" are signaling language that makes it clear to the receiver that the statement is a guess or that the communicator has uncertainty.

This is much different from the statement, "The bridge on Roberts' Road will flood during this rain event." The latter statement is more factual in nature – it is an affirmative statement with no uncertainty. The communicator is saying, under no uncertain terms, that the bridge will flood. If it turns out the bridge does not flood, then receivers may be less inclined to listen to the communicator about future events.

Consider the language that the National Weather Service uses in this Hydrologic Outlook update (an update about potential river flooding): "This outlook means that elevated water levels and potential impacts are possible, but not yet certain." This statement makes the uncertainty clear: "impacts are possible, but not yet certain." The statement also makes clear that the potential hazard is elevated water levels.

Transparency also requires that we describe how and why we came to our conclusion. In the National Weather Service example, they state that "Several rounds of rainfall will be possible from Saturday afternoon through Sunday evening. Rainfall may be moderate to heavy at times. Widespread rainfall amounts of one to three inches are possible across the region, with localized amounts of three to five inches." This makes it clear that the reason why the National Weather Service is predicting potential floods is that there may be heavy rains in the area. By explaining the rationale for the uncertain conclusion, the communicator is being transparent about the information they used to come to their conclusion.

4.5 TIMELINESS: THE RIGHT COMMUNICATION AT THE RIGHT TIME

Emergency response communications need to be given at the right time. What is the right time? The right time is when your audience can take action. For instance, telling your audience they need to evacuate an area immediately after a chemical spill has occurred will help them limit their exposure. If you know that an emergency situation is imminent in the near future, for instance, a hurricane is highly likely to make landfall in the area, then communicating the need to evacuate with sufficient time for the audience to leave in an orderly manner is appropriate. It is also important to let your audience know when they do not need to evacuate.

In some emergency situations, sheltering in place, locking doors and windows, and taking other steps to secure a home or building may be the appropriate course of action. If that is the case, getting that information out to your audience in time to minimize their exposure or risk is highly important.

Updating your audience and letting them know when to expect future updates is also necessary. People need to have updated information so that they can plan and act accordingly. Having a regular cadence of information updates makes the process predictable, and it helps your audience plan. However, it is okay to occasionally break the cadence and provide earlier updates to your audience, especially if their risk significantly changes.

For instance, if your audience is sheltering in place and the risk has significantly decreased to the point where they can open their doors and windows, then let them know out of cadence and as soon as possible. If your audience needs to continue to maintain the same level of alert, that is not a reason to break cadence.

4.6 APPROPRIATENESS: USE LANGUAGE THAT YOUR AUDIENCE UNDERSTANDS

Effective crisis communications are understandable by their audience. That means that communicators need to use words and sentences that are approachable, appropriate, and understandable to the audience. If the audience does not understand your jargon, it will be lost on them. For instance, I use 24-hour time in my daily life as my watch and phone run on 24-hour time. My children do not immediately understand when I say, "Dinner will be at 1735 tonight" – they have to do the math and translate in their head that I said, "Dinner will be at 5:35 PM tonight." If you speak in jargon, you might as well be speaking a foreign language. Jargon is helpful among technical specialists as a shortcut; however, with lay audiences, you will lose them.

I advise crisis communicators to imagine they are talking to their friends. Now, imagine you need them to take some action in a calm and orderly manner. How are you going to explain to them: 1) what you need them to do, 2) why you need them to do it, and 3) how you came to the point where you need to make this ask of them?

Following is a composite example of what I often hear in an evacuation announcement:

> At 2112 hours tonight a roller got stuck on a grain movement train. The stuck roller initiated the production of free electron sparks, causing the ignition and conflagration of biological plant materials within the grain elevator. The produced gases and heat increased the interior pressure of the grain elevator until the interior pressure overpowered the structural integrity of the grain elevator. The resulting overpressure damaged nearby homes and caused particulate pollution to inundate the locale, leading to respiratory health concerns. Therefore, we have ordered all residents within one mile to egress from their residence immediately and to find accommodations outside of the area of exclusion.

Now, you might say that this is an extreme example, and I would agree it is extreme. However, I have seen some communications similar to this. I wrote it this way because it exemplifies several of the issues I see with respect to appropriateness and approachability.

1) In the example, the "ask" (i.e., the evacuation order) is at the end of the communication. It is too late. Make your ask upfront. If your audience has trust in you, that is all they need to hear. They are already sold on the evacuation.
2) This example is full of jargon. Most of us would not speak this way with our friends. In fact, most of us would not say these words in these combinations. Most of us do not use 24-hour time in our everyday lives. Express times as

AM and PM times. The use of "conflagration of biological plant materials" is jargony. Instead, we might say, "The soybeans were on fire." I rarely use the word "overpressure" unless I am lecturing on high-yield nuclear explosives. And very few of us talk about "the structural integrity" of anything.
3) It is difficult to understand why you are asking people to evacuate.
4) It is difficult to understand who made the call that there could be respiratory health concerns.
5) It is also difficult to understand why exactly people need to leave their homes. Evacuation orders are a very tall order for people, especially families. In this case, people will need to leave their homes and find a hotel room if they do not have local family or friends who live outside of the evacuation zone.

How can we improve this emergency response communication? I recommend that emergency response communicators use this model:

1) Make the "ask" (what you need them to do) upfront.
2) Tell them why you are making the "ask" (why you need them to do this).
3) State the rationale for the "ask" (how you came to the "ask" being the best option to minimize risk).
4) End by telling them when they can expect updates (either the cadence or the time for the next update).

Next, we remove the jargon and provide clearer explanations. Here is an improved version of the emergency response communication:

> We are ordering all residents within 1 mile of the grain elevator located at 15152 Soccer Lane to evacuate their homes immediately. Chuck County Deputies are going door to door to inform residents of this evacuation order. We are asking residents to evacuate due to possible health issues that may result from breathing smoke that is in the air. At 9:12PM we received notice that the grain elevator at 15152 Soccer Lane had exploded and the grain inside was on fire. We were also told that nearby houses were damaged as a result of the explosion. The County Director of Public Safety made the decision to order the evacuation out of an abundance of caution to prevent people getting sick from inhaling the smoke from the fire. The current time is 9:45PM. We will provide an update on what is going on at 10:15PM, and every three hours thereafter. We will also provide an update just as soon as it is safe for residents to return home. Thank you.

4.7 OWNERSHIP: OWN YOUR MISTAKES AND CORRECT THEM IMMEDIATELY

Emergency response communicators are humans. That means, among other things, they will make mistakes. When mistakes happen, there is one action to take to prevent an erosion of trust: ownership.

Ownership means that you take responsibility for the mistake publicly. You clearly state that there was a mistake. You state that you are taking responsibility for the mistake, and you correct the mistake as soon as you know about it. Taking ownership allows you to fix mistakes that made you dishonest and allows you to correct the message so that you and the message are both honest. An important part of ownership is also clearly communicating how you will change the process to prevent mistakes of that type in the future.

Failing to take ownership could result in reputational damage, especially an erosion of trust. As discussed earlier, trust is key in emergency response communications. Your audience is more likely to take the actions you are requesting or ordering when there is trust. When your audience loses trust, they are less likely to believe you, even if that means they are at increased risk of harm.

Taking ownership is hard. It means admitting fault. It means admitting that you or your team made a mistake. It is a bruise to one's ego. But taking ownership is critical, especially before or during after-action reviews. Taking ownership is the first step in process improvement. Once people own their actions and recognize how they impacted team performance, the team can move on and focus on how each contributor can improve to ensure the team improves as a whole.

If your emergency response communications continue to make the same mistakes, your audience will notice. Your audience will lose trust. That means your communications will be less effective.

4.8 CASE STUDY: COVID-19, MASKS, HERD IMMUNITY, AND UNCERTAINTY

During the COVID-19 pandemic, recommendations from US public health leaders changed rapidly. Early in the pandemic, the public was asked to not wear masks as they were not very effective for the general public, and the masks were needed by public health workers. Later, the recommendations changed, and masking was either highly encouraged or required in most jurisdictions. Also, the estimates on the number of people required to reach herd immunity changed over time.

Interestingly, as pointed out in the news media (Powell and Prasad, 2021), Dr Anthony Fauci may have told two noble lies: the first about mask-wearing and the second about the number of people required to be immunized to achieve herd immunity.

Early in the pandemic, Fauci claimed that masks were not effective and the general public should not use them (March 2020: Dr Anthony Fauci talks with Dr Jon LaPook about Covid-19, 2020). A few months later, Fauci stated that "Masks are not 100% protective. However, they certainly are better than not wearing a mask" (Fauci Explains Why the Public Wasn't Told to Wear Masks When the Pandemic Began, 2020). Fauci went on to explain that the reason he said the public would not benefit from masks earlier in the pandemic was to ensure health workers had access to surgical masks and N95 masks.

Thus, based on Fauci's words, the noble lie was that the public would not benefit from masks. The benefit that Fauci sought from telling this noble lie was that healthcare workers would be able to access the surgical masks and N95 masks because the public would not create a run on the masks, which were already in short supply due to pandemic-related supply chain issues.

Fauci then corrected his noble lie a few months later and offered his reasoning. What he did not do was take ownership of the fact that he told a noble lie and acknowledge that it was a lie. Rather, he explained his reasoning for the noble lie but was not contrite about the fact that it was wrong to lie. Thus, Fauci failed to take ownership of his noble lie. As a result, he lost the trust of a large number of Americans.

The second noble lie that Fauci told was about herd immunity. Fauci is reported to have said, "When polls said only about half of all Americans would take a vaccine, I was saying herd immunity would take 70 to 75 percent. Then, when newer surveys said 60 percent or more would take it, I thought, 'I can nudge this up a bit,' so I went to 80, 85" (McNeil, 2020; Powell and Prasad, 2021). This is a noble lie as Fauci is attempting to increase the number of people who would get the COVID-19 vaccine. However, as before, the rapid change in the advice signals that the advice is not based on changes in the underlying science, as we were led to believe, but is instead someone's opinion intended to cause behavior changes. A perhaps cynical way of viewing this is that an expert is manipulating the public into behavior that the expert believes to be right, but without transparency and without the backing of scientific information.

Again, when found out, the public's trust in Fauci becomes tarnished. He failed to honestly communicate what the science said. He failed to honestly convey the uncertainty inherent in the science. In fact, he appears to have fabricated the uncertainty in the levels of population vaccination to achieve herd immunity.

One cannot help but to wonder if certain aspects of the Federal government's COVID-19 response would be viewed less politically had Fauci been more honest and transparent. Being more honest and transparent would likely have led to increased trust in America's public health leaders.

4.9 CONCLUSIONS

There are six principles that govern effective communications, regardless of the crisis and audience. These six principles are: 1) Trust, 2) Honesty, 3) Transparent, 4) Timeliness, 5) Appropriateness, and 6) Ownership. When used together, these principles will help to ensure the success of present and future communications.

REFERENCES

Badu, J. et al. (2023). Crisis communication and trustworthiness among crisis actors: Towards a typology of crisis management difficulties. *Saf Extreme Environ*, **5**, 119–130.

Brown, R. C. H. and de Barra, M. (2023). A taxonomy of non-honesty in public health communication. *Public Health Ethics*, **16**, 86–101.

Fauci Explains Why Public Wasn't Told to Wear Masks When Pandemic Began (2020).https://www.thestreet.com/video/dr-fauci-masks-changing-directive-coronavirus

March 2020: Dr. Anthony Fauci talks with Dr Jon LaPook about Covid-19 (2020).https://www.youtube.com/watch?v=PRa6t_e7dgI

McNeil, D. G. (2020). How much herd immunity is enough? *The New York Times*.https://www.nytimes.com/2020/12/24/world/how-much-herd-immunity-is-enough.html#

Miller, C. B. (2021). *Honesty: The Philosophy and Psychology of a Neglected Virtue*. Oxford: Oxford University Press.

Powell, K. and Prasad, V. (2021). The noble lies of COVID-19. *Slate*.https://slate.com/technology/2021/07/noble-lies-covid-fauci-cdc-masks.html

Reichart, J. (2003). A theoretical exploration of expectational gaps in the corporate issue construct. *Corp Reputation Rev*, **6**, 58–69.

Slovic, P. (1993). Perceived risk, trust, and democracy. *Risk Analysis*, **13**, 675–682.

Willink, J. and Babin, L. (2015). *Extreme Ownership: How U.S. Navy Seals Lead and Win*. New York: St. Martin's Press.

5 Time Is a Murderer
The Cost of Critical Path Drag in Emergency Response

Stephen A. Devaux

5.1 INTRODUCTION

In the 1953 John Huston movie *Beat the Devil,* Peter Lorre says to Humphrey Bogart: "Time is a crook!" But on many projects, Time is much more sociopathic than any mere crook. After a disaster, as victims wait for help to arrive, Time wanders through the chaos with Death at its side. With every passing hour, mortality is likely to rise at an increasing rate, as the trapped, injured, and infected slowly succumb.

As Dr Adedeji B. Badiru wrote in Chapter 15 on the Coordinated Systems Approach, emergency responses are programs consisting of both projects and operations and "require conventional planning, organization, scheduling, control, and phase-out." Benjamin Franklin's truism that time is money has long been given lip service in project work, even if the specific quantification of time in monetary units has been much more noticeable by its absence. But new techniques and metrics in critical path scheduling have allowed planners to identify the time/money impact of both specific work items and specific resource scarcities on project and program value. These allow for optimizing the work process on the basis of reducing time and thus deriving maximum value from the project. These same techniques need to be applied in planning emergency response, where the cost of time is measured in human suffering.

In this chapter, we shall see:

- How using standard business project management techniques, such as the creation of work breakdown structure templates that can be rapidly modified to specific situations, can increase agility and reduce response time.
- How using program management techniques to identify and sequence the specific value-generating projects can provide the response team with a clearer route to reduced mortality and damage.
- How new techniques in critical path scheduling, such as clear quantification of the value/cost of time and new metrics such as critical path drag and drag cost, can be used to optimize response time in such planning templates and greatly reduce response time, mortality, and damage.

DOI: 10.1201/9781003648178-6

5.2 OF PROGRAMS AND PROJECTS

The *Guide to the Project Management Body of Knowledge (PMBOK™ Guide)* (2008) defines a project as "a temporary endeavor undertaken to create a unique product, service, or result," and a program as "a group of related projects managed in a coordinated way to obtain benefits and control not available from managing them individually" (p. 442). These definitions apply to the many specific outcomes and services that must be generated in an emergency response effort. Each project, such as securing an area, searching for survivors, providing medical care and evacuation, and establishing mechanisms for delivery of food, water, and shelter, carries with it its own parcel of benefits. In Dr Badiru's Triple C model, the coordination of these projects and the operations they create is the final product of the preceding communication and cooperation, during both the planning phase and the initial actions of the implementation phase.

In managing time and its harmful side effects, for more than 50 years projects have used the technique called critical path analysis. A critical path is the longest sequence of activities, delays, and constraints through a project schedule. The two vital data inputs to this analysis are the constraints due to activity duration and precedence.

- Duration is an estimate of how long each planned task will take to complete.
- Precedence, or dependency information, is the logical order in which the work must be performed.

As much as possible, the sole delaying criterion in defining precedence constraints should be the nature of the work. We can neither paint the wall until we've plastered it, nor debug the software code until we've written it, nor search through the rubble until the building has collapsed.

Of course, resource constraints must eventually be taken into consideration. For example, the use of amphibious vehicles for supply and evacuation is only possible to the extent that they are available. However, best practice suggests postponing consideration of resource unavailability until the impact of each specific lack can be isolated and measured. As we shall see, critical path analysis will allow us to compress our schedule by altering durations ("crashing the critical path" by increasing resource usage) and precedence ("fast-tracking" by doing more work in parallel) to optimize a schedule that will give us the greatest value for our investment of time and money. The resources can then be fitted onto that schedule, and the impact of shortages measured and perhaps ameliorated.

But although critical path analysis is designed as a project-level tool, a modified version can also play a crucial role in planning the program. At the program level, the individual projects have dependencies among the other projects. Here, the precedences are based not so much on the logical nature of the work (as they are at the project and work activity level) but on the basis of the benefit that the inclusion of each project at a specific point in the program is designed to generate.

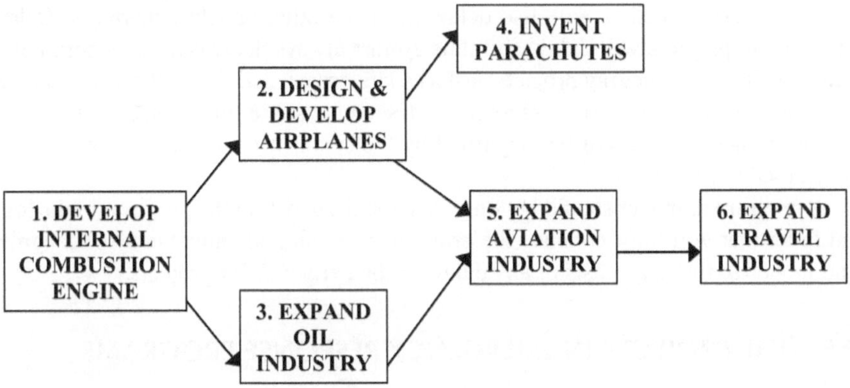

FIGURE 5.1 Sequence of aviation history

An early parachute was designed by Leonardo da Vinci, and the first successful jump was made in France in 1785. But it generated very little value prior to the success of the Wright brothers' project. The airplane was an "enabler" for the parachute (not to mention for the largest branch of the travel industry). The internal combustion engine enhanced the value of oil drilling and refining, as well as the aviation industry. If mankind had deliberately planned its aviation history in a program, the sequence would have been as shown in the diagram below (Figure 5.1):

Notice in Figure 5.1 that:

- Parachute invention did not *require* practical airplanes as in a critical path method (CPM) dependency, but…
- The benefits generated by parachutes, as well as the expanded aviation and travel industries, required airplanes as a preceding enabler.
- All the benefits generated by practical airplanes required the internal combustion engine as a preceding enabler. Therefore, from a program point of view, the internal combustion engine was the most valuable of the developments above, with a value-added approximately equal to the value of the entire "program."

The chart above displays the logical order in which the projects would have been implemented as a program in order to generate the greatest value, if only human history were properly planned. While all the items above can be seen as benefit generators in and of themselves, 1, 2, 3, and 5 are also enablers of other benefit generators, so that the cost of delay in those enablers is also magnified. In planning such a program, it would be crucial to understand that until we have a good internal combustion engine, the value of the rest of the program is close to nil. So the value-added of Item 1 (DEVELOP INTERNAL COMBUSTION ENGINE) is approximately equal to the value of the entire program.

Any delays in Item 1 will also delay all of the other benefit generators. Delays in the early projects will delay (and thus almost always decrease) the generation of value in all the succeeding projects, just as a late project activity will delay successor activities and all of their successors (i.e., "descendants") in turn. The cost of time on enabler project delays will be magnified by the cost of time on succeeding delayed project value generation.

A program manager should not only take the time to plan the program in the logical order that will most enhance the program's benefit and value but also recognize and monetize the huge costs of any delay on the early enabler projects.

5.3 THE PROJECTS IN EMERGENCY RESPONSE PROGRAMS

Emergency response planning suffers from an unfortunate dilemma. The life-and-death nature of an emergency, coupled with the enormous stress that it places on all decision-makers, makes advance preparation, including planning, optimization of processes, and rehearsing to the point of second nature, absolutely indispensable.

However, the vast variation in emergency types makes it crucial to tailor the advance preparation to a wide variety of emergencies. For just a small sample, consider the variations in the following:

- A severe hurricane in Florida.
- A severe hurricane and flooding in New Orleans.
- An EF5 tornado in a major city.
- An earthquake on the San Andreas fault.
- An earthquake and tsunami in the Puget Sound area.
- Eruption of Mt Rainier.
- Mississippi River flooding of the 1993 type.
- An Oklahoma City type of terrorist attack.
- A 9/11 type of terrorist attack.
- An emergency landing of an airliner on the Hudson River.
- A city subway chemical, biological, or radiological attack.
- A disease epidemic.
- A crippling Northeast blizzard.
- An electrical power blackout.
- The meltdown of a nuclear power plant.

These are only a tiny fraction of the potential emergencies, yet they cover a wide range in terms of the amount of advanced warning, initial lethality, potential for extended lethality, geographical isolation or expansion, accessibility to aid, hazard to emergency responders, damage to property, and many other variables. Even within a specific emergency, specific circumstances can vary tremendously. An event such as that which struck Eastern Japan in March 2011, combining as it did earthquake, tsunami, and nuclear disaster, poses more magnified issues for emergency response than would any of those events individually. If project management methods are to be used to plan responses, how do we plan for such wide-ranging catastrophes?

5.4 PROJECT TEMPLATES

In project-driven corporations that have mature processes in place, potential projects are often grouped by similar products and similar work. Template project plans are then developed for each group of projects. The template starts in the form of a work breakdown structure (WBS), with the final product decomposed into components and the components decomposed into all the work activities necessary to create those components.

Delium Training, Inc. is a company that contracts to perform the development of employee training for large corporations. An example of a template work breakdown structure for one of its training development projects is shown below in Figure 5.2. Needed resources and durations for all the work activities are then plugged into the WBS, and a schedule and budget are created. And whenever a project of this type is performed, actual durations and costs are reported and captured in each element so as to further refine the template. Both schedule and budget can be constantly honed (e.g., through critical path analysis) to shorten duration and increase efficiency.

One of the greatest values of a WBS is the ability to manage scope changes by adding, removing, or modifying a branch, a twig, or a leaf of the structure. When the structure changes, so does whatever schedule or budgetary data had been plugged into that portion of the WBS. For example, if a client decides that it does not want role plays and/or order form training, those two branches are lopped away from the template WBS, and the project plan is reduced by the amount of time, resources, and cost that would have been required for those work packages. And if another customer wants to expand the project to include training that's not part of the standard package

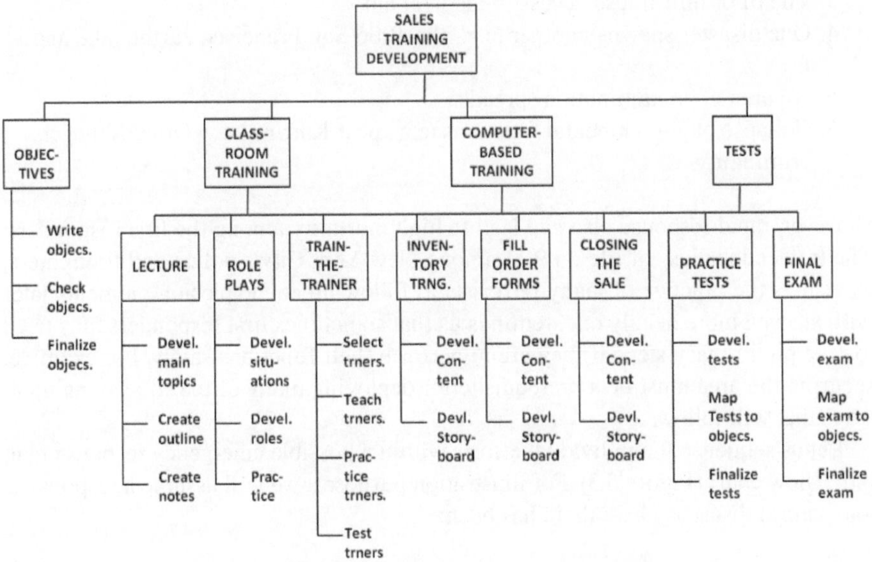

FIGURE 5.2 A WBS template for sales training on a contract basis

(e.g., telemarketing), that branch can easily be added, either planned afresh or "borrowed" from a different template that includes telemarketing training.

5.5 APPLYING TEMPLATES TO EMERGENCY RESPONSE PLANS

Just as the training development template is organized around the specific training products to be developed, emergency response templates should be organized around the products, services, and results (i.e., the outputs of each project) that are included in the response program. These outcomes should be based on the probable needs of the victim community: what things are likely, as much as possible, to decrease deaths, injuries, and property damage and establish a basis for the earliest possible recovery of the community?

As mentioned above, the specifics of the emergency often evolve as the situation develops. For example, if a major earthquake strikes near a coastline, it may be an hour or more before it becomes clear whether it will be followed by a tsunami. Response planning and rehearsals must include dealing with such a devastating byproduct. When the earthquake occurs, response teams should prepare for the aftermath of both catastrophes until the tsunami risk has been eliminated. When that happens, the tsunami-specific portions of the response template can be discarded.

Perhaps the most significant difference between a training development project (or any commercial project) and an emergency response program is the vital importance of time. There are at least six ways in which time can take on huge importance:

1. The injured begin to die.
2. The trapped are without water, food, and shelter.
3. The ill or infirm lose access to medical aid.
4. One disaster spawns another (e.g., the 1906 San Francisco earthquake and fire).
5. An area of contamination spreads.
6. Collapse of governmental functions (e.g., post-Katrina New Orleans) begets criminality.

However, rapid response also can lead to high mortality among the first responders. The tremendous loss of life on 9/11 among New York City's police and firefighters, as well as the practice of many terrorists to follow up one explosion moments later with an even more deadly one, reminds us that sometimes first responders may need to take preliminary steps if they are to perform their functions safely. For example, securing the area must be a prerequisite for deploying many of the life-saving measures that will follow.

Let us sequence the individual efforts within a possible emergency response plan into a flow chart (Figure 5.3). For illustration purposes, we will assume a response is to a natural disaster where there has been:

1. Probable injuries and loss of life.
2. Damage to property, including probable building collapses.

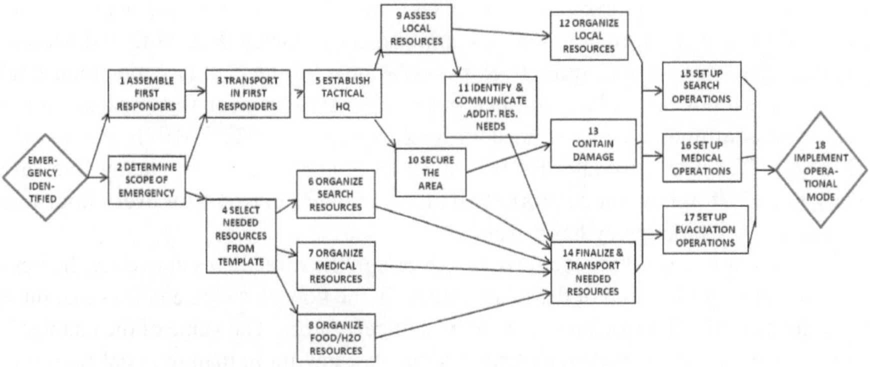

FIGURE 5.3 A flow chart for planned emergency response

Key aspects of this flow chart are:

1. Assembly of first responders occurs even before the full scope of the disaster is known. Thus, first responders should be prepared with all necessary gear (hazardous material suits, automatic weapons, etc.) unless and until the details of the emergency are known.
2. Item 2 (DETERMINE SCOPE OF EMERGENCY) should include, in quantified terms that all leaders of the operation will understand, the extent of the damage, any continued or expanding threat to life and property, and the urgency of time in establishing three particular goals, as highlighted in Figure 5.4:

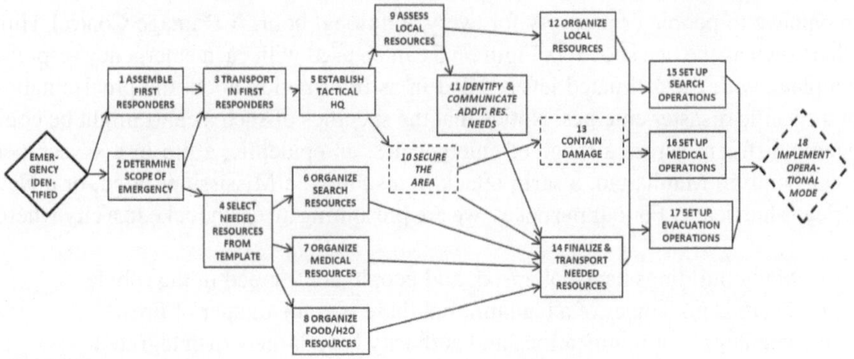

FIGURE 5.4: A flow chart highlighting the three benefit generators

Items 10, 13, and 18 are all benefit generators in that they provide benefits within themselves. For example, Item 3 (TRANSPORT IN FIRST RESPONDERS) and the setting up of specific emergency operations (Items 15, 16, and 17) are crucial to much of the rest of the emergency response, but in and of themselves, they neither save lives nor protect property. Conversely, all of the highlighted activities are designed to save lives, treat casualties, and protect property. Reaching and accomplishing these activities as quickly as possible must be the clearly understood goal of the whole team. Also, the quantified benefits of saving time in this process should have been communicated to all leaders back in Item 2 (DETERMINE SCOPE OF EMERGENCY): an estimate, for this specific emergency, of how many lives are likely to be lost or how much property damage is likely to occur for every hour that passes after the emergency has arisen.

However, it is crucial to recognize that although the three items above are the benefit generator activities, all of their "ancestors" in the flow chart are enablers that must be performed in order to even reach the benefit generators. The value of the enabler is no less than that of the benefit generator it enables, any more than the goal scored in the first minute of a 2–1 soccer victory is less valuable than the goal scored in the final minute! Indeed, as we saw in the example of the development of the internal combustion engine, the value of an enabler can often be greater than that of any single benefit generator if it is enabling more than one benefit generator. And, of course, Items 10 (SECURE THE AREA) and 13 (CONTAIN DAMAGE) are both benefit generators as well as enablers of Item 18 (IMPLEMENT OPERATIONAL MODE).

5.6 QUANTIFYING BENEFITS IN EMERGENCY RESPONSE PLANS

Planning should tie each benefit generator to the expected quantified benefits (e.g., the expected monetary value of the project investment in business project management). In the case of almost every project, time is a factor that can greatly enhance or decrease value. In the case of emergency response, the benefit of faster projects is more lives saved and more injuries and damage prevented. The benefit of completing each of the generators should therefore be stated in terms of the incremental increase in damage to people or property for every additional hour. A Damage Control Time Chart such as the one shown in Figure 5.5 can be used with each emergency response template, with the estimated levels filled in as information about the precise nature of a specific disaster emerges. Notice that the specifics of such a chart might be completely different across a range of emergencies: an epidemic, a fire in a skyscraper, a car bomb in Manhattan, a sarin attack in a subway, a Mississippi flood, or a New Orleans hurricane. For our purposes, we are presuming an earthquake in a city where:

- Many buildings have collapsed, and people are trapped in the rubble.
- There is no danger of a tsunami, but there is some danger of fires.
- Municipal communications and authority have largely disintegrated.

The chart suggests that delays in securing the area and containing the damage will result in a steadily increasing mortality rate. Delays in implementing the operational mode for searching through the rubble, setting up triage and other medical processes, and evacuating acute cases will result in the greatest number of post-event casualties, which will peak at about 9 to 12 hours after the event and then decline slowly as the number of possible rescues that are still alive declines.

HOURS	SECURE THE AREA LIVES/H.	INJURIES/H.	DAMAGE/H.	CONTAIN THE DAMAGE LIVES/H.	INJURIES/H.	DAMAGE/H.	IMPLEMENT OPERATIONAL MODE LIVES/H.	INJURIES/H.	DAMAGE/H.
0 – 2	B	B	A	C	B	C	E	B	B
3 – 4	B	B	A	B	B	D	F	B	B
5 – 6	B	B	A	B	A	D	F	B	B
7 – 8	C	B	A	B	A	D	F	B	A
9 – 12	C	B	B	C	A	D	G	A	A
13 – 24	D	B	B	C	A	B	F	A	A

A = 0 LIVES/H., 0 INJURIES/H., $0 DAMAGE/H.
B = 2 LIVES/H., 5 INJURIES/H., $500K DAMAGE/H.
C = 5 LIVES/H., 15 INJURIES/H., $1M DAMAGE/H.
D = 10 LIVES/H., 50 INJURIES/H., $5M DAMAGE/H.
E = 20 LIVES/H., 100 INJURIES/H., $20M DAMAGE/H.
F = 50 LIVES/H., 250 INJURIES/H., $100M DAMAGE/H.
G = 100 LIVES/H., 500 INJURIES/H., $500M DAMAGE/H.

FIGURE 5.5 A Damage Control Time Chart for a specific emergency

5.7 USING CRITICAL PATH METHOD TO PLAN A SCHEDULE FOR EMERGENCY RESPONSE

We shall now plan and optimize our emergency response schedule. We will start by taking our flow chart and turning it into a network logic diagram (sometimes called a Project Evaluation and Review Technique (PERT) chart) by estimating the expected durations, in hours, of each of the efforts (Figure 5.6).

In a network logic diagram, an activity may not start until *all* of its immediate predecessors are finished. (There are such things as complex precedence dependencies, called start-to-start, finish-to-finish, and start-to-finish relationships, or SS, FF, and SF relationships for short. These can be important tools for fast-tracking a schedule, and every schedule planner should be familiar with their use. However, for the purposes of this chapter, we will deal only with finish-to-start dependencies,

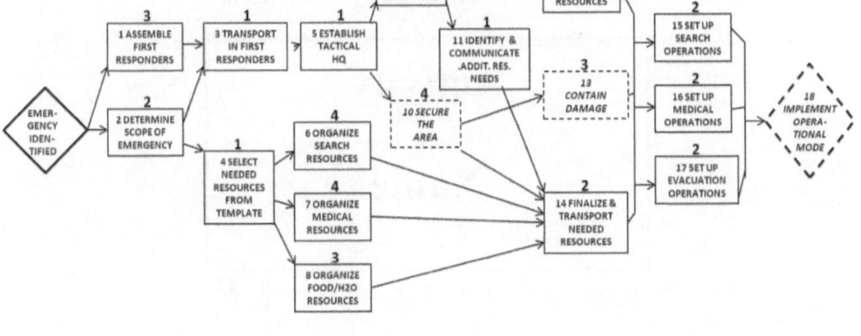

FIGURE 5.6 A network logic diagram showing the durations of the efforts for this specific emergency

where a predecessor must finish before a successor can start.) For example, Item 14 (FINALIZE & TRANSPORT NEEDED RESOURCES) cannot start until all five of its predecessors (6, 7, 8, 10, and 11) have finished. This means that whichever predecessor finishes last determines the earliest possible start of the successor.

The CPM of scheduling consists of two algorithms:

- The forward pass algorithm traces network logic and durations from the first activity to the last and determines the earliest that each activity can start (ES) and finish (EF).
- The backward pass algorithm starts at the end, with the early dates or times determined for the last activity by the forward pass, and it traces network logic and durations backward, from the last activity to the first, and determines the latest that each activity can finish (LF) and start (LS) *without delaying the last activity beyond its early dates*. These dates or times are then printed in a box for each activity using the convention illustrated in Figure 5.7:

Based on the durations and the dependencies, we can now calculate the CPM schedule as shown in Figure 5.8 below:

Our project begins as soon as the emergency is identified. Certain items have exactly the same early numbers (above the box) as late numbers (below the box). These items are on the longest path through the project, which is called the *critical path* because:

1. The duration of the longest path determines the duration of the project – every project is as long as its longest path.
2. Any delays on the longest path will make the project longer, while delays off the longest path will *only* make the project longer if the delays are so great as to make a new longest (and critical) path.
3. If we wish to shorten the total project duration, we have to shorten the longest path. This point is often overlooked but is perhaps most important, especially on a project where hundreds of lives hang in the balance.

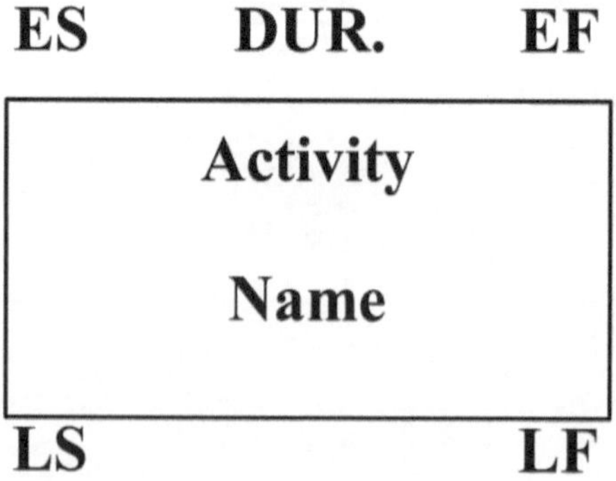

FIGURE 5.7 A network logic diagram activity box showing planned early and late starts and finishes

In Figure 5.8, we have highlighted the critical path with thick borders: Items 1, 3, 5, 10, 13, and 15 through 18. The fact that all three of our life-saving benefit generators (Items 10, 13, and 18) are on the critical path will make the upcoming optimization process easier. If one were off the critical path, we would need to optimize the path to that item separately in order to pull it in earlier and thus save more lives.

CPM, which has been around for more than half a century, also quantifies the amount of time by which an activity is removed from the critical path into a metric called *total float* (or, in Microsoft Project software, *total slack*). Total float (TF) is the amount of time an activity can slip without delaying the end of the project, i.e., without becoming critical. It is calculated using the formula TF = LF – EF. In Figure 5.9, the TF of each non-critical item is printed directly under the middle of the activity box.

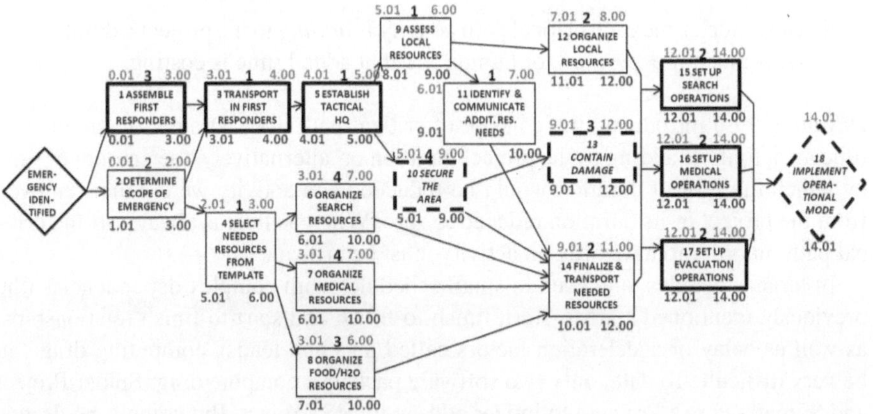

FIGURE 5.8 A CPM network logic diagram with the critical path highlighted with thick borders

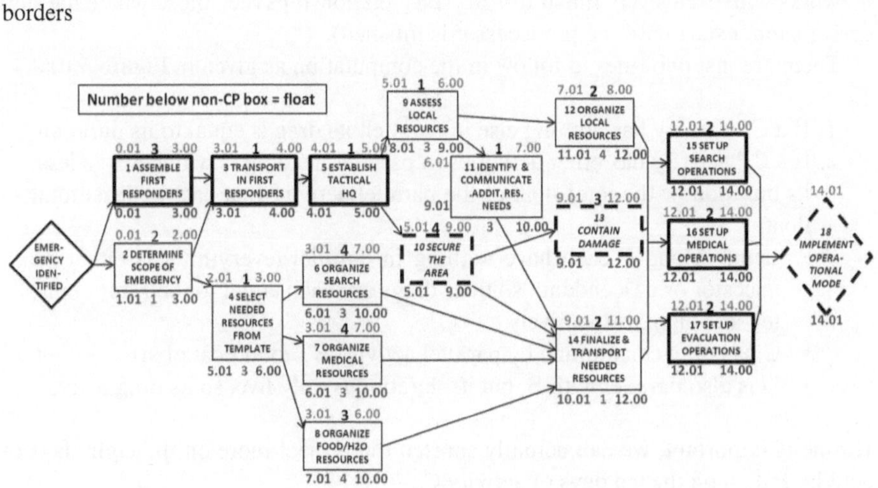

FIGURE 5.9 CPM network logic diagram with total float calculations

5.8 CRITICAL PATH DRAG: THE MISSING QUANTIFICATION ON THE CRITICAL PATH

While total float is an important metric, by itself, it does nothing to help shorten the project because as we plan the project, float is always *off* the critical path, on activities that are not delaying the project at all and thus costing us neither time nor lives. Critical path theory, and all CPM software algorithms, compute total float. But what do they say about activities that are *on* the critical path? Answer: *zero*! They tell us they have zero total float, which is approximately the same as repeating to us that the activity is critical. When activities *aren't* critical, CPM theory and the software quantify things nicely for us. But CPM tells us zero for the critical activities.

What *should* CPM theory and the software tell us about critical activities? We need to know:

1. How much time each critical path activity is *adding* to the project's duration.
2. How much money, pain, or human life that added time is costing.

Devaux (1999) introduced the concept of critical path drag. Drag is the amount of time an activity is adding to the project duration or, alternatively, the amount of time by which the project duration would be reduced if an activity were either removed from the project or its duration reduced to zero. Whereas float is always off the critical path, in order to have drag an activity must be critical.

In large schedules, and even in small schedules with complex dependencies (the previously mentioned start-to-start, finish-to-finish and start-to-finish relationships, as well as delay or acceleration factors called lags and leads), computing drag can be very difficult. To date, only two software packages compute drag: Spider Project and Sumatra.com's Project Optimizer add-on to MS Project. But computing drag is important – human lives may depend on it! So, we should learn to compute it in small networks with exclusively finish-to-start (FS) relationships (i.e., those where the successor cannot start until the predecessor is finished).

There are just two rules to follow in the computation as given in Figure 5.10:

1. If a CP activity has nothing else in parallel, its drag is equal to its duration.
2. If a CP activity has other activities in parallel, its drag is whichever is less: its duration or the total float of the parallel activity that has the least total float.
   - Items A and F each have nothing in parallel (everything is either an ancestor or descendant), so their drags are each equal to their durations, ten and eight, respectively.
   - C has drag constrained by parallel activity B's total float of six.
   - D is also parallel with B, but its duration is only five, so its drag is five.

If time is important, we can actually shorten the project more on the eight days of activity F than on the ten days of activity C.

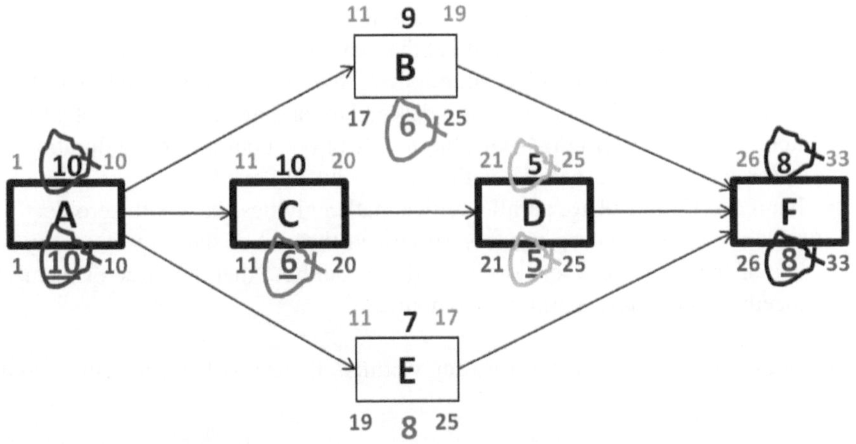

FIGURE 5.10 Simple CPM network logic diagram with drag calculations underlined

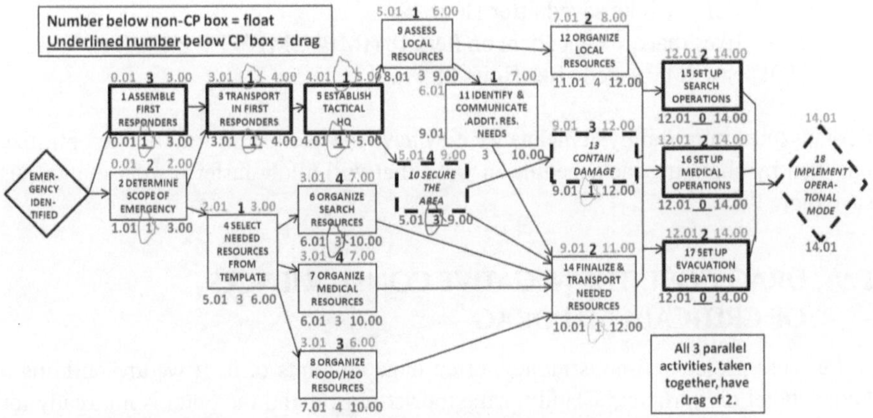

FIGURE 5.11 CPM diagram for Emergency Response with drag calculations

A network logic diagram would be much larger and more complex for an emergency response than our diagrams in Figures 5.8 and 5.9. However, let us now compute critical path drag for the simple diagram we are using in Figure 5.11:

- Item 1 (ASSEMBLE FIRST RESPONDERS) has drag of one hour as it is parallel with Item 2, which has a total float of one.
- Item 3 (TRANSPORT IN FIRST RESPONDERS) has drag of one hour. Although it is parallel with many items (4, 6, 7, and 8) that have a float of three and four hours, Item 3's drag is limited by its duration of one hour.
- Item 5 (ESTABLISH TACTICAL HQ) also has a drag of one hour for the same reasons.

- Item 10 (SECURE THE AREA) has a drag of three hours. It is parallel with many items (4, 6, 7, 8, 9, 11, and 12) that have a float of either three or four hours, and it has a duration of four hours. (Note that Item 10 is NOT parallel with Item 2 and Item 14 – it is a descendant of 2 and an ancestor of 14.)
- Item 13 (CONTAIN DAMAGE) has a drag of one hour as it has a duration of three hours and is parallel with Item 14's float of one hour.
- Items 16, 17, and 18 are parallel critical path activities, each with zero float so that each has a drag of zero. To pull in the end of the project on any one of them, we have to shorten all three. But note that the three of them together would have a drag of two hours.

What does this all mean to the disaster victims? It means that with our current schedule:

- Those lives that are dependent on the completion of Item 10 (SECURE THE AREA) will be saved after Hour 9.
- Those lives that are dependent on the completion of Item 13 (CONTAIN DAMAGE) will be saved after Hour 12.
- Those lives that are dependent on Item 18 (IMPLEMENT OPERATIONAL MODE) will be saved after Hour 14.

Perhaps most importantly, it means we now have the needed information to optimize our plan by changing the schedule in ways that will allow faster response and thus save more lives.

5.9 DRAG COST: THE NEGATIVE CONSEQUENCES OF CRITICAL PATH DRAG

In business projects, time is money, often huge amounts of it. If we are building a luxury hotel on a tropical island for the tourist season and the hotel is not ready for opening until the fourth week of the season, the extra time on our schedule has cost three weeks of revenue, worth perhaps $1 million each. It is not just the last activity or two (landscaping or electrical wiring, perhaps) that has caused the delay; *it is every activity that is on the final (or as-built) critical path.* And the *drag cost* of every critical path activity is equal to $1 million per week for up to three weeks of drag.

Similarly, it is not just the two hours required for each of activities 15, 16, and 17, setting up the search, medical, and evacuation processes, that delay the saving of many lives until after Hour 14 – it is every item on our critical path. And the drag cost of each such item is the lives, injuries, and damage that occur even as we rush to implement our life-saving processes. It is not the individuals, who are doing their best to get the work done as swiftly as possible, that cause the deaths – it is Time itself that swings the scythe.

	ITEM 10 (SECURE)	ITEM13 (CONTAIN)	ITEM 18 (IMPLMNT)	HOURLY TOTAL
HOUR 1	B=2	C=5	E=20	27
HOUR 2	B=2	C=5	E=20	27
HOUR 3	B=2	B=2	F=50	54
HOUR 4	B=2	B=2	F=50	54
HOUR 5	B=2	B=2	F=50	54
HOUR 6	B=2	B=2	F=50	54
HOUR 7	C=5	B=2	F=50	57
HOUR 8	C=5	B=2	F=50	57
HOUR 9	C=5	C=5	G=100	110
HOUR 10	C=5	C=5	G=100	110
HOUR 11	C=5	C=5	G=100	110
HOUR 12	C=5	C=5	G=100	110
HOUR 13	D=10	C=5	F=50	65
HOUR 14	D=10	C=5	F=50	65
HOUR 15	D=10	C=5	F=50	65
HOUR 16	D=10	C=5	F=50	65
TOTAL DEATHS	82	62	940	1084

FIGURE 5.12 Loss of life in the first 16 hours if there is no response

Let us look at two charts that show the loss of life in the first 16 hours after the catastrophe. Figure 5.12 shows the loss of life if there was no response, and Figure 5.13 corresponds to the response as scheduled in Figure 5.11. In Figure 5.11, the area is secured after Hour 9, the damage is contained after Hour 12, and search and rescue is fully operational after Hour 14. The information in these charts comes directly from the data in the Damage Control Time Chart in Figure 5.5.

The table in Figure 5.12 tells us that the total loss of life in 16 hours if there were no response would be 1,084. However, if we follow the CPM schedule as shown in Figure 5.11, lives that otherwise would have been lost now start to be saved as early as Hour 10 by securing the area. The result is that the total expected deaths shrink by 175, from 1,084 to 909, as shown in the table in Figure 5.13.

The highlighted cells above show how the planned response in Figure 5.11 reduces the mortality rate. Now, we can look at our critical path from Figure 5.11, see what the drag cost is of each component, and examine if there is a way to reduce the drag and, with it, the loss of life.

- The final trio of items (15, 16, and 17), setting up the search and rescue, medical, and evacuation processes, has, as a group, drag equal to its duration of two hours. One hundred lives are estimated to expire in Hours 13 and

	ITEM 10 (SECURE)	ITEM13 (CONTAIN)	ITEM 18 (IMPLMNT)	HOURLY TOTAL
HOUR 1	B=2	C=5	E=20	27
HOUR 2	B=2	C=5	E=20	27
HOUR 3	B=2	B=2	F=50	54
HOUR 4	B=2	B=2	F=50	54
HOUR 5	B=2	B=2	F=50	54
HOUR 6	B=2	B=2	F=50	54
HOUR 7	C=5	B=2	F=50	57
HOUR 8	C=5	B=2	F=50	57
HOUR 9	C=5	C=5	G=100	110
HOUR 10	*0*	C=5	G=100	***105***
HOUR 11	*0*	C=5	G=100	***105***
HOUR 12	*0*	C=5	G=100	***105***
HOUR 13	*0*	*0*	F=50	***50***
HOUR 14	*0*	*0*	F=50	***50***
HOUR 15	*0*	*0*	*0*	*0*
HOUR 16	*0*	*0*	*0*	*0*
TOTAL DEATHS	*27*	*42*	*840*	*909*

FIGURE 5.13 Loss of life in first 16 hours with planned response as in Figure 5.11

14. However, these set-up processes are necessary for future life-saving, so they cannot be eliminated. It might be possible to increase their resources and thus reduce their combined duration to one hour and their drag cost from 100 lives to 50 lives. But with three interrelated and parallel activities such as these, all efforts to shorten them will be in vain if any one of them slips back to two hours. The risk suggests that applying compression efforts elsewhere may be more beneficial. So, at least for the moment, let us accept that this trio has a drag cost of 100 lives.

- Item 13 (CONTAIN DAMAGE) is both a benefit generator in its own right and an enabler/predecessor of setting up the future life-saving operations. It has a drag of one hour, being parallel with Item 14, which has one hour of float. Being both a benefit generator and an enabler throws a wrinkle into the drag cost calculation for Item 13. In its enabler capacity, it is delaying the start of the main life-saving operations by only one hour (i.e., one hour of drag). However, as a benefit generator, if its duration could be reduced from three hours to one hour, its completion at the end of Hour 10 would save ten lives in and of itself, as well as saving 50 lives by allowing Item 18 to start one hour earlier. Thus, its drag cost as a benefit generator is 15 lives for its three days of duration and, as an enabler, its drag cost is 50 lives, for a total drag cost of 65 lives.

- Item 10 (SECURE THE AREA), like Item 13, is both a benefit generator in its own right and an enabler/predecessor of both containing damage and setting up the future life-saving operations. Its duration of four hours has a drag of three hours, being parallel with several items that have three hours of float. If the area is secure in three less hours:
  - An estimated 15 lives would be saved just by completing Item 10 three hours earlier.
  - An additional 15 lives would be saved by enabling Item 13 to be completed three hours earlier.
  - A further 200 lives would be saved by launching the life-saving processes at the beginning of Hour 12 rather than the beginning of Hour 15.

Thus, the drag cost of Item 10 is 230 lives. (Notice that Item 10, in and of itself, is a benefit generator that saves lives. But the time it takes also costs lives.)

- Item 3 (TRANSPORT IN FIRST RESPONDERS) and Item 5 (ESTABLISH TACTICAL HQ) have just one hour of drag due to their duration. But the entire path of Items 3, 5, and 10 (through SECURE THE AREA) also shares the drag-limiting parallel item float of three hours on Items 1, 6, and 7. What this means is that the combined drag on Items 3, 5 and 10 is not 1 + 1 + 3 = 5 hours, since neither float nor drag is additive along a given path between merge points in the schedule. Any time gained by shortening any one of the three will reduce the drag on the other two items, so that the total combined drag of Items 3, 5 and 10 is only three hours, which may be gained by compressing any of these three items to a total of three hours.

The drag and drag cost of each of the critical path items are shown in Figure 5.14:

ITEM	DRAG (IN HOURS)	DRAG COST IN LIVES
1	1	60
3	1	60
5	1	60
10	3	230
13	1	65
15	0	0
16	0	0
17	0	0
15, 16 & 17	2	100

FIGURE 5.14 Drag and drag cost (in loss of life) for each critical path item

5.10 USING DRAG AND DRAG COST TO OPTIMIZE THE PLAN

As we get ready to show how to use critical path drag and drag cost to optimize the emergency response plan, we must caution the reader once more that we are showing this in a greatly simplified example. Any real project would need to be doing its computation and optimization on a much more granular and complex plan, involving perhaps thousands of activities and including the complex dependencies we mentioned previously. However, for showing how the concepts are designed to work, our simple network serves the purpose nicely without introducing confusing complexity.

After carefully analyzing the network in Figure 5.12 and the table in Figure 5.15, we work with the leaders of the individual efforts and those with access to additional resources to obtain a better assembly area for the first responders, both larger and closer to the likely disaster site. The benefits are:

- The larger site allows both the assembly of a larger number of first responders and vehicles and easy-to-load storage of all needed equipment and materials, so that responders just need to report to the site and retrieve them there. This shortens the needed time for assembly from three hours to two hours. The one hour of drag on Item 1 disappears, and the project duration becomes 13 hours instead of 14 hours.
- The greater proximity of the new site to the disaster area and the easy-loading design of the equipment and materials containers reduce the time necessary for Item 3 (TRANSPORT IN FIRST RESPONDERS) from one hour to 0.5 hours. This reduces the drag on Item 3 from one hour to 0.5 hours, and the project duration becomes 12.5 hours instead of 13 hours.
- The expanded number of first responders that the new assembly site permits also reduces by half the amount of expected time necessary for Item 5

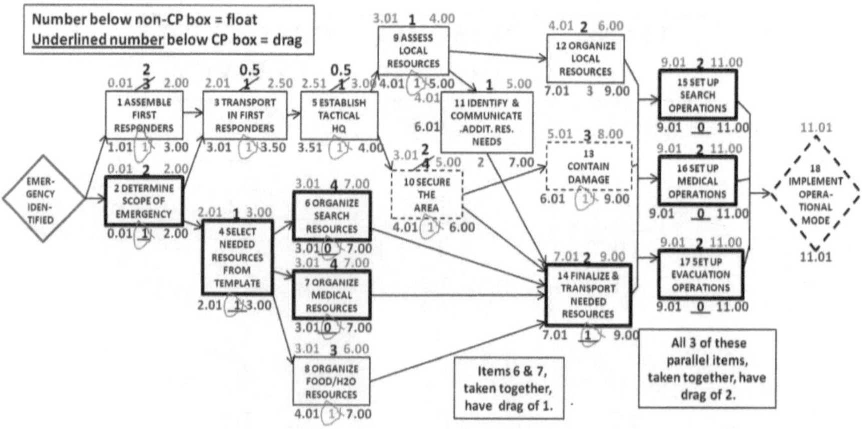

FIGURE 5.15 New durations, critical path, and drags for Emergency Response

(ESTABLISH TACTICAL HQ) from one hour to 0.5 hours. This reduces the drag on Item 5 from one hour to 0.5 hours and the project duration becomes 12 hours instead of 12.5 hours.

- Finally, the expanded number of first responders also reduces by half the amount of expected time necessary for Item 10 (SECURE THE AREA) from four hours to two hours. By this point, the earlier changes on Item 10's ancestors (1, 3, and 5) had reduced the drag on Item 10 from three hours to one hour, so this new two-hour compression changes Item 10's one remaining hour of drag to one hour of float as the critical path changes. Being a benefit generator, Item 10's earlier finish by two hours means that securing the area will start to save lives two hours earlier. Additionally, as Item 10 is the sole predecessor of benefit generator Item 13 (CONTAIN DAMAGE), it too will begin delivering its benefits two hours earlier. However, since the drag on Item 10 had previously been reduced to one hour, the end of the project and the implementation of the operational mode are only pulled in by one additional hour.

The CPM diagram for the modified schedule is shown in Figure 5.16. Notice that the critical path to the ultimate benefit generator has now changed to go through the items that involve determining, acquiring, and transporting the additional resources (Items 2, 4, 6, 7 and 14).

	ITEM 10 (SECURE)	ITEM13 (CONTAIN)	ITEM 18 (IMPLMNT)	HOURLY TOTAL
HOUR 1	B=2	C=5	E=20	27
HOUR 2	B=2	C=5	E=20	27
HOUR 3	B=2	B=2	F=50	54
HOUR 4	B=2	B=2	F=50	54
HOUR 5	B=2	B=2	F=50	54
HOUR 6	*0 (Was B=2)*	B=2	F=50	*52 (Was 54)*
HOUR 7	*0 (Was C=5)*	B=2	F=50	*52 (Was 57)*
HOUR 8	*0 (Was C=5)*	B=2	F=50	*52 (Was 57)*
HOUR 9	*0 (Was C=5)*	*0 (Was C=5)*	G=100	*100 (Was 110)*
HOUR 10	*0*	*0 (Was C=5)*	G=100	*100 (Was 105)*
HOUR 11	*0*	*0 (Was C=5)*	G=100	*100 (Was 105)*
HOUR 12	*0*	*0 (Was C=5)*	*0 (Was G=100)*	*0 (Was 105)*
HOUR 13	*0*	*0*	*0 (Was F=50)*	*0 (Was 50)*
HOUR 14	*0*	*0*	*0 (Was F=50)*	*0 (Was 50)*
HOUR 15	*0*	*0*	*0*	*0*
HOUR 16	*0*	*0*	*0*	*0*
TOTAL DEATHS	*10 (Was 27)*	*22 (Was 42)*	*640 (Was 840)*	*672 (Was 909)*

FIGURE 5.16 Loss of life in first 16 hours with optimized response schedule as in Figure 5.15

What has our schedule compression done for the lethality of the disaster?

- If the new schedule is achievable, the deaths owing directly to a lack of security in the area should cease after the end of Hour 5. That is one huge modification. Establishing security four hours earlier reduces the mortality due to lack of security from 27 to 10.
- It also enables Item 13 (CONTAIN DAMAGE) to be completed by the end of Hour 8. This reduces the mortality from spreading damage (gas fires from ruptured pipelines, for instance) by containing it four hours earlier. The result is an estimated loss of just 22 lives from spreading damage, down from 42 when Item 13 was not scheduled for completion until Hour 12.
- The big payoff comes from being able to implement operational mode for search, medical, and evacuation operations three hours earlier. That enables this benefit generator to reduce expected mortality by 200 lives, from 840 to 640.

The chart above shows a reduction in the victims of Time by a total of 235, from 909 to 672. A similar analysis could be done for injuries and property damage.

The process of schedule optimization for this planned response doesn't have to be complete at this point. Again, planning at a more detailed level often shows additional opportunities for compression through fast-tracking (i.e., doing more things in parallel) or crashing the critical path (adding resources). With the lives of hundreds of human beings on the line, we should look once more at the drag and drag cost totals on our new schedule in a chart (Figure 5.17) similar to the one in Figure 5.14.

The items that stand out are the two that have a duration of two hours *and a* drag of one hour: Item 2 (DETERMINE SCOPE OF EMERGENCY) and Item 14

ITEM	DRAG (IN HOURS)	DRAG COST IN LIVES
2	1	100
4	1	100
6	0	0
7	0	0
6 & 7	1	100
14	1	100
15	0	0
16	0	0
17	0	0
15, 16 & 17	2	200

FIGURE 5.17 Drag and drag cost (in loss of life) of each item on the new critical path

(FINALIZE & TRANSPORT NEEDED RESOURCES). In practice, activities that have both longer durations and drag often provide opportunities for compression. Would it be possible to reduce the two-hour durations of either or both of these items? If yes, then the total project duration could be reduced by up to one hour, with the operational mode starting after 10 hours. Of course, keep in mind that if we reduced Item 2 and Item 14 by one hour each, although that particular path would be reduced by two hours, the end of the project would only be pulled in by one hour, and the critical path and drag would revert to the original critical path items.

Finally, the example we have used in this chapter is based on the model of a disaster that comes without warning. However, preventable loss of life and public frustration at what seems an inadequate level of preparation often occur following predicted disasters where there were forty-eight hours or more of clear warning that *something* bad was likely to happen. In situations such as these, the template model that is chosen can often be tweaked for the known specifics of the upcoming event. For example, in the CPM schedule we are using, not only could specifics of personnel and equipment be adjusted (e.g., amphibious vehicles and scuba gear brought into the assembly area if flooding is a possible hazard), but the preparatory time could also be used to provide a "head start" that would reduce the drag and drag cost of the early efforts. By performing Item 1 (ASSEMBLE FIRST RESPONDERS) even before the event has occurred, and simultaneously performing adequately detailed preparation for Item 2 (DETERMINE SCOPE OF EMERGENCY), we could turn the latter two-hour effort into a half hour, thus starting Item 3 (TRANSPORT IN FIRST RESPONDERS) within 0.5 hours or less after the event has occurred and thereby pulling in all the benefit generators by up to an additional 1.5 hours.

5.11 CONCLUSIONS

- Employment of modern project management techniques is essential in the planning of specific genres of emergencies that seem likely to occur at some point and for which a response plan would have an ameliorating impact.
- Each of these plans should then be analyzed specifically with reference to the deleterious effects of the passage of time after the expected disaster. The impacts of time, in terms of mortality, injuries, and property, damage should be clearly quantified, hour by hour, if not in even smaller intervals, in a Damage Control Time Chart.
- Critical path analysis should then be used to assemble an initial schedule of response efforts. It should identify and focus on the specific actions/items/projects that will be the benefit generators, i.e., those that will culminate in the amelioration of some quantifiable amount of the negative impacts.
- Critical path drag and drag cost, with the latter measured in mortality, injuries and property damage as quantified earlier in the Damage Control Time Chart, should be computed for the paths leading to each benefit generator. This information should then be used iteratively to make scheduling and resourcing decisions that compress the critical path and then, when it changes, focus on the new critical path. Careful track should be kept of the

amount of benefit gained with each change until the plan seems to offer little or no further opportunity for improvement.

- In emergencies where the event is forecast in advance, all possible efforts should be made to provide the template schedule with a head start by beginning the earliest items in advance.

REFERENCES

Devaux, S. A., *Total Project Control: A Manager's Guide to Integrated Project Planning, Measuring and Tracking Systems,* John Wiley & Sons, New York, 1999.

The Project Management Institute, *A Guide to the Project Management Body of Knowledge, (PMBOK™ Guide),* 4th edition, 2008. Project Management Institute, Newton Square, PA..

6 Evacuation Planning, Analysis, and Management

Michael K. Lindell

6.1 INTRODUCTION

Evacuation is a process intended to temporarily move people from a hazardous location to a place of greater safety. It takes place frequently; an evacuation involving 1,000 people or more takes place every two to three weeks in the United States (Dotson and Jones 2005). Such movement can significantly decrease the number of deaths and injuries as well as the social impacts these casualties can cause (Lindell 2020a). Despite its frequency and success, however, evacuation should not be assumed to be an unquestionably appropriate response to all hazardous situations. In some cases, characteristics of the hazard preclude evacuation. For example, earthquakes provide no forewarning for people very close to the epicenter, so the protective action recommendation is to drop, cover, and hold instead of evacuating a building (Vinnell et al. 2022). In addition, some tornadoes, toxic chemicals, and radiological incidents have such a rapid onset and short duration that evacuation would increase the danger to people trying to evacuate. Evacuation would also be inadvisable in any hazard when the risk of movement exceeds the risk of remaining in place, as might be the case for intensive care patients. In other cases, evacuation is unnecessary because people are in structures that provide adequate protection. In such cases, shelter-in-place (SIP) provides adequate protection (Lindell 2019b). Finally, evacuation is inadvisable when the reduction in risk for residents on the periphery of the threat area is so small that it is not worth the expense and disruption involved.

The logistics of evacuation are relatively simple when authorities can provide adequate forewarning to sparsely populated risk areas where households have their own cars, so the traffic demand never exceeds the evacuation route system (ERS) capacity. This was the case in the analysis of hurricane evacuation for Willacy County, Texas (Lindell et al. 2002). Evacuation logistics are also relatively simple when people can walk to nearby safe areas, as is the case for a tsunami striking a mountainous coastal area (Wang et al. 2022). However, logistical problems increase with the size of the risk area and its population, as well as when there is a need to evacuate many residents who have limited access to transportation or even limited

DOI: 10.1201/9781003648178-7

personal mobility. In some cases, people lacking cars are sufficiently mobile that they can walk to nearby locations where they can board buses that will carry them to safety (Lindell et al. 2019a, Chapter 11). In other cases, individuals have such limited mobility that they must be picked up from their homes and transported by vans. Finally, some individuals require intensive care and thus require ambulances for transport. Although many such individuals are in institutions such as hospitals and nursing homes, others live in homes that are distributed throughout the community, and must be located through home healthcare organizations. Moreover, many households have pets, and some have farm animals that must be evacuated (Chadwin 2017). Emergency managers must take all of these conditions into account when planning for and managing evacuations.

The purpose of this chapter is to guide emergency managers and transportation planners in developing plans for vehicular evacuation from environmental hazards. It does not discuss pedestrian evacuation from buildings, aircraft, or ships because the scale and dynamics of these evacuations are quite different (Peacock et al. 2011). Moreover, this chapter's focus is on pre-impact rather than post-impact evacuations because pre-impact evacuations must be completed before the beginning of hazard exposure (in the case of natural hazards) or the accumulation of an excessive dose (in the case of toxic chemicals or radiological materials). By contrast, post-impact evacuations are usually less urgent. Specifically, even though some people decide to evacuate later because of the loss of electric power for cooling during the summer (Shen et al. 2024), there is likely to be less congestion on evacuation routes out of the impact area.

The remainder of this chapter will be divided into three major sections. The first section covers pre-impact activities involved in evacuation planning. The second section covers evacuation analysis—the activities associated with assessing the time required to evacuate a risk area and the points on the ERS where bottlenecks are most likely to occur. The third section addresses evacuation management—the activities involved in actually implementing an evacuation plan.

6.2 EVACUATION PLANNING

Disaster researchers (Perry and Lindell 2007) and evacuation analysts (Houston 2009) agree that a critical first step in evacuation planning is to establish continuing contacts among all of the organizations that will be involved in implementing an evacuation—especially emergency management, transportation, police and fire departments, social services, and the American Red Cross (or other operators of congregate care facilities—"public shelters"). In the case of regional evacuations, this includes the affected organizations in other jurisdictions—counties or states—that will also be involved in evacuation, shelter, and reentry. As will be discussed below, an effective planning process addresses a number of issues that need to be resolved by risk jurisdictions (the ones from which people are evacuating), transit jurisdictions (the ones through which they travel), and host jurisdictions (the ones in which they stay until returning to their homes).

6.2.1 Evacuation Planning Organization

Critical activities during evacuation operations include interagency communications, provisions for accepting outside support personnel (e.g., common credentialing), multichannel/multilingual public information from joint information centers, media monitoring, support for emergency responder families, en route fuel operations, traffic monitoring, transportation support for transit-dependent populations, mobile response teams, and shelter coordination. Evacuation routes need to be coordinated to ensure that plans in adjacent jurisdictions do not conflict, as happened in the Three Mile Island incident (Chenault et al. 1980). Critical activities during reentry operations include damage assessment and documentation, debris removal, infrastructure restoration, and communication with evacuees. Planning activities should include annual audits of evacuation plans to ensure that they remain current; continuing training to ensure that personnel understand their roles; periodic drills, tabletop exercises, and field exercises to test the plan under different emergency scenarios; and critiques to ensure that problems are identified and changes made to correct those problems (Lindell and Perry 2007).

Of course, evacuation planners should recognize that evacuation management, like any other emergency response activity, generally requires *improvisation* as well as *planning* (Mendonça and Wallace 2007). Improvisation is usually needed because the incidents invariably deviate from the scenarios that guide evacuation plan development. Consequently, it is essential that evacuation managers participate in drills and exercises with a variety of scenarios so they can learn how to adjust to conditions that deviate from planning assumptions (Ford and Schmidt 2000).

6.2.2 Basic Planning Concepts

The fundamental framework for evacuation planning is illustrated in the *chains of events model* and its associated formula for Evacuation Time Estimates (ETEs). As indicated in Figure 6.1, ensuring that a risk area is cleared before the arrival of hazardous conditions requires an understanding of two chains of events—the environmental hazard chain and the community response chain (Lindell and Perry 1992; Mileti 1975). The environmental hazard chain for a hurricane can be characterized by the storm's movement over time, beginning with its initial detection and continuing with its monitoring through disaster impact. This chain generally terminates when the storm makes landfall, although it sometimes continues when a stalled storm deposits intense rainfall until it dissipates (e.g., Hurricane Harvey in 2017). As the storm progresses, computer models provide exposure projections of its expected landfall time, location, intensity, and wind field. Evacuation managers, households, and businesses use these *exposure projections* to identify areas that are likely to be affected by extreme wind, storm surge, and inland flooding. In turn, this *decision information* allows them to identify a) the geographical areas and population segments that should take protective action, b) the most appropriate protective action recommendation (PAR) for each target group, and c) the time at which these PARs should be initiated (Cova et al. 2017). Once evacuation managers have decided to

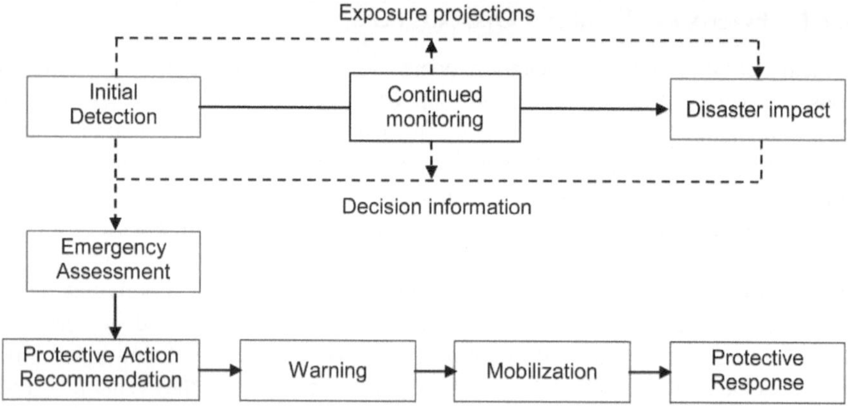

FIGURE 6.1 Chains of events model (adapted from Lindell and Perry 1992)

issue PARs, they compose warning messages (Sutton et al. 2024) and disseminate them to the risk area through channels such as broadcast media and social media. Households and businesses that have received these warnings typically mobilize by engaging in milling to confirm the warning (Wood et al. 2018), relaying warnings to others (Lindell et al. 2019b), and preparing for evacuation by packing bags and securing the home (Lindell et al. 2005). Once mobilization is complete, they begin their evacuation.

The time required to complete the four steps in the community response chain from the time authorities detect a threat until an evacuating household exits the risk area can be defined as a function of four time components (Urbanik 2000, Urbanik et al. 1980):

$t_T = f(t_d, t_w, t_p, t_e)$, Equation 6.1

where t_T = a household's total evacuation clearance time; t_d = authorities' warning issuance delay time; t_w = the household's warning receipt time; t_p = the household's preparation (mobilization) time; and t_e = the household's evacuation travel time. Authorities' warning issuance delay time (t_d) is a constant for any given jurisdiction, but household warning receipt times (t_w) and preparation times (t_p) are distributions over households that are combined to produce a departure time distribution. This departure time distribution and data on household geographic distribution are then entered into an evacuation modeling program that computes the distribution of household evacuation travel times (t_e) and thus the distribution of evacuation clearance times (t_T)—see Lindell et al. (2019a, Chapter 9).

6.3 EVACUATION ANALYSIS

There are four steps in evacuation analysis. These are to a) identify risk areas/sectors, b) identify the ERS and assess its capacity, c) forecast evacuation demand, and

d) model traffic behavior. Specific guidelines for nuclear power plant evacuation studies can be found in Smith (2021) and USNRC/FEMA (2019).

6.3.1 Identify Risk Areas/Sectors

A risk area is, as the name implies, the geographic area at risk from a given hazard. For some hazards, equivalent terms are used, such as "special flood hazard areas" (for floods), "vulnerable zone" or VZ (for toxic chemicals), and "emergency planning zone" or EPZ (for nuclear power plants). For most hydrometeorological and geological hazards, specialized agencies conduct risk analyses and provide risk area maps—e.g., hurricanes (www.nhc.noaa.gov/surge/risk/); landslides (landslides.usgs.gov/learning/nationalmap/); and tsunamis (www.conservation.ca.gov/cgs/geologic_hazards/Tsunami/Inundation_Maps/Pages/Statewide_Maps). However, the identification of risk areas for hazardous materials ("hazmat") is more difficult because the size of the risk area depends upon a number of factors, such as the quantity of material released, its volatility, toxicity (or radioactivity), and meteorological conditions such as wind speed, wind direction, and atmospheric stability (Lindell 2019a). For example, the US Department of Transportation (USDOT 2024) indicates that the risk area for a small daytime release of many toxic gases is about a half mile (800 meters) downwind, but a nighttime spill of a large quantity of methyl isocyanate has a downwind protective action distance of seven miles (11 km) or more. The US Environmental Protection Agency (www.epa.gov/oem/tools.htm) provides procedures for releases from fixed site facilities, which tend to have larger release volumes and thus larger VZs than transportation incidents. There is a standardized ten-mile plume inhalation EPZ for US commercial nuclear power plants (USNRC/FEMA 2019).

Whether for a natural (e.g., hurricane) or technological (e.g., nuclear power plant) hazard, it is unlikely that all parts of an extremely large risk area will be advised to take the same protective action in an emergency. In a nuclear power plant EPZ, for example, some areas are likely to be advised to evacuate, others to shelter in place, and still others to continue normal activities while monitoring the news media. Thus, large risk areas are often divided into smaller areas corresponding to recurrence intervals or event intensities. For example, the Federal Emergency Management Agency (www.fema.gov/flood-maps/know-your-risk/homeowners) primarily categorizes flood plains as A ("base" flood or 100-year floodplain), V (coastal 100-year floodplain subject to wave action), B (500-year floodplain or 100-year floodplain protected by a levee), C (outside the 500-year floodplain), D (outside the 500-year floodplain and protected from a 100-year flood by a levee), and X (an area with a possible flood hazard but for which there has been no flood hazard analysis). Hurricane risk areas are frequently subdivided according to their exposure to different Saffir-Simpson categories (Category 1–5). In some jurisdictions, each Saffir-Simpson category defines a different risk area, whereas in other jurisdictions, Saffir-Simpson risk areas are combined to define different evacuation zones (e.g., Category 1–3 storms define Evacuation Zone A, whereas Category 4–5 storms define Evacuation Zone B).

The most effective way to implement such protective actions is by identifying sectors—called "emergency response planning areas" in nuclear power plant emergency planning—that are areas of relatively homogeneous risk in which residents will all be advised to take the same protective action. Since these sectors should also be readily identifiable by those within them, emergency planners sometimes define these sectors in terms of postal codes (see Figure 6.2). A clear definition of each sector is important because many people have difficulty identifying their location on risk area maps (Chen et al. 2022b; Lindell 2020b) and some people lack even the basic map comprehension skills needed to interpret the map compass and scale (MacPherson-Krutsky et al. 2020).

Defining sectors by postal codes can work well in urban areas because they are relatively compact but are problematic in rural areas since they can cover large areas with heterogeneous risk levels. In such cases, sector boundaries should be defined by well-known political boundaries (e.g., county lines), geographical features (e.g., rivers), and major roads. Defining risk areas by geographical features is important because these can act as evacuation impediments that restrict the number, directions, and capacities of evacuation routes. For example, Figure 6.2 identifies multiple evacuation routes on Galveston Island and the mainland portion of Galveston County, but the bridge from the island to the mainland is a bottleneck that restricts evacuation

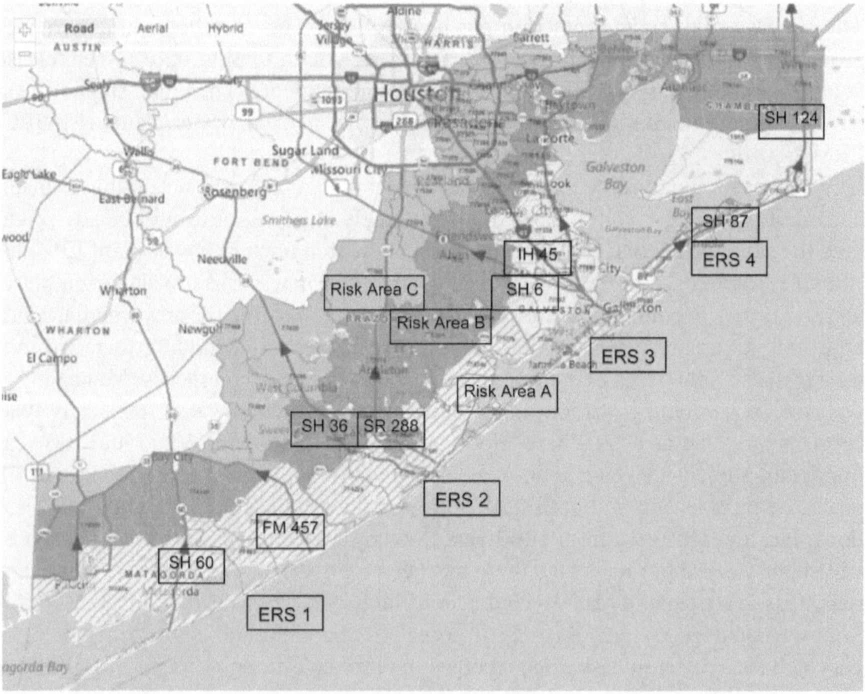

FIGURE 6.2 Risk areas and the evacuation route system for the Houston/Galveston study area

route capacity below the levels on either side. Detailed analysis indicated that the bridge approach limited ERS capacity more than the bridge itself (Urbanik 1978).

6.3.2 Identify the ERS and Its Capacity

Evacuations often result in a very large number of vehicles attempting to use the ERS simultaneously and, moreover, using those roads almost exclusively to travel in a single direction. Thus, continuing to use normal traffic control mechanisms such as stop signs and traffic signals—and especially toll booths on tollways—can substantially delay evacuating vehicles. Consequently, evacuation managers should designate the roads with the greatest capacity as the primary evacuation routes and devise traffic management strategies that maximize ERS capacity (Lindell et al. 2019a, Chapter 8).

ERS capacity can be estimated in three steps. First, analysts must identify the distinct set of links (individual road segments) that provide routes out of the risk area. For example, ERS 4 in Figure 6.2 is defined by State Highway (SH) 87 (link 1), which traverses the Bolivar Peninsula and joins SH 124 (link 2) to leave the risk area. Second, the analyst must assess the capacities of the individual links by considering each link's number of lanes, shoulder type and width, intersection characteristics (including turn lanes and signal phasing), speed limits, and surrounding land use (Dotson and Jones 2005; TRB 2022). Third, the analyst must examine the configuration of the links in the ERS to determine whether they form a serial, parallel, converging, or diverging pattern. Continuing the example of ERS 4, both SH 87 (link 1, running down the center of the Bolivar Peninsula to its base) and SH 124 (link 2, running from SH 87 inland) have capacities of 800 vehicles per hour (vph). Serial links generally are limited by the smallest capacity in the set of links for that evacuation route—as when a link with an 800 vph capacity feeds a link with a 600 vph capacity, thus reducing the overall capacity to 600 vph or less. It is also possible for the reverse to be true, as when a link with a 600 vph capacity underloads a link with an 800 vph capacity, also producing an overall capacity of 600 vph. However, there often are additional vehicles attempting to access the downstream link. In this case, SH 124 originates in Risk Area A (which is on the coast) but passes through Risk Area B (the dark-shaded area that is inland from Risk Area A), so the downstream link with greater capacity than the upstream link that feeds it is likely to reach capacity anyway.

In general, parallel links have additive capacities—as when two parallel links with capacities of 800 vph have a combined capacity of 1,600 vph (see ERS 2 for an example of two parallel evacuation routes—SH 36 and SH 288). Diverging links (a single link splitting into multiple links, see SH 6 diverging from IH 45 on the mainland just across from Galveston Island in ERS 3) generally follow the same rule as serial links because here, too, the capacity of the overall evacuation route is determined by the capacity of the link with the smaller capacity. In general, it is the upstream link feeding the diverging links that impose the capacity limit. Converging links (multiple links feeding into a single link, see Route 457 converging into SH

60 in ERS 1) are problematic because traffic cannot merge seamlessly, so the actual flow into the downstream route is likely to be lower than its nominal level.

It is important to recognize that link capacity can be degraded by various conditions, some of which are controllable and others uncontrollable. In some cases, controllable traffic impediments can be temporarily suspended (e.g., road repairs) or corrected (e.g., traffic accidents) to return link capacity to its normal level. The uncontrollable impediments (e.g., adverse weather) may require the use of compensatory actions such as additional evacuation routes or earlier evacuation initiation.

6.3.3 Forecast Evacuation Demand

Evacuation demand is the rate at which vehicles enter the ERS. It is a function of trip generation (the number of evacuating vehicles) and the departure timing distribution, which is determined by the combination of t_w and t_p. As indicated in Table 6.1, forecasting trip generation begins with an assessment of the size and distribution of four broad population segments, which are the a) vehicle-owning resident population, b) transit-dependent resident population, c) transient population, and d) institutionalized population (e.g., hospital patients). These population segments can be expected to differ in their distributions of warning receipt and evacuation preparation times, as well as their access to vehicles.

In addition, evacuation analysts must recognize that the size of each population segment within each sector varies over time. There is variation by time of day as people travel to work, school, and other daytime activities and return home at night. This diurnal variation is most pronounced during the work week, but there can also be substantial variation by time of year in some communities, as tourists and people with second homes arrive in vacation communities. Finally, there can be substantial increases in the transient population due to major festivals and sports events.

6.3.3.1 Vehicle-Owning Resident Population

The basic unit of the vehicle-owning resident population is the *household* because past research has reported that households tend to evacuate as a unit and usually seek to reunite if separated before evacuating (Tierney et al. 2001). In the past, household evacuations have been delayed if members were separated at the time of warning receipt (Perry et al. 1981). However, the widespread availability of cell phones for all household members has reduced this problem because household members can determine whether those who are absent are safe and identify a place to meet. In many cases, there are multiple vehicles and even multiple trailers per household. The number of vehicles and trailers, when divided by the ERS capacity in vehicles per hour, provides an approximate lower bound for the number of hours to complete an evacuation because it does not account for congestion. The number of evacuating vehicles is typically 65%–75% of the number of registered vehicles (Baker, 2000), but these vehicles do not necessarily leave at the same time for hurricanes (Maghelal et al., 2017). Moreover, there can be much lower vehicle use for tsunamis, with only 75% of US Pacific Coast residents expecting to evacuate by car and even smaller percentages in other countries (Chen et al. 2022a).

TABLE 6.1
Evacuation Model Parameters and Data Sources

Parameter	Data Source
Background Data Collection	
1. Risk Area and Sector definition	Hazard analysis
2. Evacuation route system (ERS) definition	Transportation department
Trip Generation	
3. Number and distribution of vehicle-owning resident households	National census data
4. Number of evacuating vehicles per residential household	Behavioral research
5. Number of evacuating trailers per residential household	Behavioral research
6. Number of persons per residential household	National census data
7. Number and distribution of the transit-dependent resident households	National census data
8. Number and distribution of transient households	Local Visitors' Bureau
9. Number of evacuating vehicles per transient household	Behavioral research
10. Size and distribution of the institutionalized population	Local records
11. Size and distribution of the non-institutionalized population with disabilities	Local records/National census data
12. Percentage of residents' PAR compliance/spontaneous evacuation	Behavioral research
13. Percentage of transients' PAR compliance/spontaneous evacuation	Behavioral research
Departure Timing	
14. Percentage of early evacuating residential households	Behavioral research
15. Percentage of early evacuating transient households	Behavioral research
16. Percentage of early evacuating institutions	Local agreements
17. Residential households' departure time distribution	Behavioral research
18. Transients' departure time distribution	Behavioral research
19. Institutions' departure time distribution	Local agreements
20. Non-institutionalized population's departure time distribution	Local agreements
Destination/Route Choice	
21. Evacuees' ultimate destinations	Behavioral research
22. Evacuees' proximate destinations/route choices	Behavioral research
23. Evacuees' utilization of the evacuation route system	Behavioral research

6.3.3.2 Transit-Dependent Population

The number of households without vehicles can be estimated by using the data available from the National Household Travel Survey (nhts.ornl.gov/tools.shtml). Although the percentage of carless households in a geographical area (derived from the NHTS) can be multiplied by the number of households in that area to estimate the number of households that will need public transit to evacuate, such estimates are only approximate. On the one hand, some households have vehicles that are in poor repair and cannot provide reliable transportation over long distances, such as those required for hurricane evacuations. On the other hand, some households that do not own vehicles will obtain rides with other households that do (Lindell et al., 2019, Chapter 6). These two effects tend to cancel each other, but the net effect is likely to vary from one jurisdiction to another.

A common procedure for evacuating transit-dependent populations is for them to walk to the nearest elementary school, where they can obtain rides on buses. This procedure produces substantial evacuation preparation times for this population segment because, unlike vehicle-owning households that can load their car(s) and leave immediately after packing their bags, transit-dependent households must walk to the nearest school, wait for their bus to arrive, and (generally) wait on the bus as it travels to the next pickup location before traveling out of the risk area (t_e). Moreover, the time to evacuate transit-dependent households can increase substantially if there is insufficient bus capacity to evacuate everyone in one trip and buses must make multiple trips.

6.3.3.3 Transients

Aside from their effect on the size of the evacuating population, transients are potentially problematic because they are likely to differ from local residents in having a lower likelihood of receiving informal warnings from peers, which is an important source of warnings in emergencies (see Lindell et al. 2019b for a review of empirical studies and Koll et al. 2023 for an agent-based model—ABM). The lower level of informal warnings may delay their departure times. However, they have no need to protect property and need less time to pack for the trip out of the risk area, which tends to decrease their departure times. In many cases, transients have their own vehicles, but those who have arrived by public transportation, especially commercial airlines, might find it difficult to reschedule their departures.

6.3.3.4 Special Needs Population

For purposes of evacuation, the special needs population comprises people with a variety of functional limitations in communication, medical health, functional independence, supervision, and transportation (FEMA 2021a, Stough and Kelman 2018). Some members of the special needs population are school children who must be evacuated directly to a safe location or who must be returned to their homes, where they will evacuate with the rest of their households. Whichever option school officials adopt must be communicated to parents during the planning phase before any incident occurs. This will reduce the number of parents seeking to pick up their children at school but will not prevent it (Murray-Tuite et al. 2012). Another important category of the special needs population is prisoners who must be evacuated under close supervision to another correctional institution—preferably before the rest of the risk area population begins to evacuate.

The third major category of the special needs population comprises those who are institutionalized in hospitals, nursing homes, group homes, or other types of facilities. Like school children and prisoners, the size and distribution of institutionalized patients are relatively easy to identify. However, the fourth special needs category is the approximately 17% of the non-institutionalized US population who have disabilities that substantially limit one or more activities of daily living (Brault 2008). Some of this segment of the risk area population will need assistance when evacuating but their location and specific needs are difficult to identify in advance. Lack of information about the number, location, and types of disabilities presents problems for determining what types of vehicles will be needed to evacuate these people and to what types of facilities (and thus, the evacuation routes and destinations) they should be sent. One solution has been for evacuation managers to identify a local service provider, such as a Visiting Nurse Association, that maintains a current contact list.

6.3.3.5 Evacuation Compliance and Shadow Evacuation

It is well-established that an official warning is the best predictor of household evacuation (Huang et al. 2016). Moreover, the level of warning compliance increases with people's perceptions of threat, which is influenced by authorities labeling an evacuation as voluntary or mandatory (Baker 1991). Even "mandatory" evacuations have less than perfect compliance, in part because the authority and resources for enforcement are often lacking (Wolshon et al. 2005a). For example, Morss and Hayden (2010) reported that 25%–40% of the population of Galveston Island failed to evacuate despite a mandatory evacuation order and a warning of "certain death" if they did not evacuate. Conversely, it is also well established that there will be *shadow evacuation*—evacuation from areas that authorities do not consider to be at risk (Zeigler et al. 1981). For example, the nuclear power plant accident at Three Mile Island produced about 150,000 evacuees in response to an evacuation advisory that applied to 10,000 people at most (Lindell and Perry 1983). Furthermore, there was an estimated 47% evacuation rate from Harris County, Texas, for Hurricane Rita (Stein et al. 2010), even though less than 10% of that county's population was in the officially designated hurricane risk area.

6.3.3.6 Household Departure Times

Household departure times can vary, depending upon the immediacy of the threat—usually days of forewarning for hurricanes but minutes for hazmat transportation accidents. A household's departure time is determined by adding its evacuation preparation time to its time of warning receipt. As Figure 6.3 indicates, the rate of warning reception and preparation times can each be represented as an exponential function, $p_t = 1 - \exp(-at^b) + c$, where p_t is the proportion of the population prepared at time t, and a and b are parameters that determine the shape of the curve. Moreover, the parameter c has recently been added to account for the fact that a significant number of households monitor an increasing threat, such as an approaching hurricane, and receive an evacuation warning as soon as it is issued (Lindell et al. 2021). Lindell et al. (2002) used parameters $a = 2.00$, $b = 0.50$ (and implicitly $c = 0$ since they did not include this term) for a representative warning time distribution (the left-hand curve in Figure 6.3) and $a = 0.085$, $b = 2.55$ for a representative scenario preparation time distribution (the middle curve). When combined, these two distributions yield a departure time distribution (the right-hand curve). These distributions

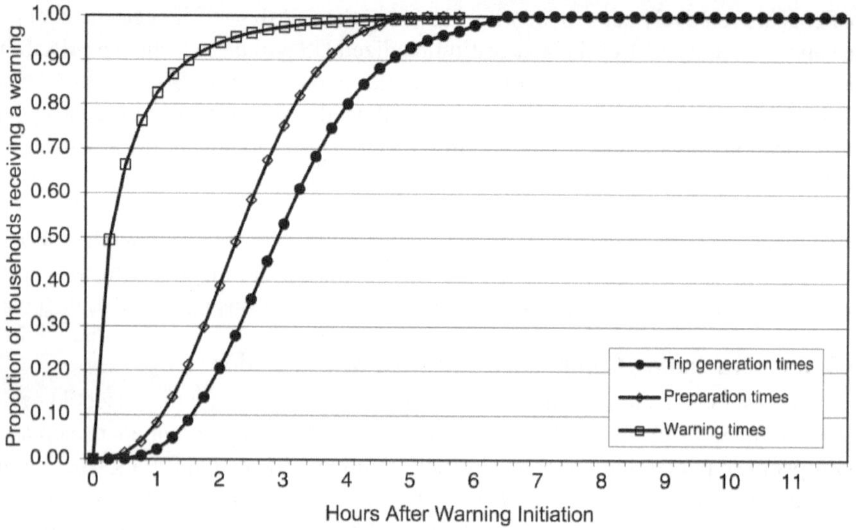

FIGURE 6.3 Generic trip generation time distribution function

would be appropriate for a rapid onset scenario, but there are two reasons why they can be inappropriate for hurricane evacuations in major metropolitan areas. First, some households that monitor news media coverage of an approaching hurricane begin evacuation preparations before they receive an official evacuation warning. Second, evacuations typically take place over two or more days, so the departure time distributions *for each day* tend to be minimal overnight (midnight–0600), rise from 0600–noon, rise further from noon–1800, and decline 1800–midnight (Huang et al., 2012, 2017, Lindell et al. 2005).

The shape of the *warning distribution* depends upon the nature of the warning system (Rogers and Sorensen 1988; Sorensen and Rogers 1989). The larger the percentage of the population that can be warned *simultaneously by broadcast systems* (e.g., sirens, tone alert radio, Emergency Alert System broadcasts through commercial TV and radio stations, and Wireless Emergency Alert broadcasts through cell phones), the sooner the warning distribution will reach asymptote (the point at which everyone who can receive a warning does so). Conversely, the larger the percentage of the population that must be warned *sequentially by contagion systems* (e.g., peers relaying the warnings they have received), the later the warning distribution will reach asymptote (Koll et al. 2023). By contrast, the shape of the *preparation distribution* depends upon warning recipients' perceptions of the urgency of the situation and their ability to respond promptly (Lindell et al. 2020). For example, people complete evacuation preparations sooner for a local tsunami that will arrive in 30 minutes than for a hurricane that is two days away. In addition, able-bodied people whose families are united and who have emergency kits already packed will be able to begin their evacuations sooner than those who lack these preparations. However, few households are prepared to evacuate immediately, even in Pacific Northwest tsunami zones (Lindell et al. 2022).

The estimation of the departure time distribution is even more complex for situations in which there is no forewarning before hazard onset—a "no-notice" evacuation. In such cases, families can be separated with, for example, two spouses working at different locations and multiple children at different schools. Families' attempts to reunify constitute an additional component of preparation time (before beginning their trip out of the risk area) that can produce inbound traffic into the risk area and cross-flows through the risk area. This can delay households' own departures from the risk area and disrupt outbound flows of traffic comprising those seeking to leave directly after receiving a warning (Murray-Tuite 2007; Murray-Tuite and Mahmassani 2003, 2004).

6.3.4 Model Traffic Behavior

In many cases, evacuations produce demand that exceeds ERS capacity, thus producing queues of vehicles waiting for access to the ERS or stuck in congestion on it. The need to incorporate queuing time into the calculations means that modeling traffic behavior for a large area with an extensive road network requires the use of a traffic modeling program (Lindell et al. 2019a, Chapter 9). In addition, Agent-Based Models (e.g., Chen et al. 2023; Siam et al. 2022) and Least Cost Distance evacuation models that use Geographic Information Systems (Wood et al. 2023) have been developed to model the evacuation of smaller areas. All of these models require input data from the previous stages discussed in this section—identifying risk areas/sectors, identifying the ERS and its capacity, and forecasting evacuation demand. Some traffic modeling programs can generate data on total traffic volume, average vehicle travel time, risk area clearance time, hourly volume, total volume, and average speed at each exit from the risk area, and queue lengths at selected intersections (Jones et al. 2011). It is important to conduct sensitivity analyses using a range of plausible values for each of the major input parameters to see how the model's output data, especially ETEs, are affected (Lindell 2008).

6.4 EVACUATION MANAGEMENT

The principal tasks involved in the management of an actual evacuation are threat detection and emergency classification, protective action selection, population warning, evacuation transportation support, evacuation traffic management, reception and care (e.g., shelter accommodations), and reentry management (Perry and Lindell 2007). There are other population protection functions that must be performed in an emergency response but are not directly related to evacuation management. These include search and rescue (finding and transporting those who are lost or injured), impact zone access control and security (keeping people out of evacuated areas and protecting the property there), hazard exposure control (protecting emergency responders from danger), emergency medical care (providing definitive care to the sick and injured), and environmental surety (monitoring and remediating hazmat contamination). These tasks can be most effective if evacuation managers use the Incident Command System (ICS) to guide their response operations. In turn, ICS will be most effective when non-emergency mission agencies such as social services and the American Red Cross have also been trained and participated in exercises using ICS (Lutz and Lindell 2008).

6.4.1 Incident Detection and Classification

Sometimes, as was the case in the 2018 Palu Indonesia tsunami, the risk area population needs no assistance from authorities in recognizing environmental conditions as immediately dangerous (Wang et al. 2022). In other cases, such as hurricanes and nuclear power plant accidents, specialized agencies are needed to detect a hazard, forecast the areas it is likely to affect, and assess the severity of the threat to people and property. The National Weather Service uses two emergency classes to communicate the certainty, severity, and immediacy of the threat at designated locations. A *Hurricane Watch* means hurricane conditions are possible in a defined section of the coast within the next 48 hours, and a *Hurricane Warning* means hurricane conditions are expected in that area within the next 36 hours. The US Nuclear Regulatory Commission has established a set of four emergency classes, together with the specific plant and environmental conditions (emergency action levels) defining each class, and specific response actions expected for each class (USNRC/FEMA 2019). The problem of incident detection and classification is much more complex for chemical facilities because there are so many different types and sizes of facilities that produce, store, and dispose of chemicals (Lindell 2019a). There appears to be no available data on chemical facilities' ability to promptly detect and accurately classify incidents requiring protective actions such as evacuation. Moreover, Sorensen and Rogers (1988) found that few communities even had adequate mechanisms for receiving notifications about incidents from chemical facilities within their jurisdiction.

6.4.2 Protective Action Selection

Authorities who seek to clear the risk area before the onset of hazardous conditions should establish a trigger for issuing evacuation warnings in less than the time it takes to complete an evacuation before hazard impact (Cova et al. 2017). In the case of hurricanes, this trigger has been known as an *evacuation decision arc*—the distance of Tropical Storm wind speed from the coast, where this distance is computed by multiplying the storm's forward speed by t_T, the jurisdiction's clearance time (Lindell and Prater 2007b). It is important to recognize that this trigger can vary from one hazard to another because some hazards are lethal as soon as exposure occurs (e.g., being overtaken by a ten-meter tsunami wave), whereas other hazards may require an extended period of exposure before unsafe doses occur (e.g., some toxic chemicals and radiological materials). In addition, triggers can vary from one jurisdiction to another, even for the same event (Sorensen et al. 2020). It is also important to realize that evacuation is unnecessary—and might be dangerous—for those who can achieve protection by SIP (Lindell 2019b). SIP within buildings is effective against floods when these structures are elevated above the flood crest, against hurricanes when they are also strong enough to withstand hurricane wind, and against radiation exposure when they are dense enough to provide shielding from external radiation or have sufficiently low air exchange rates that they delay the infiltration of contaminated air. If a hazard strikes without forewarning (e.g., railroad tank car derailment), staying indoors with all ventilation shut off (e.g., doors, windows, heaters, fireplaces, and air conditioners) can often achieve lower exposures than would result from either pedestrian or vehicular evacuation through an airborne hazmat plume. These different types of cases require an assessment of the relative risk of SIP compared to evacuation (DHS 2019). For patients in hospital intensive care wards, the risks of evacuation might be so high that SIP is the only feasible option. Advance analysis and planning, and perhaps facility retrofit, are needed to ensure that these patients and their caregivers will remain safe while others evacuate.

6.4.3 Population Warning

The findings of studies on individual responses to environmental hazards can be depicted by the Protective Action Decision Model (Lindell 2018; Lindell and Perry 2004, 2012—see also FEMA 2021b). According to this model, individuals' protective action decision making begins with environmental cues (sights such as wildfire smoke and flames, sounds such as the roar of tornado wind, and smells such as chemical odors) and social cues such as observations of other people evacuating. However, protective response is usually initiated by warnings of environmental threats received from authorities and peers. These sources transmit warning messages via one or more channels to receiving individuals in the risk area. The effects of these warnings depend on the receivers' personal characteristics. The relevant effects are changes in receivers' beliefs and behaviors, whereas the receivers' personal characteristics include their physical (e.g., strength), psychomotor (e.g., vision and hearing), and cognitive (e.g., primary and secondary languages, as well as their mental models/schemas) abilities as well as their economic (money and vehicles) and social (friends, relatives, neighbors, and coworkers) resources. In addition, people's beliefs and behaviors are related to their previous disaster experience and their demographic characteristics.

Environmental cues, social cues, and socially transmitted warnings initiate a series of pre-decision processes—exposure and attention to, and comprehension of the available information. In turn, these pre-decision processes elicit core perceptions of the environmental threat, alternative protective actions, and relevant stakeholders. These core perceptions provide the basis for information search strategies and protective action decision making. The information search strategies typically involve seeking confirmation of the threat from a different information source, such as going outside to look for a funnel cloud after receiving a tornado warning (Lindell 2012) or obtaining additional information from peers through the "milling" process (Wood et al. 2018) as well as relaying information to their peers (Lindell et al. 2019b). When there is enough information about the threat to justify protective action, people choose what they consider to be the most appropriate protective action decision, which is supported by situational facilitators and constrained by situational impediments. In general, behavioral responses can be characterized as continued information search, protective response (problem-focused coping), and emotion-focused coping. In many cases, there is a feedback loop as additional environmental or social cues are observed or information is sought.

Warnings are crucial elements in initiating evacuation, so emergency managers need to understand the best ways to construct and transmit them. First, an ideal warning message will increase PAR compliance and decrease shadow evacuation if it is provided by a credible source that describes the threat in terms of its expected impact intensity, timing, and location, provides a PAR, and indicates sources to contact for further information or obtain assistance in taking protective action. Warnings should be disseminated via multiple channels and transmitted repeatedly on each channel so people receive, heed, and understand the warning message (Olson et al. 2023; Sutton et al. 2024; Wood et al. 2018).

There are diverse channels for disseminating warnings to those at risk (Lindell and Perry 1992; Lindell and Prater 2010). These are face-to-face warnings, mobile loudspeakers, fixed sirens, commercial radio and television, NOAA Weather Radio, telephones, email, Internet websites, text messages, social media such as Twitter/X, and newspapers. In recent years, FEMA has developed the capability to disseminate emergency warnings using Wireless Emergency Alerts (WEAs) to mobile phones that supplement the Emergency Alert System (EAS) through commercial radio and television and the National Oceanic and Atmospheric Administration's Weather Radio.

Each of these channels can be evaluated with respect to eight characteristics. These are precision of dissemination (the ability to target only those at risk), penetration of normal activities (especially the ability to overcome ambient noise), message specificity and completeness (the ability to convey all of the elements of an ideal warning message), susceptibility to message distortion (a problem that arises when a warning message is passed through one or more intermediate communicators), rate of dissemination over time (the time between being issued by authorities and receipt by the last receivers), receiver requirements (especially expensive equipment or specialized knowledge and skill), sender requirements (also expensive equipment or specialized knowledge and skill), and feedback (sender verification that the receiver has received the warning). Emergency managers should consider how each warning channel will meet the demands of the hazards to which their communities are exposed (especially the amount of forewarning, the size of the impact area, and the likely impact intensity) and their communities' technological infrastructure. For example, WEAs have many desirable characteristics, such as high precision and penetration of normal activities, lack of distortion, rapid dissemination, and modest sender requirements. WEAs are limited by receiver requirements such as possession of a cell phone in an area that has adequate signal strength, the 360-character limit constraining message specificity and completeness, and the lack of feedback indicating that the warning has been received.

6.4.4 Evacuation Transportation Support

As noted earlier, some segments of the risk area population lack vehicles or have other obstacles to evacuation. For the transit-dependent, local authorities need to make arrangements with school districts or mass transit providers such as transit districts. Emergency managers need to verify that transit providers have not made arrangements with other jurisdictions that would need the same buses at the same time. Such duplicate demands could arise if the providers signed agreements with officials in two different counties on the assumption that these agreements would be activated only for very local evacuations (Daines 1991). Similar caution must be taken to review concurrent service agreements for multiple hospitals and nursing homes, which have the added requirement of ensuring that there are available beds in receiving facilities before transporting patients (Auf der Heide and Scanlon 2007). Moreover, care must be taken to ensure that the number of ambulances, buses, and other vehicles is sufficient to accommodate the maximum capacity of these facilities. In addition, criteria for transporting and sheltering pets should be made and publicized via the news media before and during an incident (Chadwin 2017).

6.4.5 Evacuation Traffic Management

There are two fundamental strategies for evacuation traffic management—ERS capacity management and evacuation demand management (Lindell et al. 2019a, Chapter 8). ERS capacity management seeks to minimize or avoid traffic jams by increasing capacity through procedures such as contraflow. Evacuation demand management seeks to regulate the number of vehicles attempting to use the ERS at any time so that demand does not exceed capacity.

6.4.5.1 ERS Capacity Management

The primary methods for maintaining ERS capacity are intersection control and prompt clearance of traffic impediments such as vehicles blocking traffic lanes (Ballard and Borchardt 2006; Jones et al. 2011; Lindell et al. 2019a, Chapter 8). Some collisions can be cleared by other evacuating vehicles that push the incapacitated vehicle off the roadway, but others require authorities to station tow trucks along the evacuation routes. In addition, stationing gasoline tankers along evacuation routes can refuel stalled vehicles.

The primary methods for increasing ERS capacity are utilizing highway shoulders as traffic lanes and implementing contraflow—reversing the direction of inbound lanes or shoulders (Jones et al. 2011). Utilizing shoulders as traffic lanes only increases capacity by about 8% (Wolshon et al. 2005b). However, the cumulative effect of even this small capacity increase could be significant if implemented over multiple evacuation routes in areas with large populations and long ETEs, such as the 34 hours required in some counties on the Texas coast (Lindell et al. 2002).

However, the use of highway shoulders for evacuation traffic has some distinct limitations, such as precluding their use for emergency vehicle access to accident sites (Ballard and Borchardt 2006). Since tow truck travel will be impaired if traffic is at a standstill and all lanes and shoulders are occupied, evacuation managers must designate specific lanes or alternate routes for emergency access. In addition, the evacuation routes must be examined carefully to ensure that any shoulders designated for evacuation traffic are not eliminated at bridges or underpasses, as was the case on I-37 North during Hurricane Bret (Prater et al. 2000).

Complete contraflow appears to be an attractive solution because it can increase link capacity by about 70%, but it eliminates the lanes needed for emergency vehicles or buses returning for additional evacuees. Partial contraflow (reversing only one of two inbound lanes) addresses this problem by maintaining one or more lanes in their normal inbound configuration, but only increases outbound capacity by about 30%. In addition, single-lane contraflow configurations increase the potential for head-on collisions. Regardless of which contraflow configuration is selected, evacuation managers need to correctly anticipate the length of time required for implementation. Estimates of the time required to staff traffic control points, install traffic control devices, and clear inbound lanes of inbound traffic range from 4 to 12 hours, depending on the length and complexity of the contraflow segment (Wolshon et al. 2005b).

6.4.5.2 Evacuation Demand Management

The primary methods of evacuation demand management are to manage the total number of people seeking to evacuate, manage the loading of the ERS, and manage the allocation of vehicles to evacuation routes. The word "manage" is crucial because it is not possible to impose complete "control" over any aspect of the evacuation process. One important method of evacuation demand management is to reduce the number of shadow evacuees entering the ERS. In addition, the need for evacuation from inside the risk area can be reduced if local structures are adequate for SIP and people believe that SIP will provide adequate protection (e.g., Lindell 2019b).

Evacuees' departure timing can be managed by phased (also called "staged") evacuations in which people in areas of lower risk are asked to delay their evacuations until after people in areas of higher risk have evacuated (Jones et al. 2007, 2011). Computer simulations of phased evacuation have produced mixed results, with Zhang et al. (2014) concluding that this strategy produces significant improvements only when an ERS is likely to have a significant amount of congestion. In that case, the effectiveness of phased evacuation would depend on the level of compliance, with Pel et al. (2010) reporting that even relatively low levels of compliance could produce greater evacuation efficiency than simultaneous evacuation. More recent survey research suggests that compliance is likely to be sufficient, with Bian et al. (2023) reporting that 66% of their survey respondents expected to comply with a phased evacuation order. Those most likely to comply are residents with longer housing tenure and those who expect longer evacuation travel delays. Conversely, those who are least likely to comply expect to evacuate to peers' homes or to bring more vehicles during evacuation. This research suggests that it would be important for evacuation managers to explicitly ask people in later phases to wait for those in earlier phases to complete their evacuations. This is because shadow evacuees from inland areas tend to begin their hurricane evacuations later than residents of coastal risk areas (Lindell et al. 2011; Wu et al. 2012). This can create traffic jams when the inland residents try to enter the ERS at the same time as coastal residents are arriving there. Fortunately, the convergence of coastal and inland evacuees from Hurricane Rita produced evacuation queues in inland areas that were beyond the impact of hurricane wind and surge. However, the stalled evacuation traffic was vulnerable to severe summer heat.

A third demand management strategy is to reroute evacuation traffic from overutilized routes to underutilized ones. This strategy could be effective because people tend to use the most familiar routes to their evacuation destinations (Lindell and Prater 2007a). Unfortunately, such habits tend to overload the freeways and underload minor highways (Dow and Cutter 2002). ERS overloading does have the potential to be self-limiting because some drivers who encounter severe traffic congestion divert to alternate routes when they are aware of feasible alternative routes (Lindell et al. 2019a, Chapter 6). In the past, improvised diversion to alternate routes has been insufficient, but currently available cell phone apps, such as Google Maps and Waze, can identify congested routes, estimate current travel times, and suggest suitable alternative routes. Evacuation managers can supplement improvised diversion by providing variable message signs (VMSs) that also support evacuation route diversion. They can also force the diversion of some lanes onto alternate routes that are planned in advance and implemented as needed during an evacuation.

Other demand management strategies include smoothing freeway traffic flows by restricting access to the ERS by closing selected freeway ramps or metering access to them. Similarly, arterial traffic flows can be smoothed by eliminating turning and crossing maneuvers, revising traffic signal timing, or instituting manual traffic control at intersections (Lindell et al. 2019a, Chapter 8).

6.4.5.3 Evacuation Safety

Lindell and Perry's (1992, Chapter 4) review of the available evidence on evacuation safety indicated that the accident rate for private vehicles is almost certain to be no higher and is quite likely to be lower than during normal driving periods. This is because traffic tends to be slow, moving at about 35 mph or less and predominately one way (outbound). Consequently, any accidents that do occur would be less serious and, therefore, less likely to produce casualties or to severely obstruct traffic flow. This conclusion is supported by recent simulation studies showing that evacuation traffic accidents have minimal impacts on overall clearance times (Bahaaldin et al. 2016; Robinson et al. 2018).

There are insufficient data to determine whether this finding can be generalized to adverse road conditions. The finding by Bastien et al. (1985) that no traffic accidents were reported during an evacuation through a volcanic ashfall suggests that a moderate degradation of road conditions would not materially alter accident rates. However, evacuation analysts should anticipate that some road conditions could be so dangerous that the traffic accident risks of the evacuation might become an important consideration. Indeed, slick road surfaces caused by sleet, snow, and rain do increase the incidence of traffic accidents (Chen et al. 2009), but the effects of reduced visibility (e.g., fog, dust, ash), high winds, or wildfire do not appear to have been studied.

The available evidence on hospital and nursing home evacuation indicates that it is possible to evacuate hospitals effectively through a combination of reducing censuses by early discharge of stable patients and by transporting the remaining patients to other hospitals. In some cases, evacuations can be accomplished in short time periods without appreciable safety risks despite significant logistical barriers (Chenault et al. 1980). More recent research has moved beyond individual case studies by identifying a variety of important factors needed in models of hospital evacuation. For example, Yazdani et al. (2021) called attention to the characteristics of hazard impact (e.g., amount of forewarning, destruction of buildings, disruption of infrastructure such as electric power); patient census (by health status, especially mobility); staffing levels (by specialty); evacuation vehicle availability (e.g., Advanced Life Support ambulances, Basic Life Support ambulances, and buses—Zane et al. 2010); and evacuation travel time to, and capacity of, receiving hospitals. Abir et al. (2022) extended this analysis by noting that hospital evacuations involve both ambulatory and non-ambulatory individuals and that the movement of the latter is also constrained by mobility assistive devices such as wheelchairs and gurneys. This limitation would also apply to nursing home evacuations. In addition, it is necessary to understand the difference between *building evacuation* (vertical evacuation to higher floors or exit to assembly areas outside the building) and *regional evacuation* (vehicular transportation to a facility that can provide an equivalent level of healthcare). Analyses using building and regional evacuation models can be used to validate requirements for hospital evacuation plans, but Khorram-Manesh et al. (2022) concluded that European Union states lack common guidance for hospital evacuation. It appears that this is true for the US as well.

6.4.5.4 Real-Time Evacuation Traffic Management

Large-scale evacuations can generate traffic that crosses municipal, county, and state boundaries. Consequently, evacuation managers can experience traffic flows that are unexpectedly large. A lack of coordination became a major problem during the 1999 response to Hurricane Floyd, which generated 3.5 million evacuees in Florida, Georgia, South Carolina, and North Carolina. Some metropolitan areas have also adopted a number of features of intelligent transportation systems. For example, Houston TRANSTAR is a regional facility that is jointly operated by state, county, city, and transit authority personnel to manage both normal and evacuation traffic. During normal operations, TRANSTAR receives traffic information from closed-circuit television cameras and embedded highway traffic sensors so it can operate dynamic message signs and a highway advisory radio to communicate with motorists, control traffic signals, and dispatch emergency vehicles to remove traffic impediments. During emergency operations, TRANSTAR staff activate an Emergency Operations Center to accommodate representatives from other regional, state, and non-governmental agencies. TRANSTAR also supports a website (www.houstontranstar.org/) that provides motorists with hurricane information, including risk area maps, evacuation route maps, and brochures explaining the contraflow procedures for the major evacuation routes.

6.4.6 Evacuation Accommodations

When evacuations last overnight or longer, people need places to stay until it is safe to return. The types of evacuation accommodations people choose are a well-studied aspect of evacuation logistics, with researchers finding consistently that only a small percentage of evacuees use public shelters in all types of disasters. The Mileti et al. (1992) review concluded that only 15% of evacuees go to public shelters, which are primarily occupied by ethnic minorities, the poor, and later departures. More recently, Lindell et al. (2019a, Chapter 6) reported that a median of 62% of hurricane evacuees stayed with friends/relatives, 27% stayed in hotels/motels, and 3% used public shelters.

6.4.7 Reentry Management

Managing evacuees' reentry after an evacuation is a major challenge for emergency managers because many evacuees fail to comply with official reentry plans (Siebeneck and Cova 2008). Evacuees generally want to return to their homes as soon as possible because they believe the benefits of immediate reentry outweigh the risks. Specifically, evacuees are concerned about looting in their neighborhoods, which they overestimate, and some are concerned about loss of income while away (Siebeneck et al. 2013). However, premature reentry can expose returnees to safety hazards from the collapse of unstable buildings and health hazards from moving back into homes that lack electric power, water, and sewer. Moreover, returnees who return before traffic control points are opened can find themselves parked there for days, waiting to return to their homes (Dash and Morrow 2000).

In some cases, evacuees are not allowed to return because their homes are in areas that must be evacuated permanently in a strategy of managed retreat from hazard zones (Hino et al. 2017). For those areas in the evacuation zone that are safe to reoccupy, officials can use one of three reentry strategies (Siebeneck and Cova 2021). The first strategy, full-scale return, allows all evacuees to return simultaneously to the entire evacuation zone. This strategy would be appropriate for a county that evacuated for a hurricane that caused no damage because it struck elsewhere. The second strategy, temporary return ("look and leave") allows evacuees to return during restricted hours, often with overnight curfews. The third strategy, phased return, allows permanent access to specific portions of the evacuation zone when they are safe to reoccupy—as when roads are cleared and electric power is restored. In practice, local officials can combine these strategies by implementing managed retreat in the most hazardous areas, full-scale return in unaffected areas, temporary return in the most severely damaged areas, and phased return to damaged areas as utilities are restored. In addition to the official return strategies, households sometimes adopt self-imposed restrictions on reentry, with the most able-bodied "return scouts" returning to assess damage and make their homes habitable for more vulnerable members (Siebeneck and Cova 2008).

A major impediment for evacuation managers is a need to communicate their reentry strategy to evacuees who might be scattered among many distant destinations (Siebeneck and Cova 2008). For example, the average evacuation distance was 429 km/266 miles during Hurricane Katrina (Wu et al. 2012). In the past, many evacuees relied on news media as a source of information about their communities while evacuated (Siebeneck and Cova 2008), such as during the 2008 Cedar Rapids, Iowa, flood (Siebeneck and Cova 2014). Similarly, Reuter et al. (2023) reported that four studies published from 2012 to 2015 found that people in multiple countries preferred news media to social media for information in all phases of an emergency. However, peers were more popular than news media as sources of reentry information in 2005 Hurricane Rita (Siebeneck and Cova 2008) and 2012 Hurricane Ike (Lin et al. 2014). This is consistent with Reuter et al. (2023), which reported that German use of social media in all phases of an emergency increased significantly from 2017 (54%) to 2021 (71%). These increases were accompanied by decreases in the use of other media, with print media decreasing from 32% to 22% from 2019 to 2021. Radio and TV decreased from 61% to 47% and 62% to 45%, respectively, in the same time period.

Despite the increasing research attention to social media in disasters, few studies have compared the use of different media in the aftermath of disasters, and there do not seem to have been any that examined the types of reentry information that were communicated. For example, Silver and Behlendorf (2023) examined the degree to which different types of users relied on Twitter before, during, and after Hurricane Dorian. Although they reported the extent of searching and sharing different types of pre-impact storm information, they did not report comparable information about post-impact information. Thus, in the absence of data on evacuees' reliance on different information channels, evacuation managers should use multiple channels to communicate information about conditions in the evacuation zone and official reentry plans. Although evacuees cannot access on-air broadcasts from their hometown radio and TV stations or obtain print copies of hometown newspapers, they can obtain official information about evacuation zone reentry through these news media sources' websites. In addition, they can also obtain this information by accessing their local emergency management agency's website and its social media posts.

6.5 CONCLUSIONS

Evacuations can be managed effectively, but the larger the scale of the evacuation or the shorter the amount of forewarning (or both), the greater the need to plan, analyze, and manage it effectively. Effective evacuation planning requires coordination among diverse agencies at different levels of government, as well as with non-governmental organizations such as the American Red Cross. Effective analysis requires identifying risk areas/sectors, defining the ERS and assessing its capacity, forecasting evacuation demand, and modeling traffic behavior. Effective evacuation management requires incident detection and classification, protective action selection, population warning, evacuation transportation support, evacuation traffic management, shelter accommodations, and reentry management. Evacuation managers can protect the risk area population from environmental hazards if they address all of these issues successfully.

6.6 ACKNOWLEDGMENTS

This research was supported by numerous grants from the National Science Foundation over the past five decades. Most recently, these include Grants IIS-1212790, IIS-1540469, CMMI-1760766, CMMI-1826455, and CMMI-1902888. In addition, it was supported by US Army Corps of Engineers Sacramento District contract W91238-16-P-0072 and Washington Emergency Management Division contract E19-192. None of the conclusions expressed here necessarily reflect views other than those of the author.

REFERENCES

Abir, I.M., Ibrahim, A.M., Toha, S.F., & Shafie, A.A. 2022. A review on the hospital evacuation simulation models. *International Journal of Disaster Risk Reduction* 77:103083.

Auf der Heide, E., & Scanlon, J. 2007. The role of the health sector in planning and response. In *Emergency management: Principles and practice for local government, 2nd ed.*, eds. K.J. Tierney and W.F. Waugh, Jr., pp. 183–206. Washington DC: International City/County Management Association.

Bahaaldin, K., Fries, R.N., Williamson, M.R., & Chowdhury, M. 2016. The impact of traffic incident locations on a metropolitan evacuation. *International Journal of Transportation* 4:81–96.

Baker, E.J. 1991. Hurricane evacuation behavior. *International Journal of Mass Emergencies and Disasters* 9:287–310.

Baker, E.J. 2000. Hurricane evacuation in the United States. In *Storms*, Vol. 1., eds. R. Pielke, Jr. and R. Pielke, Sr., pp. 308–319. London: Routledge.

Ballard, A.J. and Borchardt, D.W. 2006. *Recommended practices for hurricane evacuation traffic operations.* FHWA/TX-06/0-4962-P2. College Station, TX: Texas Transportation Institute. https://library.ctr.utexas.edu/hostedpdfs/tti/0-4962-p2.pdf.

Bastien, M.C., Dumas, M., Laporte, J., & Parmentier, N. 1985. Evacuation risks: A tentative approach for quantification, *Risk Analysis* 5:53–61.

Bian, R., Murray-Tuite, P., Trainor, J., Edara, P., & Triantis, K. 2023. Modeling evacuees' intended responses to a phased hurricane evacuation order. *Applied Sciences* 13:5194.

Brault, M. 2008. *Disability status and the characteristics of people in group quarters: A brief analysis of disability prevalence among the civilian noninstitutionalized and total populations in the American Community Survey.* Washington, DC: U.S. Census Bureau. www.census.gov/content/dam/Census/library/working-papers/2008/demo/gq-disability.pdf.

Chadwin, R. 2017. Evacuation of pets during disasters: a public health intervention to increase resilience. *American Journal of Public Health* 107:1413–1417.

Chen, C., Koll, C., Wang, H., & Lindell, M.K. 2023. An interdisciplinary agent-based evacuation model: Integrating the natural environment, built environment, and social system for community preparedness and resilience. *Natural Hazards and Earth System Sciences* 23:733–749.

Chen, C., Lindell, M.K., & Wang, H. 2022a. Tsunami preparedness and resilience in the Cascadia Subduction Zone: A multistage model of expected evacuation decisions and mode choice. *International Journal of Disaster Risk Reduction* 59:102244.

Chen, C, Wang, H., Lindell, M.K., Jung, M.C., & Siam, M.R.K. 2022b. Tsunami preparedness and resilience: Evacuation logistics and time estimations. *Transportation Research Part D: Transport & Environment* 109:103324.

Chen, S.R., Cai, C.S., & Wolshon, B. 2009. From normal operation to evacuation: Single-vehicle safety under adverse weather, topographic, and operational conditions. *Natural Hazards Review* 10:68–76.

Chenault, W.W., Hilbert, G.D., & Reichlin, S.D. 1980. *Evacuation planning in the TMI accident*. Human Sciences Research Inc, McLean, VA. https://apps.dtic.mil/sti/pdfs/ADA080104.pdf.

Cova, T.J., Dennison, P.E., Li, D., Drews, F.A., Siebeneck, L.K., & Lindell, M.K. 2017. Warning triggers in environmental hazards: Who should be warned to do what and when? *Risk Analysis* 37:601–611.

Daines, G.E. 1991. Planning, training, and exercising. In *Emergency management: Principles and practice for local government,* eds. T.E. Drabek and G.J. Hoetmer, pp. 161–200. Washington, DC: International City Management Association.

Dash, N., & Morrow, B.H. 2000. Return delays and evacuation order compliance: The case of Hurricane Georges and the Florida Keys. *Environmental Hazards* 2:119–128.

DHS—Department of Homeland Security. 2019. *Planning considerations: Evacuation and shelter-in-place guidance for state, local, tribal, and territorial partners.* Washington, DC: Author.

Dotson, L.J., & Jones, J. 2005. *Identification and analysis of factors affecting emergency evacuations: Main report.* NUREG/CR-6864, Vol. 1, SAND2004-5901. Washington, DC: US Nuclear Regulatory Commission. www.nrc.gov/reading-rm/doc-collections/nuregs/index.

Dow, K., & Cutter, S.L. 2002. Emerging hurricane evacuation issues: Hurricane Floyd and South Carolina. *Natural Hazards Review* 3:12–18.

FEMA—Federal Emergency Management Agency. 2021a. *Developing and maintaining emergency operations plans: Comprehensive preparedness guide (CPG) 101 September 2021, Version 3.0.* Washington, DC: Author. www.fema.gov/emergency-managers/national-preparedness/plan#cpg.

FEMA—Federal Emergency Management Agency. 2021b. *Improving public messaging for evacuation and shelter-in-place: Findings and recommendations for emergency managers from peer-reviewed research.* Washington, DC: Author. www.fema.gov/emergency-managers/national-preparedness/plan/evacuation-shelter-in-place.

Ford, J.K., & Schmidt, A.M. 2000. Emergency response training: Strategies for enhancing real-world performance. *Journal of Hazardous Materials 75*:195–215.

Hino, M., Field, C.B., & Mach, K.J. 2017. Managed retreat as a response to natural hazard risk. *Nature Climate Change* 7:364–370.

Houston, N. 2009. *Good practices in transportation evacuation preparedness and response: results of the FHWA workshop series*, FHWA-HOP-09-040. Washington DC: Federal Highway Administration, Office of Transportation Operations. www.ops.fhwa.dot.gov/publications/publications.htm.

Huang, S-K., Lindell, M.K., & Prater, C.S. 2016. Who leaves and who stays? A review and statistical meta-analysis of hurricane evacuation studies. *Environment and Behavior* 48:991–1029.

Huang, S-K, Lindell, M.K., & Prater, C.S. 2017. Toward a multi-stage model of hurricane evacuation decision: An empirical study of Hurricanes Katrina and Rita. *Natural Hazards Review* 18:05016008.

Huang, S.K., Lindell, M.K., Prater, C.S., Wu, H.C., & Siebeneck, L.K. 2012. Household evacuation decision making in response to Hurricane Ike. *Natural Hazards Review* 13:283–296.

Jones, J., Walton, F., & Wolshon, B. 2011. *Criteria for development of evacuation time estimate studies*, NUREG/CR-7002 SAND2010-0016P. Washington, DC: US Nuclear Regulatory Commission. www.nrc.gov/reading-rm/doc-collections/nuregs/index.

Jones, J.A., Bixler, N., Schelling, F.J., & Sullivan, R. 2007. *Review of NUREG-0654, Supplement 3, "Criteria for protective action recommendations for severe accidents"*, NUREG/CR-6953, Vol. I, SAND2007-5448P. Washington, DC: U.S. Nuclear Regulatory Commission. www.nrc.gov/reading-rm/doc-collections/nuregs/index.

Khorram-Manesh, A., Phattharapornjaroen, P., Mortelmans, L.J., Goniewicz, K., Verheul, M., Sörensen, J.L., Pereira, I., Ricklin , M.E., Faccincani, R., Dark, P.M., Carlström, E., Marzaleh, M.A., Peyravi, M.R., Al Sultan, M., Santamaria, E., Comandante, J.D., & Burkle, F. 2022. Current perspectives and concerns facing hospital evacuation: The results of a pilot study and literature review. *Disaster Medicine and Public Health Preparedness* 16:650–658.

Koll, C. Lindell, M.K., Chen, C., & Wang, H. 2023. Emergency warning dissemination in a multiplex social network. *Journal of Artificial Societies and Social Simulation* *26*(1):1–7. doi:10.18564/jasss.494

Lin C-C., Siebeneck, L.K., Lindell, M.K., Prater, C.S., Wu, H.C., & Huang, S.K. 2014. Evacuees' information sources and reentry decision making in the aftermath of Hurricane Ike. *Natural Hazards* 70:865–882.

Lindell, M.K. 2008. EMBLEM2: An empirically based large-scale evacuation time estimate model. *Transportation Research* A 42:140–154.

Lindell, M.K. 2012. Response to environmental disasters. In *Handbook of environmental and conservation psychology,* ed. S. Clayton, pp. 391–413. New York: Oxford University Press.

Lindell, M.K. 2018. Communicating imminent risk. In *Handbook of disaster research*, 2nd ed., eds. H. Rodríguez, J. Trainor, and W. Donner, pp. 449–477. New York: Springer.

Lindell, M.K. 2019a. Emergency management: HAZMAT. In *Encyclopedia of security and emergency management,* eds. L.R. Shapiro and M-H. Maras. New York: Springer.

Lindell, M.K. 2019b. Emergency management: Shelter in-place. In *Encyclopedia of security and emergency management,* eds. L.R. Shapiro and M.-H. Maras. New York: Springer.

Lindell, M.K. 2020a. Chapter 1: An overview of hazards, vulnerability, and disasters. In *The Routledge handbook of urban disaster resilience*: *Integrating mitigation, preparedness, and recovery planning,* ed. M.K. Lindell, pp. 3–32. New York: Routledge.

Lindell, M.K. 2020b. Improving hazard map comprehension for protective action decision making. *Frontiers in Computer Science.* doi: 10.3389/fcomp.2020.00027.

Lindell, M.K., Arlikatti, S., & Huang, S-K. 2019. Immediate behavioral response to the June 17, 2013 flash floods in Uttarakhand, North India. *International Journal of Disaster Risk Reduction* 34:129–146.

Lindell, M.K., Kang J.E., & Prater, C.S. 2011. The logistics of household hurricane evacuation. *Natural Hazards* 58:1093–1109.

Lindell, M.K., Lu, J.C., & Prater, C.S. 2005. Household decision making and evacuation in response to Hurricane Lili. *Natural Hazards Review* 6:171–179.

Lindell, M.K., Murray-Tuite, P., Wolshon, B., & Baker, E.J. 2019. *Large-scale evacuation: The analysis, modeling, and management of emergency relocation from hazardous areas.* New York: Routledge.

Lindell, M.K., & Perry, R.W. 1983. Nuclear power plant emergency warning: How would the public respond? *Nuclear News* 26:49–53.

Lindell, M.K., & Perry, R.W. 1992. *Behavioral foundations of community emergency planning*. Washington, DC: Hemisphere Press.
Lindell, M.K., & Perry, R.W. 2004. *Communicating environmental risk in multiethnic communities*. Thousand Oaks, CA: Sage.
Lindell, M.K., & Perry, R.W. 2007. Planning and preparedness. In *Emergency management: Principles and practice for local government*, 2nd ed., ed. K.J. Tierney and W.F. Waugh, Jr., pp. 113–141. Washington DC: International City/County Management Association.
Lindell, M.K., & Perry, R.W. 2012. The Protective Action Decision Model: Theoretical modifications and additional evidence. *Risk Analysis* 32:616–632.
Lindell, M.K., & Prater, C.S. 2007a. Critical behavioral assumptions in evacuation analysis for private vehicles: Examples from hurricane research and planning. *Journal of Urban Planning and Development* 133:18–29.
Lindell, M.K., & Prater, C.S. 2007b. A hurricane evacuation management decision support system (EMDSS). *Natural Hazards* 40:627–634.
Lindell, M.K., & Prater, C.S. 2010. Tsunami preparedness on the Oregon and Washington coast: Recommendations for research. *Natural Hazards Review* 11:69–81.
Lindell, M.K., Prater, C.S., & House, D.H. 2022. Cascadia Subduction Zone residents' tsunami evacuation expectations. *Geosciences* 12:189.
Lindell, M.K., Prater, C.S., & Wu, J.Y. 2002. *Hurricane evacuation time estimates for the Texas Gulf coast*. College Station, TX: Texas A&M University Hazard Reduction and Recovery Center. https://tamucoa.b-cdn.net/app/uploads/2021/10/02-02R-Lindell-Prater-Wu.pdf.
Lindell, M.K., Sorensen, J.H. Baker, E.J., & Lehman, W.P. 2020. Community response to hurricane threat: Estimates of household evacuation preparation time distributions. *Transportation Research D: Transport and Environment* 85:102457.
Lindell, M.K., Sorensen, J.H. Baker, E.J., & Lehman, W.P. 2021. Community response to hurricane threat Estimates of warning diffusion time distributions. *Natural Hazards Review* 22:04021007.
Lutz, L.D., & Lindell, M.K. 2008. The Incident Command System as a response model within emergency operation centers during Hurricane Rita. *Journal of Contingencies and Crisis Management* 16:122–134.
MacPherson-Krutsky, C., Brand, B.D., & Lindell, M.K. 2020. Does updating natural hazard maps to reflect best practices increase user comprehension of risk? *International Journal of Disaster Risk Reduction* 46:101487.
Maghelal, P., Peacock, W. G., & Li, X. 2017. Evacuating together or separately: Factors influencing split evacuations prior to Hurricane Rita. *Natural Hazards Review* 18:04016008.
Mendonça, D., & Wallace, W.A. 2007. A cognitive model of improvisation in emergency management. *IEEE Transactions On Systems, Man, And Cybernetics—Part A: Systems And Humans* 37:547–561.
Mileti, D.S. 1975. *Natural hazard warning systems in the United States: A research assessment*. Boulder, CO: University of Colorado Institute of Behavioral Science.
Mileti, D.S., Sorensen, J.H., & O'Brien, P.W. 1992. Toward an explanation of mass care shelter use in evacuations. *International Journal of Mass Emergencies and Disasters* 10:25–42.
Morss, R.E., & Hayden, M.H. 2010. Storm surge and "certain death": Interviews with Texas coastal residents following Hurricane Ike. *Weather, Climate, and Society* 2:174–189.
Murray-Tuite, P.M. 2007. Perspectives for network management in response to unplanned disruptions. *Journal of Urban Planning and Development* 133:9–17.
Murray-Tuite, P.M., & Mahmassani, H.S. 2003. Model of household trip-chain sequencing in emergency evacuation. *Transportation Research Record* 1831:21–29.

Murray-Tuite, P.M., & Mahmassani, H.S. 2004. Transportation network evacuation planning with household activity interactions. *Transportation Research Record* 1894:150–159.

Murray-Tuite, P. M., Schweitzer, L., & Morrison, R. 2012. Household no-notice evacuation logistics: How well do households optimize? *Journal of Transportation Safety & Security* 4:336–361.

Olson, M.K., Sutton, J., Cain, L.B., & Waugh, N. 2023. A decade of wireless emergency alerts: A longitudinal assessment of message content and completeness. *Journal of Contingencies and Crisis Management.* doi:10.1111/1468-5973.12518.

Peacock, R.D., Kuligowski, E.D., & Averill, J.D. 2011. *Pedestrian and evacuation dynamics.* New York: Springer.

Pel, A.J., Huibregtse, O.L., Hoogendoorn, S.P., & Bliemer, M.C. 2010. Optimizing evacuation instructions while anticipating traveler compliance behavior. In *13th International IEEE conference on intelligent transportation systems*, pp. 462–467. IEEE. http:doi.org//10.1109/ITSC.2010.5625233

Perry, R.W., & Lindell, M.K. 2007. *Emergency planning.* Hoboken, NJ: John Wiley.

Perry, R.W., Lindell, M.K., & Greene, M.R. 1981. *Evacuation planning in emergency management.* Lexington, MA: Heath Lexington Books.

Prater, C., Wenger, D., & Grady, K. 2000. *Hurricane Bret post–storm assessment: A review of utilization of hurricane evacuation studies and information dissemination.* College Station, TX: Texas A&M University Hazard Reduction & Recovery Center. https://tamucoa.b-cdn.net/app/uploads/2021/10/00-05R-Prater-Wenger-Grady.pdf?

Reuter C, Kaufhold M.A, Biselli T, Pleil H. 2023. Increasing adoption despite perceived limitations of social media in emergencies: Representative insights on German citizens' perception and trends from 2017 to 2021. International Journal of Disaster Risk Reduction 96:103880.

Robinson, R.M., Collins, A.J., Jordan, C.A., Foytik, P., & Khattak, A.J. 2018. Modeling the impact of traffic incidents during hurricane evacuations using a large scale microsimulation. *International Journal of Disaster Risk Reduction* 31:1159–1165.

Rogers, G.O., & Sorensen, J.H. 1988. Diffusion of emergency warnings. *Environmental Professional* 10:185–198.

Shen, J., Murray-Tuite, P., Wernstedt, K., & Guikema, S. 2024. Estimating pre-impact and post-impact evacuation behaviors: An empirical study of hurricane Ida in coastal Louisiana and Mississippi. *Journal of Transport Geography* 118:103925.

Siam, M.R.K., Wang, H., Lindell, M.K., Chen, C., Vlahogianni E.I., & Axhausen, K.W. 2022. An interdisciplinary agent-based multimodal wildfire evacuation model: Critical decisions and life safety. *Transportation Research Part D: Transport & Environment* 103:103147.

Siebeneck, L.K., & Cova, T.J. 2008. An assessment of the reentry process for Hurricane Rita 2005. *International Journal of Mass Emergencies and Disasters* 26:91–111.

Siebeneck, L.K., & Cova, T.J. 2014. Risk communication after disaster: Return entry following the 2008 Cedar River flood. *Natural Hazards Review* 15:158–166.

Siebeneck, L.K., & Cova, T.J. 2021. The disaster return-entry process: A discussion of issues, strategies and future research. *Disaster Prevention and Management* 30:369–383.

Siebeneck, L.K., Lindell, M.K., Prater, C.S., Wu, H.C., & Huang, S.K. 2013. Evacuees' reentry concerns and experiences in the aftermath of Hurricane Ike. *Natural Hazards* 65:2267–2286.

Silver, A., & Behlendorf, B. 2023. Understanding your audience: The influence of social media user-type on informational behaviors and hazard adjustments during Hurricane Dorian. *Meteorological Applications* 30:e2148.

Smith, T. 2021. *Criteria for development of evacuation time estimate studies*, NUREG/CR-7002, Revision 1. Washington, DC: US Nuclear Regulatory Commission. www.nrc.gov/docs/ML2101/ML21013A504.pdf.

Sorensen, J.H., Lindell, M.K., Baker, E.J., & Lehman, W.P. 2020. Community response to hurricane threat: Estimates of warning issuance time distributions. *Weather, Climate and Society* 12:837–846.

Sorensen, J.H., & Rogers, G.O. 1988. Local preparedness for chemical accidents: A survey of U.S. communities. *Industrial Crisis Quarterly* 2:89–108.

Sorensen, J.H., & Rogers, G.O. 1989. Warning and response in two hazardous materials transportation accidents in the U.S. *Journal of Hazardous Materials* 22:57–74.

Stein, R.M., Dueñas-Osorio, L., & Subramanian, D. 2010. Who evacuates when hurricanes approach? The role of risk, information, and location. *Social Science Quarterly* 91:816–834.

Stough, L.M., & Kelman, I. 2018. People with disabilities and disasters. In *Handbook of disaster research*, 2nd ed., eds. H. Rodríguez, J. Trainor, and W. Donner, pp. 225–242. New York: Springer.

Sutton, J., Olson, M.K., & Waugh, N A. 2024. The Warning Lexicon: A multiphased study to identify, design, and develop content for warning messages. *Natural Hazards Review* 25:04023055.

Tierney, K.J., Lindell, M.K., & Perry, R.W. 2001. *Facing the unexpected: Disaster preparedness and response in the United States.* Washington, DC: Joseph Henry Press.

TRB—Transportation Research Board. 2022. *Highway capacity manual*, 7th ed. Washington, DC: Author.

USDOT—US Department of Transportation. 2024. *North American emergency response guidebook.* www.phmsa.dot.gov/training/hazmat/erg/emergency-response-guidebook-erg.

USNRC/FEMA—US Nuclear Regulatory Commission/Federal Emergency Management Agency. 2019. *Criteria for preparation and evaluation of radiological emergency response plans and preparedness in support of nuclear power plants*, NUREG-0654/FEMA-REP-1. Washington, DC. www.nrc.gov/reading-rm/doc-collections/nuregs/staff/sr0654/r2/index.html

Urbanik, T. 1978. *Texas hurricane evacuation study.* College Station, TX: Texas Transportation Institute.

Urbanik, T. 2000. Evacuation time estimates for nuclear power plants. *Journal of Hazardous Materials* 75:165–180.

Urbanik, T., Desrosiers, A., Lindell, M.K., & Schuller, C.R. 1980. *Analysis of techniques for estimating evacuation times for emergency planning zones.* NUREG/CR-1745. Washington, DC: US Nuclear Regulatory Commission. https://inis.iaea.org/collection/NCLCollectionStore/_Public/35/053/35053342.pdf?r=1&r=1.

Vinnell, L.J., Inch, P., Johnston, D.M., & Horspool, N. 2022. Behavioral responses to earthquake shaking: Video footage analysis of the 2016 Kaikōura earthquake in Wellington, Aotearoa New Zealand. *Earthquake Spectra* 38:1636–1660.

Wang, H., Lindell, M.K., Siam, M.R.K., Chen, C., & Husein, R. 2022. Local residents' immediate responses to the 2018 Indonesia earthquake and tsunami. *Earthquake Spectra* 38:2835–2865.

Wolshon, B., Urbina, E., Wilmot, C., & Levitan, M. 2005a. Review of policies and practices for hurricane evacuation. I: Transportation Planning, Preparedness, and Response. *Natural Hazards Review* 6:129–142.

Wolshon, B., Urbina, E., Levitan, M., & Wilmot, C. 2005b. Review of policies and practices for hurricane evacuation. II: Traffic operations, management, and control. *Natural Hazards Review* 6:143–161.

Wood, M.M., Mileti, D.S., Bean, H., Liu, B. F., Sutton, J., & Madden, S. 2018. Milling and public warnings. *Environment and Behavior* 50:535–566.

Wood, N., Peters, J., Cheung, K.F., Yamazaki, Y., Calvo, D., & Guard, C. 2023. Modeling non-structural strategies to reduce pedestrian evacuation times for mitigating local tsunami threats in Guam. *International Journal of Disaster Risk Reduction* 95:103859.

Wu, H.C., Lindell, M.K., & Prater, C.S. 2012. Logistics of hurricane evacuation in Hurricanes Katrina and Rita. *Transportation Research Part F: Traffic Psychology and Behaviour* 15:445–461.

Yazdani, M., Mojtahedi, M., Loosemore, M., Sanderson, D., & Dixit, V. 2021. Hospital evacuation modelling: A critical literature review on current knowledge and research gaps. *International Journal of Disaster Risk Reduction* 66:102627.

Zane, R., Biddinger, P., Hassol, A., Rich, T., Gerber, J., & DeAngelis, J. 2010. *Hospital evacuation decision guide.* AHRQ Publication No. 10-0009. Rockville, MD: US Department of Health and Human Services Agency for Healthcare Research and Quality.

Zeigler, D., Brunn, S. and Johnson, J. 1981. Evacuation from a nuclear technological disaster. *Geographical Review* 71:1–16.

Zhang, Z., Spansel, K., & Wolshon, B. 2014. Effect of phased evacuations in megaregion highway networks. *Transportation Research Record* 2459:101–109.

7 Planning and Management of Transportation Systems for Evacuation

Brian Wolshon and Vinayak Dixit

7.1 INTRODUCTION

Emergency evacuations are defined as the prompt and rapid movement of people away from a threat or actual occurrence of a hazard. The spatial extent of an evacuation and the urgency at which an evacuation must be carried out is generally a function of the threat or hazard, including its size and spread; speed and direction of movement; and potential lethality and destructiveness. These factors also influence the behavioral response of evacuees, including how many evacuees depart an area of threat, when they leave, where they go, what routes they take, and what means of travel they take, among many other aspects of the event. Past research, observation, and experience have shown that individual decisions of whether or not to evacuate are based in large part on the level of threat perceived by that individual, both directly or sensed, based on the actions of others similarly affected. Thus, factors like the level of danger posed by a threat, one's proximity to it at present or in the near future, and the responses of others within the social network of the potential evacuee all influence decision-making.

From a transportation perspective, the hazard conditions and behavioral responses they elicit are important because they influence evacuation *travel demand*, or the number of people and/or vehicles that are expected to be moving during an event. Perhaps even more important than just the number of people are the temporal and spatial characteristics of this demand generation. Where evacuees leave from, when they leave these locations, where they travel to gain safe shelter, what routes they will select to undertake the travel, and even what modes of transportation they will use to make the trip all govern the ability of transportation networks and assets to adequately serve this demand in a timely manner. Key performance parameters such as travel time and clearance time, the formation and recovery of congestion, travel delay, and so on are all the direct result of how, when, and where evacuees load themselves on a network.

DOI: 10.1201/9781003648178-8

To illustrate this idea, Tamminga et al. (2011) used traffic simulation modeling to show that the total amount of time needed to evacuate an area, also known as *clearance time*, is increased significantly if the time window for evacuees to respond to an evacuation order is reduced. In effect, transportation networks become fully saturated and then overloaded with vehicles, similar to what might be seen in the evacuation of a crowded room or movie theater. If everyone ran to leave at the same time, the aisles and area immediately in front of the exit doors would become congested, and the smooth and orderly movement of people would break down, resulting in longer wait times for those further behind. Conversely, if the movement of people could be regulated such that there was no stopping or waiting, the overall time required to clear them would be significantly less. The daunting question then becomes how to regulate the flow in the face of danger and provide adequate capacity when threatening conditions arise.

The following sections of this chapter highlight these and other key concepts related to the planning, operation, and management of transportation systems, assets, and personnel for emergency evacuations. While written from a broad perspective that includes many key concepts from the field of emergency management, the chapter focuses on a transportation-based view of evacuations. This includes how transportation planners, engineers, and managers view and assess evacuations from the standpoint of demand generation and providing capacity within transportation systems to best serve those needs. While many aspects are quite similar to routine transportation practices, the analysis and planning for emergencies and evacuations present many unique challenges. This chapter highlights them as well as emerging, innovative, and effective practices that have been identified through recent research and experience. The purpose of this chapter is not to make readers experts in all aspects of evacuation-related transportation but rather to acquaint them (especially those with no or limited backgrounds) with the key needs, aspects, policies, and practices of transportation planning and engineering for evacuations.

7.2 MANAGEMENT AND DIRECTION OF EVACUATIONS

In terms of hazard response, evacuations are often the last step in a process that begins several minutes, hours, or even days earlier. Thanks to recent advancements in weather forecasting, threats like hurricanes, for example, can give an advanced warning time of nearly a week. This amount of lead time gives emergency response and transportation agencies a significant advantage in being able to anticipate the amount of demand that may be created and then prepare and implement responses for these conditions. Unfortunately, however, hurricanes tend to be an exception to the rule of evacuations. The vast majority of events requiring evacuations give little, if any, advanced warning.

Given the wide variation in factors that influence the scale and urgency of evacuations, it is helpful to recognize the role transportation plays in evacuations and how it influences the process. To help in that understanding, the following sections discuss the management of evacuation in the United States, how evacuation practices have evolved based on recent experiences, the types of conditions for which evacuations may be needed, and some relevant background.

7.2.1 Role of Transportation in Evacuations

What often comes as a surprise to those unfamiliar with evacuations is that, historically, they have been carried out with little input from transportation agencies and professionals. The daily activities of transportation planners, engineers, control systems managers, maintenance technicians, and others have a primary focus on providing consistent, safe, and efficient transportation to the traveling public. Traditionally, this has meant keeping up with routine needs like reducing roadway congestion, enhancing highway safety, and designing, constructing, and maintaining physical infrastructure. Given these responsibilities and the perpetually limited financial resources of transportation agencies, there has, in the past, been little time, money, or, in some cases, interest in taking on the additional responsibilities of emergency transportation management. Similarly, emergency management professionals have not always been aware of the capabilities and resources available from their transportation counterparts.

It has not been until the past decade or so that the planning and management of evacuations has moved away from the exclusive arena of emergency management agencies to involve agencies with a primary transportation focus. Since the highly publicized failings of Hurricanes Floyd, Katrina, and Rita, as well as the more recently recognized potential from threats like terrorist attacks and tsunamis, state departments of transportation, regional transit authorities, and other providers of transportation services have become key players in the planning and management of evacuations. This involvement has also been formalized through the development of the National Incident Management System (NIMS), in which the roles and responsibilities of transportation during emergencies are spelled out in Emergency Support Function 1 (ESF 1) (FEMA 2008).

7.2.2 Hazards and the Need for Evacuation

Evacuations occur more frequently in the United States (US) than is often realized. A recent US Nuclear Regulatory Commission (NRC) report showed that, on average, an evacuation involving 1,000 or more people occurs once every two to three weeks somewhere in the country (Dotson and Jones 2005). While evacuations are most often associated with hurricanes, the need to evacuate can come from many different types of hazardous events which, themselves, can be classified in numerous different ways. One method distinguishes hazards in terms of origin, *natural* or *manmade*. Common natural hazards include hurricanes, floods, earthquakes, wildfires, and tornados. Manmade hazards include technological hazards like biological, chemical and radiological (BCR) hazards like anthrax attacks, toxic chemical spills, and nuclear power plant accidental releases, as well as conditions like explosions, fires, hazardous material spills, etc. Manmade conditions may be further subclassified in terms of *intentional* or *unintentional*. Although it is likely that the majority of manmade hazards are unintended consequences of human activity, some are purposefully initiated. Occurrences such as wars and terrorist attacks are both examples of intentionally manmade events that have required evacuations.

The NRC evacuation study statistics, compiled by the Sandia National Laboratories over the ten-year period between 1993 and 2003, suggest that the vast majority of incidents requiring an evacuation tend to be small, localized events. Of the 230 evacuation events, 171 of them, or nearly 80%, involved 1,000 people or less. While wildfires and floods were the hazards for which an evacuation was most commonly required, hazardous material incidents and transportation-related events also accounted for more than a quarter of the documented evacuations over this period.

No matter their size, evacuations are, by nature, disruptive events that can have significant economic and political consequences. The costs of hurricane evacuations, for example, can exceed $1 million per mile of coastline from losses in tourism, commerce, and general productivity. Evacuation orders can also be difficult to implement because the movement and development of hazards can change over short periods of time. The scope and breadth of an evacuation must also be proportional to the threat, so evacuation orders need to be sufficiently large to protect people but not so large that they needlessly disrupt the economic activity of a region, resulting in an over- or "shadow" evacuation, or worse, leading to a "cry wolf" perception among the public.

Currently, the US is somewhat unique among countries in the world in that evacuations are used as a primary protective action during disasters and emergencies. Most countries use limited, if any, highway-based evacuation for hurricanes. One of the reasons for this is that, unlike many other countries, the US has the ability to move large numbers of people significant distances in a timely and safe manner and then shelter them at locations away from the hazard zone. This is likely to change in the future as developing countries increase their rates of automobile ownership and roadway infrastructure.

Over time, some critics of evacuation have also argued that private transportation availability has led to an over-reliance on evacuations. They contend that the need to evacuate for hurricanes could be reduced by strengthening building codes and increasing the availability of locally-based shelter facilities that do not require long travel distances. Such planning could also reduce or eliminate the inability of transportation networks to adequately serve the amount and immediacy of demand generated by a large-scale evacuation.

7.2.3 Evacuation Types

For planning and management purposes, evacuations associated with these very hazards are often categorized based on the amount of advanced warning time they give. While some hazards develop and/or move slowly, giving days or even weeks of advanced warning time, others can occur with no advanced warning. These temporal differences are important because they limit the ability to issue and receive critical evacuation information as well as allow or prohibit time to implement citizen-assisted evacuation plans and capacity-adding traffic management measures.

As part of their information on the planning and implementing transportation measures for emergency events, the US Department of Transportation (USDOT) defined several types of incidents in terms of the amount of advanced notice they give (Zimmerman et al. 2007). While the USDOT definitions are not specific in the precise amount of advanced warning time, they broadly characterize them into the general groups of "advanced notice" and "little- or no-notice."

An obvious example of an advanced-notice event is a hurricane, which can be identified and tracked up to several days in advance. The key factor is the time such hazards afford to assess options and then formulate and/or implement actions. The USDOT describes advanced-notice events in the following way (Zimmerman et al. 2007).

> With an advance-notice evacuation, information becomes available during the Readiness Phase regarding the incident that has occurred and the factors that may require an evacuation. Decision makers have time to collect the information they need to determine whether an evacuation should be ordered and, if so, the best way to carry it out.

In contrast, a no-notice event leaves no time for pre-event activity and is characterized as the following by the USDOT:

> A little- or no-notice incident is one that occurs unexpectedly or with minimal warning. The lack of warning and the quick response time required introduce distinct challenges for evacuating at-risk populations. No-notice incidents do not provide emergency responders sufficient time to prepare for a specific incident. This greatly affects agencies' abilities to pre-activate emergency protocols, pre-position needed assets, and warn and direct the public. No-notice evacuations require a significantly different approach to planning than advance-notice evacuations because they will be based on a set of capabilities and strategies that will likely be more limited in the time and resources available for implementation.

There is also a third, much more loosely defined, type of evacuation event known as "short-notice" events. Opinions range widely on what constitutes a short-notice event, but in general, they are described as lying between no-notice and long-notice events. Some define the amount of advanced notice as short as 30 minutes, while others extend it to 24 hours or more. From a transportation emergency response standpoint, short-notice events appear to permit some level of traffic management, but nothing as extensive as the implementation of regional contraflow or full transit-assisted evacuation plans. One example of a short notice is a fast-moving wildfire or nuclear power plant emergency in which one to several hours may be available to issue orders and give route and destination guidance to evacuees.

7.2.4 Evacuation Guidance and Directives

Once an evacuation is deemed necessary, the extent and type of evacuation must be determined and then communicated to the affected populations. The nature of the evacuation guidance and level of urgency is dependent on the characteristics of the hazard and clearance times described earlier. Currently, there is no formalized language or standards that govern the ordering or communication of evacuations in the United States.

Reviews of evacuation policies and practices (NCHRP 2009) show that nationwide, evacuations are most often classified as *recommended* or *mandatory*. Recommended evacuations are typically used to warn people when a threat to life and property exists or will likely exist in the immediate future. Although people who receive such warnings are not required to evacuate, it is to their advantage to do so. In hurricane scenarios, recommended evacuation orders are targeted toward people most vulnerable to hurricane storm surges and extreme winds, including offshore workers, persons on coastal islands, and other special populations having particularly long lead-time requirements. From a traffic perspective, recommended evacuations are also used as a way to motivate the most threatened people to move first and clear more heavily populated areas before later, more urgent evacuation orders have the potential to cause congestion and delays along the travel routes. No special traffic control or transportation measures are usually taken during recommended evacuations, and people may remain if they so choose.

Past experience has shown that mandatory evacuation orders are considered to be the most serious by potential evacuees. Realizing this, public officials charged with emergency management use this for the most threatening of conditions. During a mandatory evacuation, authorities put maximum emphasis on encouraging evacuation and limiting ingress into threatened areas. Mandatory orders are also made when many evacuation transportation network management plans (like contraflow and transit-assisted evacuation) go into effect.

Although people are "required" to leave under mandatory evacuation orders, such orders are difficult to enforce, and most government agencies lack both the resources and the legal authority to compel threatened individuals to leave. In the past, many people have resisted government officials' orders to leave their homes and property. Under such conditions, emergency management officials acknowledge that if a person wants to stay, the state will not physically remove them even if it is absolutely certain that they would be harmed. In discussions with county law enforcement officials in California, it was found that some deputies were able to encourage mandatory evacuations by compelling parents to release minor children to authorities under child endangerment laws. Once children were taken into protective custody, parents would make the decision to leave as well.

Prior study has also shown that other, more ambiguous, evacuation terminology is also common in the US. Words like "voluntary" and "precautionary" are also used in some locations, and the terms "recommended" and "precautionary" are often used interchangeably and are not necessarily as clearly defined as the previous two. One agency described their precautionary evacuations as "pre-voluntary" and thought of them as a way to get people or entities in need of long preparation times or those in recognized at-risk areas to move toward action. Again, decisions of whether or not to leave are left to individuals, and few special transportation arrangements are made.

The definition and terminology of evacuation declarations are important because they impact peoples' decision of whether or not to leave. Prior research has shown that people who said they heard mandatory evacuation orders are the most likely to evacuate, while recommended evacuation orders are met with less urgency (PBS&J 2000). The type of evacuation order and how it is communicated is also critical to avoid spontaneous or shadow evacuation.

Shadow evacuations occur when people who believe they are at risk evacuate even though they have not been officially advised or recommended to do so (Gunter 2001). Shadow evacuees most often leave because of concern about safety but could also leave for other reasons. Authorities in Florida and Texas feel that one of the reasons for the extreme number of evacuees during Hurricane Floyd, then later in Rita, was the result of shadow evacuations. However, it has been suggested that the over-evacuation problem in Houston also resulted from vague and inconsistent instructions provided by the authorities.

7.3 EVACUATION TRANSPORTATION PROCESSES

The last 25 years have seen tremendous advances in the way that evacuations are planned, implemented, managed, and analyzed. Techniques such as contraflow, staged and phased evacuations, cross-state regional coordination, special needs and transit-assisted evacuation, as well as planning and analysis techniques like regional multimodal traffic simulation, have come about due in large part to a series of high-profile failures. There is also now a recognition of a greater list of hazards for which evacuations are now required to serve as a protective action. This fact, coupled with changing population demographics and changing climatological patterns, have also resulted in natural hazards like hurricanes that are being forecast to occur both with higher frequency and increasing levels of severity in the future.

The need for, size of, and urgency at which evacuations are carried out can vary widely based on a number of key variables associated with the timing, coverage area, and movement of a threat. These spatio-temporal variables largely dictate, most notably, the extent of the hazardous conditions that are created and the amount of time until they arrive. This can be further complicated by whether the source of the hazard is also known in advance (known as a fixed-site hazard like a nuclear power plant) or whether the hazard location can occur in a random location as is predominantly the case for wildfires, train derailments, highway chemical spills, etc. In turn, all of these conditions come together to influence the implementation of protective actions and the guidance of evacuees, including how many evacuees need to leave, how far they will need to travel, and the types of traffic control and emergency pro-active actions can be taken to expedite the evacuation process.

Hazards and their effects, however, are just one part of the equation. Two other important considerations in planning and implementation of evacuations are the demographics and behavioral response of the people who will be evacuating as well as their access to transportation resources. Prior research has shown that socioeconomics can play a significant role in both the decision of when to evacuate (if at all) and how this travel will be accomplished. This dictates when and how fast the network will load as well as the need, amount, and type of additional supporting transportation assistance (shared rides, buses, trains, shelter in place, etc.). Transportation resources also go beyond providing buses for assisted evacuations and the personnel to carry them out. The ability to evacuate is also a function of the network configuration and coverage (e.g., where roads are and where they are not) and the capacity of the routes within it.

In the United States, much of the knowledge about evacuations, particularly those carried out on a mass scale, has come from experiences associated with hurricanes. However, the conditions necessitating evacuations extend beyond this single threat. They also include a wide spectrum of naturally occurring and manmade occurrences that occur with and without notice, and can be as localized as a single building or city block or as large as a multi-state region. Although each of these hazards brings with it a unique set of challenges and preparedness action needs, the evacuation processes used for all of them are actually surprisingly similar. What changes are the scale of implementation and the timing at which it occurs.

The following sections discuss the key spatial and temporal considerations that are considered in evacuation planning and analysis, as well as how various hazard conditions impact the planning process. The discussion also includes examples of how these various parameters and systems have been applied, adapted, and modified for use in evacuation. Knowledge of these processes and being able to frame them in terms of time and space are also quite valuable in modeling from two perspectives. First, it makes it possible to disaggregate the often enormously complicated and interrelated processes of the evacuation into separate, smaller components that are easier to observe and record. Then, it permits each of these key components to be represented quantitatively as equations or as a distribution of continuous data so that they can be described and analyzed using computer model representations.

7.3.1 Temporal Parameters

Among the temporal evacuation variables, one of the most critical is the amount of advanced notice available prior to the onset of hazardous conditions discussed earlier. Advanced warning time is also important because it dictates the amount of notice that response agencies have to implement control and management measures like contraflow, road closures, and emergency signal timing plans, as well as the time to activate assisted evacuation plans like evacuation bus services, medical special needs evacuations for the elderly, infirm, and disabled. It can also limit or extend the amount of time that evacuees have for pre-evacuation mobilization activities, such as picking up children from school, coordinating with mobility-limited friends and relatives, closing homes and businesses, gathering materials and supplies, and so on. Although it may seem that there is little time for these types of time-consuming activities during short-notice hazmat incidents; for example, there are numerous cases where they could still be used. Nuclear power plant emergencies, in particular, are commonly planned assuming that several hours will be available between the time a reactor emergency occurs and the time a containment breech begins to pose a risk to persons within the plume exposure area. This could permit, among other activities, police control checkpoints and contraflow lane reversals to be implemented and school and other assisted evacuation plans to be initiated.

Advanced warning time also affects the ability of officials to issue evacuation orders because they must be communicated through various formal (e.g., media releases, reverse 911 calls, etc.) and informal means, including social networks (e.g., friends, family, co-workers, neighborhoods, etc.). This lead time is particularly important for non-resident transient populations who may be within the evacuation zone for work, shopping, and other recreational activities. Research and development work, particularly related to hurricane evacuations, in modeling behavioral responses under the various advanced-notice conditions is available in the literature. This information has been quantified and adapted to create evacuee departure times and response distributions, which can be used in simulation models of evacuation. With additional calibration or adjustment, it is expected that even hurricane evacuation behavioral responses could be adapted for use in analyzing short- to no-notice events such as those commonly associated with hazmat incidents.

Once an evacuation is underway, there are numerous other temporal parameters that can be used to evaluate the performance of evacuation processes. From a transportation analysis perspective, these can include evacuation travel time and delay as well as the time needed to implement and/or remove evacuation traffic management and control measures like contraflow, road and bridge closures, and police control points. From an emergency management perspective, key temporal parameters may include onset time and duration of hazard conditions, time to issue evacuation orders, evacuee mobilization time, and so on. Again, these processes have been quantified in prior work for use in planning and evaluating evacuation alternatives.

7.3.2 Spatial Parameters

Like the temporal parameters described previously, evacuations also encompass a range of spatial parameters that also influence the manner in which evacuations are planned and carried out. They can also be used to evaluate the effectiveness of evacuation plans and identify areas of need and improvement.

Among the most essential spatial parameters that dictate the size of the evacuation protective action zone is the spatial extent of the hazard. Obviously, the larger the area of threatening conditions, the larger the area that must be evacuated. However, the spatial distribution of the resident and transient populations within the threatened population is what actually influences the amount of people and vehicles that would be in the evacuation. In the past, large storms threatening thousands of square miles have made landfall in sparsely populated areas of south Texas, for example, did not require major evacuations. Alternatively, while the 9/11 terrorist attacks in New York affected several city blocks, it required the evacuation of several million people. Although most hazmat incidents would be expected to be considerably smaller in scale than a hurricane, there are many hazmat hazard scenarios that could affect hundreds of square miles.

Two other hazard parameters that influence the urgency, extent, and direction of the evacuation are the approach direction and movement of threatening conditions.

An illustrative example of the effect of moving hazards on an evacuation is wildfires in urban-wildland interface areas. Because of the highly variable development and movement of wildfires, which are themselves a function of weather and fuel conditions, it is not possible to develop specific detailed evacuation plans. In Southern California, for example, emergency preparedness and response agencies find it more effective to work from a general evacuation framework, rather than a plan, to permit greater flexibility to respond to rapidly changing fire conditions. This includes designating the geographic extent of the threat region, the amount of available advanced warning time, the available routes, and even the shelter destinations. With the exception of nuclear power plant facilities, which are typically planned to assume a fixed-site emergency, the majority of hazmat incidents would be expected to create evacuation conditions that are more similar to wildfires where the locations of the protective action zone and urgency at which the evacuation need to be conducted is not known in advanced and can change rapidly based on wind strength and direction.

Other important spatial parameters that affect evacuation processes are the location and required travel distance to safe shelters, arrangement and access to transportation networks, and the location and frequency of downstream bottlenecks. For hazards like nuclear power plant emergencies and hurricanes, shelters are planned well in advance of the emergency and, as such, all evacuation travel is planned to reach them. However, for wildfires, safe shelter destinations as well as the routes recommended to reach them may change from event to event or even several times within a single event. Similarly, the available road network, including intersections, merges, terminal points, and capacity restrictions (e.g., bridges, tunnels, etc.), influence the direction of movement away from the threat.

7.4 EVACUATION TRAVEL BEHAVIOR AND RESPONSE

Understanding the evacuation behavior of the population is critical for devising traffic management strategies to safely evacuate people from the path of a major hurricane. Literature on evacuation behavior suggests that the common perception of irrational evacuation behavior during hurricanes (possibly due to panic) is not accurate (Quarantelli 1985; Tierney et al. 2006). In fact, people collectively act rationally during evacuations, and their decision to evacuate depends on factors such as direct perception of threat (Mikami and Ikeda 1985) and issuance of evacuation notice (Mikami and Ikeda 1985; Fitzpatrick and Mileti 1991; Sorenson and Mileti 1988). With the premise of rational evacuation behavior there should be models that can explain evacuation behavior based on certain environmental and demographic factors. Baker (1991) found that housing and storm-specific threat factors also affected evacuation behavior. Hultaker (1983) noted that families tend to make decisions about evacuation collectively and not on an individual basis. In a study of parishes in Southeastern Louisiana, it was found that people whose homes were damaged by an earlier hurricane were more likely to heed the official recommendation to evacuate (Howell and Bonner 2005).

The evacuation behavior studies can be categorized based on the questions they attempt to answer. Drabek (1983) referred to the research problem of trying to understand why some subjects evacuate while others do not as the "Shall we leave?" question. Another critical group of questions categorized by Sorenson (1991) was the "When shall we leave?" question. This question relates to the variations in departure times during a single hurricane or any short-notice disaster, for that matter. An important component of these variations, in the context of a short-notice disaster, is the time spent preparing for the evacuation after making the decision to evacuate. This duration is referred to as mobilization time in this study and relates to the "Why do we leave when we do?" question (Sorenson 1991). Understanding these variations can be used to generate empirical data based on traffic loading rates that can, in turn, be used for evacuation planning. According to Sorenson (1991), the relationship between mobilization time and the characteristics of the evacuees is critical for developing improved evacuation plans. Studies attempting to understand the mobilization time, sometimes also referred to as "evacuation delay," has found that households with older members and pets have higher mobilization time due to the need for appropriate transportation (Sorenson 1991; Vogt 1991; Heath et al. 2001).

The time it takes to decide to evacuate has been found to be affected by the time of issuance of the "order to evacuate." However, the use of individual households' decision time to evacuate to define the mobilization time accounts for not only the time at which orders to evacuate were first issued for an area but also the time the evacuating households received the information. Hence, the effect of these external factors is already incorporated in the mobilization time since it is obtained by subtracting the decision times (affected by *external conditions*) from the departure times. Therefore, the authors are of the opinion that *mobilization time* for individual households may be better defined using the time the households actually decided to evacuate.

A study conducted by the US Army Corps of Engineers (USACE) (2000) showed that the evacuation response rates follow an S-curve and that 10% of all evacuees had left by the time evacuation orders were delivered. The evacuation patterns are different if the evacuation is due to a hurricane that was recently preceded by another hurricane. Based on data from Hurricanes Charley and Frances that hit Florida in 2005, Dixit et al. (2008a) found that the number of evacuees that left at the end of the first day was 10% higher during a recent subsequent hurricane as compared to those observed during an earlier one. They found that home ownership, number of individuals in the household, income levels, and level/risk of surge were significant in the USACE model explaining the mobilization times for the households during a subsequent hurricane. While pets, the elderly, and children in households are known to increase the mobilization times during isolated hurricanes, they were not significant in the model.

Alsnih et al. (2005) summarized the research on evacuation demand, illustrating both a general model of evacuation behavior and the response curves. Fu and Wilmot (2004) developed a sequential logit model to estimate evacuation response. An attractive aspect of this model is that it is able to predict not only when people will leave but also how many will leave. Later, Fu et al. (2006) suggested a survival analysis based on evacuation response models. Continuing this work, Fu et al. (2007) calibrated an evacuation response curve model for Hurricane Floyd (1999) in South

Carolina from 1999 and used the model to predict evacuation behavior for Hurricane Andrew in Southeastern Louisiana from 1992. In both regions, these were the first hurricanes of the corresponding seasons, and the populations in these regions were not affected by recent prior hurricanes. Their study did not find any statistically significant difference between the predicted response curve and the actual response curve for Hurricane Andrew. Also, the model developed by Fu et al. (2007) was shown to transfer reliably across different regions and hurricanes. The sequential logit model (Equations 7.1 and 7.2) proposed by Fu et al. (2007) is recommended for use in evaluating departure time choice. L_i denotes the probability of the number of evacuees leaving, while S_i denotes the probability of evacuees staying till time i. CL_i is the cumulative probability of leaving at time i (Equation 7.3), where S_1 is equal to one and Table 7.1 explains the parameters which were calibrated by Fu (2004).

$$L_i = \frac{e^{0.555Flood+0.267Mob+0.008Speed_i+1.543TOD1_i+1.721TOD2_i+1.681dorder1_i+1.998dorder2_i+5.247Gamdist_i-8.18}}{1+e^{0.555Flood+0.267Mob+0.008Speed_i+1.543TOD1_i+1.721TOD2_i+1.681dorder1_i+1.998dorder2_i+5.247Gamdist_i-8.18}} S_i$$

Equation 7.1

$$S_i = \prod_{j=2}^{i-1} \frac{1}{1+e^{0.555Flood+0.267Mob+0.008Speed_i+1.543TOD1_i+1.721TOD2_i+1.681dorder1_i+1.998dorder2_i+5.247Gamdist_i-8.18}}$$

Equation 7.2

$$CL_i = \sum_{j=1}^{i} L_j$$

Equation 7.3

TABLE 7.1
Dynamic Evacuation Departure Time Model

Evacuation Response Model (Fu 2004)

Covariate	Definition	(Coefficient)
Intercept	Model constant	-8.18
Flood	1 if the residence is believed very likely to be flooded, 0 otherwise	0.555
Mobile	1 if residence is a mobile home, 0 otherwise	0.267
Speed	Hurricane wind speed (mph)	0.008
TOD(1)	Time-of-Day, 0 for night (from 6 p.m. to 6 a.m.) as reference	1.543
TOD(2)	category, 1 for morning (from 6 a.m. to 12 p.m.), 2 for afternoon (12 to 6 p.m.). Two Dummy Variables	1.721
dorder(1)	Evacuation order. 1 for voluntary, 2 for mandatory, and 0 for	1.681
dorder(2)	none. Two Dummy Variables.	1.998
Gamdist	Transformation of distance (mi), with gamma distribution. The parameters selected for the model were 8 and 0.6 for shape and scale, respectively	5.247

It is important to note that the model was developed based on six-hour time intervals, and therefore, the resulting response curve should have the same resolution. To highlight the use of this model, an example hurricane is considered in Table 7.2. To further demonstrate the model, the evacuation response curve is developed for the case when the residences in the region are believed to be flooded, as shown in Table 7.3.

The cumulative probability of leaving that was calculated in the last columns of Table 7.2 and Table 7.3 were plotted in Figure 7.1.

The total probability of evacuating increases when the residences are under flood risk. As mentioned earlier, this model not only captures evacuation departure rates but also captures how many people will evacuate. The probabilities, when multiplied by the total population of the area, will predict the total number of people who have evacuated in a given time period.

More recently, there have been more advanced statistical models, such as Hasan et al. (2011) and Dixit et al. (2012), that have used more sophisticated modeling paradigms but, as of yet, have not been able to demonstrate transferability (Fu 2004).

From a modeling perspective, the next question that needs to be answered is that of the destination choice of the evacuees. Modali (2005) used a gravity model to predict evacuation destinations and found that the traditional trip purpose stratification needs to be modified based on destination type (hotel, friend, relative). Chen (2005) used an intervening opportunity model to model evacuation destination choice, since it incorrectly placed the most importance on travel impedance instead of the hurricane path or availability of shelter. In this model, the destinations are considered sequentially based on travel time. Though the model performed reasonably, there was scope for significant improvements.

Cheng et al. (2008) use a discrete choice model to predict evacuation destination choice. The model is based on a logit modeling process and assigns a probability for each destination city based on a destination's distance from the origin city, whether the destination is likely to be in a hurricane landfall zone, destination population, and destination's ethnicity. The model is shown in Table 7.4 and Equation 7.4. The parameters shown in Table 7.4 are from the study conducted by Cheng et al. (2008).

$$PD_i = \frac{e^{-4.655*10^{-2}*DIST_i+1.66*10^{-7}*POP_i-0.5171*DANGER_i+1.5562*MSA_i+0.6711*ETHPCT_i}}{\sum_j e^{-4.655*10^{-2}*DIST_j+1.66*10^{-7}*POP_j-0.5171*DANGER_j+1.5562*MSA_j+0.6711*ETHPCT_j}}$$

Equation 7.4

To highlight the use of this model, an example hurricane is considered in Table 7.5. The probability is calculated using the coefficients in Table 7.4 and the formula shown in Equation 7.4.

The total number of people leaving at any given time (t) to a particular destination (i) is given by N_i^t in Equation 7.5, where PD_i is the probability of choosing destination i, and L_t is the probability of leaving at time t.

$$N_i^t = POP * PD_i * L_t$$

Equation 7.5

TABLE 7.2
Example Dataset with No Flood

Time	Flood	Mobile	TOD1	TOD2	dorder1	dorder2	Speed	Distance	gammadist	CI_i
12:00 a.m.–6:00 a.m.	0	0	0	0	0	0	105	543	0.193	0.002
6:00 a.m.–12:00 p.m.	0	0	1	0	0	0	115	484	0.231	0.013
12:00 p.m.–6:00 p.m.	0	0	0	2	1	0	130	445	0.245	0.334
6:00 p.m.–12:00 a.m.	0	0	0	0	1	0	145	394	0.245	0.345
12:00 a.m.–6:00 a.m.	0	0	0	0	1	0	165	334	0.209	0.356
6:00 a.m.–12:00 p.m.	0	0	1	0	0	2	175	273	0.141	0.599
12:00 p.m.–6:00 p.m.	0	0	0	2	0	2	160	202	0.056	0.878
6:00 p.m.–12:00 a.m.	0	0	0	0	0	2	145	129	0.008	0.884

TABLE 7.3
Example Dataset with Flood

Time	Flood	Mobile	TOD1	TOD2	dorder1	dorder2	Speed	Distance	gammadist	CI_i
12:00 a.m.–6:00 a.m.	1	0	0	0	0	0	105	543	0.193	0.003
6:00 a.m.–12:00 p.m.	1	0	1	0	0	0	115	484	0.231	0.022
12:00 p.m.–6:00 p.m.	1	0	0	2	1	0	130	445	0.245	0.468
6:00 p.m.–12:00 a.m.	1	0	0	0	1	0	145	394	0.245	0.484
12:00 a.m.–6:00 a.m.	1	0	0	0	1	0	165	334	0.209	0.499
6:00 a.m.–12:00 p.m.	1	0	1	0	0	2	175	273	0.141	0.756
12:00 p.m.–6:00 p.m.	1	0	0	2	0	2	160	202	0.056	0.951
6:00 p.m.–12:00 a.m.	0	0	0	0	0	2	145	129	0.008	0.96

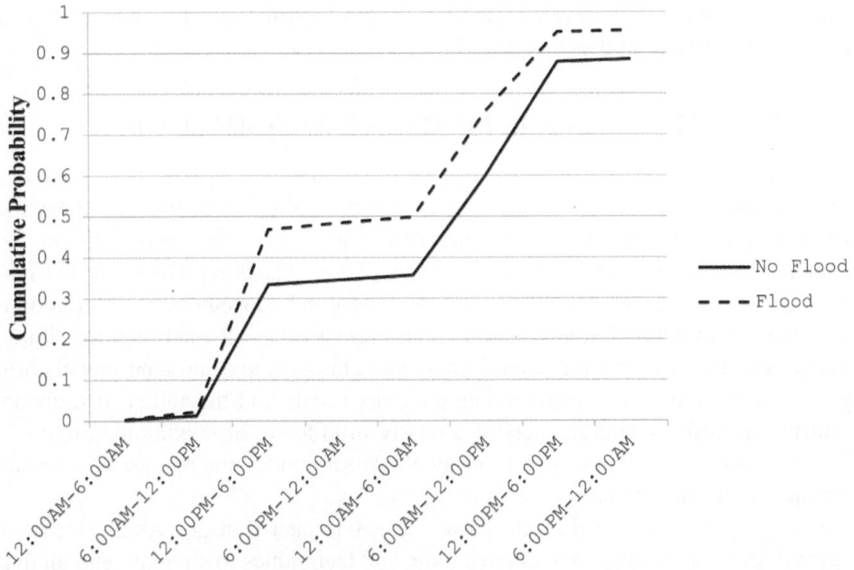

FIGURE 7.1 Comparison of cumulative probability of departure of evacuees in an area at risk of flood and those that are not

TABLE 7.4
Logit Model Variables and Their Coefficients

Destination Choice Model (Cheng et al. 2008)

Covariate	Definition	Coefficient
DIST	O-D Distance (mi)	–0.004655
POP	Destination City Population	1.66E-07
DANGER	Risk Indicator (Dummy Variable)	–0.5171
MSA	Metro Area Indicator (Dummy Variable)	1.5562
ETHPCT	White Percentage	0.6711

TABLE 7.5
Example Dataset for Destination Choice

	Distance	Population	Danger	MSA	ETHPCT	PD_i
City 1	80	400,000	1	0	16	0.070
City 2	200	500,000	0	0	15	0.035
City 3	160	600,000	0	1	17	0.780
City 4	280	500,000	0	1	15	0.115

This can then be used to develop temporal Origin-Destination tables which are used in traffic simulation models.

7.5 EVACUATION TRAFFIC MODELING AND SIMULATION

As traffic simulation models have grown in computational speed and analytical detail, it has become easier to apply them for the evaluation of large roadway networks with increasingly larger amounts of traffic. Today, simulation systems like DynaSmart, TRANSIMS, VISSIM, and even older platforms like CORSIM have the ability to create and track the second-by-second movements of hundreds of thousands of individual vehicles over thousands of miles of roadways for simulation periods that can last for several days. Such massive and intricate models offer the capability to produce detailed data on a large scale and the ability to study and evaluate the system-wide impacts of a nearly infinite set of conditions. Figure 7.2 shows the spectrum of modeling tools available for conducting analyses on evacuation operations and planning.

Since it is recognized that mass evacuations impact transportation systems on regional levels, it is necessary to have tools and techniques to simulate and analyze traffic conditions at these high levels while maintaining the ability to focus on specific areas of concern. Figure 7.3 presents the process for developing and analyzing a simulation model to study evacuation operations and plans.

Regional-scale evacuation simulations have several key requirements that need to be addressed, including the ability to model vast geographical areas with an enormous number of vehicles and time durations that cover multiple days. In addition, individual vehicular dynamics must be coupled with the ability to calibrate and validate the results so that the spatial and temporal patterns of traffic observed in the simulation reflect realistic conditions. Until recently, the ability to achieve any one – let alone all – of these requirements has been difficult, if not impossible.

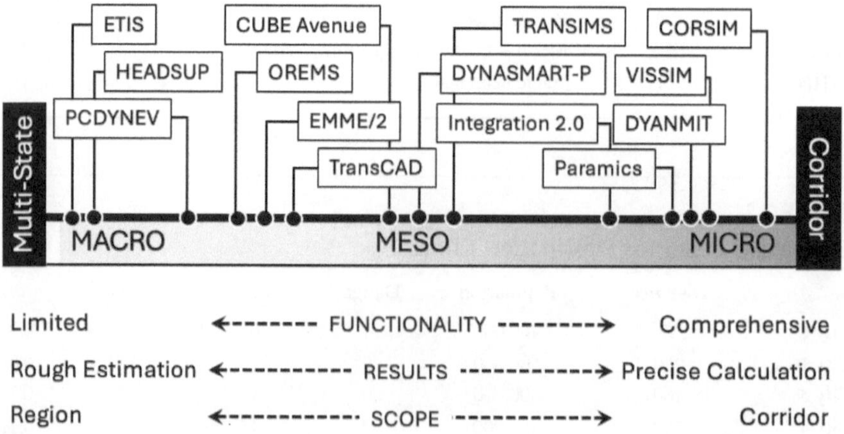

FIGURE 7.2 Evacuation modeling spectrum (adapted from Hardy and Wunderlich, 2007)

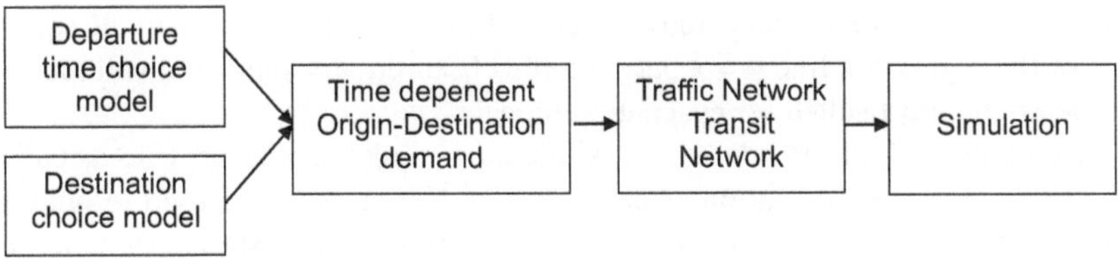

FIGURE 7.3 Process to develop and analyze evacuation operations and plans

Early studies on applying traffic simulation for evacuation were limited in their geographical scales and time durations. Evaluation studies conducted with high-fidelity microscopic simulation could only be achieved on small networks over time durations of 12 to 20 hours. Several of the earliest focused on the design and traffic operations at contraflow crossovers (Theodoulou 2003; Lim and Wolshon 2005), the evaluation of evacuation routing (Theodoulou 2003; Williams et al. 2007; Dixit et al. 2008b), and the impact of evacuation-level demand on small urban signal networks (Jha et al. 2004; Sbayti et al. 2006). The simulation of larger regional networks was limited to aggregate-level analyses using macroscopic traffic modeling (Hobeika et al. 1985; KLD 1984; Kirschenbaum 1992). From this, only approximate evacuation clearance time and delays could be made, but no understanding of bottlenecks and traffic impacts could be achieved because of the low resolution of the models.

The problems associated with the current state of practice for the planning and management of transportation systems during evacuations have been:

1. Myopic small-scale modeling of evacuation operations.
2. Lack of calibration and validation of simulation models with actual data collected during evacuation.
3. Lack of modeling of the movement of low-mobility populations during evacuations.

Recently, Chiu et al. (2008) conducted a regional scale simulation study using DynusT to evaluate the regional impacts of various evacuation strategies for the Houston-Galveston, Texas, metropolitan region during Hurricane Rita. This model represented a significant advance over prior work in that it was among the first to evaluate the traffic impacts of an evacuation at a regional scale.

In fact, several earlier studies have utilized survey data or normal day traffic to calibrate and validate their simulation models. While this may not be a realistic representation of what actually occurs during a mass evacuation, previous modelers have had little choice due to a lack of observed traffic data during evacuations. The calibration and validation of the traffic simulation models are a critical aspect of the modeling process and are needed to ensure that the traffic simulation model replicates the real world with reasonable accuracy.

The Federal Highway Administration's Volume III: Guidelines for Applying Traffic Microsimulation Modeling Software (2004), as well as an in-depth study by Barcelo and Casas (2003), identified various statistics for calibrating and validating simulation models. In a recent study conducted by Dixit et al. (2011), the R-squared value of the regression line y = x between the observed and simulated volumes was considered the most suited for evacuation models.

Once calibrated and validated, the simulation model should provide a realistic representation of the evacuation process. This model can then be used to quantitatively and qualitatively examine the spatio-temporal characteristics (speed, volume, density, queuing, and congestion formation/recovery) of the evacuating traffic and evaluate transit evacuation plans.

To visualize the output results of the simulation, color-coded maps of speed were used to graphically represent traffic patterns over space and time. This method was found to be useful to display data in an easy-to-understand manner for analysis. The color maps were particularly valuable for the identification of bottlenecks and understanding the spatio-temporal distribution of speed and volume along various routes. For example, in a study conducted by Dixit et al. (2011), the spatio-temporal graphs were used to identify locational bottlenecks, indicated within the boxes, and the dynamics of queue formation, represented by the black sloped lines in Figure 7.4.

After the failure to effectively coordinate the movement of low- and non-mobile populations prior to Hurricane Katrina, there has been an increased interest in developing methods to create and evaluate transit evacuation plans. The New Orleans transit evacuation plan that was developed, also referred to as the New Orleans City-Assisted Evacuation Plan , calls for a two-tiered system of buses to circulate locally within the city to pick up evacuees, then transport them to regional coaches for movement to more remote shelter destinations Bian and Wilmot (2018).

To model transit evacuation plans, it is critical to understand:

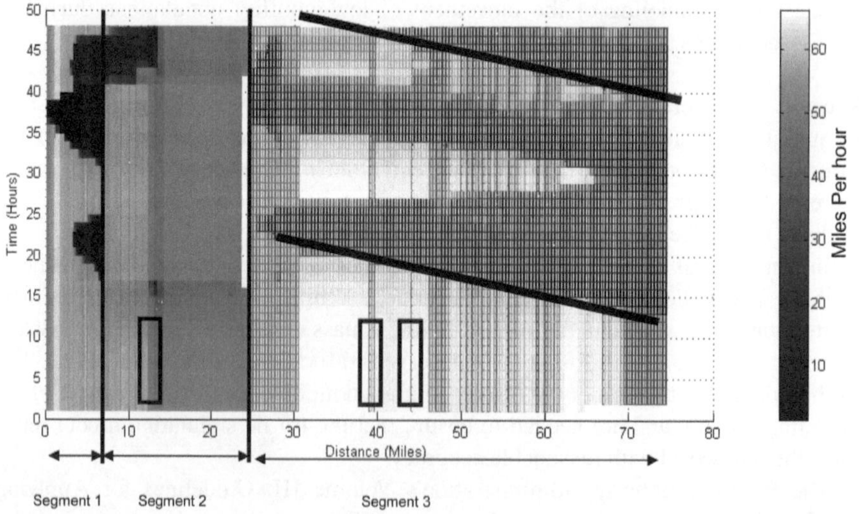

FIGURE 7.4 Spatio-temporal distribution of speed (adapted from Dixit et al. 2011)

- The percentage of the population expected to utilize this assisted evacuation.
- The temporal demand profile, which is based on the departure time distribution, can be reasonably assumed to have a model the same as those discussed earlier in this chapter.
- A slightly modified response curve and separate bus routes were assumed for tourists seeking transport to the airport.
- The simulation network model can then be used to test scenarios and determine the trips that would be required by bus transit to evacuate all low-mobility populations to their intended destinations.

A more detailed analysis can be found in Naghawi and Wolshon 2011a and 2011b, as well as Abdelgawad and Abdulhai (2010), who developed a multimodal evacuation plan for cities. Though Naghawi and Wolshon's (2011a,2011b) study was for a hurricane evacuation of New Orleans, Abdelgawad and Abdulhai (2010) study was for a "no-notice" evacuation event in the city of Toronto.

7.6 CONCLUSIONS

The history of mass evacuation practice has shown that evacuation traffic management plans have been based largely on lessons learned from failures identified in prior events. This approach has resulted in evacuation plans that cater to "failures of the last evacuation." Unfortunately, this does little to address the future and may leave the public vulnerable to unforeseen conditions. The use of simulation modeling to evaluate evacuation plans provides somewhat of a "crystal ball" and holistic view of the entire evacuation operation that can also be used to test any contingency that can be imagined and has not been experienced in the past. For this reason, simulation can help develop more robust and effective evacuation plans.

The simulation models provide spatio-temporal distribution of traffic, and color-coded maps of speed and volume help to identify bottlenecks. The benefit of using such large models lies in their usefulness to emergency management officials in evaluating evacuation plans, the duration of the contraflow operations, and identifying bottlenecks. The spatio-temporal speed graphs can also be utilized to determine travel times and locations to place fuel containers for vehicles running out of fuel. The insights gained through the regional modeling of evacuation were found to be useful in determining bottlenecks several miles downstream and can be used to develop a more holistic regional evacuation plan. When combined, models and concepts such as those demonstrated here provide a significant resource for policy decisions, both large and small. Simulation models could be used to test other policy scenarios, such as providing incentives for people to shelter in certain locations, such as secure hospitals and schools, or to test the feasibility of encouraging evacuees to leave their cars at home and evacuate via transit with the option of designating certain routes as bus-only evacuation corridors. In the future, plans are also being developed to incorporate other modes of traffic, such as air and rail, to provide an even more robust illustration of evacuation operations.

It is also important to recognize that evacuations vary based on the characteristics of hazards, and therefore, it is critical to develop plans that consider various types of hazards and the consequent evacuations. For evacuation plans to be robust, there is a need to develop scenario-based evacuation plans that are flexible and adaptive to a hazard type, making the evacuation plans more efficient.

REFERENCES

Abdelgawad, H., and Abdulhai, B. (2010) "Managing Large-Scale Multimodal Emergency Evacuations." *Journal of Transportation Safety and Security*, Vol. 2, No. 2, pp. 122–151.

Alsnih, R., Rose, J., and Stopher, P. (2005) "Understanding Household Evacuation Decisions Using A Stated Choice Survey – Case Study Of Bush Fires." Presented at the 84th Annual Meeting of the Transportation Research Board, Washington, DC, January 9–13.

Baker, E. J. (1991) "Hurricane Evacuation Behavior." *International Journal of Mass Emergencies and Disasters*, Vol. 9, No. 2, pp. 287–310.

Barcelo, J., and Casas, J. (2003) "Methodological Notes on the Calibration and Validation of Microscopic Traffic Simulation Models." (CD-ROM) 84th Annual Meeting of the Transportation Research Board, Washington, DC, January 9–13.

Bian R, Wilmot CG. (2018). An analysis on transit pick-up points for vulnerable people during hurricane evacuation: A case study of New Orleans. International Journal of Disaster Risk Reduction 31:1143-1151.

Chen, B. (2005) *Modeling Destination Choice in Hurricane Evacuation with an Intervening Opportunity Model.* Master's Thesis, Department of Civil and Environmental Engineering, Louisiana State University, Baton Rouge, LA.

Cheng, G., Wilmot, C., and Baker, E. (2008) "A Destination Choice Model for Hurricane Evacuation." Presented at 88th Annual Meeting of the Transportation Research Board, Washington, DC.

Chiu, Y., Zheng, H., Villalobos, J. A., Peacock, W., and Henk, R. (2008) "Evaluating Regional Contra-Flow and Phased Evacuation Strategies for Texas Using a Large-Scale Dynamic Traffic Simulation and Assignment Approach." *Journal of Homeland Security and Emergency Management*, Vol. 5, No. 1, Article 34

Dixit V. V., Montz, T., and Wolshon, B. (2011) "Validation Techniques for Region-Level Microscopic Mass Evacuation Traffic Simulations." *Transportation Research Record: Journal of Transportation Research Board*, Vol. 2229, pp. 66–74.

Dixit V. V., Pande, A., Radwan, E., and Abdel-Aty, M. (2008a) "Understanding the Impact of a Recent Hurricane on Mobilization Time During a Subsequent Hurricane." *Transportation Research Record*, Vol. 2041, pp. 49–57.

Dixit, V. V., Ramasamy, S., and Radwan, A. E. (2008b) "Assessment of I-4 Contraflow Plans Microscopic vs. Mesoscopic Simulation." *Transportation Research Record*, Vol. 2041, pp. 89–97.

Dixit VV, Wilmot C, Wolshon B. (2012). Modeling risk attitudes in evacuation departure choices. Transportation Research Record 2312(1):159-163.

Dotson, L. J., and Jones, J. (2005) "Identification and Analysis of Factors Affecting Emergency Evacuations, Main Report." Sandia National Laboratories/U.S. Nuclear Regulatory Commission Report No. NUREG/CR-6864, Vol. 1 / SAND2004-5901, Washington, DC, January, p. 61.

Drabek T. E. (1983) "Shall We Leave? A Study of Family Reactions When Disaster Strikes." *Emergency Management Review*, Vol. 1(Fall), pp. 25–29.

Federal Emergency Management Agency (2008) "National Incident Management System." Department of Homeland Security, Washington, DC, December. http://www.fema.gov/pdf/emergency/nims/NIMS_core.pdf (accessed May 7, 2012).

Federal Highway Administration (2004) "Traffic Analysis Toolbox Volume III: Guidelines for Applying Traffic Microsimulation Modeling Software." http://ops.fhwa.dot.gov/trafficanalysistools/tat_vol3/Vol3_Guidelines.pdf (accessed November 15, 2010).

Fitzpatrick, C., and Mileti, D. S. (1991) "Motivating Public Evacuation." *International Journal of Mass Emergencies and Disasters*, Vol. 9, No. 2, pp. 7–18.

Fu, H. (2004) "Development of Dynamic Travel Demand Models for Hurricane Evacuation." PhD Dissertation, Louisiana State University. http://etd.lsu.edu/docs/available/etd-04092004-081738/unrestricted/Fu_dis.pdf (accessed June 4, 2012).

Fu, H., and Wilmot, C. (2004) "Sequential Logit Dynamic Travel Demand Model for Hurricane Evacuation." *Transportation Research Record*, Vol. 1882, pp. 19–26.

Fu, H., and Wilmot, C. (2006) "Survival Analysis Based Dynamic Travel Demand Models for Hurricane Evacuation." Transportation Research Record 1964(1):211-218..

Fu, H., Wilmot, C., and Zhang, H. (2007) "Modeling the Hurricane Evacuation Response Curve." Transportation Research Record 2022(1):94-102..

Gunter, P. (2001) "Emergency Planning for Nuclear Power Accidents." Reactor Watchdog Project, NIRS. http://www.nirs.org/reactors/emergencyplanning71301.html (accessed February 24, 2003).

Hardy, M., and Wunderlich, K. (2007) "Evacuation Management Operations (EMO) Modeling Assessment: Transportation Modeling Inventory." FHWA Contract No. DTFH61-05-D-00002. Washington, DC: U.S. Department of Transportation.

Hasan, S., Ukkusuri, S. V., Gladwin, H., and Murray-Tuite, P. (2011) "A Behavioral Model to Understand Household Level Hurricane Evacuation Decision Making." *ASCE Journal of Transportation Engineering*, Vol. 137, No. 5, pp. 341–349.

Heath, S. E., Kass, P. H., Beck, A. M., and Glickman, L. T. (2001) "Human and Petrelated Risk Factors for Household Evacuation Failure during a Natural Disaster." *American Journal of Epidemiology*, Vol. 153, No. 7, pp. 659–665.

Hobeika, A. G., and Jamei, B. (1985) "MASSVAC: A Model for Calculating Evacuation Times under Natural Disasters." Computer Simulation in Emergency Planning, Society of Computer Simulation, La Jolla, CA.

Howell, S. E., and Bonner, D. E. (2005) "Citizen Hurricane Evacuation Behavior in Southeastern Louisiana: A Twelve Parish Survey." http://poli.uno.edu/unopoll/Summary%20Report%20July%2019%202005%20(2).pdf (accessed June 4, 2007).

Hultaker, O. (1983) "Family and Disaster." *International Journal of Mass Emergencies and Disasters*, Vol. 1, No. 1, pp. 7–18.

Jha, M., Moore, K., and Pashaie, B. (2004) "Emergency Evacuation Planning with Microscopic Traffic Simulation." *Transportation Research Record,* Vol. 1886, pp. 40–48.

Kirschenbaum, A. (1992) "Warning and Evacuation during a Mass Disaster: A Multivariate Decision-Making Model." *International journal of Mass Emergencies and Disasters,* Vol. 10, No. 1, pp. 91–114.

KLD (1984) "Formulations of the DYNEV and I-DYNEV Traffic Simulation Models Used in ESF." Federal Emergency Management Agency, Washington, DC.

Lim, E., and Wolshon, B. (2005) "Modeling and Performance Assessment of Contraflow Evacuation Termination Points." *Transportation Research Record,* Vol. 1922, pp. 118-128..

Mikami, S., and Ikeda, K. (1985) "Human Response to Disasters." *International Journal of Mass Emergencies and Disasters*, Vol. 3, No. 1, pp. 106–132.

Modali, N. (2005) *Modeling Destination Choice and Measuring the Transferability of Hurricane Evacuation Patterns.* Master's Thesis, Department of Civil and Environmental Engineering, Louisiana State University, Baton Rouge, LA.

Naghawi, H., and Wolshon, B. (2011a) "Operation of Multimodal Transport Systems during Regional Mass Evacuations." *90th Transportation Research Board Meeting*, Washington, DC. January 23-27.

Naghawi, H., and Wolshon, B. (2011b) "Performance of Multi-Modal Evacuation Traffic Networks: A Simulation Based Assessment." *90th Transportation Research Board Meeting*, Washington, DC.January 23-27.

National Cooperative Highway Research Program (NCHRP) (2009) *Transportation's Role in Emergency Evacuation and Reentry*, Synthesis of Highway Practice Report No. 392, Transportation Research Board, National Research Council, Washington, DC, p. 142.

PBS&J Inc. (2000) "Hurricane Floyd Assessment – Review of Hurricane Evacuation Studies Utilization and Information Dissemination." Post, Buckley, Schuh & Jernigan, Inc., Tallahassee, FL.

Quarantelli, E. L. (1985) "Realities and Mythologies in Disaster Films." *Communications: The European Journal of Communication*, Vol. 11, pp. 31–44.

Sbayti, H., and Mahmassani, H. S. (2006) "Optimal Scheduling of Evacuation Operations." *Transportation Research Record,* Vol. 1964, pp. 238–246.

Sorenson, J. H. (1991) "When Shall We Leave? Factors Affecting the Timing of Evacuation Departures." *International Journal of Mass Emergencies and Disasters*, Vol. 9, No. 2, pp. 153–165.

Sorenson, J. H., and Mileti, D. S. (1988) "Warning and Evacuation: Answering Some Basic Questions," *Industrial Crisis Quarterly*, Vol. 2, pp. 195–209.

Tamminga, G., Tu, H., Daamen, W., and Hoogendoorn, S. (2011) "Influence of Departure Time Spans and Corresponding Network Performance on Evacuation Time." *Transportation Research Record: Journal of the Transportation Research Board*, Vol. 2234, pp. 89–96.

Theodoulou, G. (2003) *Contraflow Evacuation on the Westbound I-10 Out of the City of New Orleans.* Master Thesis, Louisiana State University, Baton Rouge, LA.

Tierney, K., Bevc, C., and Kuligowski, E. (2006) "Metaphors Matter: Disaster Myths, Media Frames, and Their Consequences in Hurricane Katrina." *ANNALS, AAPSS*, Vol. 604, No. 1, pp. 57–81.

US Army Corps of Engineers (2000) "Alabama Hurricane Evacuation Study Technical Data Report: Behavioral Analysis." Final Report.

Vogt, B. M. (1991) "Issues in Nursing Home Evacuations." *International Journal of Mass Emergencies & Disasters*, Vol. 9, pp. 247–265.

Williams, B. M., Tagliaferri, A. P., Meinhold, S. S., Hummer, J. E., and Rouphail, N. M. (2007) "Simulation and Analysis of Freeway Lane Reversal for Coastal Hurricane Evacuation." *ASCE Journal of Urban Planning and Development*, Vol. 133, No. 1, pp. 61–72.

Zimmerman, C., Brodesky, R., and Karp, J. (2007) "Using Highways for No-Notice Evacuations: Routes to Effective Evacuation Planning Primer Series," United States Department of Transportation Report No. FHWA-HOP-08-003, Washington, DC, November.

8 Modeling and Simulation of Fuel Availability at Gas Stations during Extreme Events

Olufemi A. Omitaomu,
Brandon A. Miller, and Nagendra Singh

8.1 INTRODUCTION

When disaster strikes, effective fuel supply management and coordination are essential to meet heightened fuel demand due to intensified relief and evacuation activities. However, the retail fuel supply chain, like other supply chains, is fragile; it is sensitive to economic trends, bottlenecks, and natural disasters. The inherent complexity of the retail fuel supply chain often means that short-term disruptions can have far-reaching downstream consequences. Thus, the retail fuel supply is regularly disrupted by hurricanes, winter storms, cyber-attacks, and other disasters. Natural disasters in particular pose a substantial threat not only to the fuel supply chain but also to the individuals who rely on it in the critical hours and days that follow. For instance, during the 2021 winter storm Uri in Texas, approximately 4.8 million affected individuals had to resort to using gas for both electricity and heat due to the widespread power outages caused by damaged electrical infrastructure. This situation posed the risk of carbon monoxide poisoning (Donald, 2021). Moreover, according to the National Oceanic and Atmospheric Administration (NOAA), Florida has encountered ten hurricanes of Category 3 or higher since 2000 (NOAA, 2023). The evacuations before these hurricanes make landfall, combined with challenges in delivering fuel caused by road damage and hazardous conditions, frequently result in significant fuel shortages that can persist for weeks (GasBuddy, 2019). These shortages pose a risk of impeding emergency responders in the area and causing delays for individuals evacuating late.

According to the Energy Information Administration (EIA), the retail fuel supply chain in the United States involves multiple steps and entities. The major steps in the supply chain can be described as follows:

DOI: 10.1201/9781003648178-9

- **Exploration and Production:** Oil companies explore and extract crude oil from domestic and international sources. The extracted crude oil is transported via pipelines, ships, or trucks to refineries.
- **Refining:** Crude oil is processed at refineries, where it undergoes various refining processes like distillation, cracking, and treatment to separate it into different petroleum products such as gasoline, diesel, jet fuel, and others. Refineries mix different components to create various grades of gasoline and diesel that meet regulatory standards and consumer demand. According to the Homeland Infrastructure Foundation-Level Data (HIFLD), there are some 155 refinery locations across the United States (HIFLD, 2019).
- **Distribution:** Refined products are transported from refineries to distribution terminals via pipelines, trucks, trains, and ships. These terminals act as storage hubs and distribution points. At distribution terminals, fuels are stored in large tanks before being loaded onto trucks or trains for further transportation to retail outlets.
- **Wholesale Supply:** From distribution terminals, fuel products are sold to wholesalers or jobbers, who then distribute them to retail outlets such as gas stations. Wholesalers often contract with multiple retailers to supply fuel.
- **Retail Supply:** Gas stations and convenience stores purchase fuel from wholesalers or refiners. They store the fuel in underground storage tanks and dispense it to consumers via pumps.
- **Consumer Demand and Sales:** Consumers purchase fuel for vehicles or other uses at gas stations. The price of fuel is influenced by factors such as crude oil prices, refining costs, taxes, and market demand.

Throughout the retail fuel supply chain, there are numerous logistical and regulatory considerations, including safety standards, transportation logistics, pricing fluctuations based on market conditions, environmental regulations, and competition among different entities in the supply chain. Government agencies and oversight bodies, such as the Environmental Protection Agency (EPA), the Department of Transportation (DOT), and state regulatory agencies, ensure compliance with safety, environmental, and quality standards. Additionally, market dynamics, geopolitical factors, technological advancements, and economic conditions significantly impact the fuel supply chain in the United States.

Based on the steps in the supply chain, it is evident that disruptions and congestions can arise at various points in the supply chain, leading to downstream ripple effects. However, the magnitude of these effects fluctuates depending on the region and the specific event. For example, the state of Florida, used as a case study in this chapter, lacks its own oil refineries and interstate pipelines, and instead relies on imports via its ports (EIA, 2022). As such, Florida's fuel supply vulnerabilities exist primarily in its upstream distribution system. This susceptibility intensifies during periods of heightened demand caused by events like hurricanes or other natural disasters. Nevertheless, it is crucial to acknowledge that Florida's bulk terminal facilities can store an inventory lasting between 11 and 16 days, theoretically adequate to withstand short-term crises such as hurricanes (DeCorla-Souza, 2018;

Florida Department of Transportation, 2018). Consequently, the primary areas of disruption center around the interactions involving tanker trucks, retail gas stations, and consumers at the culmination of the supply chain. At this stage, bottlenecks are more probable due to a combination of increased demand at gas stations and the hindrance faced by trucks in replenishing stations due to impassable roads and hazardous conditions. This chapter introduces a modeling and simulation framework designed to estimate the duration until fuel depletion at gas stations. This framework leverages a queueing model to assess demand at the retail fuel facility level and examines the impact of disruptions caused by extreme events on this specific subsystem.

The significance of gasoline during crises often goes unnoticed by most people. Yet, when severe weather causes the power grid to fail, having immediate access to fuel can be the determining factor between survival and vulnerability. Whether it is fueling a generator to help a family endure a winter storm or enabling a swift evacuation during an unrelenting hurricane, gasoline frequently becomes crucial for the survival and welfare of those caught in catastrophic situations. With the escalating intensity and impact of storms due to ongoing global climate shifts, the reliability of fuel access during crises becomes increasingly pivotal. This underscores the significance of the fuel supply chain responsible for distributing gasoline to retail outlets nationwide.

Addressing and preventing disruptions within these supply chains is challenging even under normal circumstances, let alone during extreme weather events. Consequently, shifting focus to the demand aspect might be advantageous. Predicting potential disruptions and informing consumers about the status of nearby fuel facilities could facilitate quicker evacuations and reduce the risk of harm to individuals facing severe weather events.

To achieve this goal, we implement a data-driven queueing model engineered to simulate demand patterns and forecast remaining fuel levels in retail fuel stations. Additionally, we present a case study using this simulator, to analyze fuel stations affected by Hurricane Ian in 2022. The model presented in this chapter is part of the STATIONS (Situation-Temporal Awareness Tool for Integrated Oil and Natural Gas Systems) project (Kar et al., 2021). In addition to the fuel availability simulation in this work, the STATIONS project also models the accessibility of retail fuel facilities using the number of roads connected to a station and its proximity to major roadways, among other models.

8.2 RELATED LITERATURE

While no literature appears to exist on specifically forecasting fuel shortages and outages through queueing models, many existing supply chains follow an analogous structure of production, processing/refinement, bulk storage, and retail sale for public consumption. These can provide an alternative view of shortages due to supply chain disruptions, and even how they are modeled through queueing theory. Additionally, much research has attempted to model various disaster scenarios using queueing theory, including fuel management and evacuation strategies during hurricane events.

As discussed previously, retail fuel facilities play a key role in evacuations and can also serve as significant bottlenecks due to "range anxiety" and uncertainty in conditions on the road ahead (Sabbaghtorkan et al., 2022). By analyzing how queueing theory has been applied in the various perspectives of a disaster alongside the existing methods for simulating and mitigating disaster scenarios at retail fuel facilities, we can determine how best to apply queueing theory to the problem at hand.

8.2.1 Simulation of Disruption in Analogous Supply Chains

Most research on supply chain disruption focuses on strategies for mitigating the impacts of upstream disruptions (Zheng et al., 2021). Among these, multi-sourcing strategies (Schmitt and Tomlin, 2012; Wang et al., 2010), holding inventory for disruption (Tomlin and Wang, 2011), and facility location strategies (Snyder and Daskin, 2007) are the most common approaches. This bias towards supply-side modeling is understandable, given the inherent difficulty in attempting to model the complex, individualistic decision-making strategies that drive demand. There is, however, a body of research dedicated to understanding and mitigating problematic demand-side phenomenon, such as panic buying. Zheng et al. (2021), for instance, attempt to model the impact of what is known as the "social learning (SL) effect" on panic buying. The SL effect is the influence of one individual's decision to panic buy or "hoard" a product on another individual's purchasing decisions. Simply put, if one sees a group of people panic buying, or reads about a potential shortage on social media, the likelihood that one will, in turn, purchase more of a product than they need increases. This effect is known to cascade and can result in a premature shortage if enough individuals take part in panic buying behavior. Zheng et al. (2021) attempt to quantify this phenomenon in order to enable demand-informed stocking/purchasing strategies on the part of retail facilities when a supply disruption is anticipated.

The model presented in this work only tangentially touches upon human behavior to the extent that it is intended to mitigate what Zheng et al. (2021) refer to as the "social learning effect" through increased situational awareness. Even still, incorporating this effect into the STATIONS model would almost assuredly increase the robustness of its predictions, but it is presently outside the scope of this work.

8.2.2 Extreme Weather Impacts on Fuel Supply Chains

When analyzing the effects of extreme weather events on fuel distribution, two major themes emerge: damage to infrastructure and increase in demand. While the former is somewhat dependent upon the location of the event, it is important to note that significant percentages of the nation's oil refineries and associated liquid fuel infrastructure are located either offshore or in low-lying coastal regions (Wilbanks et al., 2007). As such, these sections of the fuel supply chain are at a significantly increased risk for damage due to extreme weather events, and hurricanes in particular. Additionally, port closures and traffic congestion frequently cause delays in fuel deliveries down the supply chain (Florida Department of Transportation, 2018).

Then, there are the inevitable spikes in demand for liquid fuel that occur during and after extreme weather. This occurs for a myriad of reasons. When extreme weather warrants an evacuation, the resulting uptick in driving and road congestion places an enormous burden on the local fuel supply. Even when there is no evacuation, widespread power outages may force individuals and critical facilities such as hospitals to rely on gas-powered backup generators (Abbey et al., 2014).

8.2.3 Queueing Theory in Disaster Management

Broadly speaking, disaster management occurs in four phases: mitigation, preparation, immediate response, and recovery/reconstruction (Baxter et al., 2019). The simulation presented in this work is focused primarily on the immediate response phase through increased situational awareness and, to a lesser extent, preparation. Much of the other studies in the disaster management space (e.g., Caunhye et al., 2016; Balcik et al., 2008; Yi & Kumar, 2007) focus on the distribution and pre-allocation of supplies, rather than on spreading out demand to ease the burden on existing supplies, which is the intended result of this work. When we examine works on applications of queueing models in disaster management, they tend to focus on relief/recovery efforts in the wake of disaster (Masoumi et al., 2022; Krishnamurthy et al., 2013).

The study by Sun et al. (2022), however, does speak to situational awareness by providing a queueing model intended to make real-time routing recommendations to evacuees experiencing disasters. The model itself is intended to be driven and informed by real-time traffic data acquired from weight-in-motion sites and various other proposed sources. Given that no reliable analogues exist for real-time monitoring of retail fuel storage levels, we introduce a method for estimating this parameter through a combination of static data sources and stochastic processes.

8.2.4 Disaster Management and Simulation of Downstream Fuel Distribution

In this instance, the bulk of the research dedicated towards optimizing fuel distribution in the downstream supply chain is focused on standard operating conditions (Lima et al., 2016). More recently, in coordination with FEMA, the MIT Center for Transportation and Logistics has begun to address this gap through the development of an intricate and data-driven model of the downstream fuel supply chain to help mitigate bottlenecks during disasters (Russell et al., 2020). While the development of some of the model parameters is not dissimilar to those presented in this work, the demand on individual retail stations appears to be a static value calculated from census statistics and inflated to simulate increased demand during emergency situations. While the current work does utilize census statistics for demand – opting to only count individual drivers rather than all residents of the state of Florida – the end parameters are used to drive and fine-tune a queueing model to estimate time-varying demand, rather than to pass a static parameter to queues upstream in the supply chain.

One of the most recent studies applying queueing theory to the simulation of fuel distribution in disasters is that of Sabbaghtorkan et al. (2022). Like much of the literature preceding them, the authors focus in part on modeling a location-allocation problem by determining the optimal refueling location for individuals attempting to utilize gas stations along evacuation routes (e.g., Gao et al., 2010). However, we hypothesize that rather than waiting until they arrive at an evacuation route, evacuees are more likely to attempt to obtain fuel from the *nearest* accessible retail facility. Given that the progression of vehicles in the STATIONS simulator is not tracked, we interpret this concept by including all available retail fuel facilities in the study area. Moreover, our proposed implementation seeks to reduce range anxiety by providing situational awareness without prescription of evacuees' fuel requirements.

The primary contribution of this study is the robust and time-varying simulation of the demand side of the fuel distribution system for emergency and evacuation events through a combination of data-driven parameters and stochastic processes. Additionally, this work serves as one of the, if not the only, attempts in the existing literature to forecast outages in retail fuel facilities based on demand upsurge, rather than optimizing the reaction to a pre-existing/known outage or attempting to mitigate outages through supply chain interventions.

8.3 METHODOLOGY

8.3.1 Study Site

There are multiple reasons for selecting the state of Florida as the site for this case study, with Florida's frequent exposure to extreme weather events being one of the primary driving factors. With most of the state's infrastructure and 21.5 million residents located along its coasts, evacuations due to hurricanes are a regular occurrence (US Census, 2020). Additionally, financial losses due to weather have accumulated to around $230 billion since 1980 (Florida Department of Agriculture and Consumer Services, 2021). With populations and frequency of extreme weather anticipated to increase in the coming years, the cost in both infrastructure and human life could rise significantly without intervention (Florida Department of Agriculture and Consumer Services, 2021). Combine this with a fragile fuel supply chain and high tourist population, and it is clear that Florida is in urgent need of tools to improve situational awareness of fuel availability for both evacuees and emergency responders.

8.3.2 Fuel Availability Simulator

The STATIONS Fuel Time to Empty (FTE) simulator comprises a set of independent queueing models employing a First-Come, First-Served (FCFS) scheduling algorithm and uses the First-In, First-Out (FIFO) queueing method, simulating the flow of fuel through individual retail fuel facilities. The queues employ data-informed uniform distributions, G, to randomly select inter-arrival times and vehicle service times, and each queue has a varying number of servers/connections c. As such, they are considered to be G/G/c queues in standard notation. Each model execution mirrors the fuel movement within a single facility, symbolized by a resource container and a set number of connections *c* that determine the resource availability. These elements correspond to the underground storage tank and fuel pumps at the respective station. The capacity of the tank, number of pumps, and station locations are derived from various data sources consolidated into the Florida Gas Stations Dataset. The process of assembling this dataset is detailed in the subsequent section.

The behavior of the STATIONS FTE model encompasses two primary processes: fuel supply to the station and the demand on its finite resources. The demand simulation, detailed in the preceding paragraph, is more dynamic and comprises the queueing model. A visual representation of the demand aspect is outlined in Figure 8.1. Fluctuations in demand over time hinge partly on inter-arrival times – periods between vehicles arriving – which are randomly chosen but derived from estimated driver numbers in the vicinity and the count of other fuel facilities in the region. The calculations for these intervals are expounded upon in the following section. Essentially, the model assumes a linear correlation between potential drivers on the road and the frequency of vehicles arriving at the station. Hence, the simulation's selection of arrival times is calibrated to match each station's unique potential arrival time range.

The fuel demand is influenced by the specific fuel needs of each vehicle. Consequently, within the simulation, a tank size is allocated to each entering car by randomly selecting the vehicle type based on a user-defined distribution. This setup grants the user control over the frequency of different vehicle types appearing in the simulation. Currently, the model operates with five vehicle categories: sedans, midsize SUVs/vans, large SUVs/trucks, offroad vehicles, and heavy trucks. Once a vehicle category is chosen, the quantity of fuel dispensed to the vehicle becomes a

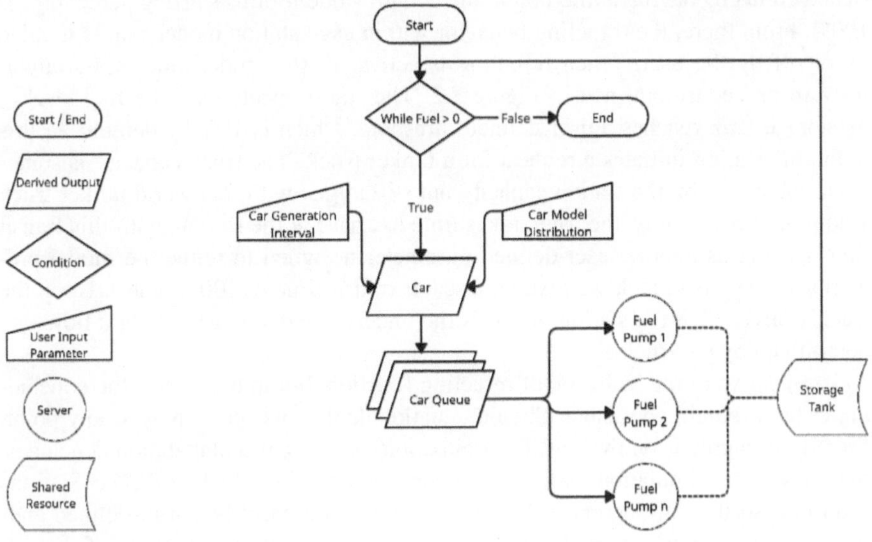

FIGURE 8.1 Flowchart for the demand simulation of a single station

random percentage between 5% and 95% of the total vehicle tank capacity, as evacuees with any room in their fuel tank are going to want to fill up in anticipation of congestion on a potentially lengthy trip. This amount of fuel determines the duration the vehicle spends at the fuel pump, calculated simply as the required fuel multiplied by a flow rate of ten gallons per minute, adhering to the EPA regulation's maximum flow rate (40 CFR 80). Additionally, an extra 1.5 minutes per vehicle is included to accommodate transitions.

As vehicles enter the simulation, their inter-arrival times and desired fuel amounts are established, following which they are assigned to an available fuel pump. The fuel is then dispensed from the underground tank, after which the vehicle exits the simulation. However, if no pump is free, the vehicle waits until a pump becomes available. In instances where all pumps at a station are occupied, additional vehicles will only seek fuel if the queue length is fewer than three. This rule aims to prevent excessively lengthy queues from slowing down the simulation when inter-arrival times are short. While this rule is not necessarily indicative of actual customer behavior, the impact on the gas station in question should be minimal once the queue length exceeds the number of pumps.

Regarding fuel supply determinations, the STATIONS model offers relatively straightforward functionality for two main reasons. Firstly, extreme events often impede fuel shipment from bulk terminal facilities to retail stations due to factors like inaccessible roads, hazardous driving conditions, or supply chain bottlenecks caused by cyber-attacks. Secondly, integrating data-driven supply calculations would necessitate incorporating the upstream segments of the fuel supply chain, which currently lies beyond the scope of this study but could be a focal point for future endeavors.

At the beginning of each simulation, the station starts off with a user-defined percentage of its total capacity. Given that most stations attempt to prepare for hurricane events by having a filled tank, the default value for this starting percentage is 100%. From there, the refueling behavior within each station model can be toggled on or off by the user. When refueling is activated, the model follows a straightforward procedure outlined in Figure 8.2. The station waits until the fuel level in its storage tank reaches a user-defined threshold, which is 15% by default. At this point, the station initiates a request for a tanker truck. The truck capacity is somewhat influenced by the station capacity but still aligns with real-world tanker truck volumes. Subsequently, the truck takes time to arrive at the station, with this transit time serving as another user-defined parameter designed to refine the model predictions. For this model, we assume a scalar transit time of 100 minutes. Upon the truck's "arrival" at the station, it refills the underground storage tank at a flow rate determined by the truck size.

Irrespective of the inclusion of refueling functionality in the model, the concluding criteria remain consistent. Should a station deplete its fuel supply at any point, even if the supply is on the way, the simulation for that particular station concludes, initiating a new simulation for the subsequent station within the Florida Gas Stations Dataset described in Section 0 (Kar et al., 2021). Alternatively, a user-defined end-time parameter exists, capable of terminating the simulation regardless of the stations' operational status. The eventual outcome of a simulation run is a geospatial

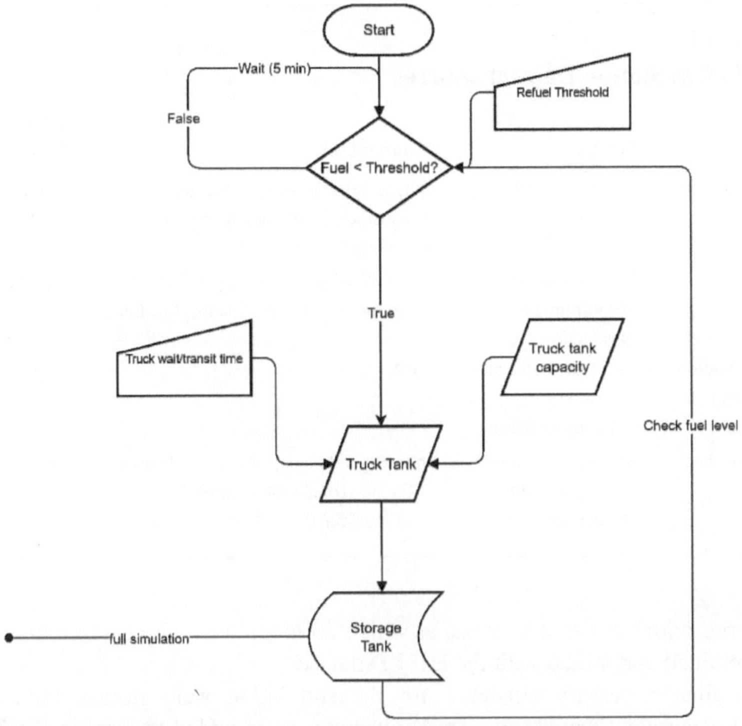

FIGURE 8.2 Flowchart for fuel supply simulation

dataset containing predictions for the fuel time to empty for each station, alongside the user-input parameters used in the simulation.

8.4 DATA PROCESSING

8.4.1 Florida Gas Stations Dataset

Due to the variety of data attributes necessary to perform this simulation, the Florida Gas Stations Dataset is an amalgamation of several data sources. The attributes in this dataset used directly in the simulation consist of station locations, the number of pumping stations, capacity and number of underground storage tanks, and access to a generator. Station locations were primarily derived from the HIFLD website. This was then combined with a dataset of active fuel facilities and licenses in Florida to eliminate inactive gas stations. These datasets also contained information on the number of pumps and storage tanks. Unfortunately, not all of the stations in the Florida Active Fuel Facilities dataset corresponded to a station in HIFLD. As such, the ArcGIS Online Geocoding Service was employed to generate geolocations for the remaining stations. The geocoding match score for each station was then

TABLE 8.1
Florida Gas Station Dataset Sources

Name	Source	Source URL	Date of Acquisition
FL Active Fuel Licenses	FL Department of Revenue	https://floridarevenue.com/taxes/taxesfees/Pages/fuel_active.aspx?Filter=1	October 2020
FL USTs	FL Department of Environment Protection	https://prodlamp.dep.state.fl.us/www_stcm/publicreports/FacilityLocTank	October 2020
FL Gas Station Generator Dataset	FL Department of Agriculture Consumer Services	N/A	August 2020
FL Active Fuel Facilities	FL Department of Environmental Protection	https://geodata.dep.state.fl.us/datasets/5a25461b4f6a4903a1b398255765a05a_0 (No longer active)	October 2020

compared with the listed address, at which point stations with a score above 98% were retained and joined with the HIFLD dataset.

The final necessary attributes for the simulation were storage tank capacity and generator accessibility. These attributes were added by joining the Florida Underground Storage Tanks (USTs) and Florida Gas Station Generator datasets to the geolocated fuel facilities dataset to generate the final Florida Gas Stations Dataset. Table 8.1 below lists all the above datasets as well as their sources.

8.4.2 Vehicle Ownership Data

Each year, the American Community Survey (ACS) publishes a table that maps vehicle ownership by household size for every census tract in the US. This takes the form of the number of one-person households with one vehicle, one-person households with two vehicles, and up to four-or-more-person households with four or more vehicles. The Vehicle Ownership Dataset was pulled for the year 2019 in order to match up with the census tract geometries that existed prior to the 2020 census. As mentioned previously, this data is used to calculate the range of inter-arrival times for each station in the simulation by estimating the maximum and minimum possible number of drivers assigned to the station of interest. In this work, the maximum number of possible drivers is calculated for each census tract as Equation 8.1:

$$\sum_{i/C} \min(P_i, V_i) * H_i \qquad \text{Equation 8.1}$$

where C is the set of all household categories i (1-person 1-vehicle, 2-person 1-vehicle, etc.), H_i is the number of households in category i, and P_i and V_i represent the number of persons and vehicles in each household in i, respectively. Behind this value is the assumption that all individuals in a given household will make one trip during the simulation time, either to evacuate the area or to purchase fuel for cars/generators in the event of a power outage. This assumption may not hold for non-emergency scenarios, in which the fear of a fuel shortage may spur individuals to make multiple trips to fill up additional vehicles. In this scenario, the maximum number of drivers in a census tract would be the number of vehicles multiplied by the number of households. In this work, however, the assumption is that the simulation is taking place in an emergency scenario, and therefore Equation 8.1 is utilized in all models to determine the maximum number of drivers.

The minimum number of drivers in each census tract is simply the total number of households in each census tract that own at least one vehicle. Once the range of possible drivers is established for each tract, they must then be associated with a retail fuel facility. To do this, the Vehicle Ownership Dataset is joined with existing census tract geometry from the 2019 census, and the tract geometry is overlaid with the Florida Gas Stations Dataset to associate each station with its tract. In this study, the drivers in a census tract are assigned to each station by equal association, i.e., the number of drivers is simply divided by the number of stations in the tract.

It is important to note that the number of possible drivers is not a direct input to the simulations but is instead used to calibrate a range of inter-arrival times. This association is assumed to be linear, and a demand weight is calculated from the full driver dataset such that the minimum arrival time – 30 seconds – corresponds to the station with the largest (non-outlier) assigned maximum driving population, and the maximum arrival time – about five minutes – corresponds to the station with the smallest minimum driver count. Outliers here are defined as exceeding three standard deviations of the mean driver count. Stations with an assigned driving population flagged as an outlier simply use the minimum arrival time value. The range of possible inter-arrival times is calculated for each census tract as Equation 8.2:

$$\left[W * D_{max,t} + int, W * D_{min,t} + int\right] \qquad \text{Equation 8.2}$$

where W and int are the demand weights and time intercepts for all models in the simulation, respectively, and $D_{max,t}$ and $D_{min,t}$ are the maximum and minimum number of drivers for census tract t. The current demand weight and time intercept are -1.09038×10^{-3} and five minutes, respectively. The five-minute intercept value is somewhat arbitrary but is intended to account for census tracts in the ACS dataset that have "0" minimum drivers.

8.5 CASE STUDY

On September 28, 2022, Hurricane Ian made landfall as a Category 4 hurricane in southwestern Florida at approximately 4:35 PM EST. The storm hovered over Florida for more than two and a half days, claiming over 150 lives either directly or indirectly and causing $112 billion in damage across the state. In an attempt to

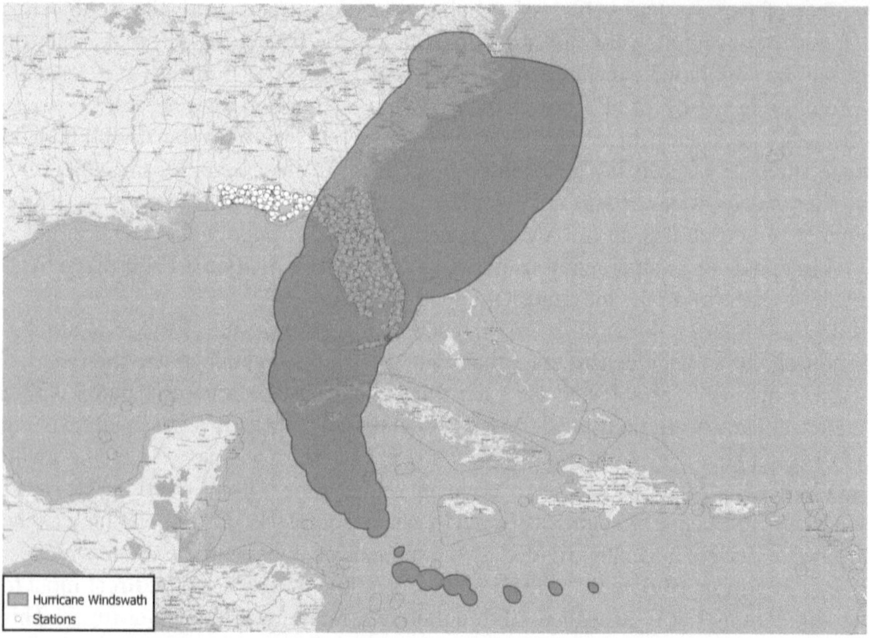

FIGURE 8.3 Overlay between Hurricane Ian wind-swath and the Florida Gas Stations Dataset

simulate the impact of the hurricane on Florida's fuel supply, we have retrieved geospatial wind-swath shapefiles from the National Hurricane Center (NHC) to narrow the scope of the simulation to only those fuel stations directly impacted by Ian (National Hurricane Center, 2022). The overlay used to select fuel stations for use in the simulation can be seen in Figure 8.3. A total of 5,115 gas stations were selected from the Florida Gas Stations Dataset based on this overlay.

To simulate the landfall event, the test simulations presented in this section last a total of 72 hours, slightly longer than Ian remained over the state of Florida. For the duration, the refueling functionality is disabled, as accelerating wind gusts would have forced drivers to halt deliveries due to safety concerns. In this scenario, each station is assumed to be cut off from the rest of the supply chain, and its status is determined solely by the amount of demand placed upon it.

At present, there is no reliable source of time-varying fuel station outages that could be used to verify the output of the STATIONS simulator. As such, output validation must be performed subject to reality-based constraints. First and foremost is a steady-state constraint; that is, parameter configurations representing ideal conditions should not predict a significant number of outages. To this end, the simulation for each station is again allowed to run for a total of 72 hours using the default values for each of the user-defined parameters: car model prevalence, demand weight, vehicle fuel levels, and the starting fuel level for all stations. It should be noted that some outages may occur due to the fact that the default demand parameters are inflated to calibrate for an evacuation event.

Determining appropriate behavior outside of the steady-state condition is far less straightforward without validation data. As such, rather than determining whether an outcome is "appropriate" or not, we test the impact of the user-defined parameter values on the resulting number and distribution of outages occurring in the simulation. Of these parameters, those governing the behavior and attributes of the simulated vehicles are considered to have the most uncertainty. These parameters consist of the demand weight (which controls inter-arrival time), the per-vehicle fuel demand, and the car model distributions. The fine-tuning of the demand weight is done by reassessing the desired absolute minimum and maximum inter-arrival times, symbolized as $1/\lambda$, and recalculating the demand weight and time intercept accordingly. As discussed in Section 0, the default values are 30 seconds and 5 minutes for the minimum and maximum inter-arrival times. To isolate the impact of each end of the distribution, a total of six tests are carried out with the parameter variations and corresponding demand weights shown in Table 8.2. The shaded entry designates the "control" parameter configuration run using default values.

The per-vehicle fuel demand tests follow a similar routine by varying the distribution of tank capacity percentages selected in the simulation. In this case, however, the variation will be in the ratio of high-demand vehicles – 5% to 50% of tank capacity – and low-demand vehicles – 51% to 95% capacity. The default value for this ratio is 1:1, or a uniform distribution between 5% and 95% capacity. Given that evacuees are more likely to stop when their tank is less than halfway filled, the proportion of customers with less than 50% remaining fuel capacity will be increased during testing. Thus, the test ratios will be 2:1, 3:1, and 4:1. This also helps to represent the variation in fuel demands over the course of a standard week, assuming that individuals operating under a standard 40-hour work week prior to the evacuation order are most likely to refuel on Sunday. Therefore, the closer the event occurrence is to Sunday, the fewer individuals there will be with significant fuel requirements.

TABLE 8.2
Governing Parameters for Inter-Arrival Time (1/λ) with the Default Configuration Highlighted in Gray

Minimum $1//\lambda$ (Seconds)	Maximum $1//\lambda$ (Minutes)	Demand Weight ($\times 10^{-3}$)
10	5	–1.171149
20	5	–1.130765
30	5	–1.090380
30	10	–2.301914
30	20	–4.724982
30	30	–7.148049

Finally, we must test the impact of the vehicle model distributions on the simulator outage predictions. As discussed in Section 8.3 , there are five vehicle categories used in this work: sedans, midsize SUVs/vans, large SUVs/trucks, offroad vehicles, and heavy trucks. Each vehicle category has a predefined tank capacity representative of the standard capacity for the respective category. The prevalence of each category in the simulation is relative and is a user-defined parameter. The default prevalence values are loose estimates based on US vehicle registration statistics acquired from the Bureau of Vehicle Statistics and the Department of Transportation. These values have been adjusted to match the categories defined in this study and to account for discrepancies in statistic years for each category. For each vehicle type, the default prevalence values are as follows: sedan: 25%, midsize SUV/van: 20%, large SUV/truck: 50%, offroad: 2%, heavy truck: 3%. Given the uncertainty present in these estimates, testing the impact of each vehicle's prevalence on the simulation is necessary. In order to isolate these impacts, extreme values for each vehicle category, along with a default configuration, are tested according to the procedure in Table 8.3. Once again, the shaded entry designates the default configuration or "control" run.

The results of each of the tests described above are summarized by the distribution of outages over the course of 72 simulation hours, as well as the percentage of stations out of fuel at the end of the simulation.

8.6 RESULTS AND DISCUSSION

8.6.1 Steady-State Behavior

The results of the steady-state analysis are encouraging. While there appears to be plenty of fluctuation in fuel levels for the stations over the course of the simulation, only six stations ultimately failed under the elevated demand conditions. Upon closer

TABLE 8.3
Vehicle Model Probabilities with the Default Configurations Highlighted in Gray

Variation	Sedan	Midsize SUV/Van	Large SUV/Truck	Offroad Vehicle	Heavy Truck
Control	25%	20%	50%	2.0%	3.0%
Sedan Dominant	90%	2.5%	2.5%	2.5%	2.5%
Midsize SUV/Van Dominant	2.5%	90%	2.5%	2.5%	2.5%
Large SUV/Truck Dominant	2.5%	2.5%	90%	2.5%	2.5%
Offroad Vehicle Dominant	2.5%	2.5%	2.5%	90%	2.5%
Heavy Truck Dominant	2.5%	2.5%	2.5%	2.5%	90%

inspection, five of the six stations ran out of fuel around the twelve-hour mark. The sixth emptied around two days after the simulation start time. Perhaps unsurprisingly, these stations all had the lowest fuel capacities in the Florida Gas Stations Dataset, with five having a 2,000-gallon capacity and the sixth having a 3,000-gallon capacity.

8.6.2 Unstable System Configurations

In order to establish a baseline, let us first take a look at the control configuration. Figure 8.4 below shows the spatial-temporal distribution of outages for the simulation run on the default/control parameters. The resultant outages appear to have an even spatial distribution throughout the state and seem to increase in frequency towards the end of the simulation, with an average simulation end time of 55 hours. Most notable is the sharp increase in the number of outages compared to the steady-state configuration, with the control run predicting a total of 413 outages, or about 8% of the 5,115 selected stations.

Now that we have established the steady-state case and the impacts of the baseline configuration, we can contextualize the results of the parameter variations described in Section 8.5. Table 8.4 displays the summary statistics for each of the test simulation runs alongside the steady-state and control configuration results. Of the three parameters tested in this case study, the vehicle model prevalence seems to have the

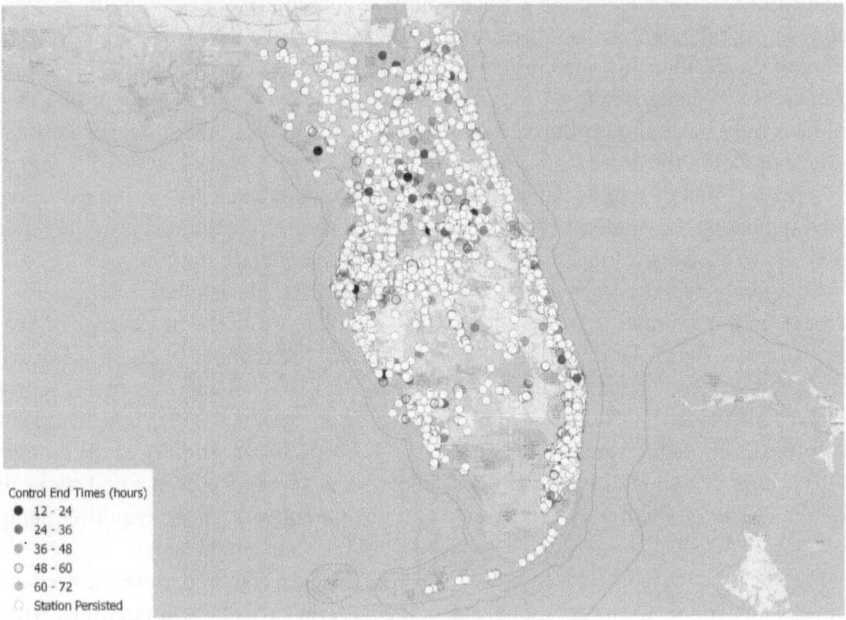

FIGURE 8.4 Predicted time to empty status (in hours) for stations in the control simulation configuration

TABLE 8.4
Summary Statistics for Steady-State, Control, and Test Configurations

Variation	Number of Outages	Outage Percent	Average End Time (Hours)
Steady-State	6	0.117%	20
Control	413	8.07%	56
Sedan Dominant	105	2.05%	53
Midsize SUV/Van Dominant	311	6.08%	55
Large SUV/Truck Dominant	698	13.6%	55
Offroad Vehicle Dominant	475	9.28%	56
Heavy Truck Dominant	1,402	27.4%	54
Minimum $1//\lambda = 10$ Seconds	484	9.46%	54
Minimum $1//\lambda = 20$ Seconds	445	8.70%	55
Maximum $1//\lambda = 10$ Minutes	67	1.31%	48
Maximum $1//\lambda = 20$ Minutes	29	0.567%	48
Maximum $1//\lambda = 30$ Minutes	14	0.274%	43
66% of vehicles < half tank	660	12.9%	55
75% of vehicles < half tank	754	14.7%	54
80% of vehicles < half tank	808	15.8%	54

most significant impact on the outage counts. Specifically, the simulation in which the Heavy Truck vehicle model occurred 90% of the time saw triple the number of outages. Given that this vehicle model has the largest tank capacity (35.5 gallons), an increase in outages is to be expected. However, it is intriguing to note that these vehicles only have about nine more gallons of capacity than the most predominant vehicle model in the control simulation – Large SUVs and Trucks, with 26.5 gallons. This implies that even modest variations in vehicle tank capacities will have an outsized impact on the prediction of fuel outages and should, therefore, be studied more carefully to ensure accurate assumptions of vehicle model distributions.

Comparatively, the impact of shifting the ratio of high-demand to low-demand vehicles in the simulation is straightforward. An increase in the percentage of vehicles with less than half a tank of fuel will increase the number of outages linearly. For instance, looking again at Table 8.4, we can see that a 9% increase in half-empty vehicles results in a 14% increase in outages – from 660 to 754. Further increasing the prevalence of half-empty vehicles to 80% results in an additional 50 outages. With access to validation data, this parameter may prove useful in fine-tuning the simulation, given the highly predictable nature of its impact on the resulting outage counts.

Finally, we come to the parameters governing inter-arrival time. Here, we see some significant changes in the prevalence of outages, primarily in the simulations with a larger maximum inter-arrival time. The disparity between these results and those of the simulation runs with smaller minimum arrival times is likely one of scale, in that the changes to the upper bounds can be far more drastic without reaching impossible

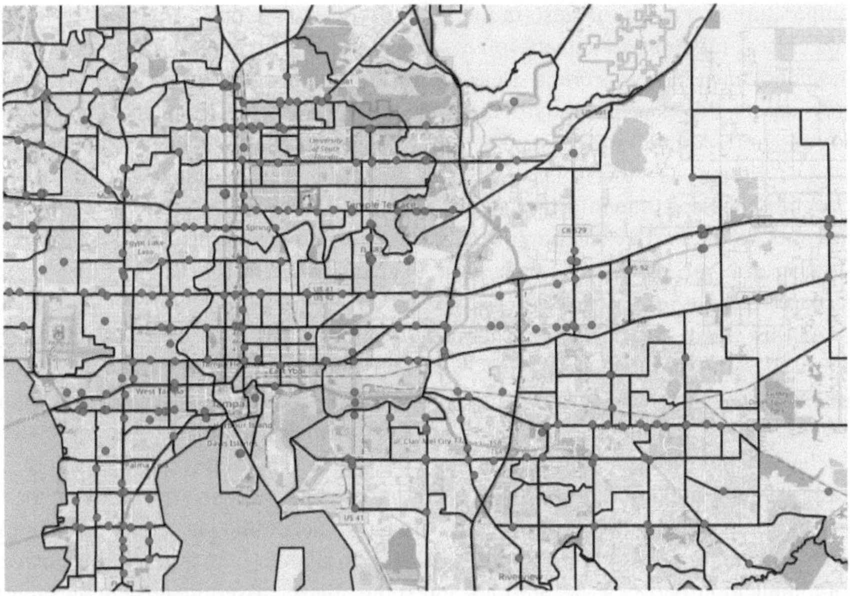

FIGURE 8.5 Gas stations (gray) overlaid with census tract borders (black) and OpenStreetMaps (background) near Tampa, FL

values. There are, of course, other factors at play that may potentially limit the impact of the minimum inter-arrival time parameter. For instance, the queue limit of three vehicles means that stations with high assigned driving populations may be reaching their vehicle capacity, at which point further increases in arrival rate will have no impact. Additionally, the significant variation in the estimated number of drivers assigned to the stations could be limiting the frequency of arrivals and, therefore, reducing the impact of lowering the minimum $1/\lambda$ value.

There is additional cause for concern when analyzing the procedure for assigning drivers in a census tract to the fuel stations within it. Figure 8.5 shows a section of the overlay of the census tract geometry used to assign drivers to stations by equal allocation. Here, we can see that it is far from uncommon for fuel stations to fall on or near the boundaries of their respective census tracts. This is because, as evidenced by the underlying OpenStreetMap, census tract boundaries are frequently drawn along major roadways. This has significant implications for the validity of an equal assignment procedure, as gas stations further from one another are far less likely to be servicing the same subset of the population. Any future extensions of the functionality of the STATIONS FTE model should account for this discrepancy through a more robust assignment procedure.

8.7 SUMMARY

The types of extreme weather events this study was performed to aid in have played out time and time again over the years. With the anticipated steady rise in ocean temperature comes an increase in the intensity of these events. Their power to disrupt critical functions of society follows doggedly. While generations of researchers and policymakers have worked tirelessly to slow and possibly even reverse this progression, its effects are already making themselves known. Climate change prevention and mitigation efforts must be paired with tools that allow society to better brace itself and recover in the wake of disaster. Situational awareness is one of the key tools for this. Real-time information on fuel availability not only empowers individuals to make the best evacuation decisions for themselves but also reduces the kind of uncertainty and panic that leads some to abandon their vehicles and others to fill garbage bags with gasoline.

At this stage of development, there is significant testing, functionality expansion, and validation that the STATIONS FTE simulator must undergo before it can fill such a critical role. However, the study presented here is a solid stepping-stone towards an accurate predictive model for fuel availability during extreme events. We have demonstrated that the existing model performs more than adequately for steady-state simulations. Additionally, the parameters that govern the behavior of this model can be readily and intuitively tuned to accommodate other regions and types of events, provided the requisite data is available. Functional gains such as communication between gas stations and robust driver assignment, among others, will only serve to improve the robustness of the model predictions.

8.8 ACKNOWLEDGMENTS

This material was based upon work supported by the US Department of Energy's Office of Cybersecurity, Energy, Security, and Emergency Response. The authors acknowledge Nicholas Roberts and Bandana Kar for their contributions during the early stage of the STATIONS project while they worked at Oak Ridge National Laboratory.

This work was sponsored by the US Department of Veterans Affairs. This manuscript has been authored by UT-Battelle, LLC, under contract DE-AC05-00OR22725 with the US Department of Energy (DOE). The US government retains, and the publisher, by accepting the article for publication, acknowledges that the US government retains a nonexclusive, paid-up, irrevocable, worldwide license to publish or reproduce the published form of this manuscript, or allow others to do so, for US government purposes. DOE will provide public access to these results of federally sponsored research in accordance with the DOE Public Access Plan (http://energy.gov/downloads/doe-public-access-plan).

REFERENCES

Abbey, C., Cornforth, D., Hatziargyriou, N., Hirose, K., Kwasinski, A., Kyriakides, E., Platt, G., Reyes, L., & Suryanarayanan, S. (2014). Powering through the storm: Microgrids operation for more efficient disaster recovery. *IEEE Power and Energy Magazine, 12*(3), 67–76.

Balcik, B., Beamon, B. M., & Smilowitz, K. (2008). Last mile distribution in humanitarian relief. *Journal of Intelligent Transportation Systems, 12*(2), 51–63.

Baxter, A. E., Lagerman, H. W., & Keskinocak, P. (2019). Quantitative modeling in disaster management: A literature review. *IBM Journal of Research and Development, 64*(1/2), 1–3.

Caunhye, A. M., Zhang, Y., Li, M., & Nie, X. (2016). A location-routing model for prepositioning and distributing emergency supplies. *Transportation Research Part E: Logistics and Transportation Review, 90*, 161–176.

DeCorla-Souza, K. (2018). *Feasibility Analysis for Petroleum Distribution Centers.* Tech. Rep., ICF Incorporated, LLC. https://oppaga.fl.gov/Documents/Reports/18-PETRO.pdf.

HIFLD (2019). *Oil Refineries.* Homeland Infrastructure Foundation-Level Data (HIFLD). hifld-geoplatform.opendata.arcgis.com/datasets/oil-refineries/explore. Date of Access December 2023.

Donald, J. (2021). Winter storm uri 2021. *FiscalNotes; A Review of the Texas Economy.* comptroller.texas.gov/economy/fiscal-notes/2021/oct/winter-storm-impact.php. Date of Access December 2023.

EIA (2022). Hurricane Ian temporarily disrupts Florida's gasoline supply chain. *Today in Energy.* www.eia.gov/todayinenergy/detail.php?id=54099. Date of Access December 2023.

Florida Department of Agriculture and Consumer Services (2021). *2021 Office of Energy Annual Report.* https://ccmedia.fdacs.gov/content/download/104182/file/2021-OOE-Annual-Report.pdf. Date of Access December 2023.

Florida Department of Transportation (2018). *Hurricane Irma's Effect on Florida's Fuel Distribution System and Recommended Improvements.* Tech. Rep., Florida Department of Transportation. fdot.gov/docs/default-source/info/CO/news/newsreleases/020118-FDOTFuel-Report.pdf.

Gao, Y., Chiu, Y. C., Wang, S., & Küçükyavuz, S. (2010). Optimal refueling station location and supply planning for hurricane evacuation. *Transportation Research Record, 2196*(1), 56–64.

GasBuddy (2019). This is how quickly gas stations run out of fuel and get replenished in the United States during major hurricanes. *GasBuddy News.* www.gasbuddy.com/go/this-is-how-quickly-gas-stations-run-out-of-fuel-and-get-replenished-in-the-united-states. Date of Access December 2023.

Kar, B., Brewer, J., Omitaomu, O., Iyengar, A., Roberts, N., & Hoesly, R. (2021). *Accessibility and Availability of Gas Stations for Liquid Fuel Supply During Severe Weather Events.* Oak Ridge National Lab (ORNL), Oak Ridge, TN.

Krishnamurthy, A., Roy, D., & Bhat, S. (2013). Analytical models for estimating waiting times at a disaster relief center. In Vasileios Zeimpekis, Soumia Ichoua, Ioannis Minis (eds) *Humanitarian and Relief Logistics: Research Issues, Case Studies and Future Trends.*. (pp. 21–41). Springer, New York.

Lima, C., Relvas, S., & Barbosa-Póvoa, A. P. F. (2016). Downstream oil supply chain management: A critical review and future directions. *Computers & Chemical Engineering, 92*, 78–92.

Masoumi, M., Aghsami, A., Alipour–Vaezi, M., Jolai, F., & Esmailifar, B. (2022). An M/M/C/K queueing system in an inventory routing problem considering congestion and response time for post-disaster humanitarian relief: A case study. *Journal of Humanitarian Logistics and Supply Chain Management, 12*(2), 182–219.

National Hurricane Center (2022). Advisory wind field and forecast radii. *NHC Data in GIS Formats.* https://www.nhc.noaa.gov/gis/. Date of Access December 2023.

NOAA (2023). Detailed list of continental united states hurricane impacts/landfalls. *Hurricane Research Division*. www.aoml.noaa.gov/hrd/hurdat/UShurrs_detailed.html. Date of Access December 2023.

Russell, T., Boutilier, J., Kleinmann, S. & Goentzel, J. (2020). Actionable analysis: Simulating and visualizing fuel distribution during disasters. Tech. Rep., MIT Humanitarian Supply Chain Lab, MIT Center for Transportation & Logistics, Cambridge, MA. http://hdl.handle.net/1721.1/126737.

Sabbaghtorkan, M., Batta, R., & He, Q. (2022). On the analysis of an idealized model to manage gasoline supplies in a short-notice hurricane evacuation. *OR Spectrum, 44*(3), 911–945.

Schmitt, A. J., & Tomlin, B. (2012). Sourcing strategies to manage supply disruptions. In Haresh Gurnani, Anuj Mehrotra, Saibal Ray (eds) *Supply Chain Disruptions* (pp. 51–72). Springer, London.

Snyder, L. V., & Daskin, M. S. (2007). Models for reliable supply chain network design. In: Alan T. Murray, Tony H. Grubesic. (eds) *Critical Infrastructure: Reliability and Vulnerability,* (pp. 257–289) Springer Berlin, Heidelberg.

Sun, T., Lin, J., Xiong, K., & Xiao, C. (2022). Route recommendation for evacuation networks using MMPP/M/1/N queueing models. *Computer Communications, 185*, 23–39.

Tomlin, B., & Wang, Y. (2011). Operational strategies for managing supply chain disruption risk. In Panos Kouvelis, Lingxiu Dong, Onur Boyabatli, Rong Li (eds) *The Handbook of Integrated Risk Management in Global Supply Chains* (pp. 79–101). John Wiley & Sons, Inc., Hoboken, New Jersey.

U.S. Census. (2020). *Florida Was Third-Largest State in 2020 With Population of 21.5 Million*. Florida: 2020 Census. https://www.census.gov/library/stories/state-by-state/florida-population-change-between-census–decade.html. Date of Access December 2023.

Wang, Y., Gilland, W., & Tomlin, B. (2010). Mitigating supply risk: Dual sourcing or process improvement? *Manufacturing & Service Operations Management, 12*(3), 489–510.

Wilbanks, T. J., Bhatt, V., Bilello, D. E., Bull, S. R., Ekmann, J., et al. (2007). *Effects of climate change on energy production and use in the United States*. U.S. Climate Change Science Program. https://digitalcommons.unl.edu/usdoepub/12/. Date of Access December 2023.

Yi, W., & Kumar, A. (2007). Ant colony optimization for disaster relief operations. *Transportation Research Part E: Logistics and Transportation Review, 43*(6), 660–672.

Zheng, R., Shou, B., & Yang, J. (2021). Supply disruption management under consumer panic buying and social learning effects. *Omega, 101*, 102238.

9 Deciphering the Code of False Alarms to Understand Public Response to Emergency Warnings

Ann Marie Major

9.1 INTRODUCTION

Over the past 40 years, the worldwide economic cost of natural disasters has reached $6 trillion, with costs quadrupling between 1980 and 2023 (World Bank, 2023). According to the National Centers for Environmental Information (NCEI), the cost of natural disasters in the US since 1980 is estimated at $2.655 trillion, with costs reaching $228 billion in 2022 (NOAA National Centers for Environmental Information, 2023). Between 2001 and 2010, the global loss of human life from natural disasters exceeded 1.1 million and left 33% of the world's 8.1 billion people impacted by the damage and destruction (UNISDR 2012; US Census Bureau 2023).

Prepared and educated citizens with an emergency plan and basic provisions reduce the cost of disasters. In fact, according to Healy and Malhotra (2009), every dollar invested in preparedness results in a $15 reduction in damage costs. However, a Wells Fargo survey of US adults reported nearly seven out of ten respondents lacked an emergency plan, and 75% did not consider planning or having the time to plan (Ramirez 2021).

Public response to emergency warnings is a critical concern for emergency managers and responders, given the potential for loss of life, economic loss, and social disruption that follow disasters. Preparedness and mitigation programs optimize public response to disaster warnings by encouraging public compliance with national and local emergency plans and procedures, including evacuation. Researchers suggest that the lack of public preparedness results from inadequate financial resources, lack of preparation and planning, as well as issues with emergency warning systems (Major 1999). One major issue with emergency warning systems is the frequency of false alarms. Three out of four tornado warnings issued by the National Weather Service are false alarms (Lim et al. 2019).

DOI: 10.1201/9781003648178-10

This chapter summarizes research examining the influence of false alarms in natural disaster warnings. According to Lim et al. (2019), the National Weather Service issues one authentic warning for every four warnings disseminated. When an emergency agency issues a warning, it is considered a false alarm when it does not occur, occurs at a different time, or occurs at a different location. False alarms result due to problems with the technology and accuracy of emergency warnings. Because false alarms are a product of the emergency warning system, it is important for emergency managers and planners to understand how people perceive and understand false alarms.

9.2 THE PROBLEM OF FALSE ALARMS

The prediction of phenomena is at the core of the scientific method in the social and natural sciences, yet the science of prediction requires that hypotheses are falsifiable (Popper 2002). The study of public response to disaster warnings brings with it an understanding that false alarms and "near misses" are part of the scientific equation. Huppert and Sparks (2006) argue that "disastrous outcomes can only increase unless better ways are found to mitigate the effects through improved forecasting and warning, together with more community preparedness and resilience."

From a scientific perspective, a false alarm is the prediction of an undesirable event that fails to occur. The false alarm effect, according to psychologists, holds that every failure of the predicted event to occur reduces the credibility of the alarm and, over time, the public's willingness to respond appropriately (Breznitz 1984). A second aspect of the false alarm effect (FAE) introduces an effect of fear caused by the initial prediction. Breznitz (1985) argued that a greater level of fear associated with the initial threat will result in a stronger false alarm effect when the threat is canceled.

Although the research literature examining public response and behavior in disasters is extensive, support for the false alarm exists only in experimental literature and a limited number of field studies. The difficulties social scientists face in studying false alarms in the field are the short time frame surrounding false alarms and the prohibitive financial and personal requirements for conducting field research following warnings that do not occur. The limited funding available is more likely to be directed to follow up on disasters that do occur.

Further complications arise in studying and understanding false alarms because of what defines a disaster. Chapman (2005) argues that the scientific community, in general, does not view technological disasters as predictable and has not developed the prediction systems largely because of a lack of understanding of the complexity of the socio-technological and natural events that cause disasters. One difference between technological and natural disasters is the complexity of the triggering events, which can be extremely complex in technological disasters because of the human-technology interaction (Chapman 2005). Applebaum (1997) defined socio-technical systems in terms of the interaction of human actions and relationships with technological tools and practices.

Challenges to human decision-making in socio-technological systems occur when key players work from outdated models that no longer apply to the situation and interpret information as reliable when it originates from unreliable sources. This then results in a dearth of information within the organization. A key concern that arises in technological disasters is overconfidence or a "false sense of security" because warnings are a means of testing the system itself (Reason 1997). Chapman (2005) points to the issue of cognitive factors, including "overconfidence," which can be viewed as unrealistic optimism, where people believe they are not vulnerable to a threat and therefore do not prepare emergency plans.

Another problem arises when an automatic alarm system is considered an inconvenience or a hindrance to smooth system operations and is turned off. This was the case on the Deepwater Horizon, an oil-drilling platform in the Gulf of Mexico, on the night of April 20, 2010. The automatic gas and fire detection alarm had been disengaged at management's direction. Management was reported to have said that an automatic system is less safe than a manual system. Workers on the platform said that the alarm had been switched to manual operation to avoid false alarms awakening crew members and corporate officials who were sleeping (Barstow et al. 2010; Lin 2010).

A different issue arises when there are calls for more and earlier alarms, especially regarding tornadoes and hurricanes, while at the same time, other emergency managers are calling for fewer alarms to reduce the number of false alarms. The rationale for earlier alarms is that longer lead times will result in fewer deaths and injuries. In their analysis of more than 18,000 tornadoes covering a period of 17 years, Simmons and Sutter (2009) found that the decrease in fatalities and injuries owing to longer lead times was equivalent to the increase in fatalities and injuries resulting from the increase in false alarms. Those who argue for fewer alarms argue that fewer will reduce the number of false alarms and decrease the reinforcement of the FAE. In a classic summary of human response to alarms, Janis (1962) argued that a sufficiently high number of false alarms will lead the public to disregard any warning that does not have attached to it additional reasons for compliance.

In theory, a false alarm decreases public attention and response to future alarms because the occurrence of the false alarm reduces the credibility of the warning system, which results in the false alarm effect (Baker 1993; Davenport 1993; Levy and Salvadori 1995; Mileti and Fitzpatrick 1993; Mitchell 1993). Warning systems exist for all sorts of disasters, including residential, commercial, wildlands, and forest fires; mass casualty incidents (e.g., a train derailment); explosions from terrorist acts or industrial accidents; weather disasters such as hurricanes and tornadoes; natural disasters such as volcanic eruptions and earthquakes; and technological disasters. In fact, many of these types of disasters overlap. For example, an earthquake can result in an explosion that then results in fire.

Simmons and Sutter (2008), in their study of tornadoes that occurred between 1986 and 2002, found that a warning, compared with no warning, reduced injuries by 32%, but that fatalities were only reduced by 1.0%. The researchers suggest that the lack of reduction in fatalities results from the few powerful, atypical tornadoes that touch down. Just 300 of the more than 18,000, or less than 1% of the tornadoes in their analysis produced fatalities, and of those, 15 killed more than ten persons each (Simmons and Sutter 2008).

Hurricanes offer another problem in that the longer the timespan between the prediction of a hurricane's point of landfall and its occurrence, the more likely the prediction is to be a false alarm (Regnier 2008). Because of their size, hurricanes can extend over hundreds of miles of coastal front and can change course unexpectedly, as was the case with Hurricane Rita in 2005. A hurricane's storm track may follow a more-or-less straight line, wander in a series of sharp turns, or even turn back on itself as it responds to pressures from other systems that steer it. For example, an estimation of where Hurricane Rita would make landfall, made 120 hours (5 days) in advance, was 197 nautical miles in error. An estimation made 12 hours in advance had an error of only 27 nautical miles (Knabb et al. 2006). Thus, the longer the officials delay an evacuation order, the smaller the population area that requires evacuation.

The problem of hurricane false alarms is not a question of whether there is or will be a hurricane but where the storm is likely to cross land. This information is critical to the question of evacuation decisions and how long officials can wait before they run out of time and evacuation is no longer an option. A small city needs up to 45 hours for an evacuation (Regnier 2008). For Hurricane Rita, the error in identifying the 48-hour position prediction was 93 nautical miles; that is, Rita would most likely make landfall somewhere within that area. The 36-hour prediction reduced that distance to 76 miles, and the 12-hour prediction error cut the distance to 27 miles. As noted earlier, Rita made landfall near the east edge of the 27-mile landfall line.

9.2.1 Frequency of False Alarms

Three out of every four tornado warnings are "false" (Brotzge et al. 2011; Lim et al. 2019). If an alarm is issued and there is no report of the predicted twister, as is the case for 75% of tornado warnings in the United States, the alarm is defined as a false alarm. This does not mean that no tornado existed; however, if the tornado was not verified, either by radar or observation in the field, it is classified as a false alarm (Barnes et al. 2007). Thus, it is important to understand that the causes of false alarms are not entirely the fault of the NWS but are a combination of NWS prediction accuracy and the performance of the distribution systems—mass media and interpersonal communication—over which the NWS has no control. Table 9.1 provides the proportions of false alarms by weather events, where the false alarm ratio (FAR) is calculated by dividing the number of false alarms by the number of disaster predictions (Wilks 2006).

9.2.2 Types of False Alarms

An alarm is a double-edged sword. A disaster can occur without warning, resulting in no warning. In addition, the public is subject to missed alarms, false alarms, near misses, close calls, and direct hits. If a warning is inaccurate and the event does not occur, it is clearly a false alarm. If a warning is accurate and no alarm is given, it is

TABLE 9.1
FARs for Ten Weather Events

FAR	Year	Event
0.75	1992	Tsunamis[a]
0.76	2003	Tornadoes in the United States
0.32	2003	Hurricanes
0.46	2005	Flash floods
0.31	2005	Winter storms
0.31	2005	High wind warnings
0.48	2005	Severe thunderstorms
0.48	2005	Combined tornadoes and severe thunderstorms
0.43	2003	Tropical cyclone genesis, North Pacific Basin
0.32	2004	Tropical cyclone genesis, North Atlantic Basin

[a] Morrison (2007, 12).
All other events: Barnes et al. (2007, 1–2).

a missed alarm, and a disaster may result. To the extent that any warning reinforces a false alarm effect created by previous false alarms, fewer people in the danger zone are expected to heed the next warning. An important finding from field studies that is relevant for emergency managers is that the false alarm effect is not the only likely outcome of a failed prediction. To date, the research indicates that there may be no measurable effect on the beliefs of some of the residents of the threatened area, and there also may be a mobilization effect in which some people believe they must make better preparations for a potential future disaster. Research shows that all three effects can result from a single false alarm: the false alarm effect, the mobilization effect, and no effect (Atwood and Major 1998; Farley 1998).

9.2.3 When False Alarms Happen

Earthquakes provide no reliable warning of when, or if, they will occur. Observed slippages and tremors in a fault line may indicate imminent danger, but the date, time, or magnitude of a potential event is never announced. In late 1989, an earthquake false alarm with a 50-50 chance for a "tidally triggered," 6.5–7.5 magnitude tremor in the New Madrid Seismic Zone (NMSZ) was predicted for December 3, 1990, plus or minus 48 hours (Davis 1990). Iben Browning, an Arizona businessman with no training in seismology, issued that prediction on December 12, 1989, at the Missouri Governor's Conference on Agriculture in Osage Beach. Although Browning did hold a doctorate in zoology, the news media made him an "earthquake expert" by uncritically reporting his false claims to have predicted other earthquakes (Showalter 1993). The NMSZ prediction was not Browning's first experience with earthquake forecasting.

Browning's false alarm for a December 3, 1990, earthquake was reinforced by an unpredicted 4.6 magnitude earthquake on September 26, 1990 (Farley 1993). The news media provided extensive coverage of Browning's prediction, and between September 1 and December 3, 1990, the local newspaper printed 147 news stories about the prediction; 46% were front-page stories (Gao 1991). Not one of those stories provided an explanation that the ambiguous 50-50 chance provided *no* information about the likelihood of the earthquake appearing on schedule. An estimate by two geologists (Johnson and Nava 1985) of the likelihood of a 6.3 magnitude quake in the next 50 years placed the likelihood of a damaging quake as between 86% and 97%, not quite as precise as the estimate of the businessman from Arizona, but far more realistic (Atwood and Major 1998). None of the news media stories pointed out that geoscientists are still unable to predict earthquakes.

9.2.4 No Warning and a Missed Alarm

If there is no warning followed by a missed warning or the warning arrives too late, a double disaster can result, as was the case on March 27–28, 1964. At 5:36 p.m. (Alaska Daylight Time), on Good Friday, March 27, 1964, a 9.2 magnitude earthquake, with the epicenter 12 miles north of Prince William Sound on Alaska's south coast, generated a tsunami. The earthquake lasted four minutes and caused damage estimated between $300 million and $400 million (1964 US dollars). The tsunami caused 11 deaths and $8 million in damage 3,000 miles away in Crescent City, California (Brocher et al. 2014). Known as "Tsunami City," Crescent City has been hit by 34 tsunamis since 1931, including the one generated by the deadly 9.2 magnitude Great East Japan Earthquake of March 11, 2011. The seismic wave struck Crescent City about ten hours after the earthquake, with a maximum wave height of about 8.1 feet. Sixteen fishing boats were sunk in the harbor (Nishijima 2011).

In 1964, the first three of the four seismic waves that struck Crescent City, though modest in comparison with the fourth wave, damaged or destroyed businesses along the waterfront, as well as docks and boats. On March 28, the fourth and most destructive wave struck Crescent City at about 1:45 a.m. and inundated the city (Anderson 1969). The California Disaster Office (CDO) issued two tsunami alarms based on information received from disaster officials in Alaska. The first alarm was issued at 11:08 p.m. and the second at 11:50 p.m., ten minutes before the tsunami was predicted to reach the Crescent City area at 12:00 a.m. local time (Anderson 1969).

Crescent City emergency officials did not respond to the first warning (Anderson 1969), and when the second CDO warning arrived, it probably appeared to local disaster officials to be too late for an effective local warning. Instead of reaching the Crescent City area at midnight, as predicted, the deadly fourth wave hit the city nearly two hours late at 1:45 a.m. on March 28). The harbor was destroyed, the city was underwater, and 11 people were killed.

9.2.5 A Near Miss and a Direct Hit

Near misses by hurricanes come in various measures of what is "near." Two pairs of hurricanes are used here to illustrate the false alarm problem and public response.

In 1996, Hurricanes Bertha and Fran were predicted to make landfall in South Carolina: Hurricane Bertha on July 12, 1996, and Hurricane Fran on September 5, 1996. Both storms struck the US East Coast, not in South Carolina, where they were initially predicted to strike, but farther north in North Carolina, just above the border between the two states (Dow and Cutter 1998). In South Carolina, 41% of the residents evacuated for Bertha, a Category 1 hurricane, and 59% evacuated for Fran, a weak Category 3 storm (Dow and Cutter 1998). According to the Saffir-Simpson Hurricane Scale, a Category 1 storm yields winds up to 74 to 95 miles/h (119 km/h). A Category 3 storm can yield 111 to 130 miles/h or 178 to 208 km/h (Schneider 2012). The final paths of the two storms crossed as they made landfall on or near the southern edge of Cape Fear (Dow and Cutter 1998, Fig. 1, 241). An estimated 750,000 people evacuated for the storms, and for many, if not most, of the evacuees, it was a false alarm. A survey of evacuees following their return home found that the respondents said they would evacuate again if advised to do so. Overall, there was no substantial false alarm effect (Dow and Cutter 1998).

9.2.6 A Too-Close Call and a Direct Hit

Hurricane Rita certainly was not a near miss for Galveston, and it may have been too close to Galveston to be a "close call" as the eye wall tracked along the northern shore of the island (Knabb et al. 2006), but it does provide a clear track, so to speak, to the problems associated with evacuations that are not well planned and controlled. Hurricane Rita made landfall on the Texas coast about 85 miles (straight line estimate) north-northeast of Galveston and caused one of the largest evacuations in United States history (Knabb et al. 2006). More than two million Texans tried to evacuate. An unknown number of evacuees were trapped in miles-long lines of stalled traffic, and 120 people died before Hurricane Rita made landfall (Casselman and Campoy 2008). One news story reported the experience of two people who had tried to follow the evacuation directive. A young woman who reported sitting in traffic for 16 hours trying to leave Galveston ahead of Rita said, "I'd rather drown than wait in traffic." A young man who had tried to evacuate gave a clear false alarm effect belief when he said, "I've heard about so many hurricane warnings before, and nothing ever happened." He did not evacuate for Hurricane Ike in September 2008, and rode out the direct hit in his Galveston apartment (Casselman and Campoy 2008).

There is a myth that hurricanes turn away at the last minute, and this myth is both supported and refuted by the experiences of Galveston's residents. Hurricane Allen in 1980 was a Category 5 hurricane when it encountered a dry air mass in the western Gulf of Mexico and turned south before reaching Galveston, making landfall north of Brownsville as a Category 3 hurricane. Hurricane Ike made no such concession to the estimated 90% of Galveston's residents not following the official evacuation order, and Ike made a direct hit on the island. Hurricane Rita turned northwest shortly before reaching Galveston and made landfall near the Texas-Louisiana border, but the "last minute" was a bit late, and Rita moved along the north shore of the island as a Category 3 hurricane before turning north-northeast. Table 9.2 presents the monetary damages (in US dollars) for 11 selected natural disasters.

TABLE 9.2
Damage Losses for Selected Natural Disasters

Year	Category	Estimated Losses (US Dollars)[a]	Event
1964	9.2	300 to 400 million	Alaska "Good Friday" earthquake[b]
1964	n.a.	8.0 million	Crescent City, CA tsunami[c]
1992	5	125.0 billion	Hurricane Andrew
2005	5	200.0 billion	Hurricane Katrina[d]
2005	3	12.037 billion	Hurricane Rita[e]
2006	1	270.0 million	Hurricane Bertha
2006	3	1.6 billion	Hurricane Fran[c]
2008	4	4.3 billion	Hurricane Gustav[c]
2008	5	24.9 billion	Hurricane Ike[c]
2011	5.8	200–300 million	East Coast earthquake[f]
2022	5	112 million	Hurricane Ian[g]

[a] Not adjusted for inflation.
[b] Alaska Earthquake Information Center.
[c] Knabb, Brown, and Rhone (2006).
[d] Adeola, F. O. (2009).
[e] Knabb, Brown, and Rhone (2006).
[f] Morello and Wiggins (2011).
[g] Mulligan and Chesnes (2023).

9.3 PUBLIC RESPONSE AND THE FALSE ALARM EFFECT

From experimental research, what is known about the false alarm effect is that people who experience the highest level of fear before the warning's cancellation are assumed to be the least likely group to attend to a future warning. They are the most likely to downgrade the credibility of the warning, and they are the least likely to take protective actions to save their lives and property (Breznitz 1984, 1985). A psychological explanation for these findings is that respondents experience a "loss of face" because of an initial belief in the warning and a belief that the preparations they had undertaken were a waste of time because the warning did not materialize (Breznitz 1984).

Drabeck (1986) pointed out that the experimental findings where Breznitz (1984) confirmed a false alarm effect did not consider the role of social interaction and news media coverage of the warning. Survey research does, in fact, provide some evidence of a false alarm effect; however, it is certainly not far-reaching in large measure, perhaps because of the complexity of interacting factors. In a panel mail survey of residents living in Marked Tree and Wynne, Arkansas, and New Madrid and East Prairie, Missouri, Showalter (1993) found no decline in residents' concern about future earthquake predictions in view of a false alarm. This might be because residents of the NMSZ region had experienced earthquakes, given that they resided in an active seismic zone.

Public response following two earthquake false alarms in California provides limited support for a false alarm effect. On April 21, 1976, Dr. James Whitcomb of the California Institute of Technology's Seismology Laboratory issued a prediction that a 5.5 to 6.5 Richter magnitude earthquake would occur before April 1977 in the Los Angeles area. Whitcomb made public that his prediction was a hypothesis as a part of his efforts to study predictions; however, in December 1976, he withdrew the prediction. In that same month, on December 2, 1976, a geophysicist with a doctorate named Henry Minturn issued a prediction for an earthquake on December 20 in the Los Angeles area. Minturn was not affiliated with any scientific organization, although he claimed previous success in earthquake forecasting. United States Geological Survey scientists refuted his methods. December 20, 1976, came and went, and no earthquake occurred.

In a longitudinal analysis of the withdrawn prediction and the prediction that did not happen, Turner et al. (1986) found that approximately one-third (27%) of their Los Angeles respondents recalled that a warning had been retracted, and 4 out of 10 (43%) recalled that an earthquake that had been predicted, in fact, had not occurred. Although these data provide limited indirect evidence for a false alarm effect, it is important to note that nearly three-fourths (72.7%) of their respondents did not recall the Whitcomb prediction two years after it was issued, and the majority (57%) of Los Angeles respondents did not recall the Minturn prediction.

A panel study in southern Illinois and southeastern Missouri communities provided insight into what happens when a disaster prediction fails (Atwood and Major 1998). Iben Browning's 50-50 chance of at least a 6.5 Richter magnitude earthquake for December 2-3, 1990, plus or minus 48 hours, failed to materialize. This study found support for the false alarm effect, with 45.8% of the pre- and post-prediction panel respondents reporting a decrease in their perceptions of the importance of future earthquakes (Table 9.3).

However, nearly 1 in 5 (16.8%) respondents reported what Mileti and Fitzpatrick (1993) described as a mobilization effect, where the respondents attribute greater importance to future warnings based on their experience with the false alarm. Nearly 4 in 10 (37.4%) respondents reported no change in the level of importance that they attributed to future earthquake predictions because of the false alarm. What is important is that nearly half of the respondents in the panel study remained consistent in their perceptions about future earthquake warnings. That is, the false alarm had no impact on their view about future warnings.

Respondents who reported no change in their views about how important they felt the earthquake problem was in the NMSZ were more likely to have thought about the earthquake prediction than were respondents who were characterized by a mobilization effect. Nearly 40% (37.4) of respondents who were consistent in their beliefs reported greater confidence in news stories about the earthquake prediction than did respondents who were more likely to report greater attention to future warnings (i.e., the mobilization effect). The "no change" respondents reported that preparations and

TABLE 9.3
Percentages of Respondents Characterized by the Mobilization Effect, No Change, and FAE Following a False Alarm

Problem Importance	%	n
Mobilization effect	16.9	44
No change	37.4	98
False alarm effect	45.8	120
Total	100.0	262

Note: These outcomes are from a 1990 survey conducted in Cape Girardeau, Missouri, following a predicted earthquake's failure to materialize at the appointed time (Atwood and Major 1998).

mitigation were very important and reported greater confidence in information from other people and experts (Atwood and Major 1998).

What this field study demonstrates is that respondents' reactions to a warning differ. Indeed, as Breznitz (1984, 1985) argued from his experimental data, there does appear to be a false alarm effect. However, survey research from panel studies points to a mobilization effect, where respondents are more likely to pay attention to future warnings, as well as a "no change" effect, where respondents maintain the same interest in attending and responding to false alarms following a warning.

9.4 DISCUSSION

A key concern about public response to disaster warnings is what the public learns from them, whether the events occur or not. In one of the few field studies exploring the false alarm effect (Atwood and Major 1998), many respondents were characterized by the false alarm effect because the mean for the majority of respondents who believed the earthquake prediction after the false alarm decreased from 3.57 to 2.29 ($t = 13.95$, $p < 0.001$). Respondents who did not think that the emergency warning was important maintained their belief that there was no concern to worry about; however, those respondents still reported undertaking mitigation behaviors. Nearly 1 in 5 respondents (16.8%) reported being more likely to believe a future warning. Disaster warning messages that refer in some way to the public's previous experience with disaster events will be more likely to gain the attention of the public and may encourage public preparations for a future disaster.

Once emergency management officials decide to issue a disaster warning, the mass media play a key role in disseminating the warning to the public and establishing a chain of events from the initial warning to public response. If a disaster warning fails to materialize, then research indicates the public will continue to attend to and respond to future warnings if emergency managers provide a coherent explanation of why the disaster warning did not transpire (Mileti and Fitzpatrick 1993).

However, post-cancellation explanations disseminated through the news media are not guaranteed to reach the same public who heard the initial warning and cancellation, and there is no guarantee the public will accept the official explanation for a warning cancellation or false alarm (Baker 1993; Ledingham and Masel-Walters 1985; Lindell and Perry 1993; Tonn et al. 1990). In the chain of events that follows a prediction, amplified news media coverage of the warnings leads to public interest and discussion, as well as information seeking about the warning (Mileti and Fitzpatrick 1993; Turner et al. 1986).

Communication problems, including warning delays and interpretations, result from differing levels of coordination among federal, state, and local agencies, as well as different policies, procedures, and equipment. The California Disaster Office's warnings and coordination with local emergency offices, described earlier in the chapter, provide an example of warning delays during the 1964 Alaska earthquake and subsequent tsunami in Crescent City, California. The mass media are seen as helpful in disseminating warnings, but after the event, the media rarely report information that would help survivors put their lives back together. Instead, reporters focus on "human interest" stories that highlight past events and hold interviews with survivors focusing on the emotional aspects of the events.

Research has examined the differences in terms of demographics in disaster preparedness and gender. For example, Morrow and Enarson (1996) found that women of minority backgrounds and those from lower socio-economic status do not have the power and resources to respond adequately to disaster warnings. Despite their lack of resources, women often assume the role of caregivers and have an interest in risk reduction because of their caregiver roles (Enarson 2001; Major 1999). In a study of Hurricane Andrew, Morrow and Enarson (1996) reported that women take on the responsibility of preparing family members by gathering supplies and undertaking protective actions if those protective actions are affordable.

Post-disaster analyses make clear that those members of the public with the least financial resources suffer the greatest losses because they live in mobile homes or dwellings that have not been constructed to withstand damage when weather disasters strike. They are less likely to own a car and are unable to evacuate from an area following a warning because they have no means of transportation, nor do they have the money to establish themselves in temporary housing in another city. They often lack the financial resources to purchase and store additional food and water. In a study of tornadoes, Lim et al. (2019) found false alarms to be only one reason people failed to prepare despite emergency warnings. The respondents who believed the tornado warnings were more likely to take precautions than those who did not believe the warnings.

The false alarm effect is a real-world outcome that has at least three characteristics. False alarms may reduce public belief in the warning system. At the same time, false alarms may increase attention to and belief in future warnings, which is the mobilization effect. The FAE may have no effect on the credibility of the warning system. The five most important reasons people act or do not act on a warning are the following: (1) the amount and quality of the information they have regarding the threat; (2) the extent to which they believe they are at risk from the threat; (3) their ability to afford preparations and evacuation; (4) the strength of their belief that they must remain in their homes to protect their belongings and property; and (5) their previous experience in taking shelter in their own homes during previous disasters and the belief that they can repeat the experience with no ill effects.

Human-technological interaction adds additional factors to the equation regarding the role of decision-making and the wisdom of deciding to turn off the automatic alarm system to eliminate false alarms, when those very false alarms may have prevented disasters resulting in a substantial loss of life and billions of dollars in property destruction. When the Deepwater Horizon platform sank and the fires had been extinguished, the world's attention turned to a disaster of unknown proportions, because oil had been escaping from the well and polluting a large area of the Gulf Coast and Gulf of Mexico.

Perhaps the most important lesson to be learned is that false alarms are a blessing and a bane for remaining vigilant in the face of disasters, and that the public, researchers, and emergency managers and responders need to remind themselves that false alarms are essential to disaster prediction, preparation, and mitigation.

The research reported here, and the outcomes of many other studies, support the false alarm and mobilization hypotheses, and it appears that over the past dozen years, sufficient evidence has accumulated to remove these two variables from the hypothesis category and treat them as permanent members of the sets of variables used in the assessment of natural and human-made hazards. It is no longer a question of whether they operate during events, but of how they impact other variables directly and indirectly and are themselves influenced by other variables in the equation. For many years, at least in political communication campaign research, the "no-apparent-effect" respondents tended to be ignored by researchers because "nothing happened." Understanding people who perceive no change in how they view warnings and how they prepare or do not prepare for emergencies is as important as understanding people who are affected by the false alarm effect and the mobilization response.

Would there have been fewer casualties in Joplin, Missouri, if there had been no sirens for the city's residents to ignore on the afternoon of Sunday, May 22, 2011, as the EF-5 tornado that killed 158 people in just a few minutes approached the city? The critics of warning sirens and the frequency of their use seem to believe so.

Respondents who reported they were less likely to pay attention to a future earthquake warning (i.e., the false alarm effect) were also more likely to have believed the prediction than those who reported a mobilization effect. In addition, respondents characterized by a mobilization effect, that is, those who indicated they would pay more attention to a future warning, initially were less likely to believe the prediction. Breznitz (1985) noted this outcome and commented that when one who has been "fooled" or "made the fool," there is likely to be the temptation to downgrade the importance of the situation as a matter of "saving face." There also is the likelihood that some people at risk from disaster—flash floods, hurricanes, tornadoes, blizzards—because they are convinced they are in danger, are more likely to be concerned about future disasters.

The false alarm effect, indeed, does occur, and its effects need to be considered when communicating with the public about disaster preparation. A substantial proportion of the public is neither more nor less likely to believe future emergency warnings. However, these no-effect respondents, who tend to be ignored in favor of those characterized by the false alarm effect, are much more likely to understand preparations for the event and are more likely to communicate with members of their social networks. The no-effect respondents may be a critical public to target with information, given that they are undertaking preparations, perhaps because they understand that false alarms are a fact of life in the face of potential disasters. Warning officials may remove the sting of false alarms by praising community performance because, in the final analysis, no one knows if any warning will become a false alarm until the danger has passed. After all, false alarms are a critical part of the emergency warning system.

REFERENCES

Adeola, F. O. 2009. Katrina cataclysm: Does duration of residency and prior experience affect impacts, evacuation, and adaptation behavior among survivors. *Environment and Behavior* 41(4): 459–489.

Anderson, W. A. 1969. Disaster warning and communication processes in two communities. *Journal of Communication* 19: 92–104.

Applebaum, S. H. 1997. Socio-technical systems theory: An intervention strategy for organizational development. *Management Decision* 35: 452–463.

Atwood, L. E., and A. M. Major. 1998. Exploring the "cry wolf" hypothesis. *International Journal of Mass Emergencies and Disasters* 16: 279–302.

Baker, E. J. 1993. Empirical studies of public response to tornado and hurricane warnings in the United States. In *Prediction and perception of natural hazards*, eds J. Nemec, J. M. Nigg, and F. Siccardi, 65–73. Dordrecht: Kluwer Academic Publishers.

Barnes, L. R., E. C. Gruntfest, M. L. Hayden, et al. 2007. False alarms and close calls: A conceptual model of warning accuracy. *Weather and Forecasting* 22: 1140–1147.

Barstow, D., D. Rohde, and S. Saul. 2010. Deepwater Horizon's final hours. *The New York Times,* December 25, A1.

Breznitz, S. 1984. *Cry wolf: The psychology offalse alarms.* Hillsdale, NJ: Lawrence Erlbaum Associates.

Breznitz, S. 1985. False alarms: Their effect on fear and adjustment. *Issues in Mental Health Nursing* 7: 335–348.

Brocher, T., J Filson, G. Fuis, et al. 2014 March. *The 1964 great Alaska earthquake and tsunamis: Modern perspective and enduring legacies.* Earthquake Science Center. Menlo Park, CA: U.S. Geological Survey. http://dx.doi.org/10.3133/fs20143018, https://pubs.usgs.gov/fs/2014/3018/pdf/fs2014-3018.pdf.

Brotgze, J., S. Erickson, and H. Brooks. 2011. A 5-yr climatology of tornado false alarms. *Weather and Forecasting* 26: 534–544.

Casselman, B., and A. Campoy. 2008. Many weren't scared enough to flee. *The Wall Street Journal*, September 10, A3.

Chapman, J. 2005. Predicting technological disasters: Mission impossible? *Disaster Prevention and Management* 4: 343–352.

Davenport, A. G. 1993. The impact of structural damage due to hurricanes and the prospects for disaster reduction. In *Prediction and perception of natural hazards*, eds J. Nemec, J M. Nigg, and F. Siccardi, 12–31. Dordrecht: Kluwer Academic Publishers.

Davis, J. F. 1990. *The ad hoc working group on the December 2-3, 1990, earthquake prediction: Evaluation of the December 2-3, 1990*, New Madrid Seismic Zone Prediction. Sacramento, CA: Report of the State of California, Division of Mines and Geology.

Dow, K. and S. Cutter. 1998. Crying wolf: Repeat responses to hurricane evacuation orders. *Coastal Management* 26: 237–252.

Drabeck, T. E. 1986. *Human systems responses to disaster. An inventory of sociological findings*. New York: Springer-Verlag.

Enarson, E. 2001. What women do: Gendered labor in the Red River Valley flood. *Environmental Hazards* 3: 1–18.

Farley J. E. 1993. Public, media, and institutional responses to the Iben Browning earthquake prediction. *International Journal of Mass Emergencies & Disasters* 11(3):271-277.

Farley, J. E. 1998. Down but not out: Earthquake awareness and preparedness trends in the St. Louis metropolitan area, 1990-1997. *International Journal of Mass Emergencies and Disasters* 16(3): 303–319.

Gao, D. 1991. *Content analysis of earthquake coverage in two local newspapers: Southern Illinoisan and Southeast Missourian*. Carbondale, IL: Unpublished manuscript, School of Journalism, Southern Illinois University.

Healy, A. and Malhotra, N. 2009. Myopic voters and natural disaster policy. *American Political Science Review* 103: 387–406. https://doi.org/10.1017/S0003055409990104.

Huppert, H.E., and S. J. Sparks. 2006. Extreme natural hazards: Population growth, globalization, and environmental change. *Philosophical Transaction of the Royal Society A: Mathematical, Physical & Engineering Sciences* 364: 1875–1888.

Janis, I. L. 1962. Psychological effects of warnings. In *Man and society in disaster*, eds. G. Baker and D. Chapman, 55–91. New York: Basic Books.

Johnson, A. C., and S. J. Nava. 1985. Recurrence rates and probability estimates for the New Madrid Seismic Zone. *Journal of Geophysical Research* 90: 6737–6753.

Knabb, R. D., D. P. Brown, and J. Rhone. 2006. *Tropical cyclone report: Hurricane Rita*, March 18–26, 2005, National Hurricane Center. Miami, FL: NOAA National Weather Service.

Ledingham, J. A., and L. Masel-Walters. 1985. Written on the wind: The media and hurricane Alicia. *Newspaper Research Journal* 6: 50–58.

Levy, M., and M. Salvadori. 1995. *Why the earth quakes*. New York: W. W. Norton.

Lim, J. K., B. F. Liu, and M. Egnoto. 2019. Cry wolf effect? Evaluating the impact of false alarms on public responses to tornado alerts in the southeastern United States. *Weather, Climate, and Society* 11: 549–563. http://dx.doi.org/10.1175/WCAS-D-18-0080.1.

Lin, R. G. II. 2010. Alarms, detectors disabled so top rig officials could sleep. *Los Angeles Times*, July 23. Available at: https://www.latimes.com/archives/la-xpm-2010-jul-23-la-oil-spill-disabled-alarms-20100723-story.html. (Accessed November 16, 2023).

Lindell, M. K., and R. W. Perry. 1993. Risk area residents' changing perceptions of volcano hazard at Mt. St. Helens. In *Prediction and perception of natural hazards*, eds. J. Nemec, J. M Nigg, and F. Siccardi, 159–166. Dordrecht: Kluwer Academic Publishers.

Major, A. M. 1999. Gender differences in risk and communication behavior: Responses to the New Madrid earthquake prediction. *International Journal of Mass Emergencies and Disasters* 17: 313–338.

Mileti, D. S., and C. Fitzpatrick. 1993. *The great earthquake experiment: Risk communication and public action*. Boulder, CO: Westview Press.

Mitchell, J. 1993. Natural hazard prediction and responses in very large cities. In *Prediction and Perception of Natural Hazards*, eds. J. Nemec, J. Nigg, and F. Siccardi, 29–37. Dordrecht: Kluwer Academic Publishers.

Morello, C., and O. Wiggins. 2011. Region tallies earthquake damage, mostly uninsured. *The Washington Post*, August 24. Available at: https://www.washingtonpost.com/local/region-tallies-earthquake-damage-mostly-uninsured/2011/08/24/gIQAFdxScJ_story.html. (Accessed December 28, 2023).

Morrison, W. A. 2007. *Tsunamis; monitoring, detecting, and early warning systems*. Washington, DC: Congressional Research Service.

Morrow, B. H. and E. Enarson. 1996. Hurricane Andrew through women's eyes: Issues and recommendations. *International Journal of Mass Emergencies and Disasters* 14: 5–22.

Mulligan, M. and M. Chesnes. 2023. Hurricane Ian costliest storm in Florida history, Reached Cat 5, new report states. *Tampa Bay Times*, April 23. Available at: https://www.tampabay.com/hurricane/2023/04/03/hurricane-ian-florida-landfall-damage-estimate-total-deaths/ (Accessed December 22, 2023).

Nishijima, T. 2011. U.S. town learned from tsunami. *Daily Yomiuri Online*. Available at: http://www.youmiuri.co.jp/dy/national/T120315004995.html.

NOAA National Centers for Environmental Information (NCEI). 2023. *U.S. billion-dollar weather and climate disasters*. https://www.ncei.noaa.gov/access/billions/, http://dx.doi.org/10.25921/stkw-7w73.

Popper, K. R. 2002. *The logic of scientific discovery*. London: Routledge.

Ramirez, K. 2021. Wells Fargo study shows most Americans are not ready for natural disasters: How you can prepare? *Fox Business*, October 1. Available at: https://www.foxbusiness.com/personal-finance/wells-fargo-study-americans-not-ready-natural-disasters-how-to-prepare (Accessed December 17, 2023).

Reason, J. T. 1997. *Managing the risks of organizational accidents*. Surrey: Ashgate Publishing.

Regnier, E. 2008. Public evacuation decisions and hurricane track uncertainty. *Management Science* 54(1): 16–28.

Schneider, B. 2012. *Extreme weather: A guide to surviving flash floods, tornadoes, hurricanes, heat waves, snowstorms, tsunamis, and other national disasters*. New York: Palgrave Macmillan.

Showalter, P. 1993. Prognostication of doom: An earthquake prediction's effect on four small communities. *International Journal of Mass Emergencies and Disasters* 11: 279–292.

Simmons, K., and D. Sutter. 2008. Tornado warnings, lead times, and tornado casualties: An empirical investigation. *Weather and Forecasting* 23: 246–258.

Simmons, K., and D. Sutter. 2009. False alarms, tornado warnings, and tornado casualties. *Weather, Climate, and Society* 1: 38–53.

Tonn, B. E., C. B. Travis, R. T. Goeltz, et al. 1990. Knowledge-based representations of risk beliefs. *Risk Analysis* 10: 169–184.

Turner, R. H., J. Nigg, and P. D. Heller. 1986. *Waiting for disaster: Earthquake watch in California*. Berkeley and Los Angeles, CA: University of California Press.

United National International Strategy for Disaster Reduction (UNISDR). 2012. Disaster losses top one trillion dollars as donors underfund risk reduction, March 20. Available at: http://www.unisdr.org/archive/25831 (Accessed December 28, 2023).

U.S. Census Bureau. 2023. World population clock. Available at: https://www.census.gov/popclock/world (Accessed December 31, 2023).

Wilks, D. S. 2006. *Statistical methods in the atmospheric sciences*. 2nd ed. Burlington, MA: Academic Press.

World Bank. 2023. Disaster risk management, October 16. Available at: https://www.worldbank.org/en/topic/disasterriskmanagement/overview (Accessed December 28, 2023).

10 Damage Assessment and the Use of Technology after Disasters

Implications for Emergency Managers and Others Involved in an Important Function

Natasha Byrd, Melanie Robison, and David McEntire

10.1 INTRODUCTION

Natural, technological, and anthropogenic disasters are occurring more frequently and affecting people in many ways. The factors contributing to the increased hazardous events may be diverse, including new and more intense hazards, climate change, increased civil and political unrest, and widening socioeconomic disparities. The combination of hazards and unique vulnerabilities creates serious consequences for communities and nations. For example, natural disasters cause nearly USD 500 billion in economic damage annually and kill approximately 45,000 people worldwide each year (Ritchie, 2022; Statista, 2023). Innovative strategies are critical to our efforts to successfully deal with the challenges disasters present to communities and nations.

The research presented in this chapter examines the vital function of damage assessment after disasters and explores different technological platforms that have been utilized in real-world applications (apps). While there have been numerous advancements in technology relating to damage assessment over the past decade, there is insufficient knowledge about this topic. For this reason, this chapter will review what is known about damage assessments and discuss the role of technology in this essential activity in emergency management. It will first present various concepts related to damage assessment and provide general background information

 DOI: 10.1201/9781003648178-11

on this function. At this point, the methodology used in this study will be identified. The chapter will then discuss our findings on the various types of technologies utilized and explore their benefits and other challenges. The chapter concludes with recommendations to help emergency managers and others who participate in the essential damage assessment function.

10.2 OVERVIEW OF CONCEPTS AND LITERATURE REVIEW

After a disaster, first responders, emergency managers, public officials, and many other professionals and departments will seek to understand the degree to which the hazard has affected the community. These personnel and their associated organizations will be interested in identifying what has happened, determining how bad the disaster is, exploring what post-disaster actions will be required, and applying for federal funding (if it is justified) to facilitate response and recovery operations. These activities are conducted by assessing broad impacts and evaluating specific damages and economic losses.

An **impact assessment** provides a broad evaluation of the consequences, including injuries, deaths, damaged and destroyed homes and buildings, economic losses, environmental destruction, social disruption, and the relation of the situation to the quality of life (McEntire et al., 2012). Thus, an impact assessment is comprehensive and examines the big-picture consequences of a disaster.

Closely related to an impact assessment is a more specific assessment. The common understanding of a **damage assessment** is surveying landscapes, buildings, and infrastructure to determine the extent of damage and identify pressing financial needs after a disaster (McEntire, 2022; McEntire et al., 2012). Damage assessments serve two purposes when communities seek federal aid: 1) gathering information from residents/businesses for individual and family assistance programs and 2) obtaining information about losses sustained by the affected jurisdiction for public assistance.

The existing literature on damage assessment has identified many different methods undertaken to evaluate impacts and losses. It also mentions the various stakeholders involved in this function, along with numerous challenges encountered. More recently, research has started to examine the impact of technology on damage assessment. Each of these topics will be mentioned in turn.

10.2.1 Types and Methods of Damage Assessment

There are various types of damage assessments. These include rapid, preliminary, and technical assessments (McEntire, 2022). There are also diverse methods of accomplishing damage assessments, such as drive-by, flyover, and site visits.

A **rapid damage assessment** is typically the first assessment performed during a disaster. Depending on the type of disaster, the rapid damage assessment is often initiated while the event is occurring or immediately after. These assessments help leaders comprehend the event's scope and begin to understand what resources must be deployed internally and requested from the outside.

The **preliminary damage assessment** (PDA) is a more thorough damage assessment performed by local, state, and federal administrative agencies. This type of assessment is more accurate and complete than rapid assessments and is a necessary step in applying for and receiving federal funding. However, jurisdictions are not guaranteed to be awarded federal disaster assistance funds. Depending on the disaster type and the amount of aid requested, local and county emergency managers must contact the Federal Emergency Management Agency (FEMA) to notify this government organization about the consequences of the event (FEMA DAOM, 2016). As a result, FEMA and emergency managers will coordinate with joint PDA leadership and Other Federal Agencies (OFAs) as needed to complete the PDA.

Engineering or technical assessments are "conducted by engineers, insurance agents, FEMA employees, and contractors" (McEntire, 2022). While these assessments are performed, those involved determine the exact costs of cleanup, demolition, repair, and rebuilding. Engineers can also evaluate the safety of buildings and notify residents if and when they can return to their homes or businesses. During or after these assessments, the professionals involved also outline a plan of action to repair damaged infrastructure.

There are also diverse means of accomplishing the three different types of assessments discussed earlier. One strategy employed during the initial assessment phase is an **aerial assessment**, historically via plane or helicopter. These flyovers are often used in large-scale events, such as tsunamis, hurricanes, tornadoes, earthquakes, or major wildland fires. The aerial perspectives can give a general understanding of the damages. Aerial assessments can also allow politicians and emergency management officials to have direct images without entering unsafe ground areas.

However, the most frequently used assessment technique is **direct visualization**. Direct visualization, whether by **windshield scans** or **by foot** (i.e., a **site visit**), gives damage assessment personnel and emergency managers a better sense of the location and scale of damages. This method often allows the collection of specific details to guide the response and aids in decision-making to identify and implement recovery priorities.

10.2.2 Participants and Stakeholders Involved in Damage Assessment

Many organizations are involved in the damage assessment process. First responders will arrive on the scene to assist in rescues, save lives, fight fires, and protect property. They also verify damages and report relevant information to their departments and other community leaders. Building officials and others in charge of infrastructure will also participate in damage assessment. Their goal is to assess the impact of disasters on residential/commercial edifices and other community structures. Additional entities are also required to fulfill this crucial disaster function. Those associated with voluntary organizations active in disaster (VOADs), such as the Red Cross and Salvation Army, may gather information about residential losses. Other entities, including the Chamber of Commerce, may tally numbers pertaining to damages sustained by businesses. This information will typically be submitted to emergency managers, who will compile the findings. If the scope of the event warrants further involvement, state and federal levels of government may also participate. Each stakeholder performs various roles in damage assessment, from physical surveys and structural assessments to data collection in different sectors.

10.2.3 Challenges in Damage Assessment

Research reveals that damage assessments must be performed as early and accurately as possible to obtain federal declarations, guide response and recovery operations, and facilitate financial reimbursements. It is also essential to understand that damage assessments may be performed multiple times after a disaster as conditions unfold and as data is gathered. Damage assessment is, therefore, not a single action but often a continuous and dynamic process that must be updated, repeated, and verified numerous times (McEntire et al., 2012; McEntire, 2022). Therefore, emergency managers can face challenges when performing this function and seeking assistance from state and federal sources. These challenges include timeliness, accuracy, and politics.

10.2.3.1 Timeliness

Timeliness is a critical factor in damage assessment, especially in the earliest stages post-disaster when life rescues are being performed. However, the initiation of damage assessment can be delayed due to limited personnel and a lack of resources needed to track losses. Access to affected areas may also delay damage assessments due to damaged roads, street debris, flooding, and other impacts.

10.2.3.2 Accuracy

Studies on damage assessments reveal that the personnel collecting information for the PDA are responsible for being as accurate as possible about impacts and then sharing pertinent data with FEMA. This is no easy task because the number of homes, businesses, government buildings, roads, bridges, and other infrastructure damaged can be overwhelming. Many mistakes can be made while damage assessments are being undertaken and compiled (e.g., missing certain locations, double counting homes, committing numerical errors when tallying results, etc.). Therefore, giving careful attention to this function and having accurate information about damages is vital after a disaster. For instance, once a jurisdiction has submitted the request for a joint preliminary damage assessment (JPDA), a representative from FEMA will follow up with local and county emergency managers to verify information remotely or conduct in-person site visits (FEMA DAOM, 2016). If the data is questionable, a disaster declaration at the state or federal levels may be delayed or rejected altogether.

10.2.3.3 Politics

The complexity of disaster management has led some people to call the PDA process a "political process" (McEntire et al., 2012). This can be demonstrated in different ways. First, local, state, and federal governments may be accused of a lack of preparedness or an ineffective response to disasters (Nelson, 2016). However, more specifically, there can be disagreements about damage assessment findings. Local and state government officials may exaggerate findings or attempt to pressure the federal government to accept damage assessment numbers in order to obtain as much financial aid as possible or receive it in an expedited manner. Disagreements can, therefore, arise about damage assessments, leading to public condemnation or adverse decisions that underscore the urgent need to help those impacted.

Once FEMA analyzes the applications for assistance, the organization will send the approval to the White House for consideration. The President may sign and approve federal assistance per the 1988 Stafford Act for presidential disaster declarations (FEMA, 2021). If the damages do not meet the expected thresholds, the President will instruct FEMA to reject the application or instruct those involved to provide further information. This can result in frustration among the affected community and state. Thus, politics may factor into the damage assessment process in various ways.

10.2.4 Evolution of Damage Assessment Techniques and Technology

The prior information provides what has historically been known about damage assessments. However, techniques for damage assessment have changed in dramatic ways over the past decade as new technology has been introduced. Researchers have increasingly focused on the new hardware available, such as imaging capabilities and sensors (Myint et al., 2008). McEntire (2022) also notes that "advances in technology are making the assessment of disaster damages far easier and more accurate than in the past" (p. 281). Innovative technologies used in damage assessments today include spatial video, remote sensing/satellite imagery, drones, social media and crowdsourcing, new software programs and mobile applications, and artificial intelligence (AI). Descriptions of these technological tools are included below.

10.2.4.1 Spatial Video

Spatial video utilizes GPS-enabled video cameras mounted on vehicles that are driven through disaster areas, whether the drivers are experts or civilian volunteers (Lue, 2014). Damage surveys that utilize spatial video are conducted faster and more efficiently than surveys performed without this technology (Kocaman et al., 2018). This technology also allows a more rapid confirmation of damages, so the process of applying for aid may be sped up considerably.

10.2.4.2 Remote Sensors and Satellite Imagery

Remote sensors are devices that can be placed in affected areas to capture measurement data without anyone being in direct contact. Some of these technologies, such as rain or flood gauges, may be physically present in the monitored location. In other cases, distant means of assessment, like radar or satellite imagery, are utilized to comprehend the scope and extent of damages (Munawar et al., 2022).

Various types of remote sensors have been used for decades to predict and assess damage in different areas. For example, the United States Geological Survey installs and monitors sensors all over the United States to measure floods in waterways, seismic activity, volcanic lava flows, wind, precipitation, and more (US Geological Survey, n.d.). The information on rising water levels or the strength and duration of seismic events can be utilized by emergency managers to estimate or predict damage.

High-resolution satellite images have long been employed in damage assessments using passive and active technologies (Havivi, 2022; Myint, 2008). Passive strategies are constantly monitored from a distance and require little human input. Active technologies require requests for information and surveillance on demand to seek out specific areas in question (Eguchi et al., 2008). In either case, by comparing pre-existing baseline images of a region to new photos taken immediately after a disaster, damage to buildings, roads, and geographical landscapes can be visualized and compared. Using high-resolution Digital Elevation Models (DEMs) or Digital Surface Models (DSMs), emergency managers and others can also assess the levels of floodwaters when contrasting them with previous images (Muhadi et al., 2020).

10.2.4.3 Drones

Types of aerial assessments that may achieve the best images are also extensively studied. Drones are additional tools for emergency management and aerial damage assessments (Zwęgliński, 2020). The Federal Aviation Administration (2021) defines a drone as "an aircraft operated without the possibility of direct human intervention from within or on the aircraft" (para. 7). These drones often weigh less than 100 lbs. and are operated from the ground using handheld controllers. They are often maneuvered within a visual line of sight to increase the safety of others nearby (Federal Aviation Administration, 2021). However, other drones can be operated from airports, offices, or other remote locations. Drones can be equipped with high-resolution cameras and transmit real-time pictures or video to the operator.

Drones have been utilized for damage assessment when aircraft are unavailable. Drones can access areas that could pose a risk to personnel on the ground. Unlike regular aircraft, drones may be launched from makeshift pads, which is a considerable benefit when airfields are closed due to damage or overburdened by other vehicles. However, research and practical experience illustrate that drone operators must be trained and that airspace regulations must be understood and followed (Greenwood et al., 2020).

Engineers in Colorado utilized imaging data collected by drones immediately following the devastating Marshall Fire in late 2021. Observations from these efforts were performed, and various data were used to evaluate long-term impacts, such as learning how the infrastructure would withstand a disaster. Drones allowed for higher quality data collection and improved visualization in areas affected by the fire compared to attempting to go on foot (Strain, 2022).

10.2.4.4 Social Media and Crowdsourcing

Numerous researchers are now focusing on data mining utilizing **social media**, which can be performed with various software programs, volunteers, and even artificial intelligence (Kankanamge et al., 2020; Nguyen et al., 2017; Shan et al.,

2019). According to one definition, "social media is a collective term for websites and applications that focus on communication, community-based input, interaction, content-sharing, and collaboration" (Lutkevich & Wigmore, 2021). As of 2023, it is estimated that over 60% of the worldwide population uses social media, including Facebook, X (formerly known as Twitter), Instagram, TikTok, WhatsApp, YouTube, Snapchat, Sina Weibo, Telegram, Reddit, and others (Shewale, 2023). The data generated from these platforms can be beneficial when conducting damage assessments.

For instance, **crowdsourcing** is a strategy of soliciting information from large numbers of users of these platforms for a specific purpose. Various case studies have shown how utilizing data from these methods can be used for damage assessment (Cheng et al., 2021; Imran et al., 2022). Based on experiences in the 2010 earthquake in Haiti, Nelson et al. (2010) concluded that crowdsourcing could be helpful with openly sourced mapping, as many countries worldwide do not have up-to-date maps. Assessments and responses may be expedited by combining openly sourced maps with reports confirmed by software volunteers cross-referencing the geocached data.

A crowdsourcing method was also evaluated during the 2013 Emilia earthquake by collecting information from smartphone users and utilizing it in the government's damage assessment and subsequent response. According to Cimellaro et al. (2014), "the idea is to consider residents that have a smartphone as a network of mobile sensors," who would then submit the photos and geospatial information systems (GIS) information to a central command (p. 523). This information can be pieced together for initial damage assessments and to prioritize responses.

In 2017, researchers in China likewise evaluated and compared social media posts to official assessment reports from government sources during two typhoons (Chen, 2021). They found that it is possible to assess damages to affected areas with a relatively high degree of accuracy by utilizing objective photos and the associated coordinates obtained from social media posts. This supports prior research in Australia with similar results when using social media tweets during the 2010–2011 South East Queensland flooding events (Kankanamge et al., 2020).

10.2.4.5 Software Programs and Mobile Applications

Numerous software programs and associated mobile applications and extensions are now available to utilize in damage assessment (see Table 10.1). This means that various electronic tools can capture and relay damages by using computers, tablets, smartphone devices, or any combination thereof. These programs and applications often rely on information collected before an event (e.g., property addresses and property values). However, local governments can create customized damage assessment platforms after disasters, while others may purchase proprietary mobile applications to assist in reporting after an event.

Some software systems allow assessors to take pictures, videos, and other images of damaged locations on any electronic device (e.g., smartphones, iPads, or tablets). Responders and other assessment personnel can input information as they perform evaluations or combine that data collected from other sources, such as social media or AI.

TABLE 10.1
Sample Software Programs and Mobile Applications

AskRail	An application available to first responders showing real-time data on hazardous materials carried by railcars on all Type I railroads in North America. In the event of a disaster, responders can access this information to assess the potential severity of damages and the types of response needed (RailInc Corp. 2024).
ArcGIS, Survey123	This application from Esri includes FEMA templates and allows easy access to its damage assessment forms (Using FEMA's Survey123, 2020). Esri also creates mapping and analytics software available on computer, cloud, and mobile applications (Esri, n.d.). The ArcGIS Survey123 program has pre-made reporting templates that can be used by civilians and rescuers or damage assessment responders. The damage reports completed by civilians during the initial assessments can then be confirmed as soon as feasible. Templates within this program can be completed and submitted via mobile app available on various mobile phone operating platforms, which has been a weakness in other application programs.
Orion	Another mobile application is available on various smartphone operating systems. It is designed to collect and organize FEMA damage assessment data. This allows users to upload photos and complete forms and includes the FEMA cost calculator to help estimate damage costs (Futurity IT, 2021).
Crisis Track	This software is a multi-functional application tool used in multiple situations. This program was created by a technical engineer and a GIS specialist, with input from an emergency manager. It can be used early in damage assessment to collect photos and GPS locations, coordinate response teams, and provide real-time maps. Other functions may be used for situational reporting, tracking response needs, managing resources, and accessing incident action plans, among other uses. As incidents progress, the program can assist in collecting and submitting documentation to FEMA, even directly from responders in the field (Crisis Track).
Veoci	A final example of software is available for both computers and mobile applications. This program also allows for ease of response planning, resource tracking, access to incident action plans, and up-to-date weather reports. Damage assessment forms are available to complete remotely, including instant photograph uploads. This program also facilitates responder communications with mass SMS notifications, check-in requests, and voice SMS messages that can immediately be sent to other users on the platform (Veoci, 2023).

10.2.4.6 Artificial Intelligence

Artificial intelligence is now being utilized to help predict and identify damage patterns, among other uses in emergency management (Cheng et al., 2021). **Artificial Intelligence** is a rapidly developing form of computer technology. As one author states, "AI is a machine's ability to perform the cognitive functions we associate with human minds, such as perceiving, reasoning, learning, interacting with an environment, problem-solving, and even exercising creativity" (McKinsey & Company, 2024). AI allows significant amounts of information to be analyzed faster than before and can even help predict specific outcomes (Imran et al., 2014). Artificial intelligence in damage assessment is a rapidly evolving and growing subset of technological advances (Bao, 2022). Many damage assessment studies involving social media and crowdsourcing utilize AI algorithms to mine real-time data (Hu et al., 2023; Nguyen et al., 2017). Additionally, artificial intelligence is also being used to model and compare images obtained via satellite or other means to assess the damage from disasters (Syifa et al., 2019).

10.3 STUDY METHODOLOGY

As mentioned earlier, this study aims to verify what is known about damage assessment and also identify how technology has transformed this function in recent years. The authors, therefore, applied to the Utah Valley University Institutional Review Board and obtained approval to conduct the study mentioned here. The authors then contacted several individuals in their professional network to question them about recent disaster events, processes, and technologies used in their experiences with damage assessments. In addition, the authors asked their professional contacts if they had any other recommendations for interviews through the process of snowball sampling.

Overall, ten participants working in emergency management agreed to be interviewed (see Table 10.2). These individuals include emergency managers, directors of emergency management organizations, and chief building officials in Colorado, Utah, and Texas. Interviewees also included two employees of FEMA: one at Region VIII and one individual at FEMA headquarters in Washington, DC.

Each participant was asked if they had experienced recent disasters, and the disasters examined in this study are presented in Table 10.3. Those interviewed were also questioned about how their damage assessments were conducted, what challenges

TABLE 10.2
Individuals Interviewed for This Study

Study Participants
Salt Lake County chief building official
Salt Lake County City Council representative/emergency manager
Texas director of disaster management
Colorado director of emergency management
Washington County emergency operations manager
FEMA integration team lead
Utah State mitigation planner/intern
Salt Lake County program manager
Project lead for geospatial damage assessments
Utah state liaison

TABLE 10.3
Types of Disasters Explored in This Study

Floods	On September 9, 2013, Boulder, Colorado experienced a major flood. According to Castellani (2023), the amount of rain the region received the week of the flood was equal to a year's worth of rainfall. With 17.24 inches of precipitation and recent wildfires, the rivers in the area reached record-breaking flood levels due to mudslides and flash flood activity.
	Winter 2022–2023 was a record year for snowfall for Utah, enabling counties to put funds aside for emergency purposes. As a result of the snowfall record since 1983, one county claimed a state of emergency due to the damages caused within the county (Fox, 2023; Brophy, 2023).
Windstorms	On March 13, 2019, a windstorm hit parts of Amarillo, Texas. The winds caused semi-trucks to blow over on the interstate, trees to fall onto homes, and breaking windows in historic buildings. Amarillo is considered the windiest city since it gets winds from Colorado, Kansas, and the panhandles (National Weather Service, 2019).
	On September 8, 2020, hurricane-level straight-line winds from the canyon hit Northern Utah from Logan to Salt Lake City, causing multiple trees to fall over and damaging the city's sidewalks, homes, and parks. Their top priority was getting trees off houses, roads, and sidewalks. Then, clearing trees from parks, city buildings, and private properties (Gonzalez et al., 2020). This was the third disaster in 2020, including the COVID-19 pandemic, the earthquake, and the windstorm in the Salt Lake Valley.
Earthquake	In March 2020, the COVID-19 pandemic caused an emergency order for everyone to quarantine in their homes; shortly after the shutdown, a 5.7 earthquake hit Magna, Utah. That resulted in 2,590 aftershocks in the same area from March 18, 2020–February 28, 2021, which were felt across the Wasatch Front Mountain range (earthquakes.utah.gov).
Wildfires	On December 30, 2021, the Marshall Fire was ignited and soon became the largest wildfire in Colorado's history in impact and devastation in urban areas (Dougherty & Johnson, 2023). The wildfire was a combination of two fires, Eldorado Springs and the Marshall Fire in Boulder County, Colorado – the area is known for downslope winds with plenty of fuel to feed the spread of the fire (Dougherty & Johnson, 2023). Doughtery and Johnson explained, "The Marshall Fire destroyed or damaged more than 1,000 homes and dozens of commercial structures, [it] burned over 6,000 acres, and deeply affected the lives of thousands of Boulder County residents" (Dougherty & Johnson, 2023, p. 1).
	The August 8, 2023, fire in Maui County, Hawaii, was considered the deadliest fire within a century, killing 97 people (EPA, 2024; Omer, 2023). The island had dry conditions, and high winds spread the fires quickly and displaced over 2,000 people. The Governor of Hawaii estimated the damage costs to be around USD 6 billion (worldvision.org). The island received aid from surrounding islands and the mainland.

they encountered, and what types of technologies were used to gather data to send reports to the state and FEMA.

The interviews about the aforementioned disasters were semi-structured, allowing for further commentary and insights. Interviews were digitally recorded and transcribed to ensure accurate information was documented for this study.[1] The list of questions asked in the interviews included:

1. Have you participated in damage assessment in a recent disaster?
2. Who was involved in the damage assessment function?
3. What process was utilized to conduct the damage assessment?
4. Was technology used in assessments? If so, which ones?
5. What challenges were witnessed during the damage assessment process?
6. What successes did you witness in this process?
7. What lessons were learned?
8. Do you have any other comments or observations about damage assessment that we have not covered in our interviews?

The information collected was then reviewed to look for important topics and trends, and the various subjects were subsequently integrated into an outline for this chapter.

During the data collection phase, the authors also examined other outside articles to learn about the disaster events and websites from various vendors who market damage assessment software, including many of the technology products discussed in these interviews. Preliminary drafts of this document were provided to and reviewed by those interviewed for this article to reduce errors. Edits and corrections have been made to the draft chapter where appropriate.

10.4 FINDINGS

While reviewing the interviews, we identified common themes, including the importance of impact assessment, the purpose and process of damage assessment, the diverse participants involved in the damage assessment process, the use of technology, the accompanying benefits, and the challenges of damage assessment. The findings section discusses the experiences the participants had during the damage assessment process and the obstacles that came with it.

10.4.1 Impact Assessment

The interviews reiterated the importance of impact assessments in determining what assessors should focus on during the initial hours of the incident or disaster. The findings revealed that completing impact assessments provides vital situational awareness and essential information about life safety concerns. This information can be collected within minutes and hours after a disaster event, helping incident commanders and emergency managers identify priorities and deploy resources.

One emergency manager mentioned that "most emergency managers or programs are seeing that the impact assessment is so important early on with many disasters."

If jurisdictions start with an impact assessment, they can obtain a baseline of the situation and then focus more on their damage assessment needs.

Another reason to start with an impact assessment is to quickly view the impact on residents' homes. One participant mentioned:

> I think the initial phase really is about housing because we get about 24 hours… grace period. And then after that, the community is just coming off the chain on being upset… They want to know when they're going back.

Assessment teams must evaluate the broader impact first so they can identify subsequent priorities and actions.

10.4.2 The Purpose and Process of Damage Assessment

When discussing the damage assessment process, those interviewed stressed the purpose of this function. One of the participants mentioned that "[a major purpose of damage assessment is to] get us the damage level that we need to file [for] state and federal relief programs." Thus, the data gathered after each disaster is used to see if those jurisdictions qualify for cost reimbursement from FEMA. This goal impacts the strategies for creating damage assessment teams, the time required to gather data, and the methods of collecting information.

10.4.2.1 Setting up Teams

According to those we interviewed, it is essential that those in charge of damage assessment identify and appoint appropriate teams to conduct this function and carefully assign these groups to evaluate specific sectors or to cover different areas (e.g., residential properties, businesses, infrastructure, government facilities, neighborhoods, downtown, etc.). In one case in northwest Texas, individual strike teams were created and assigned quadrants to ensure appropriate coverage after a devastating windstorm. However, in other cases, those interviewed noted the importance of creating broader strike teams with mixed disciplines. This approach can help the damage assessment teams see a bigger picture and have more accurate and complete data.

10.4.2.2 Time Required to Gather Data

Depending on the type and extent of the disaster and its location, the time required to complete damage assessments varied dramatically. An emergency manager in northwest Texas mentioned that his community could collect "56 jurisdictional assessments – 337 on the residential side, and 66 [on the commercial side]" within five hours. A community in Utah identified 225 locations where damage had occurred (consisting of 896 panels of sidewalks affected by the event) within three days of a major windstorm. Other participants noted that they were able to finish damage assessments within three to fifteen days, with some submitting up to a total of 4,500 individual damage assessments. Alternatively, some cases took much longer to complete the damage assessments – up to weeks or even months. This was particularly the case when historic buildings required extra attention and examinations from experts in this area.

In any case, damage assessments were a laborious process. Individuals sometimes worked 10–12 hours or more each day immediately after a disaster. One participant said, "[I would] get up early, pack myself a lunch, throw three bottles of water in the car," and leave for the assigned location. His only break was to "stop at a gas station to find a restroom." This same program manager mentioned that damage assessors on his team used a variety of means to gather information: driving in their vehicles, riding scooters, and traveling on foot. The participant in our study mentioned that he would drive his truck to different neighborhoods, where he would unload and ride his bike to view damages and then recharge his phone each time he drove to the following location.

10.4.2.3 Methods Used to Gather Data

Besides physically visiting affected areas, other methods were utilized to gather information about damages. In some cases, and depending on the disaster, centralized disaster recovery centers were set up to allow individuals to report damages in person. In other cases, local Emergency Operation Centers (EOCs) created internet-based surveys allowing residents to self-report their property damage from their cell phones or home computers. In these situations, solicitations were sent out through social media, phone applications, local news and radio stations, and a link for residents to report any damages resulting from a disaster. When this information was collected, personnel would need to review the data, clarify self-reports via phone calls to those impacted, and compile the overall numbers. These steps aim to ensure the reports are as accurate as possible before submitting the initial damage assessment (IDA) packages to the state and FEMA. Once FEMA receives the information, this national government organization will clarify the data's accuracy as part of their procedures to see whether the jurisdiction will get approval (FEMA PDA guide, 2021).

10.4.2.4 The Various Participants Involved in Damage Assessment

Those interviewed for this study indicated their use of diverse personnel to conduct thorough damage assessments. Our interviews reiterated that first responders, building officials, and emergency managers at all levels of government were typically involved in performing this function. However, other personnel played essential roles in damage assessment. For instance, the Civil Air Patrol was tasked with damage assessment activities after certain disasters. This helped to provide an aerial view of the locations impacted by disasters. There were also computer experts and others with unique specialties who helped to gather, process, or distribute data. These individuals and professional teams are mentioned below.

10.4.2.5 Satellite and GIS Experts

According to those interviewed, experts in GIS aided in creating surveys for either residential self-reporting or government officials involved in conducting community damage assessments. In some cases, links were created by GIS specialists to allow these individuals to enter data. In other cases, a mobile app could be downloaded, allowing personnel to enter information, take pictures, and submit reports 24/7. In either situation, the data could be visually represented (with different color-coded damages) and tabulated in spreadsheets. Those working with the US Geospatial Resource Center at FEMA encourage damage assessors to collect GIS information on different types of structures: agricultural, commercial, educational, governmental, industrial, residential, utility, and more. The role of the US Geospatial Resource Center is regarded as essential, as they help train FEMA officials to utilize powerful technology like satellites and geospatial programs.

10.4.2.6 Engineering, Historic, and Other Specialists

Some of the disasters required other unique skills. For instance, engineers who specialize in earthquake repairs were relied upon to analyze damages to structures and estimate costs for repairs and rebuilding. After the Salt Lake area windstorm in 2020, historical archaeologists were called upon to assess the damage to the tombstones and caskets that were displaced when trees were uprooted. These individuals had the ability to geospatially locate where remains were buried to ensure tombstones were placed in the correct locations. In another situation, one FEMA official noted that a particular damaged structure contained historical art pieces that needed evaluation. He noted that "there [are only] two people in the world that [are specialized to] assess the value of… the artwork." Since this was a very specific circumstance, it was not the building that was the biggest concern but the cultural pieces within the building itself.

10.4.3 Damage Assessment Platforms

Several technologies were mentioned as essential tools for damage assessment among study participants. These systems included Crisis Track, Esri/ArcGIS Survey123, the situational awareness section (SAS) viewer, Google Drive, aerial imagery analysis, and drones. This section will describe how these systems were used during the damage assessment process.

10.4.3.1 Crisis Track

An emergency management Director in Colorado noted that his jurisdiction uses Crisis Track, which he helped develop with a colleague who is an expert in computer programming and IT. After a prior disaster, this director and his colleague met in the emergency management office and started to customize the new software according to their needs. Over time, the software has gradually evolved into the system people utilize today. The emergency management director mentioned, "The Crisis Track version you're seeing is [based on the needs of our jurisdiction] related to… damage [and impact]." This allowed them to proactively improve for future disasters.

10.4.3.2 Esri/ArcGIS/Survey123

Several jurisdictions use Esri products, including ArcGIS and Survey123. One jurisdiction utilized these programs and sent out a link for residents to fill out a survey or self-report damages. One building official mentioned, "Our staff couldn't handle the volume of calls and different things, so our… GIS [specialists] and IT team actually… stepped in and built the Survey123." Residents could go online to report their damages by answering various questions (e.g., name, address, damage, insurance, etc.). When that information was received, personnel in the office would triage and follow up on the reports. Departments could return phone calls to clarify answers, hold video conferences, or assign inspectors to complete physical visits. Another participant stated that in addition to Survey123, his state has also developed its own data systems called I-Stat and P-Stat to gather damage assessments related to FEMA's individual and public assistance programs. At the federal level, a FEMA team lead stated, "There's Survey123… that our folks are now… encouraging many people to use." Esri's ArcGIS suite of products has allowed many damage assessment professionals to combine specific applications and extensions to customize their particular needs.

This program was used extensively after a particularly bad windstorm that occurred in late 2020. Four city engineers and two data analysts performed field surveys and damage assessments over three days. While these individuals were in the field discussing their software needs, they were able to piece together a combination of Esri ArcGIS programs and software extensions to best meet those needs.

One engineer described how it is common for data to be tracked in a tabulated list but suggested that there might be a better way to visualize the data. He stated,

> If you were to look at it like a heat map, you can see windstorms flow out of canyons and you see the data is centralized around these canyon corridors. Looking at a tabulated list, you would never know that…. Geospatially, it's a very data-rich way to take a look at what's happening here.

In response to the storm, the officials decided to use a combination of ArcGIS Survey123 for location tracking, ArcGIS Field Maps, ArcGIS Dashboards, and StoryMaps to allow for notes and stories to go along with the photos and locations they were collecting.

The data analysts were able to activate and combine these tools for use in just a few hours, with beta testing to take place that very afternoon. By the following day, their programs were ready for field use. Combining these different programs and extensions allowed data layers to present a more complete picture of damage, facilitating recovery needs.

10.4.3.3 SAS Viewer

One of the participants used what is called the situational awareness section viewer. A director of emergency management mentioned, "In that geospatial [system]… [we create a picture of what we call] a 'SAS pie'…. [It is an image drawn] on your impact area." The jurisdiction created its SAS viewer to improve situational awareness right after the event. This tool allows emergency managers to organize assessment teams and focus on the impacted areas. It enabled this director's team to analyze the various layers of the images and utilize that data to understand where teams were needed to initiate the impact assessment.

10.4.3.4 Google Drive

Some organizations use Google Drive to track information for various events. One mitigation planner mentioned that an organization she worked for used Google Drive and Google Sheets – a spreadsheet program – to track information. The spreadsheet was shared with everyone on her team so they could input the data together. The participant added, "[with the recent] spring flooding, we did a huge damage assessment push," and the Google Sheet helped compile the information. In addition to the Google Drive, the mitigation planner mentioned that her organization had a fax/email cover sheet with all the questions that jurisdictions in the state needed to complete damage assessments. She sent this document to jurisdictions so they could fill it out and fax/email it back to them.

10.4.3.5 Aerial Imagery Analysis

Another piece of technology used by those involved in damage assessment was aerial imagery. With this tool, assessors could see damage to rooftops and whether homes were taken off their foundations. A participant mentioned that when the wildfires in Maui, Hawaii, occurred, FEMA could not get an aerial view of the island and had no ability to go to the site in person. The organization had to rely on videos posted on social media to get an aerial imagery analysis.

However, aerial imagery is not always helpful in providing situational awareness. A project lead in geospatial damage assessments mentioned the downside of the "Nadir view – [or] the top-down [satellite] view." He stated, "I am unable to see [the] sides of the structure… [so his estimates are] going to be a little more conservative." Therefore, site visits by damage assessors may be required in addition to aerial imagery to see the sides of the houses and the condition of basement structures.

10.4.3.6 Drones

Immediately following the March 2020 Magna Earthquake in Utah, one emergency manager was able to utilize a drone for the first time. He stated that a law enforcement officer happened to have a drone in his vehicle and offered to use it to assist in visualizing damage to various buildings on Main Street. As these responders walked down the street and deployed the drone, they retrieved several photos of damaged buildings, which were then used to formulate the response and inform development of the recovery plan. This manager stated that by using the drone, "we could get a better visual of the damage that had actually happened." Since then, their department has purchased its own drone and trained two unmanned aerial vehicle (UAV) operators for future use.

Drones were also utilized during the Marshall Fire. The images collected from these devices were used for the IDA. However, one participant noted that he preferred helicopters over drones as they can go higher than a drone. Nevertheless, if no aircraft were available, a drone was regarded as an effective tool to obtain situational awareness.

10.4.4 Benefits

As technology continues to evolve, so do the benefits that enhance the ability to gather information for preliminary damage assessments. Those interviewed frequently discussed the benefits of filling out assessment forms with a smartphone in one's hand and automatically attaching images with the camera on the device. The capabilities of various technological services have provided jurisdictions with the ability to have multiple people enter data, while others monitor the GIS mapping dashboard and compile reports coming in from residents and public officials. The interviews touted the advantages of software features, user accessibility, and documentation.

10.4.4.1 Software Features

The software systems mentioned previously allow multiple users to access the damage assessment data. One of the individuals noted that with the technology, we can "have a lot of people conduct these damage assessments." He mentioned this is important because "time is of the essence." The nature of the technology allows multiple team members to sign in at one time to gather data. One participant added that technology has allowed us to "go out and respond quickly, track our teammates,... and collect the data within days of the event [is] real success." This allows jurisdictions to pool damage assessments, enhancing the richness of data in reports, which will help the affected jurisdictions meet FEMA disaster thresholds.

With modern technology, EOCs can also monitor data being recorded in real time. Each individual involved in damage assessment can capture pictures, record videos, and upload other information needed for documentation. The systems allow teams to see where members are conducting assessments in different panels on a map indicating where people have traveled. Geolocated reports enable teams to label properties surveyed with color-coded dots indicating residential, business, or public structures.

The EOC officials were able to identify who uploaded the information and, when necessary, occasionally communicated with personnel in the field. This allowed conversations to verify information while they were still in the area or to go back to clarify with photos from different angles.

10.4.4.2 User Accessibility

Software systems often require extensive training before they can be used. However, those interviewed noted that it is essential to have user-friendly software to allow anyone to use these systems when a disaster occurs. One participant stated that his "[technology is] so flexible and easy... that people can use it." The technology was so intuitive that users could easily apply the program's menus and processes to find what they needed. Another participant in the study agreed that it was easy for their community residents to report damages through their city app at the palm of their hand. He observed that residents were already familiar with submitting reports on a city mobile app they use. The program manager stated, "I feel like we have better systems in place [now] to work with our constituents on things or to pass information." Jurisdictions also offered resources to aid those unfamiliar with the technology.

Although many systems are intuitive and easy to utilize, one person interviewed commented on the value of "just-in-time training." He stated that training right after a disaster could also be provided to damage assessors to help them understand assignments, responsibilities, forms, assessment methods, and any other pertinent information related to their role in this critical function.

10.4.4.3 Improved Documentation

According to those interviewed, the technology also improved the ability to document, track, approve, and follow up on damage levels throughout the PDA process. One participant observed, "I think it [the technology] forced people to actually document better than we have in the past." The program manager then demonstrated a visual of how to go into the system and complete a report. The digital forms with dropdown menus helped assessors enter the required information and ensure that all relevant data was captured.

Another benefit of the damage assessment technology is that local leaders had access to various screens to see the impact of damages and assessors' progress in real time. A program manager mentioned, "This is great information for our leadership because they are able to understand the impacts very quickly and are able to understand resourcing requirements based on these impacts." Once that information is gathered, it can be utilized to create the PDA for the state and FEMA.

The detailed documentation speeds up the review and approval process. For instance, when FEMA personnel came to Utah to verify jurisdiction damage assessment reports, one of the emergency managers noted that they could see that "we had everything mapped out like this [and] they knew that we had the rates dialed in. They had our engineering estimates for how much this was going to cost." In another jurisdiction, a director of emergency management pointed out that "our data was so exact that FEMA had no problems or delay in approving it." Because the technology guides personnel to input data more accurately, FEMA spends less time clarifying damaged labels. In addition, it was mentioned that careful documentation of damages also allows personnel to track repairs. For instance, the location of damages to sidewalks helped city personnel find panels destroyed by falling trees, repair them, and note that the job was completed.

10.4.5 Challenges of Damage Assessment

Despite the advantages of technology in speeding up the damage assessment process, those interviewed for this study mentioned some underlying concerns about this critical activity. Some common problems encountered included communication between organizations, misconceptions about reporting damages, misunderstandings about FEMA disaster programs, and difficulty distinguishing between pre-existing conditions and damage from the disaster itself. Technological challenges included the inability of some devices to function outside of cell service, incorrect reports, and other unique situations.

10.4.5.1 Communication between Organizations

Depending on the type of disaster, multiple people were involved in the damage assessment process. This fact, along with different purposes for documentation and diverse means of collection, sometimes made it difficult to share information.

When multiple entities are involved in damage assessment, it can be challenging to communicate with other organizations. An emergency manager mentioned that "there wasn't a centralized authority [to] say… 'National Guard has been in here…. They've collected [information on] all the tree stumps…. Contractor 'A,' you won't need to track [this area].'" In addition, it was revealed that the way information was collected was chaotic at times because there were "multiple people… doing the same work over again… [which was] then disseminated to different organizations [instead of a single collective]."

The use of different platforms was related to the challenge mentioned above. An emergency manager stated, "Instead of using WEBEOC, [we] wanted to use [Microsoft] Teams. So, we were gathering situational awareness in Teams…. Other departments would use Google Sheets or Google Docs, and it was like… 'what is the plan here?'" Some participants mentioned how challenging it was to collect and evaluate data because there was a lack of information regarding whether an area was assessed or when a task was completed. One participant commented, "We get information out, but it doesn't always get to the right people. And that really became apparent as we were trying to track down this [data]." It was difficult at times to communicate effectively about damage assessments.

While collecting damage assessments to share with FEMA officials, a mitigation planner at the state level mentioned that her organization collected information from counties and local municipalities. She said, "Sometimes counties choose [to] collect all of their cities' information and then send it up to us in a big packet. Other cities just send it directly, and we don't really care which way it comes." The uncertainty of how information arrives often challenges people as they try to compile data to improve the possibility of receiving federal financial support.

10.4.5.2 Public Misconceptions about Reporting Damages

Some residents did not understand whom to contact to report home damages. State emergency management departments often received calls from disaster victims, and these individuals were directed to communicate with their city representatives on the matter. Participants commonly heard that people were trying to submit their damage assessments to state or federal authorities, not understanding that their local government required this information to tally damages, seek outside assistance, and begin the process of recovery.

Similarly, some individuals were unaware of how to report damages to the local government. One community was overwhelmed with residential calls, so the emergency management office created a link so people could report damages online. A community in Amarillo also issued public notifications to clarify that disaster victims could report damages through Instagram, Facebook, and X (formerly known as Twitter).

In addition, a challenge associated with self-reporting systems was accuracy and the need for assessors to verify damage levels. One participant noted, "[emotions may]... not accurately represent damages." For example, local damage assessment teams in one area received reports of significant sand on their driveway, while another resident reported that their basement was on the top floor. Those teams would go inspect the reports to document what they were seeing and clarify the claims.

10.4.5.3 Not Understanding FEMA Disaster Programs

Study participants noted frequent encounters with residents who did not understand the process to receive funds. "We were getting a lot of inquiries from locals wanting their money." An operations manager mentioned that a common challenge was that property owners may have misunderstood why public servants were coming to assess damages. One interviewee said that citizens often thought, "'Oh, you're from the government, [you're] here to help.' We'd be like... 'We're just trying to collect damage information in the hopes that this could provide individual assistance. But we can't guarantee that.' The people did not understand [how FEMA assistance works]." The damage assessment personnel and teams had to educate residents about the FEMA disaster programs.

Similar occurrences happened for local authorities after the PDA had been submitted. Mistakes included a misunderstanding of terminology in the packets. For example, FEMA would reject a claim because of the incorrect terminology, causing some pushback. A team lead recounted, "The state [had] to push back and say... it's right over here, and we called it this instead." FEMA's standards were not always met when the data was compiled and shared with those at the federal level.

10.4.5.4 Pre-existing Conditions

A challenge some jurisdictions faced was not having pictures of structures or locations demonstrating what they looked like before the incident. When FEMA clarifies PDAs, they say they need additional data, which seemed like a common occurrence among study participants. An operations manager mentioned there was scrutiny from FEMA officials when the integrity of the jurisdiction was addressed. "[They would say], 'We don't know what the pond looked like before'... [making it seem like]... they're not trusting what you've submitted." It was difficult for FEMA officials to approve funds when there was no evidence of precondition.

In other cases, the homes were so old that it was difficult for building inspectors to know what was pre-existing disrepair versus new disaster damage. The complexity behind this factor is that some constituents may see a disaster as an opportunity to claim pre-existing damage as damage resulting from the disaster. Some believed they could get money from the government and have their homes fixed for free. Nevertheless, the building inspector would say, "It was a challenge because you would see damage... then... realize... weeds [were] growing out of it.... that is not new." Those assessing the situation would be required to report that the damage consisted of pre-existing conditions.

10.4.5.5 Functionality Outside of Cell Service

Some of the participants in the study mentioned similar complications with the technologies used to evaluate damage assessment. An operations manager noted that his teams could not access some of the forms or dropdown boxes associated with their damage assessment programs because they were surveying the more rural areas of the jurisdiction. Another participant had a similar issue with cell service. If the cell phones were out of the range of service, "the application would fail to connect [and prevent real-time data collection]." Fortunately, when some of the damage assessors were back in the cell service range or could connect to the internet, the application would back up the data collected offline.

10.4.5.6 Incorrect Reports

Although technology can often improve accuracy, another issue presented during the interviews was that some applications would incorrectly mislabel damaged sites. During an interview, one building engineer showed us a screenshot of a map of plotted damages. Most of the damages were clustered in certain areas, but he pointed out a couple of points plotted far outside this location. Those outliers were clearly marked incorrectly and provided a false report of damages in an unaffected area. The building engineer spoke briefly about his team's efforts to resolve the problem. During the damage assessment, he instructed his crews to ensure the address was marked correctly at each site.

Another situation included incorrect labeling across two different software platforms. An operations manager indicated that one particular software program would often mislabel something with minor damage as having been destroyed. This jurisdiction decided to switch to a different system after FEMA pointed out the discrepancies. Once the software was switched, those collecting damage assessment reports had less trouble with mislabeling.

10.4.5.7 Unique Circumstances

There were other unique situations that presented challenges for damage assessors, many of which were out of anyone's control. In the case of the Magna earthquake, a participant mentioned that the PDA process had to start over after each aftershock. Questions arose about the possibility of damage being aggravated by the new tremors.

In addition, the Magna earthquake occurred during the COVID-19 pandemic. One individual said his organization was leery of sending people out and inspecting residential homes. They did not want people to get sick and risk spreading the virus to their families. Residents did not want to allow people into their homes for the same reason. This required emergency managers and other personnel to collect evidence of damages in a digital (photographic and video) format, which was reviewed by FEMA personnel in regional offices rather than in the field.

After a major flood incident, an emergency management director mentioned the amount of detail teams needed to collect. He said that some were able to gather information quickly while others were moving at a slower pace due to the amount of detail they were collecting. When discussing the different types of multi-disciplinary teams that are in the field, one participant mentioned, "You get these teams… that are slowed down, and it's not that [their work is] more important, but they're just slowed down because [of] a different focus [in the assessment process]." For instance, some departments involved in the damage assessment look into issues that pose a risk to public safety and monitor floods or other hazards that can potentially threaten community health. Collecting that data may take more time than other information gathered through the normal PDA process.

Another challenge that participants noted was public involvement in cleanup before damage assessments were completed. An operations manager mentioned, "I think this is a Utah phenomenon, and it was very much prevalent here. By the time we got there to do the assessments, there had been neighbors… coming by to help [the victims] already." It was common for local religious groups to help others start the recovery and repair process, not understanding that pictures of the affected structures could help the municipality receive additional aid.

10.5 SOLUTIONS AND RECOMMENDATIONS

Based on the findings of our study, several important recommendations for damage assessment became apparent. The participants who were interviewed offered great insight into what worked for them, what did not work, and ways that processes might be improved in the future. Using this information, we suggest improvements relating to after-action reviews and proactive measures, training for damage assessment, and finding alternatives for jurisdictions that may not have the budget to purchase technology.

10.5.1 After-Action Reviews and Proactive Measures

In order to prevent some of the problems encountered during damage assessments or to improve preparedness for this function, it was revealed that emergency managers could and should conduct an after-action review to review successes and lessons learned. Some organizations struggle to understand the importance of implementing an after-action review. One participant added, "You would think that we would learn from previous [experience with damage assessments], and we don't." The purpose of having after-action reviews is to activate proactive measures for the next disaster.

Another one of the lessons is the need to have a pre-existing record of properties and their estimated values before disasters occur. However, one operations manager mentioned, "How do you know what to go take pictures of? [Do you need photographs of] every road… and every piece of infrastructure?" Such pictures could prove useful for damage assessment. Therefore, personnel should determine if and to what extent they may take pictures of critical infrastructures within the jurisdiction boundaries, store those somewhere, and update those files frequently.

Planning scenarios should also be run proactively to predict and prepare for the impacts of potential disasters that may occur in their jurisdictions. One individual suggested: "Instill in [the residents and local leaders] that it is... one of their main priorities... to plan for these things." For example, the people in Utah have been told for the past few decades that they are overdue for "the big one" – an earthquake that would widely impact the community – along with the plea to be prepared for any disaster that may occur. One participant added that people would go to emergency preparedness expos, then gradually lose interest, and that would become a cycle. The participant added, "I would go to... preparedness fairs and people would be like, 'I've lived here my whole life... What are you guys talking about? I've heard that since I was a kid, and nothing's ever happened.'" If there is a sense of disinterest, then people tend not to be prepared ahead of time.

Another suggestion was extended by a FEMA team lead, who recommended having mutual aid agreements in place ahead of disaster events to ensure enough personnel are trained in time. One building official mentioned that one of the lessons they learned from not being prepared was that "I probably would have involved the county and state levels quicker." Some study participants noted their concerns about not having enough personnel to aid in damage assessments. Based on the interviews, participants showed appreciation for any help they received from any level of experience in damage assessment, and luckily, they had the resources to implement just-in-time training for those people.

10.5.2 Damage Assessment Training

Another part of preparedness is incorporating training into the action review process. One community in Colorado does all of its training through its PDA team. A director of emergency management noted that their organization trains, "Twice a year, they... bring the damage assessment team together. They will review the plan, and they'll do an exercise... [making] sure that everyone is trained and feels good connected." They also mentioned ensuring that impact assessment is included during the training exercises.

Some participants' common theme was a lack of preparedness or training. One participant mentioned, "So few people test recovery capabilities in their exercise network that you never really get to know what your true capacity is." Other participants mentioned that one of the lessons they learned after a disaster was to assign multidisciplinary teams immediately following a windshield assessment. An emergency manager recommended "[practice] pre-defining strike teams... and practice the idea of a windshield assessment." It is good practice to establish frequent training exercises to get the practice into "muscle memory."

Still, certain communities have incorporated training sessions into their schedules to instill knowledge of the damage assessment process and to ensure all other departments (e.g., the police department and fire services) understand their roles in the damage assessment process. One community trained over 500 people to participate in damage assessments and noted the recommendation to use the FEMA Preliminary Damage Assessment Guide as a reference when starting a training program (www.fema.gov/sites/default/files/documents/fema_2021-pda-guide.pdf).

10.5.3 Technological Alternatives for Jurisdictions

A final concern participants brought up was the cost of damage assessment technology. Some software charges are based on the size of the population, costing $15,000 or more per year for municipalities with a smaller population. Many communities do not have the funds available to purchase such systems. A couple of recommendations were discussed as a result. An operations manager mentioned the need to have government officials address getting a budget approved to either purchase a system or to task an in-house team of IT specialists to create their solutions. An operations manager in Utah and an emergency manager in Colorado mentioned that both states purchased licenses for their jurisdictions to use ArcGIS Survey123 (Utah) and Crisis Track (Colorado).

10.6 CONCLUSIONS

As illustrated in our literature review and the findings of this study, the damage assessment function is complex and dynamic. Different people and organizations are involved in damage assessments, requiring input from numerous professionals and civilians. Assessment is not a single event but a continuous process detailing the impacts of a type of disaster. Technology has transformed damage assessments, including tools such as SAS viewers, sensors, aerial imagery systems (i.e., drones, helicopters, and other aircraft). In addition, software programs (e.g., Esri/ArcGIS Survey 123 and Crisis Track) as well as social media and artificial intelligence resources can assist in the collection and evaluation of damages. These technology options have rapidly assisted in data collection and interpretation. This, in turn, facilitates immediate rescue operations, helps in ongoing response efforts, creates daily action plans, secures additional funding, and supports long-term recovery.

The accounts of study participants provided some useful details needed to demonstrate how the damage assessment process has transitioned from paperwork to electronic storage processes to accumulate the reports needed to potentially receive aid from FEMA. We recommend further research to learn how other jurisdictions implement damage assessment methods. In addition, we encourage emergency managers to explore ways technology can improve this function and ensure participants are trained on the latest and greatest advances in this area.

NOTE

1. The "views expressed in the [study] do not necessarily represent the views of the agency, [organizations], or the United States" (see 5 CFR 2635.807(b)(2)) since this study reflects the experiences of various professionals in emergency management and includes anecdotal accounts of the damage assessment process.

REFERENCES

Bao, H., Zeng, C., Peng, Y., & Wu, S. (2022). The use of digital technologies for landslide disaster risk research and disaster risk management: Progress and prospects. *Environmental Earth Sciences*, *81*(18). https://doi.org/10.1007/s12665-022-10575-7.

Brophy, A. (2023, March 24). 2022-23 statewide snowpack breaks the 40-year-old record. *ABC4 Utah.* https://www.abc4.com/news/top-stories/2022-23-statewide-snowpack-expected-to-break-40-year-old-record-friday/.

Castellani, B. (2023, September 14). The 2013 Boulder flood: Ten Years and three billion dollars later. *BoulderCAST.* https://bouldercast.com/the-2013-boulder-flood-two-years-and-three-billion-dollars-later/.

Chen, Z., & Lim, S. (2021). Social media data-based typhoon disaster assessment. *International Journal of Disaster Risk Reduction, 64,* 102482. https://doi.org/10.1016/j.ijdrr.2021.102482.

Cheng, C., Behzadan, A. H., & Noshadravan, A. (2021). Deep learning for post-hurricane aerial damage assessment of buildings. *Computer-Aided Civil and Infrastructure Engineering, 36*(6), 695–710. https://doi.org/10.1111/mice.12658.

Cimellaro, G. P., Scura, G., Renschler, C. S., Reinhorn, A. M., & Kim, H. U. (2014). Rapid building damage assessment system using mobile phone technology. *Earthquake Engineering and Engineering Vibration, 13*(3), 519–533. https://doi.org/10.1007/s11803-014-0259-4.

Dougherty, M. T., & Johnson, C. (2023, June 8). *Marshall fire investigative summary and review – Boulder County, Colorado.* Marshall Fire Investigative Summary and Review. https://assets.bouldercounty.gov/wp-content/uploads/2023/06/marshall-fire-investigative-summary.pdf.

Earthquakes.utah.gov. (2020). *Magna quake.* https://earthquakes.utah.gov/magna-quake/.

Eguchi RT, Huyck CK, Ghosh S, Adams BJ. (2008). The application of remote sensing technologies for disaster management. The 14th World Conference on Earthquake Engineering, October 12-17, 2008, Beijing, China.

Environmental Protection Agency. (2024). *Maui wildfires.* https://www.epa.gov/maui-wildfires.

Esri. (n.d.). *GIS mapping software, location intelligence, spatial analytics.* https://www.esri.com/en-us/home#carousel-banner-item-efd7fb457b-tabpanel.

Federal Aviation Administration. (2021). *14 CFR § 107.3 – Definitions.* Code of Federal Regulations. https://www.law.cornell.edu/cfr/text/14/107.3.

Federal Emergency Management Agency. (2021, August). *Preliminary damage assessment guide.* https://www.fema.gov/sites/default/files/documents/fema_2021-pda-guide.pdf.

FEMA. (2016, April 5). *Damage assessment operations manual.* FEMA.gov. https://www.fema.gov/sites/default/files/2020-07/fema_damage-assessment-manual_4-5-2016.pdf.

Fox, D. (2023, May 31). Utah County declares state of emergency after over $10m in flooding damages. *ABC4 Utah.* https://www.abc4.com/news/top-stories/utah-county-declares-state-of-emergency-after-over-10m-in-flooding-damages/.

Fox 13 News Utah (KSTU) (2021, August 2). *Enoch under state of emergency as 10 percent of population deals with flooding aftermath. FOX 13 News Utah (KSTU).* https://www.fox13now.com/news/local-news/enoch-under-state-of-emergency-as-10-percent-of-population-deals-with-flooding-aftermath.

Futurity IT. (2021, March 29). *Orion - Futurity IT.* Futurity IT. https://futurityit.com/orionprotected/.

Greenwood, F., Nelson, E. L., & Greenough, P. G. (2020). Flying into the hurricane: A case study of UAV use in damage assessment during the 2017 hurricanes in Texas and Florida. *PLOS ONE, 15*(2), e0227808. https://doi.org/10.1371/journal.pone.0227808.

Gonzalez, N., Stevens, T., & Means, S. P. (2020, September 9). Utah declares state of emergency after windstorm knocked down thousands of trees. *The Salt Lake Tribune.* https://www.sltrib.com/news/2020/09/09/utahs-winds-are-dying/.

Havivi, S., Rotman, S. R., Blumberg, D. G., & Maman, S. (2022). Damage assessment in rural environments following natural disasters using Multi-Sensor Remote Sensing data. *Sensors*, *22*(24), 9998. https://doi.org/10.3390/s22249998.

Hu, Y., Mai, G., Cundy, C., Choi, K., Lao, N., Liu, W., Lakhanpal, G., Zhou, R. Z., & Joseph, K. (2023). Geo-knowledge-guided GPT models improve the extraction of location descriptions from disaster-related social media messages. *International Journal of Geographical Information Science*, *37*(11), 2289–2318. https://doi.org/10.1080/13658816.2023.2266495.

Imran, M., Castillo, C., Lucas, J., Meier, P., & Vieweg, S. (2014). AIDR: Artificial intelligence for disaster response. In *Proceedings of the ACM Conference on WWW,* Seoul, 7-11 April 2014, 159-162..

Imran M, Qazi U, Ofli F, Peterson S, Alam F. (2022). AI for disaster rapid damage assessment from microblogs. Proceedings of the AAAI Conference on Artificial Intelligence 36(11):12517-12523.

Juvare. (2023, August 9). *Crisis track*. https://www.juvare.com/crisis-track/.

Kankanamge, N., Yigitcanlar, T., Goonetilleke, A., & Kamruzzaman, M. (2020). Determining disaster severity through social media analysis: Testing the methodology with South East Queensland Flood tweets. *International Journal of Disaster Risk Reduction, 42*, 101360.

Kocaman, S., Anbaroğlu, B., Gökçeoğlu, C., & Altan, O. (2018). A review on citizen science (CITSCI) applications for disaster management. *The International Archives of the Photogrammetry, Remote Sensing and Spatial Information Sciences, XLII-3/W4*, 301–306. https://doi.org/10.5194/isprs-archives-xlii-3-w4-301-2018.

Lue, E., Wilson, J. P., & Curtis, A. (2014). Conducting disaster damage assessments with Spatial Video, experts, and citizens. *Applied Geography*, *52*, 46–54. https://doi.org/10.1016/j.apgeog.2014.04.014.

Lutkevich, B., & Wigmore, I. (2021, September 3). Social media. *WhatIs.com*. https://www.techtarget.com/whatis/definition/social-media.

McEntire, D. A. (2022). *Disaster response and recovery: Strategies and tactics for resilience*. Hoboken, NJ: John Wiley & Sons.

McEntire, D. A., Souza, J., Collins, M., Peters, E. J., & Sadiq, A. (2012). An introspective glance into damage assessment: challenges and lessons learned from the Paso Robles (San Simeon) earthquake. *Natural Hazards*, *61*(3), 1389–1409. https://doi.org/10.1007/s11069-011-0071-7.

McKinsey & Company. (2023, April 24). *What is AI?* https://www.mckinsey.com/featured-insights/mckinsey-explainers/what-is-ai.

Muhadi NA, Abdullah AF, Bejo SK, Mahadi MR, Mijic A. (2020). The use of LiDAR-derived DEM in flood applications: A review. Remote Sensing 12(14):2308.

Munawar, H. S., Hammad, A. W. A., & Waller, S. T. (2022). Remote sensing methods for flood prediction: A review. *Sensors*, *22*(3), 960. https://doi.org/10.3390/s22030960.

Myint, S. W., Yuan, M., Cerveny, R. S., & Giri, C. (2008). Categorizing natural disaster damage assessment using satellite-based geospatial techniques. *Natural Hazards and Earth System Sciences*, *8*(4), 707–719. https://doi.org/10.5194/nhess-8-707-2008.

National Weather Service. (2019). March 13, 2019 High Wind Event. Available at: https://www.weather.gov/ama/March13_2019_HighWinds (accessed June 15, 2025).

Nelson A, Sigal I, Zambrano D. (2010). Media, information systems and communities: Lessons from Haiti. John S. and James L. Knight Foundation. Available at: https://www.academia.edu/419632/Media_Information_Systems_and_Community_Lessons_from_Haiti (accessed June 15, 2025).

Nelson, T. (2016). The United States stands ready to be of assistance: On the politics and humanitarianism of natural disaster. *Global Society, 30*(4), 540–557. https://doi.org/10.1080/13600826.2016.1158698.

Nguyen, D. T., Ofli, F., Imran, M., & Mitra, P. (2017). Damage assessment from social media imagery data during disasters. *ASONAM '17.* https://doi.org/10.1145/3110025.3110109.

Omer, S. (2023, October 10). Maui wildfires: Facts, FAQs, and how to help. *World Vision.* https://www.worldvision.org/disaster-relief-news-stories/maui-wildfires-facts-faqs-how-to-help.

Railinc Corp. (2024). *AskRail.* https://askrail.us/.

Ritchie, H. (2022, December 7). *Natural disasters.* Our World in Data. https://ourworldindata.org/natural-disasters#natural-disasters-kill-tens-of-thousands-each-year.

Shan, S., Zhao, F., Wei, Y., & Liu, M. (2019). Disaster management 2.0: A real-time disaster damage assessment model based on mobile social media data—A case study of Weibo (Chinese Twitter). *Safety Science, 115*, 393–413. https://doi.org/10.1016/j.ssci.2019.02.029.

Shewale, R. (2023, September 12). *Social media users — Global demographics (2023).* https://www.demandsage.com/social-media-users/.

Statista. (2023, August 22). Cost of natural disaster per year globally 2000-2022. *Statista.* https://www.statista.com/statistics/612561/natural-disaster-losses-cost-worldwide-by-type-of-loss/.

Strain, D. (2022, February 14). *Engineers deploy drones to survey Marshall Fire, gather Lessons for.* CU Boulder Today. https://www.colorado.edu/today/2022/marshall-fire-drones.

Syifa, M., Kadavi, P. R., & Lee, C. (2019). An artificial intelligence application for Post-Earthquake damage mapping in Palu, central Sulawesi, Indonesia. *Sensors, 19*(3), 542. https://doi.org/10.3390/s19030542.

U.S. Geological Survey. n.d. *Real-time data.* https://www.usgs.gov/products/data/real-time-data.

Using FEMA's Survey123 Preliminary damage assessment templates. (2020, September 21). Esri Community. https://community.esri.com/t5/arcgis-survey123-blog/using-fema-s-survey123-preliminary-damage/ba-p/898150.

Veoci. (2023). *Veoci - Emergency management.* https://veoci.com/emergency-management/.

Zwęgliński, T. (2020). The use of drones in disaster aerial needs reconnaissance and damage Assessment – Three-Dimensional Modeling and Orthophoto map study. *Sustainability, 12*(15), 6080. https://doi.org/10.3390/su12156080.

11 Revisiting Human Behavior after Disasters

The Possibility of Anti-Social Activity and Its Relation to Disaster Assistance

Amy Eddington, Natasha Byrd, and David McEntire

11.1 INTRODUCTION

When considering the concept of disasters, it is easy to think of hurricanes, tornadoes, and wildfires. In addition, human-caused disasters such as terrorist attacks are physically hazardous agents that trigger events and cause injuries, death, and disruption. There is also a human element to disasters, where various political, economic, and cultural factors combine to produce social vulnerability in complex ways. Many sociologists have studied why people are prone to experience disaster impacts or cannot adequately prepare, respond, and recover effectively or efficiently. Such scholars have also studied human behavior in disasters, concentrating on the prevalence of altruism instead of anti-social behavior. While research has consistently shown that community members and outsiders demonstrate incredible compassion for the victims and survivors of disasters, there are numerous reports in the media of fraud during disasters. This situation raises two important questions for those dealing with disasters: Are these statements about fraudulent behavior accurate? If so, what are the implications of this type of anti-social behavior for emergency management and our nation as a whole?

This chapter addresses these and other questions by examining various types of fraud committed after disasters. First, it explores the literature on human behavior, defines the concept of fraud, and identifies what is known about this activity after disasters. Then, it discusses the methodology for this study, provides findings about this topic, and shares recommendations for the emergency management profession and others who are involved in disasters and the provision of recovery assistance. The authors found that altruism is a prevalent behavioral response to disasters. However,

DOI: 10.1201/9781003648178-12

fraud may indeed occur, and this should be taken into consideration by those who are providing financial assistance.

11.2 LITERATURE REVIEW

The literature produced by disaster researchers covers a variety of topics that are relevant to this discussion. Scholars have examined human behavior, emergence, convergence, altruism, anti-social behavior, and fraud. This section delves deeper into the main points of these concepts and further clarifies their importance in the context of this chapter.

11.2.1 Human Behavior

Behavior is a topic that has fascinated researchers for decades. However, there is limited literature regarding behavior during disasters compared to behavior in general. Holguín-Veras et al. (2022) discussed barriers to researching behavior after disasters, which ranged from predicting human behavior in the aftermath of an event to the complexities of fulfilling disaster response and recovery functions. Holguín-Veras and his associates observed that collecting data about human behavior after disasters can be challenging because emergency management personnel prefer to focus more on their post-disaster activities and have limited time to participate in research studies (Holguín-Veras et al., 2022). This means that emergency management personnel are often more focused on the job at hand and doing the best they can to serve the people of the affected area, rather than spending their time answering questions for scholarly pursuits. Such a situation sheds light on some of the difficulties researchers face in obtaining accurate data about people's behaviors in emergency management's response and recovery phase.

11.2.2 Emergence

Although obtaining information about human behavior can be problematic, scholars have discovered that disasters may bring out both the best and worst in people. Researchers have come to understand the typical features of human behavior when extreme events occur. First responders – police, fire, and emergency medical service personnel – will most often faithfully fulfill the roles they train for. This includes warning others, helping them to evacuate, putting out fires, engaging in search and rescue operations, and providing emergency medical care.

Another group of official responders includes those working in healthcare in hospital emergency departments. Healthcare providers work together to treat the victims of mass casualty events through triage with various designations: Red (not treatable), Yellow (urgent care needed), and Green (minor injuries). Emergency medical providers are also trained regularly to ensure they can address the massive challenges disasters present (Hughes et al., 2021). This is vital since some patients may require up to seventeen medical providers to care for the symptoms they are experiencing and resolve any other needs during their visits. For patients to receive high-quality care, healthcare provider teams also require access to appropriate experts as needed. Hughes et al. mention, "Effective teams require… requisite attitudes, behaviors, and cognitions (ABCs) to act as a team. Teamwork ABCs are necessary for team members to work effectively together and include factors such as psychological safety, communication, situation monitoring, and transactive memory" (Hughes et al., 2021, p. c812). Employees can take care of patients and increase performance within the hospital unit by having these elements in a team.

There are many other individuals who become involved in disaster response and recovery operations: citizens, neighbors, community groups, and even the victims themselves. During a disaster, individuals will take on new roles and responsibilities, while groups of people will organize themselves in new ways to meet unfolding challenges. This phenomenon is known as emergence.

Emergence is an easy-to-understand and intuitive concept, as it simply means that an action or organization appears and comes into existence. Therefore, emergence involves novelty, formation, and growth in rapid and consequential ways (Seidel and Greve, 2017). In other words, "disasters stimulate spontaneous responses – before formal organizations can mobilize – by self-organizing, voluntary groups and individuals from within and outside disaster-affected communities. These "emergent" groups and spontaneous volunteers are a common feature of disasters" (Twigg and Mosel, 2017, p. 443). Saban (2014) discussed the importance of these spontaneous responses. "Many of the most innovative and effective initiatives to address disaster relief and recovery efforts have been designed and implemented by civil society groups" (Saban, 2014, p. 2). Hierarchical groups can provide significant resources and organizational efforts. Nevertheless, the statement made by Saban indicates that some of the best relief efforts and methods of assisting have come from smaller, self-organized groups.

Along these lines, the family unit becomes an essential place and resource for mental healing and support (Wang et al., 2021). As a foundational unit in society, family members help each other in post-disaster physical and economic recoveries. The experiences they have become a bonding element that helps mitigate anxiety and provides methods to take care of overall well-being (Wang et al., 2021). The familial example of emergence within a community impacts individuals' well-being.

11.2.3 Convergence

The post-disaster assistance process provides several opportunities for people to help the victims in various ways. First responders, public officials, and local government employees arrive at the disaster scene to assess visible impacts. These individuals and groups begin life-saving measures, endeavor to protect property, provide information to the public, clean up debris, and facilitate the process of rebuilding. Businesses will also arrive to help those in need, either to advance their financial well-being or to be good corporate citizens (McEntire, 2022). In addition, faith-based organizations, volunteer groups, and individuals will descend on the disaster site to perform any acts of service they can render to disaster victims. Abualkhair et al. (2020, p. 2) note that "volunteer convergence, which specifically refers to the influx of spontaneous volunteers, can be a valuable source of labor for carrying out various relief tasks." Such corporations, nongovernmental organizations (NGOs), charities, and citizens play a significant role during disaster assistance and recovery.

Volunteer organizations continue to provide supplies needed to meet basic needs. Schwirplies (2023, p. 53) added, "among others, they support victims finding available monetary, non-monetary, medical, and psychological assistance, rebuilding homes, and by providing appliances, food, fuel, clean water, hygiene products, and shelter." In addition, material resources will also be sent to the location of a disaster to help resolve pressing needs. At the same time, other donations may be related to funds provided to assist in recovery and repair efforts. This "material convergence produces an abundance of much-needed supplies and equipment for disaster survivors and first responders" (Abualkhair et al., 2020, p. 2). During disaster response and recovery, the most critical items individuals need are for basic survival.

Disaster relief centers (DRCs) are essential hubs for distributing relief supplies. "DRC operations, which include activities such as storage, retrieval, and distribution of relief supplies, are carried out by a combination of professional responders and volunteers" (Abualkhair et al., 2020, p. 1). While material convergence can be helpful, some challenges come with the donated materials, such as how to collect them, where to store them, how to allocate them, and who should monitor the flow of such resources. This can be a significant problem. According to Holguín-Veras et al. (2022):

> In the case of local church leaders, local disaster responders and fire departments, their staff and volunteers may not be aware of the enormous problems produced by physical donations in extreme events. The reason is that, since their experience is primarily with local emergencies and minor disasters, where the flows of non-priority supplies are only a manageable nuisance, they are not likely to identify material convergence as a significant problem that they should prepare for or devote their energy towards mitigating.
>
> **(p. 17)**

Therefore, having the human resources necessary to address donation management requirements is essential. However, monetary donations can be even more valuable in disaster relief efforts because they allow those involved to get what is required to address the needs of the affected community and disaster victims.

Financial supplies allow those overseeing the response and recovery efforts to allocate funds quickly to where they see the most need. Holguín-Veras et al. (2022, p. 15) stated, "Touting the donor-focused benefits of cash donations is essential because, notwithstanding their good intentions, at the moment of deciding what to donate, individual donors take into account factors other than those that are purely survivor-focused."

Looking at a few disasters, we can see how much individual and charity financial aid can assist those in need. For instance, "nearly $1.1 billion in generous donations were used to fund massive relief and recovery efforts and help more than 59,000 families affected by the terrorist attacks" on September 11, 2001 (American Red

Cross, 2021). After a Category 5 hurricane hit Louisiana in 2005, "two-thirds of the $3.27 billion raised by private nonprofit organizations [and tracked by the newspaper The (Washington)] Post went to help evacuees and other Katrina victims with immediate needs" (Salmon and Smith, 2006, p. 1). Three months after Hurricane Irma, the American Red Cross (2017, p. 3) noted, "the Red Cross has raised $89 million, including the value of critical donated goods and services, to help people impacted by Hurricane Irma." These acts of charity provided survivors with the supplies needed for their families.

11.2.4 Altruism

Considering the concepts of emergence and convergence, it is evident that altruistic behaviors are frequently witnessed after disasters. The word altruism was inspired by the French philosopher Auguste Comte as "altruisme," rooted in the Italian word "altrui," which was derived from the Latin term "alteri," meaning other people, others, or someone else (Jenkins, 2021). Jenkins (2021, p. 85) asserted that "altruism is the moral practice of concern for the happiness of other people, and such appears as a virtue in many cultures." Fultz and Schafer (2023) explained that altruism includes a paradox as individuals sometimes engage in self-sacrificial acts that benefit another. The altruism paradox is another term that describes prosocial behavior when someone performs acts of kindness for the benefit of others. These actions demonstrated in the paradox counteract egoistic motivations, serving for the benefit of self (Fultz and Schafer, 2023). Jenkins (2021) mentioned that this virtue can be demonstrated in different cultures, and sometimes people are not willing to go out of their comfort zone to help others in need after a disaster.

This phenomenon can be seen in various aspects of life. Unfortunately, little real conceptual progress seems to have been made toward understanding or explaining altruism (Inoue et al., 2023). While examining the impact of effective altruism (EA), Kassirer et al. (2023, p. 372) mentioned, "the EA philosophy calls for people to use evidence and reason to figure out how to benefit others as much as possible with their limited time and resources." Thus, for centuries, scientists have asked if people do things for others out of altruistic tendencies or if they do it for self-serving purposes. One argument could be that when people do something for others, they also act to feel good about themselves.

At the root of altruism is empathy, which allows individuals to have the motivation to help others without expecting something in return (Russell and Mentzel, 1990). Uttervall et al. (2013) found that people saw a positive view of the world after witnessing acts of altruism following major disasters. One of the participants in that study survived the 2004 tsunami in Indonesia and mentioned they witnessed complete strangers arriving at the hospital to talk, hug, and provide emotional support to those in need. At the same time, others brought in the last bit of their food despite not having any food, family, or shelter to go home to. Uttervall et al. (2013, p. 41) mentioned, "in most cases, [people may have experienced shock], but that did not prevent them from acting in an altruistic way nor from taking on responsibility for other family members." Those individuals observed that they would rather act to gain control of what matters most to them and do what they can to be reunited with their families again.

Regardless of the possible self-serving nature of altruistic behaviors, researchers recently found that charitable donations increase post-disasters. Okuyama and Fukushige (2021) reported that individuals who work in the public sector are more likely to donate to charity than those working in the private sector. However, they did notice "a gap between the decision to donate and determination of how much [people have] a willingness to donate" (Okuyama and Fukushige, 2021). In other words, public employees are more accommodating and flexible with their donations, even if their contribution is small (Okuyama and Fukushige, 2021).

Acts of altruism are not always self-serving, nor is it solely prosocial behavior. Altruism is instinctively shutting out any shock experienced from the disaster and taking responsibility to save and serve the lives of one's family members and others. It provides a way to positively persevere through the negative impacts of the disaster.

11.2.5 Anti-Social Behavior

To be sure, not everyone exhibits charitable behavior in regular times or when disasters occur. For this reason, it is essential to review what is known about anti-social behavior. Anti-social behavior shows a disregard for the norms of society and other people. The origins of anti-social behavior are typically demonstrated in early childhood behaviors, leading to aggressive and destructive behaviors. Calkins and Keane (2009) explained that such people experience deficits in emotional self-regulation from basic functioning to cognitive development, putting children at risk of worsened behaviors in adulthood. Crafton Hills College notes that people dealing with anti-social personality disorder fail to conform to social norms by repeating aggressive behaviors, leading to an arrest (Crafton Hills College, 2024). Anti-social behavior can be overt (e.g., an outward showing, such as abuse or fighting and other types of aggressiveness) or covert (e.g., behaviors that are hidden from others, such as alcohol or drug abuse) (Mayo Clinic, 2023).

There are some interesting discussions about anti-social behavior in the context of disasters, such as those mentioned by McEntire (2022). Hollywood and news reporters often give a very biased view of human behavior in disasters. Three crucial assumptions must be understood in relation to their portrayals. The first assumption is the concept of looting. The belief here is that people who find a damaged home or business with broken windows believe that the contents found in the debris are free for the taking. No matter the damage, it is assumed that others will take the food, electronic equipment, and other necessary supplies for various reasons (McEntire, 2022). The second assumption is that people will resort to violence with the belief that they have to defend their property. For instance, after the 1906 San Francisco earthquake, the mayor "issued 5,000 handbills telling citizens he had ordered federal troops and local police to shoot looters" (McEntire, 2022, Ch. 3, p. 9). This example asserted that people needed to arm themselves in defense of their properties.

The third belief that McEntire (2022) shared was the belief that people would take advantage of disaster victims to make money. In other words, people are assumed to engage in fraudulent behavior after disasters to seek financial advantage.

11.2.6 Fraud

Fraud is an act of deception to get money or goods illegally (Cheliatsidou et al., 2023). Fraud can be seen in many forms and may be prevalent in and after disasters. On July 16, 2023, the Federal Emergency Management Agency (FEMA) released a public statement warning about fraud and scams on their site.

> Disasters bring out criminals looking to prey on survivors who appear to be easy targets for their scams… Common tactics used by scam artists include phone calls from people claiming to work for FEMA. The caller may ask for the survivor's Social Security number, income, or banking information.
>
> **(FEMA, 2023)**

While these are not the only methods criminals use to target individuals, businesses, or other groups, it is good to remember them and understand variations in such behavior. With this in mind, it might be wise to consider if and the degree to which fraud occurs after a disaster and what, if anything, can be done about it.

11.3 METHODS

This study's primary source of information was secondary sources based on searches for news articles, journals, books, government reports, and websites. Keywords and phrases such as "human behavior during a disaster" and "disaster assistance fraud" were entered into the Utah Valley University's library search engine to locate articles and journals. In addition, these terms were entered on Google to locate additional material for this study. These sources included newspaper articles from across the country, books and articles found by searching library records, and various documents on government websites.

Ultimately, the authors collected and reviewed information from 25 sources to produce their findings and recommendations. Researchers examined human behavior in various disasters resulting from floods, hurricanes, wildfires, tornados, and the terrorist attacks of September 11, 2001.

11.4 FINDINGS

Our search for information on the topic of fraud revealed that fraudulent behavior can be witnessed among victims themselves as well as government officials and may occur at any given point in the disaster assistance process. We categorized this anti-social behavior as business and individual assistance fraud, charity fraud, and embezzlement. The following are a few examples of fraud during disaster assistance.

11.4.1 Business and Individual Assistance Fraud

There are various ways that people may seek to enrich themselves during disasters. Several examples of individuals committing fraud against the government are noteworthy. A contractor may "attempt to get more reimbursement than they are entitled to by misrepresenting their work. Companies removing debris have falsified the number of fallen trees they removed after a major ice storm in Oklahoma" (McEntire, 2022, p. 334). In some cases, such individuals have been sentenced for committing fraud during disaster assistance.

In a second case, the US Department of Justice published a report describing a Texas grand jury charging a hotel owner with seventeen counts of fraudulent claims and charging him for wire transferring $232,000 in lodging reimbursements (Department of Justice, 2006). In a similar case in Florida, a 47-year-old Jacksonville man submitted applications for assistance during Tropical Storm Debby, Hurricane Matthew, and Hurricane Irma. The case brief mentioned, "[he] falsely claimed that his primary residence in Jacksonville was damaged due to a storm … [and he therefore] had to relocate and was in need of disaster assistance" (Department of Justice-Florida, 2019). This man was sentenced to 21 months in federal prison and was ordered to pay $57,689.19 to the United States for wire fraud involving illegally obtained FEMA benefits.

Two different groups of 10 and 11 individuals were charged with fraud related to disaster assistance. Each defendant made false statements claiming that their only mode of transportation was damaged by flooding and was, therefore, inoperable. The individuals provided false estimates from a repair shop that did not exist. The defendants, ages 24 to 65, were said to be collaborating on the hoax and were each individually ordered to pay around $6,215 to $9,042 in restitution (Department of Justice-Louisiana, 2021a, 2021b).

11.4.2 Charity Fraud

Some cases involved individuals working together to steal from organizations or falsely claiming they were raising donations for the Salvation Army during relief efforts. In one case, a Red Cross volunteer and his sister stole over 100 debit cards intended for survivors of Hurricane Katrina, amounting to over $230,000. The young man reportedly took the debit cards with the help of security guards. Then, he gave his sister some debit cards and purchased jewelry for himself as well as a car for his girlfriend, friends, and family (Department of Justice, 2005). This case was a team effort between the two siblings and a guard at the DRC who aided them in accessing where the debit cards were stored.

Another case described two brothers involved in donation efforts who were caught by the teams working in the Hurricane Katrina fraud task force, which operated for three years. The task force's role in this effort was to deter, detect, and prosecute individuals who took advantage of disaster-related funds, and it also included individuals who attempted to commit fraud in the aftermath of Hurricanes Rita, Wilma, Gustav, and Ike (Department of Justice, 2008).

One notable example of charity fraud occurred in November 2007 when two brothers were sentenced to 105 to 111 months in prison for their role in creating a false donation website on behalf of the Salvation Army (Department of Justice, 2008). Their website had a link to allow contributors to donate through PayPal, an online money transfer service provider. The transferred funds were sent to various accounts with aliases and Social Security Numbers of people who were not involved in the activity. It was later discovered that the accounts were connected to the two brothers. Their website collected $48,000 before the accounts were frozen (Department of Justice, 2008).

The task force also caught a man embezzling money from a Baptist church that needed financial aid to repair its building. Since the church did not have flood insurance, the congregation applied for a Small Business Administration (SBA) loan and grants from the Bush-Clinton Katrina Fund. The church was awarded $252,000 from the SBA and $35,000 from the grant. One member of the congregation chose to keep the awards for himself. He had the check mailed to his house and then transferred the SBA loan wire to an account he created. By the time of his arrest, he had already spent $10,000 on a new car (Department of Justice, 2008).

11.4.3 Embezzlement

While private citizens commit fraud, government officials can be charged with fraud too. However, the number of government officials who commit fraud is far fewer than those who do not. Nonetheless, government officials have access to considerable sums of money and are responsible for keeping records. This may encourage some public servants to consider engaging in fraudulent behavior. The following are examples of fraud by government officials.

The first example is of a public adjuster who was sentenced in 2017 "to seven years in prison for embezzling $400,000 from Los Angeles County fire victims by cashing insurance claim checks that were meant to help rebuild homes" (Fraud Alerts/PSAS, 2018). According to the California State Law Enforcement Association (CSLEA, 2018), the public adjuster told to his clients that he would take care of the contractors and "help them rebuild." While fraud alerts did not go into additional detail, they provided examples of how public adjusters may scam the public. "Dishonest adjusters can take advantage of people in vulnerable situations by charging exorbitant fees, stealing personal information, or referring them to a shoddy contractor for a kickback" (Fraud Alerts/PSAS, 2018).

A second example describes the actions of a New Orleans mayor who accepted payoffs for contracts and was convicted of twenty fraud charges. The case summary mentioned, "Prosecutors described a pattern of transactions in which a company would come to [the mayor] after trying to get city work, and he would ask them for a favor, most often in the form of a payment [including perks, trips, and gifts]" (Department of Justice-Louisiana, 2014). The mayor embezzled over half a million dollars, while the contractors gained millions from city work.

The final example was a group of government workers falsely claiming incorrect hours worked. McEntire (2022, Ch. 9, p. 334) stated, "some city leaders have filed erroneous paperwork to bring additional monies to their communities or enrich themselves. After Hurricanes Rita and Gustav, a woman, a mayor, and a police chief filled out fraudulent time sheets. The woman sought approval and payment for her services even though she was not working at the time." As a result of their choices, the city council agreed to end the dispute by repaying FEMA $163,102.60 out of the $268,668.70 that was paid relating to Hurricanes Rita and Gustav (FBI, 2011).

In response to this kind of fraud, a law was enacted that punishes individuals with imprisonment for 30 years and a $1 million fine for committing fraud related to a presidentially declared emergency involving transferred funds (Public Law 110–179, 2008). Similar laws are expected to deter other fraud as well.

11.5 RECOMMENDATIONS

Fraud in any situation is frustrating, but it is even more irritating when monies have been allocated to help those impacted by natural, technological, or anthropogenic hazards. Fraud can add further financial or emotional trauma to disaster victims. It can also cause unnecessary and wasteful expenses for charities and government agencies involved in disasters. For these reasons, it is essential to explore recommendations to reduce fraudulent situations, including prevention before a disaster, detection of fraud and scams during a disaster, and resolution of the crime during or after recovery. This section provides recommendations on how to help prevent fraud, points to consider, and what to look for to help protect the community. This portion of the chapter also discusses how government officials can discover fraud and find ways to prevent its occurrence or respond effectively.

11.5.1 Individual Protection

One of the best recommendations is prevention by monitoring and detecting potential fraud threats. Kutz (2006) mentioned, "upfront preventive controls can help screen out the majority of fraud, and are the most effective and efficient means to minimize fraud, waste, and abuse" (p. 3). A method to monitor potential fraud is to set up a command center that screened calls regarding fraud and other activities (Department of Justice, 2008). While prevention is the preferred method for mitigating fraud, there are other options as well. Some "key elements of the detection process include data-mining for fraudulent and suspicious registrants, reviews to establish the accountability of funds, and establishing hotlines to receive tips of potential fraud" (Kutz, 2006, p.9). Spammers use keywords and phrases, and it is critical for people to be aware of them to avoid financial harm.

Educating vulnerable individuals so they may better understand the resources available to them and the signs of fraud is encouraged. For instance, fraud may include scammers who "might pretend to be safety inspectors, government officials trying to help you, or utility workers who say immediate work is required" (Puig et al., 2023). Some groups engage in rental scams. "Scammers know people need a place to live while they rebuild. They will advertise rentals that don't exist to get your money and run" (Puig et al., 2023). This is a good reminder for those affected by disasters to "never wire or give money for a deposit or rent before you've met or signed a lease" (Puig et al., 2023).

There are other recommendations to help victims protect themselves from the nefarious behavior of others. When looking for contractors, homeowners should "get three written bids, check contractors' referrals and online reputation, get a well-written contract, and never pay in full until the job is done" (Washington State Department of Labor & Industries, 2023).

11.5.2 Government Officials

This section describes tips to aid organizations in their efforts to avoid fraud. Remembering these tips from FEMA is an essential tool to help public sector officials prevent and react to fraud, too. For instance, the World Bank advises public organizations to:

1. Promote a strong ethical culture across the organization.
2. Set the tone from the top.
3. Implement annual ethical compliance declarations from employees, suppliers, and other stakeholders.
4. Establish audit committees and boards with oversight roles within public sector organizations.
5. Implement a robust anti-fraud environment.
6. Focus on fraud during ongoing reviews.
7. Establish and keep updated the internal audit fraud risk policy.
8. Invest appropriately in the resources and capacity of internal audit departments.
9. Emphasize fraud-specific training.
10. Implement organization-wide fraud awareness activities.
11. Establish appropriate channels for reporting fraud.
12. Implement procedures for responding to and investigating fraud (The World Bank, 2017).

This source therefore recommends public leaders lead by example and implement systems to aid municipalities in preventing fraud within their boundaries.

People must become aware of the types of crimes that may be committed after a disaster, along with the methods criminals implement for financial gain. It is also crucial for organizations to train their employees to be aware of different types of fraud methods that may arise while at work, no matter when the activity occurs.

11.6 CONCLUSION

The impact of disasters cannot be understated, and the assistance that follows is critical to help those affected recover and rebuild. Most disasters witness emergent and convergent behavior with an incredible outpouring of altruism. However, there are also reports of anti-social behavior, such as fraud.

Because of the potential risks of fraud, communities must be aware of the signs that fraudulent behavior is being committed. Awareness is the first step, but it is not enough to handle fraudulent activities alone. Providing education and training, before a disaster occurs is necessary to effectively monitor fraud during and after disasters. Fraud can be prevented or caught sooner if these measures had been in place. Individuals and government officials must understand what to do if they suspect related behaviors and where to report the possible fraud.

Ultimately, those involved in emergency management are encouraged to pay close attention to the possibility of fraud during and after disasters. While there are limitations to monitoring behavior during disasters and recovery assistance, having tools in place can lessen the likelihood of this anti-social behavior happening. This is vital in countering fraudulent behavior and utilizing mitigation techniques, including protecting businesses, individuals, and charities and preventing embezzlement.

REFERENCES

Abualkhair H, Lodree EJ, Davis LB. (2020). Managing volunteer convergence at disaster relief centers. International Journal of Production Economics 220:107399.

American Red Cross. (2017, December). *Red cross delivers relief and comfort in devastating storm's wake.* American Red Cross | Help Those Affected by Disasters. https://www.redcross.org/content/dam/redcross/about-us/publications/Irma_Three-Month_Update.pdf.

American Red Cross. (2021). *20th anniversary of the September 11 response.* Red Cross of Missouri. https://www.redcross.org/local/missouri/about-us/our-work/20th-anniversary-of-september-11-response.html.

California Statewide Law Enforcement Association (CSLEA). (2018). *Public adjuster sentenced to 10 years for embezzling from fire victims.* https://cslea.com/2018/03/public-adjuster-sentenced-to-10-years-for-embezzling-from-fire-victims/.

Calkins, S. D., & Keane, S. P. (2009). Developmental origins of early antisocial behavior. *Development and Psychopathology, 21*(4), 1095–1109. https://doi.org/10.1017/s095457940999006x.

Cheliatsidou, A., Sariannidis, N., Garefalakis, A., Azibi, J., & Kagias, P. (2023). The international fraud triangle. *Journal of Money Laundering Control, 26*(1), 106–132. https://doi.org/10.1108/jmlc-09-2021-0103.

Crafton Hills College. (2024). *Anti-social behavior indicators.* https://www.craftonhills.edu/faculty-and-staff/behavior-intervention-team/anti-social-behavior-indicators.php.

Department of Justice. (2005, December 6). *Red cross volunteer and his sister charged with stealing more than 100 red cross debit cards intended for hurricane evacuees.* https://www.justice.gov/sites/default/files/criminal-disasters/legacy/2012/07/30/09-04-07AG2ndyrprogrpt.pdf.

Department of Justice. (2006, March 2). *Galveston's flagship hotel owner charged with defrauding FEMA Hurricane Evacuee Programs.* Justice.Gov. https://www.justice.gov/sites/default/files/criminal-disasters/legacy/2012/07/30/09-04-07AG2ndyrprogrpt.pdf.

Department of Justice. (2008, October 1). *More than 900 defendants charged with disaster related fraud by Hurricane Katrina fraud task force during three years in operation.* #08-877. https://www.justice.gov/archive/opa/pr/2008/October/08-crm-877.html.

Department of Justice-Florida. (2019, October 16). *Jacksonville man sentenced for disaster assistance fraud involving tropical storm Debby, Hurricane Matthew, And Hurricane Irma.* Middle District of Florida. https://www.justice.gov/usao-mdfl/pr/jacksonville-man-sentenced-disaster-assistance-fraud-involving-tropical-storm-debby.

Department of Justice-Louisiana. (2014, November 19). *C. Ray Nagin, former New Orleans mayor, convicted on federal bribery, honest services wire fraud, money laundering, conspiracy, and tax charges.* Eastern District of Louisiana, U.S. Department of Justice. https://www.justice.gov/usao-edla/pr/c-ray-nagin-former-new-orleans-mayor-convicted-federal-bribery-honest-services-wire.

Department of Justice-Louisiana. (2021a). *Second round of individuals charged with disaster assistance fraud.* Western District of Louisiana, U.S. Department of Justice. https://www.justice.gov/usao-wdla/pr/second-round-individuals-charged-disaster-assistance-fraud.

Department of Justice-Louisiana. (2021b). *Ten individuals charged with disaster assistance fraud.* Western District of Louisiana, U.S. Department of Justice. https://www.justice.gov/usao-wdla/pr/ten-individuals-charged-disaster-assistance-fraud.

Federal Bureau of Investigation (FBI). (2011, June 9). Town of Ball mayor sentenced for FEMA fraud. *FBI.* https://archives.fbi.gov/archives/neworleans/press-releases/2011/town-of-ball-mayor-sentenced-for-fema-fraud.

Federal Emergency Management Agency (FEMA). (2023). *Beware of fraud and scams.* https://www.fema.gov/press-release/20230716/beware-fraud-and-scams.

Fraud alerts/PSAS. (2018, January 12). Crooked public adjusters target wildfire victims. *Los Angeles County District Attorney's Office.* https://da.lacounty.gov/community/fraud-alerts/Crooked-Public-Adjusters-Target-Wildfire-Victims.

Fultz, J., & Schafer, E. D. (2023). Altruism, cooperation, and empathy. In *Salem Press encyclopedia of health.* https://research-ebsco-com.ezproxy.uvu.edu/c/er7pa4/viewer/html/5hx5t53u6n.

Holguín-Veras, J., Encarnación, T., Van Wassenhove, L. N., Pokharel, S., Cantillo, V., Amaya, J., Wachtendorf, T., & Rilling, J. (2022). Reducing material convergence in disaster environments: The potential of trusted change agents. *Transportation Research Part E: Logistics and Transportation Review, 162.* https://doi.org/10.1016/j.tre.2022.102736.

Hughes, A. M., Sonesh, S. C., Mason, R. E., Gregory, M. E., Marttos, A., Schulman, C. I., & Salas, E. (2021). Trauma, teams, and telemedicine: Evaluating telemedicine and teamwork in a mass casualty simulation. *Military Medicine, 186*(7–8), c811–c818. https://doi.org/10.1093/milmed/usaa434.

Inoue Y, Mifune, Saijo T. (2023). Positive reputation for altruism toward future generations regardless of the cost for current others. Frontiers in Psychology 13:2022.

Jenkins, M.. (2021). *Expert humans: Critical leadership skills for a disrupted world.* Emerald Publishing Limited.

Kassirer, S., Levine, E. E., & Kouchaki, M. (2023). A call to maximize the social impact of our research: An effective altruism approach. *Academy of Management Perspectives, 37*(4), 371–382. https://doi.org/10.5465/amp.2022.0045.

Kutz, G. (2006, July 12). *Individual disaster assistance programs: Framework for fraud prevention, detection, and prosecution.* https://www.govinfo.gov/content/pkg/GAOREPORTS-GAO-06-954T/html/GAOREPORTS-GAO-06-954T.htm.

Mayo Clinic. (2023). *Antisocial personality disorder.* https://www.mayoclinic.org/diseases-conditions/antisocial-personality-disorder/diagnosis-treatment/drc-20353934.

McEntire, D. A. (2022). *Disaster response and recovery: Strategies and tactics for resilience.* John Wiley & Sons, Inc.

Okuyama, N., & Fukushige, M. (2021). Limited prosocial response: Post-disaster charitable behavior of public sector workers. *Kyklos, 74*(1), 77–102. https://doi.org/10.1111/kykl.12252.

Public Law 110-179. (2008). *Emergency and Disaster Assistance Fraud Penalty Enhancement Act of 2007.* https://www.congress.gov/110/plaws/publ179/PLAW-110publ179.pdf.

Puig, A., Tressler, C., Fair, L., Heras, G. de las, Specialist, C. E., Dee, Bright, S., Weikel, T. A., & Luner, E. (2023, May 31). Avoid scammers trying to profit from a deadly tornado. *Consumer Advice.* https://consumer.ftc.gov/consumer-alerts/2023/03/avoid-scammers-trying-profit-deadly-tornado.

Russell, G. W., & Mentzel, R. K. (1990). Sympathy and altruism in response to disasters. *The Journal of Social Psychology, 130*(3), 309–316. https://doi.org/10.1080/00224545.1990.9924586.

Saban, L. I. (2014). *Disaster emergency management.* The State University of New York Press.

Salmon, J. L., & Smith, L. (2006, February 27). Two-thirds of Katrina donations exhausted charities faced with difficult decisions and countless requests as they spend what is left. *The Washington Post.* https://www.washingtonpost.com/archive/politics/2006/02/27/two-thirds-of-katrina-donations-exhausted-span-classbankheadcharities-faced-with-difficult-decisions-and-countless-requests-as-they-spend-what-is-leftspan/81b6c737-eb84-4aa2-b913-1b1a3f2ee54e/.

Schwirplies, C. (2023). Does additional demand for charitable aid increase giving? Evidence from Hurricane Sandy. *Journal of Economic Behavior & Organization, 209*, 53–73. https://doi.org/10.1016/j.jebo.2023.01.018.

Seidel, M.-D. L., & Greve, H. R. (2017). Emergence: How novelty, growth, and formation shape organizations and their ecosystems. *Emergence-Research in the Sociology of Organizations*, 1–27. https://doi.org/10.1108/s0733-558x20170000050020.

Twigg, J., & Mosel, I. (2017). Emergent groups and spontaneous volunteers in urban disaster response. *Environment & Urbanization, 29*(2), 443–458. https://doi.org.ezproxy.uvu.edu/10.1177/0956247817721413.

Uttervall, M., Hultman, C. M., Ekerwald, H., Lindam, A., & Lundin, T. (2013). After the flood: Resilience among Tsunami-afflicted adolescents. *Nordic Journal of Psychiatry, 68*(1), 38–43. https://doi.org/10.3109/08039488.2013.767373.

Wang, W., Foutz, N. Z., & Gao, G. G. (2021). Huddling with families after disaster: Human resilience and social disparity. *SSRN Electronic Journal*, 1–14. https://doi.org/10.2139/ssrn.3892399.

Washington State Department of Labor & Industries. (2023, September 18). *Beware of contractor scams when rebuilding from wildfire damage.* https://www.lni.wa.gov/news-events/article/23-24.

The World Bank Group. (2017) *What are the most common types of fraud in the public sector? Why is there an increased focus on fraud worldwide?* https://www.worldbank.org/en/search?q=Common%2Btypes%2Bof%2Bfraud.

12 Current Threats to Biosecurity

C Raina MacIntyre, Damian Honeyman, and David Heslop

12.1 A CHANGING LANDSCAPE

Human biosecurity and biosafety are rapidly changing. The emergence of CRISPR-Cas9 in 2012 has revolutionized genetic engineering (Jinek et al. 2012). Synthetic biology has been part of the landscape since researchers created a poliovirus in 2002 (Wimmer 2006). More recently, synthetic Ebolavirus (McMullan et al. 2019) and horsepox virus (Noyce et al. 2018) have created controversy. Gain-of-function research has also evolved since 2012, when two groups of scientists engineered avian influenza viruses to be transmissible in mammals by repeated passage through animal models, resulting in a temporary moratorium on such research and a risk-benefit analysis in both the US and European Union (Casagrande et al. 2016; Fears et al. 2015). A 2023 report on the landscape of gain-of-function research combined both gain and loss-of-function research in the same analysis, thus obfuscating the risk of the former (Schuerger et al. 2023).

The acceleration of these technologies increases the risk associated with laboratory accidents and deliberate release, especially since much of such research is published in open-access journals with the methods available publicly. The risk of unnatural epidemics may, in fact, be higher than that of natural ones (MacIntyre 2015).

12.2 BIOLOGICAL WEAPONS

Biological weapons have been used throughout human history. The technology for synthetic biology and genetic engineering is vastly more accessible today (MacIntyre et al. 2015). The cost of synthetic biology has decreased exponentially in the last decade (Noyce and Evans 2018). When bioweapons are used by nation-states, this is referred to as biological warfare, and when used by non-state actors, it is referred to as bioterrorism. From prehistoric times to the present, 42 known instances of biological warfare have been recorded, 11 of which involved the category "A" agent *Bacillus anthracis*. Early examples of the use of a biological weapon include what is now Vanuatu, where Melanesian tribesmen used arrowheads contaminated with *Clostridium tetani* to attack their enemies (Carus 1998). *Francisella tularensis* was

DOI: 10.1201/9781003648178-13

the first category "A" agent used in warfare in the 14th century BC, when the Hittite army sent infected rams to their enemies, effectively poisoning their food supply (Trevisanato 2007). Between the 14th century BC and the Second World War in 1939, biological weapon attacks were largely undertaken by contaminating food, water, wells, wine, clothing, and animals, and by attacking enemies with corpses infected with *Yersinia pestis*, *Mycobacterium leprae*, variola virus, rabies lyssavirus, yellow fever virus, *Plasmodium falciparum*, and *Clostridium botulinum* (Smart 1997, Kaufer et al. 2020, Riedel et al. 2004, Noah et al. 2002, Frischknecht 2003). The first known assassination attempt with a biological weapon was with the category "B" agent ricin, when Bulgarian exile Georgi Markov was assassinated after being injected with a ricin-encapsulated pellet in 1978 (Kaufer et al. 2020). Post-1980 saw targeted attacks by groups, first in 1984, when the Rajneesh community sought to manipulate local county elections by deliberately using category "B" agent *Salmonella typhimurium* to poison salad bars in local restaurants (Török 1997), and then between 1990 and 1995, the Aum Shinrikyo sect had several failed attempts at disseminating *Bacillus anthracis*, the nerve agent sarin, and *Clostridium botulinum* (Carus 1998; Trevisanato 2007; Smart 1997; Kaufer et al. 2020). Since the turn of the century, *Bacillus anthracis* and *ricin* have been mailed to intended targets in the United States, Pakistan, and Tunisia (Kaufer et al. 2020; Riedel 2004; Noah et al. 2002; Frischknecht 2003; Török et al. 1997; Ashraf 2002). Only one of these attacks, in 2001 in the United States, proved successful, with 17 people infected and five lives lost (Kaufer et al. 2020).

Throughout history, state and non-state actors have proliferated biological weapons. The covert USSR biological warfare program "Biopreparat" pursued offensive research between 1920 and 1992 and was arguably the world's largest and most sophisticated while also operating for the longest period of time. The program attempted to weaponize a range of pathogens, including *Bacillus anthracis*, *Yersinia pestis*, *Francisella tularensis*, *Burkholderia mallei*, *Brucella* sp., *Coxiella burnetii*, Venezuelan equine encephalitis virus, botulinum toxin, staphylococcal enterotoxin B, marburg virus, variola virus, and other orthopoxviruses (Alibek et al. 1999). Japan's infamous "Unit 731" covertly researched and developed biological and chemical weapons between 1934 and 1945. The unit successfully infected fleas with *Yersinia pestis* and disseminated them over Chinese cities between 1940 and 1941 while also spreading *Salmonella typhi* and *Salmonella paratyphi* in wells, marshes, and houses (Gold and Totani 2019). Wartime human experimentation involved testing *Yersinia pestis*, *Rickettsia prowazekii*, *Vibrio cholerae*, variola virus, and botulinum toxins on Japanese prisoners (Gold and Totani 2019). Between 1940 and the late 1950s, the United Kingdom developed a biological weapons program involving research into the weaponization of *Yersinia pestis*, *Vibrio cholerae*, *Salmonella typhi*, *Salmonella paratyphi*, paramyxovirus, asfivirus, Coxsackievirus A16, *Bacillus anthracis*, brucellosis, *Francisella tularensis*, and equine encephalomyelitis (Guillemin 2005). The 1948 Arab-Israeli war saw the emergence of the Israeli biological weapons operation "Cast Thy Bread." Though shrouded in secrecy, evidence points to the poisoning of drinking water with *Salmonella typhi* in Arab communities by Israel (Morris and Kedar 2023). The Iran-Iraq war led to the revival of Iraq's biological warfare research in the 1960s, where *Bacillus anthracis*, *Clostridium perfringens*, aflatoxin, botulinum toxin, ricin, *Picornaviridae*, human *Reoviridae*, and camel pox virus were investigated as potential weapons (Spiers 2021). The United States also conducted secret biological weapons research, including Operation Seaspray, which involved spraying bacteria over San Francisco, as well as other experiments releasing trillions of spores of *Bacillus globigii* in the New York subway (MacIntyre 2022).

Other research on animal pathogens occurred on Plum Island in "Lab 257" between 1954 and 2004 on *Borrelia burgdorferi* and West Nile virus (Carroll 2009). During these infamous years, outbreaks of Dutch Duck Plague in 1967, *Borrelia burgdorferi* in 1975, and West Nile virus in 1999 occurred in the United States mysteriously, with some suggestion they may be associated with the research on Plum Island (Carroll 2009). Although not exhaustive, other countries that reportedly had active biological weapons programs include China, Libya, Syria, Taiwan, and North Korea (Atlas 1999). With vastly greater technology and increased accessibility of biological agents today, we can assume the use of bioweapons is greatly enabled. Yet without systematic tools to differentiate natural and unnatural epidemics (Chen et al. 2017 2019), identifying unnatural ones can be exceedingly difficult, as creating terror may not be a motive and public health authorities tend to assume all epidemics are natural (MacIntyre 2022).

12.3 LABORATORY ACCIDENTS

Laboratory accidents are common and often due to human error. There has been debate about the origin of the Severe Acute Respiratory Syndrome Coronavirus 2 (SARS-CoV-2) pandemic and whether it may have arisen from an accident at the Wuhan Institute of Virology (Harrison and Sachs 2022; Andersen et al. 2020). Human error and accidents are common in laboratories and sometimes result in catastrophic epidemics (Wilkening 2006). A lab accident involving a highly transmissible pathogen may result in a widespread epidemic or a pandemic. The 1971 Aral variola virus incident saw aerosols released from a bioweapons installation on the island, resulting in ten cases and three deaths (Lane and Summer 2009). Coincidentally, the last known person to die of the variola virus in 1978 was a photographer from an office above a laboratory working on the variola virus in Birmingham, England; it is not known how the photographer caught the virus (Walker 2018; Rozo and Gronvall 1977). In 1977, the influenza H1N1 virus, also known as the "Russian Flu," was thought to have leaked from a Chinese laboratory. However, speculation points toward the virus being shared between Russia and China for vaccine experiments, leading to a major accident (Nakajima et al. 1978), though the genetic sequence was nearly identical to sequences from decade-old strains (Rozo and Gronvall 1977). The American Biosafety Association catalogs laboratory accidents (Gillum et al. 2016), which occur even at the highest levels of safety. Aerosol plumes of *Bacillus anthracis* were accidentally released from the covert USSR biological warfare facility at Sverdlovsk in 1979, resulting in environmental contamination and at least 79 infections and 68 deaths. Three accidents involving the transmission of Severe Acute Respiratory Syndrome Coronavirus 1 (SARS-CoV-1) in laboratories in Singapore,

Taiwan, and China occurred between 2003 and 2004, deemed to be laboratory misconduct (Senior 2003; Orellana 2004; Walgate 2004), shortly after the SARS epidemic appeared. An ongoing leak of *Brucella* in 2019 from a pharmaceutical company in China resulted in massive environmental contamination and human and animal disease (Lina et al. 2019). A leading military lab, the US Army Medical Research Institute of Infectious Diseases (USAMRIID), had untreated wastewater accidentally sprayed into the environment in 2018 and 2019 (Young 2023).

12.4 BIOHACKING AND UNDOCUMENTED LABORATORIES

Do-it-yourself (DIY) biology and community biohacking have been widely practiced for over a decade and should have prompted intelligence agencies to improve biodefense preparedness (Engells and MacIntyre 2016). DIY labs are only allowed to operate at the BSL-1 level, but there is no monitoring or independent regulation of this. Lab-in-a-box kits can be purchased on the Internet, and biohacking may occur in private homes, not laboratories. A greater problem is undocumented or illegal labs for which there is no method for detection or monitoring. A historical example is the clandestine lab of the Rajneesh cult in Oregon, which was responsible for the largest known bioterrorist attack in the United States (MacIntyre 2015). The Rajneesh lab was discovered almost a year after the attack and long after public health authorities declared the epidemic of salmonella to be accidental, due to poor hygiene.

The finding of a warehouse containing mice, microorganisms, reagents, and laboratory equipment in Reedley, California, in late 2022 highlights the potential for illegal labs to fly under the radar (MacIntyre 2023). It was discovered accidentally by a local code enforcement officer in December 2022, but the warehouse was not searched until March 2023, at which time a large number of genetically modified mice and a range of BSL-3 level viruses such as SARS-CoV-2 and HIV were reportedly found at the warehouse. One refrigerator was labeled "Ebolavirus" (Smith 2023). The company Prestige Biotech was operating without a license and had no need for any of these test animals or biological materials based on their business, which was to import test kits from China (Smith 2023). Prestige acquired a bankrupt Chinese predecessor company, Universal Meditech Inc., which had its SARS-CoV-2 rapid antigen test recalled in 2022 by the Food and Drug Administration. Allegedly, Prestige Biotech was storing equipment in the warehouse until it could be moved to a new location. A House Select Committee on the Chinese Communist Party Hearing in the US revealed that US agencies, including the Centers for Disease Control and Prevention, did not test any of the samples present in the lab, including ones labeled "Ebolavirus" (@TexasLindsay 2023). The entire episode shows a failure of US biosecurity and national security, and it is highly unlikely that China would have made a similar mistake if a US company had set up a biotech company on their land.

Illegal labs pose a safety risk, may involve inhumane or unethical animal research, or may result in undocumented waste disposal into the community. Infection of personnel in undocumented laboratories or unsafe waste disposal may result in a community outbreak. Waste from labs may enter waterways, accumulate in soil, or become aerosolized, affecting humans, animals, or the environment. A Trojan Horse attack may be perpetrated by a state or non-state actor by establishing an undocumented lab or even a documented biotech company used as a front to launch a biological attack. Most governments do not have a systematic method to track or identify such labs. The Reedley case shows how easily undocumented labs can be established in the community and highlights a weakness in US biodefense. Decreasing costs of gain-of-function and synthetic biology (Noyce and Evans 2018) make illegal labs more accessible than ever. It is entirely conceivable that many illegal labs may exist in the community in the same way that drug labs do.

12.5 NEW FRONTIERS

The intersection of synthetic biology, artificial intelligence, geopolitics, and military competition has resulted in new and unanticipated risks and opportunities for military organizations and civilian populations. While technology such as CRISPR-Cas9 and its derivatives is revolutionizing treatments and prevention of previously untreatable conditions, particularly the potential to alter the impact of polygenic diseases and cure monogenic diseases, the risks of their use for harm are significant (Cyranoski and Ledford 2018; Cyranoski 2018; Winblad and Lanner 2017). Germline editing, previously confined to animal research, was controversially conducted in humans by Chinese scientist Dr He Jiankui, who announced germline modification of two embryos that were subsequently carried to term and born in 2016. This was met with uproar, despite the United Kingdom and Sweden having commenced such research on embryos in 2016, but other countries soon followed. By 2019, the World Health Organization (WHO) had issued a policy on human genome editing, with recommendations issued in 2021 (WHO 2021). Human genome editing, which is now widespread and being conducted by all superpowers, highlights the broader research efforts into germline editing concurrently occurring around the world both for the purpose of preventing and treating disease and also, significantly, for augmentation, enhancement, and non-medical purposes.

Previously confined to works of fiction, the age of augmented or enhanced humans, designed with "superior" genetic characteristics, has now arrived. The potential utility of germline editing and related genetic modifications – permanent or temporary – has won the attention of military and non-military organizations around the world, offering a new route for gaining a strategic edge over an adversary. It is now theoretically possible to engineer enhancements into humans that would allow higher exposures to various kinds of biological agents or toxins, render humans immune to certain kinds of transmissible agents, or alternatively be used as a weapon to weaken a target population. Augmentation of innate abilities such as cognition, memory, strength, muscle bulk, nutritional regulation, and many other physiological, neural, and humoral characteristics are also theoretically possible, with technical proof of concept already demonstrated in animal studies (Heslop and MacIntyre 2019). This extends already decades-long efforts and substantial investment into the enhancement and augmentation of innate capabilities of warfighters in most major militaries.

These same technologies can also be used for deliberate attack, influence, disruption, and psychological operations. Using technology such as CRISPR-Cas9, subtle modifications can be introduced into economically critical crops and species, resulting in unexpected and impactful changes. This "grey zone" type of warfare is more frequently being employed by major powers and offers far greater impact for the investment without the risks and costs of conventional warfare (Atlantic Council 2022). Additionally, rapid analytics and desktop protein and nucleic acid synthesis technologies are far more accessible now and allow rapid prototyping of new threat vectors with significantly less investment of personnel or requirement for background knowledge and know-how. Hypothetically, economic competitors may be confronted with pests that are suddenly resistant to all known pesticides or preventive interventions, leading to profound economic and social impact, or pathogens resistant to all available antimicrobials. Another example could be military organizations deploying enhanced soldiers who are resistant to the effects of biological toxins, chemical weapons, infectious agents, and even the effects of radiation exposure. Furthermore, enhancements and augmentations such as improved reaction times, improved light sensitivity (night vision), rapid wound healing, reduced need for nutrition and sleep, reduced fatigue, and improved cognition are all possible capabilities that could be addressed by using current or emerging synthetic biology techniques.

Even direct targeting of human populations for military purposes or "grey-zone" operations is not outside the realm of possibility, such as a larger-scale version of the salmonellosis attacks by the Rajneesh cultists in Oregon for political purposes. Such actions are currently extremely difficult to detect and have a high degree of plausible deniability – that is, the attribution of deliberate action to a particular party cannot be achieved. This new approach to conflict – to influence and shape populations, economies, and opinions rather than conquer in the traditional military sense – is predicted to become more and more prominent as competition for limited resources occurs against a background of climate change impacts and overpopulation.

Other technologies are again intersecting in unexpected or concerning ways. The emergence of advanced artificial intelligence (AI) technologies such as ChatGPT has been shown to be able to be used to optimize planning for a biological attack (Dixon et al. 2020; Hassoun et al. 2021; Service 2023). In a closely related field, a recent study demonstrated how a chemical synthesis algorithm similar to ChatGPT could be used to generate thousands of novel candidate chemical warfare agents with predicted toxicity profiles far more potent than the already highly toxic VX nerve agent (Urbina et al. 2022a, 2022b). AI technologies have the potential to empower individuals and organizations in unexpected ways and lower the barriers to accessing technology and know-how, and to enable information that can be used to develop threats. At this time, there is no international framework for regulating this emerging area of risk despite significant concerns from within and outside the AI and biological weapon research community, but calls are growing for AI to be regulated in much the same way as current chemical, biological, radiological, nuclear, and explosive (CBRNE) threats through initiatives like the Australia Group (Heslop and Keep 2023).

Mirroring the potential for AI and emerging biological technologies to cause harm, there is a significant opportunity for AI tools to contribute to reducing the likelihood of proliferation of biosecurity threats and their potential use (Heslop and Keep 2023). AI has the potential to allow for substantial automation of threat detection, intelligence gathering, early warning systems (Pfaff 2020), monitoring, and regulatory compliance activities. Equally, exploration of possible future threat vectors using generative AI techniques may provide insights into how existing risk controls can be improved by identifying possible new threat vectors and pathways. Additionally, AI tools have the ability to examine large datasets produced from simulation modeling and scenario-based examination of risk – offering data insights unachievable through human analytics – honing down competing threats and priorities more efficiently (Hynek and Solovyeva 2022). Developing frameworks around areas such as CBRNE, synthetic biology, and AI to ensure humanity realizes the benefits of these emerging dual-use technologies while avoiding the harms is becoming an ever more pressing need.

12.6 CONCLUSIONS

There have been quantum advances in technology, including gain-of-function, synthetic biology, human genome editing, and AI, as well as an ever-expanding array of enhanced potential pandemic pathogens (MacIntyre 2020). This poses an increasing threat to biosafety and a greater risk than ever of unnatural epidemics and pandemics. This means the scope and scale of biological warfare are far greater today. Yet public awareness of even biological dual-use research of concern (DURC) – let alone the implications of other technologies – is low (MacIntyre et al. 2020). The public is the most important stakeholder, as both the beneficiary of such research and also the unwitting victim of harms caused by the same research. Yet the public has not been informed or engaged in the debate about such research, which has focused mostly on the rights of scientists and the potential benefits of such research (MacIntyre et al. 2020).

There is also a need for better methods for the regulation and oversight of biological technology, including private and DIY labs. There is a role for law enforcement agencies, who could apply lessons learned from detecting illegal drug labs toward identifying illegal biolabs. Legal frameworks, including the Biological Weapons Convention, should also be reviewed as they are not fit for purpose, being unauditable and unenforceable. A pathogen of pandemic potential can spread around the world in a matter of weeks, yet legal processes fit for responding to the urgency of this threat are not available. The FBI took seven years to develop a case to charge a suspect in the anthrax attacks of 2001 (MacIntyre 2015). In the Reedley case, it took about three months to obtain a warrant to search the warehouse, and there was no consequential action by the FBI or any other agency that resulted. If an investigation involves a highly contagious pathogen that could cause a pandemic in a matter of weeks, such processes are inadequate. Furthermore, there are policy gaps in the regulation of DIY and private biolabs, human genome editing, AI, and other technologies, and a failure to consider the associated risks. There are many available methods to harness textual, image, video, and other open-source and non-open data streams to improve threat detection and identify potential illegal biolabs. Mapping of documented laboratories globally would also assist in managing risk. Currently, no comprehensive map or database of global laboratories exists, although attempts to do so have been made. A map of global laboratories could be linked to epidemic early warning systems to red-flag epidemics arising in the perimeter of unknown laboratories. Broader consideration of emerging and converging technologies such as AI, cybertechnology, and human genome editing is altogether absent, with systems, processes, and policies still siloed in individual areas (MacIntyre et al. 2018). We need better cross-disciplinary methods, involving health sciences, law enforcement, intelligence, defense, emergency response, AI, and community members. Without new approaches to biosafety, we cannot adequately mitigate the very real and increasing risk to humanity.

REFERENCES

Alibek K, Handelman S. *Biohazard: The Chilling True Story of the Largest Covert Biological Weapons Program in the World--Told from the Inside by the Man Who Ran It*: Random House Publishing Group 1999.

Andersen KG, Rambaut A, Lipkin WI, et al. The proximal origin of SARS-CoV-2. *Nat Med* 2020;26(4):450–2. doi: 10.1038/s41591-020-0820-9.

Ashraf H. Europe's response to bioterrorism starts slowly but gathers pace. *Lancet* 2002;360(9335):733–4. doi: 10.1016/s0140-6736(02)09943-9.

Atlantic Council. Today's wars are fought in the 'gray zone.' Here's everything you need to know about it. 23 February 2022. https://www.atlanticcouncil.org/blogs/new-atlanticist/todays-wars-are-fought-in-the-gray-zone-heres-everything-you-need-to-know-about-it/.

Atlas RM. Combating the threat of biowarfare and bioterrorism: defending against biological weapons is critical to global security. *BioScience* 1999;49(6):465–77. doi: 10.2307/1313554.

Carroll MC. *Lab 257: The Disturbing Story of the Government's Secret Germ Laboratory*: HarperCollins 2009.

Carus WS. *Bioterrorism and Biocrimes: The Illicit Use of Biological Agents Since 1900.* Center for Counterproliferation Research, National Defense University, Washington, D.C. 1998.

Casagrande R, et al. *Risk and Benefit Analysis of Gain of Function Research.* NIH Office of Policy. In: Scientific G, ed. 2016.

Chen X, Chughtai AA, MacIntyre CR. A systematic review of risk analysis tools for differentiating unnatural from natural epidemics. *Mil Med* 2017;182(11):e1827–e35. doi: 10.7205/milmed-d-17-00090.

Chen X, Chughtai AA, MacIntyre CR. Recalibration of the Grunow-Finke assessment tool to improve performance in detecting unnatural epidemics. *Risk Anal* 2019;39(7):1465–75. doi: 10.1111/risa.13255.

Cyranoski D. CRISPR-baby scientist fails to satisfy critics. *Nature* 2018;564(7734):13–14. doi: 10.1038/d41586-018-07573-w.

Cyranoski D, Ledford H. Genome-edited baby claim provokes international outcry. *Nature* 2018;563(7733):607–8. doi: 10.1038/d41586-018-07545-0.

Dixon TA, Curach NC, Pretorius IS. Bio-informational futures: the convergence of artificial intelligence and synthetic biology. *EMBO Rep* 2020;21(3):e50036. doi: 10.15252/embr.202050036.

Engells TE, MacIntyre R. Do it yourself biology--committed hobbyists or dangers to the public safety? *J Healthc Prot Manage* 2016;32(2):39–54.

Fears R, ter Meulen V. European academies advise on gain-of-function studies in influenza virus research. *J Virol* 2015;90(5):2162–4. doi: 10.1128/jvi.03045–15.

Frischknecht F. The history of biological warfare. Human experimentation, modern nightmares and lone madmen in the twentieth century. *EMBO Rep* 2003;4 Spec No(Suppl 1):S47–52. doi: 10.1038/sj.embor.embor849.

Gillum D, Krishnan P, Byers K. A searchable laboratory-acquired infection database. *Appl Biosafety* 2016;21(4):203-7.

Gold H, Totani Y. *Japan's Infamous Unit 731: Firsthand Accounts of Japan's Wartime Human Experimentation Program*: Tuttle Publishing 2019.

Guillemin J. *Biological Weapons: From the Invention of State-Sponsored Programs to Contemporary Bioterrorism*: Columbia University Press 2005.

Harrison NL, Sachs JD. A call for an independent inquiry into the origin of the SARS-CoV-2 virus. *Proc Natl Acad Sci U S A* 2022;119(21):e2202769119. doi: 10.1073/pnas.2202769119.

Hassoun S, Jefferson F, Shi X, et al. Artificial intelligence for biology. *Integrative and Comparative Biology* 2021;61(6):2267–75. doi: 10.1093/icb/icab188.

Heslop D, Keep J. AI, arms control and the new cold war: *The Strategist,* 16 November 2023. https://www.aspistrategist.org.au/ai-arms-control-and-the-new-cold-war/.

Heslop D, MacIntyre C. Germ line genome editing and the emerging struggle for supremacy in the Chemical, Biological and Radiological (CBR) balance of power. *Glob Biosecurity* 2019;1:169. doi: 10.31646/gbio.18.

Hynek N, Solovyeva A. *Militarizing Artificial Intelligence: Theory, Technology, and Regulation*: Taylor & Francis 2022.

Jinek M, Chylinski K, Fonfara I, et al. A programmable dual-RNA-guided DNA endonuclease in adaptive bacterial immunity. *Science* 2012;337(6096):816–21. doi: 10.1126/science.1225829.

Kaufer A, Theis T, Lau K, et al. Biological warfare: The history of microbial pathogens, biotoxins and emerging threats. *Microbiol Australia* 2020;41. doi: 10.1071/MA20031.

Lane JM, Summer L. Smallpox as a weapon for bioterrorism. In *Bioterrorism and Infectious Agents: A New Dilemma for the 21st Century* 2009:147–67. doi: 10.1007/978-1-4419-1266-4_5.

Lina S, Kunasekaran M, Moa A. Brucellosis outbreak in China, 2019. *Glob Biosecurity* 2021;3. doi: 10.31646/gbio.108.

MacIntyre CR. Biopreparedness in the age of genetically engineered pathogens and open access science: an urgent need for a paradigm shift. *Mil Med* 2015;180(9):943–9. doi: 10.7205/milmed–d-14-00482.

MacIntyre CR. *Dark Winter: An Insider's Guide to Pandemics and Biosecurity*: NewSouth Publishing 2022.

MacIntyre CR. Illegal biolabs in the community - is Reedley a one-off? *Glob Biosecurity* 2023;5 doi: 10.31646/gbio.237.

MacIntyre CR. Reevaluating the risk of smallpox reemergence. *Mil Med* 2020 doi: 10.1093/milmed/usaa084.

MacIntyre CR, Adam DC, Turner R, et al. Public awareness, acceptability and risk perception about infectious diseases dual-use research of concern: a cross-sectional survey. *BMJ Open* 2020;10(1):e029134. doi: 10.1136/bmjopen-2019-029134.

MacIntyre CR, Chen X, Kunasekaran M, et al. Artificial intelligence in public health: the potential of epidemic early warning systems. *J Int Med Res* 2023;51(3). doi: 10.1177/03000605231159335.

MacIntyre CR, Engells TE, Scotch M, et al. Converging and emerging threats to health security. *Environ Syst Decis* 2018;38(2):198–207. doi: 10.1007/s10669-017-9667-0.

McMullan LK, Flint M, Chakrabarti A, et al. Characterisation of infectious Ebola virus from the ongoing outbreak to guide response activities in the Democratic Republic of the Congo: a phylogenetic and in vitro analysis. *Lancet Infect Dis* 2019;19(9):1023–32. doi: 10.1016/S1473-3099(19)30291-9.

Morris B, Kedar BZ. 'Cast thy bread': Israeli biological warfare during the 1948 War. *Middle Eastern studies* 2023;59(5):752–76. doi: 10.1080/00263206.2022.2122448.

Nakajima K, Desselberger U, Palese P. Recent human influenza A (H1N1) viruses are closely related genetically to strains isolated in 1950. *Nature* 1978;274(5669):334–39. doi: 10.1038/274334a0.

Noah DL, Huebner KD, Darling RG, et al. The history and threat of biological warfare and terrorism. *Emerg Med Clin North Am* 2002;20(2):255–71. doi: 10.1016/s0733-8627(01)00002-5.

Noyce RS, Evans DH. Synthetic horsepox viruses and the continuing debate about dual use research. *PLoS Pathog* 2018;14(10):e1007025. doi: 10.1371/journal.ppat.1007025.

Noyce RS, Lederman S, Evans DH. Construction of an infectious horsepox virus vaccine from chemically synthesized DNA fragments. *PLoS One* 2018;13(1):e0188453. doi: 10.1371/journal.pone.0188453.

Orellana C. Laboratory-acquired SARS raises worries on biosafety. *Lancet Infect Dis* 2004;4(2):64. doi: 10.1016/S1473-3099(04)00911-9.

Pfaff CA. The ethics of acquiring disruptive technologies: artificial intelligence, autonomous weapons, and decision support systems. *Prism* 2020;8:128.

Riedel S. Biological warfare and bioterrorism: a historical review. *Proc (Bayl Univ Med Cent)* 2004;17(4):400–6. doi: 10.1080/08998280.2004.11928002.

Rozo M, Gronvall GK. The reemergent 1977 H1N1 strain and the gain-of-function debate. *mBio* 2015;6(4) doi: 10.1128/mBio.01013-15.

Schuerger CB, Quinn S, Kinoshita K, Daniels R, Puglisi OA. *Understanding the Global Gain-of-Function Research Landscape*: Technology CfSaE, ed. 2023.

Senior K. Recent Singapore SARS case a laboratory accident. *Lancet Infect Dis* 2003;3(11):679. doi: 10.1016/s1473-3099(03)00815-6.

Service RF. Could chatbots help devise the next pandemic virus? *Science* 2023;380(6651):1211. doi: 10.1126/science.adj3377.

Smart JK. *Chapter 2: History of Chemical and Biological Warfare: An American Perspective.*In: Medical Aspects of Chemical and Biological Warfare. In: Zajtchuk R, Bellamy R. Textbook of Military Medicine. Washington, DC: Borden Institute; 1997: 30, 36.

Smith E. *Congressional Investigation: Ebola at Reedley Biolab? CDC Response 'Nothing Short of Malfeasance'*: GVWire 2023.

Spiers EM. *Agents of War: A History of Chemical and Biological Weapons, Second Expanded Edition*: Reaktion Books 2021.

@TexasLindsay_. WATCH: The most damning exchange from the CDC Hearing was from Dr. Neal Dunn (R-FL). Dunn pressed Cohen on the shocking revelations of the CDC's handling of the Bio Lab found in California. "Despite vials being labeled as Ebola, HIV, etc—CDC opted to NOT test a SINGLE vial": X 2023.

Török TJ, Tauxe RV, Wise RP, et al. A large community outbreak of salmonellosis caused by intentional contamination of restaurant salad bars. *Jama* 1997;278(5):389–95. doi: 10.1001/jama.1997.03550050051033.

Trevisanato SI. The 'Hittite plague', an epidemic of tularemia and the first record of biological warfare. *Med Hypotheses* 2007;69(6):1371–4. doi: 10.1016/j.mehy.2007.03.012.

Urbina F, Lentzos F, Invernizzi C, et al. Dual use of artificial-intelligence-powered drug discovery. *Nat Mach Intell* 2022a;4(3):189–91. doi: 10.1038/s42256-022-00465-9.

Urbina F, Lentzos F, Invernizzi C, et al. A teachable moment for dual-use. *Nat Mach Intell* 2022b;4(7):607. doi: 10.1038/s42256-022-00511-6.

Walgate R. SARS escaped Beijing lab twice. *Genome Biol* 2004;4. doi: 10.1186/gb-spotlight-20040427-03.

Walker AM. The last days of smallpox: tragedy in Birmingham. *J Hos Infect* 2018;100(4):478. doi: 10.1016/j.jhin.2018.07.029.

Wilkening DA. Sverdlovsk revisited: modeling human inhalation anthrax. *Proc Natl Acad Sci U S A* 2006;103(20):7589–94. doi: 10.1073/pnas.0509551103.

Wimmer E. The test-tube synthesis of a chemical called poliovirus. The simple synthesis of a virus has far-reaching societal implications. *EMBO Rep* 2006;7 Spec No(Spec No):S3–9. doi: 10.1038/sj.embor.7400728.

Winblad N, Lanner F. At the heart of gene edits in human embryos. *Nature* 2017;548(7668):398–400. doi: 10.1038/nature23533.

World Health Organization (WHO). *Human Genome Editing: Position Paper.* Health Ethics & Governance (HEG) Research for Health (RFH), ed. 2021.

Young A. *Pandora's Gamble: Lab Leaks, Pandemics, and a World at Risk. Center Street,* New York 2023.

13 An Integrated Approach to Planning for and Responding to Ionizing Radiation Incidents

LeeAnn Racz and Alan Hale

13.1 INTRODUCTION

Despite the unavoidable exposure to background ionizing radiation, there are few hazards that are as poorly understood and therefore more feared. Although there is some debate about the validity of the assumption (Calabrese and Selby 2023), it is generally recognized that radiation is carcinogenic with a linear non-threshold (LNT) model, meaning that any radiation dose increases the risk of cancer for humans (Yanovskiy et al. 2019). However, emergency radiation incidents can often be anticipated based on the likelihood of the presence of radioactive material, and therefore response plans can be developed.

Known radiation in the workplace is typically highly regulated with closely monitored exposures. There also is the potential for unexpected radiation releases, such as in the case of an improvised nuclear device (IND), radiological dispersion device (RDD), or radiation exposure device (RED) events. Nuclear detonations result in significant explosions as well as radioactive contamination. RDDs, however, use conventional explosives or mechanical means to disperse radioactive material or emit radiation, thereby denying the use of an area. REDs are intended to expose people to radiation without their knowledge (US Department of Homeland Security 2023). Radiation incidents can also occur at hazardous waste sites, scrap metal reprocessing facilities, or during transport (USEPA 2017a). Nuclear power facilities already have robust planning, training, and exercise protocols. Regardless of the probability of occurrence, community emergency responders can develop plans, procure the required equipment, train on their equipment and plans, and exercise the plans to gain confidence in their ability to respond to radiation incidents.

This chapter provides a high-level overview of considerations for planning and preparing for responses to emergency radiation incidents. Response plans for radiation emergencies can be complex and require significant coordination and resources from multiple agencies, even at the local level. Thus, this chapter does not cover

 DOI: 10.1201/9781003648178-14

details on every aspect regarding planning for and responding to radiation incidents. Rather, it describes concepts that should be given careful thought and research prior to a radiological incident. Organizations and communities embarking on developing response plans should consult additional resources in earnest for guidance.

13.2 PLAN

Although effective containment measures may be in place, unexpected events can trigger radiation releases. Where radiation is known to be used, plans should be developed for the range of possible scenarios. The USEPA (2017b) has defined three protective action phases for responses to radiation incidents: early, intermediate, and late.

The early phase occurs immediately following an incident when little or no information about the extent of the radiological hazards may be available. Early-phase protective actions focus on avoiding radioactive gases or particulates, minimizing external exposure, and limiting the spread of contamination. The intermediate phase occurs after exposure measurements have been made, which can inform decisions. Intermediate-phase protective actions are aimed at reducing public and worker exposures to radiation, limiting the spread of contamination, and preparing for late-phase cleanup. During the late-phase response, cleanup and remediation strategies are developed to reduce environmental radiation levels to acceptable levels (US Department of Homeland Security 2023).

A radiation incident will likely draw attention from responders from outside the local area. In the US, federal agencies have plans to assist with such events, especially those that exceed the capabilities of the state and local community. However, it will take time for these agencies to mobilize and become operational at any given site. In fact, state and local governments have the primary responsibility for protecting the public during a radiation emergency (USEPA 2017a). Therefore, communities should plan for radiation incidents as well, especially during the early stages of a response, until additional resources become available.

13.2.1 Local Plans

Given the LNT model, yet the unavoidable truth that no one can escape background radiation, radiation risk management approaches attempt to reduce and maintain radiation exposures to levels as low as reasonably achievable (ALARA). The ALARA concept aims to keep radiation doses as low as can be reasonably achieved, taking into account economic and social factors, while not exceeding regulatory dose limits (Hendee and Edwards 1986).

13.2.1.1 Exposure Pathways

There are three general mechanisms for potential radiation exposure from radiation incidents: direct external exposure, inhalation, and ingestion. Specifically, these general mechanisms correspond to seven exposure pathways (Table 13.1, adapted from US Department of Homeland Security 2023).

Depending on the type of radiation and the conditions surrounding the release, some potential exposure pathways may be ruled out. For instance, in the response to a sealed radioactive source, if the source is no longer in a shielded configuration but the integrity of the source's encapsulation remains, ingestion or inhalation would not be of concern. Additionally, a response worker and a member of the public may not have the same exposure pathways. For example, long-term effects on groundwater and affected residents must be considered in late-phase operations; however, these may not be relevant to the responders. How to control and mitigate radiation doses are discussed in section 13.3.1.

13.2.1.2 Radiation Dose Limits

The Occupational Safety and Health Administration (OSHA) has set radiation dose limits that apply to both routine and emergency response operations. Routine occupational whole-body radiation doses are generally limited to 1.25 rem (12.5 millisieverts [mSv]) per calendar quarter and 5 rem (50 mSv) per year (OSHA 2024b). However, during the early stages of response actions, incident commanders may refer to the Total Effective Dose Equivalent (TEDE) guidelines (Table 13.2), which are the sum of the effective dose equivalent from external radiation exposure and committed effective dose equivalent from internal radiation exposure. TEDE guidelines may be regarded as flexible for early response stages since a single maximum dose limit cannot be established for all emergencies. Note that a dose of 25 rem (0.25 Sv) is not expected to result in acute health effects but could increase the risk of chronic effects, such as cancer (USEPA 2017b). Incident commanders may use TEDE guidelines to understand risks associated with different radiation doses and to inform their decisions about when to have personnel stop response actions. These dose guidelines are used for workers, and there may be additional considerations for employers who have Nuclear Regulatory Commission (NRC) or state-regulated material.

While public exposure is also important, the concept of avoidable dose is utilized. USEPA (2017b) offers guidance on what projected dose to the population warrants specific public health actions (e.g., relocation).

TABLE 13.1
Exposure Pathway Considerations

Specific Exposure Pathways	General Mechanism(s) of Exposure
External radiation from facility/incident site	Direct external exposure
External radiation from plume	Direct external exposure
Inhalation of radioactive particles from plume	Inhalation
Contamination of skin and clothing	Direct external exposure, inhalation, and ingestion
External radiation from ground deposition	Direct external exposure
Ingestion of contaminated food and water	Ingestion
Inhalation of re-suspended radioactive particles	Inhalation

TABLE 13.2
Total Effective Dose Equivalent (TEDE) Guidelines (Adapted from OSHA 2024b)

Activity	TEDE Guideline	Conditions
Annual limit for all occupational exposures, including for radiation workers	5 rem (0.05 Sv)	• All reasonably achievable actions must be taken to minimize dose.
Infrastructure protection and restoration necessary for public welfare (e.g., a power plant), in lower-hazard areas such as the Light Damage zone and fallout areas around a nuclear detonation site, excluding the Dangerous Fallout zone and elevated radiation areas	10 rem (0.10 Sv)	• All appropriate actions and controls must be implemented. • Appropriate respiratory protection and other personal protection is provided and used. • Monitoring is available to project or measure dose.
Life-saving, medical response, infrastructure restoration, or protection of populations in medium-hazard areas, such as the Moderate Damage zone around a nuclear detonation site, and fallout areas excluding the Dangerous Fallout zone	25 rem (0.25 Sv)	• All appropriate actions and controls must be implemented. • Appropriate respiratory protection and other personal protection is provided and used. • Monitoring available to project or measure dose.
Life-saving and critical infrastructure missions (i.e., missions that directly protect significant populations from substantial risks of injury, illness, or death) in high-hazard zones, including the Dangerous Fallout zone, to include missions that critically enable the larger response effort, such as fire suppression and critical infrastructure engineering missions	Greater than 25 rem (>0.25 Sv)	• All appropriate actions and controls must be implemented. • If life-saving emergency responder doses approach or exceed 50 rem (0.5 Sv), emergency responders must be made fully aware of both the acute and the chronic (cancer) risks of such exposure. • Appropriate respiratory protection and other personal protection is provided and used. • Monitoring is available to project or measure dose. • Life-saving and critical infrastructure engineering missions are least likely to be successful in the Severe Damage zone and may subject responders to lethal doses of radiation. • All missions are evaluated and justified by the Incident Commander, including assessment of hazards, value of the mission, and likelihood of success.

13.2.2 Medical Management of Radiation Emergency Victims

Acute radiation syndrome or sickness (ARS) is a chief concern among healthcare workers who treat patients exposed to radiation. There are four phases in ARS that are associated with four subsyndromes (hematopoietic, cutaneous, gastrointestinal, and neurovascular) which manifest over a period of hours to weeks as listed below (OSHA 2024b). Table 13.3 describes the likelihood of effects of whole-body irradiation by percentage of people exposed according to the dose ranges in units of rad and gray (Gy) as well as by time of onset after exposure and duration (adapted from Bushberg 2022 and OSHA 2024b). Note that whole-body irradiation of up to about 100 rad (1 Gy) is unlikely to cause symptoms (Bushberg 2022).

- Prodromal phase – Immediately following exposure, symptoms may include loss of appetite, nausea, vomiting, fatigue, and diarrhea. Higher doses may result in fever, prostration, respiratory distress, and hyper-excitability. If death does not occur, the symptoms typically subside within 1–2 days.
- Latent phase – Following the prodromal period, the latent period is free of symptoms, and the duration can vary depending on the radiation dose.
- Illness phase – After the latent period, illness can include infection, electrolyte imbalance, diarrhea, bleeding, cardiovascular collapse, and short periods of unconsciousness, depending on the radiation dose.
- Mortality – Following illness, victims will either recover or experience death.

Both the public and emergency workers may become injured from non-radiation hazards in an emergency. When they need medical assistance, they should be monitored for radioactive contamination and then decontaminated if needed prior to being transported to a medical facility. However, it may be more important to treat such injuries before full decontamination if decontamination would aggravate the injury. In such cases, decontamination may be limited to removing outer clothing and shoes. If outer clothing cannot be removed, even covering a person with a blanket can help to minimize the spread of radioactive material during transport (OSHA 2024b).

13.2.3 Coordination with Federal Agencies

In accordance with the National Response Framework, federal and state resources may be called upon when response to an emergency requires resources beyond what is available at the local level. The complexity of a radiological incident will likely mean that such additional resources will become involved. Table 13.4 lists the primary federal response authorities for various types of incidents. However, multiple agencies may become involved, and the Department of Homeland Security/Federal Emergency Management Authority (FEMA) may lead or coordinate support for the primary authority for complex incidents. Additional federal authorities not listed in Table 13.4 may also assist. For example, the Federal Radiological Monitoring Assessment Center (FRMAC), whose operational readiness is maintained by the

TABLE 13.3
Whole-body Irradiation Effects (Adapted from Bushberg 2022 and OSHA 2024b)

		Whole-Body Absorbed Dose				
ARS Phase	**Symptom**	**100–200 rad (1–2 Gy)**	**200–600 rad (2–6 Gy)**	**600–800 rad (6–8 Gy)**	**800–3,000 rad (8–30 Gy)**	**>3,000 rad (>30 Gy)**
Prodromal (Immediate)	**Nausea and vomiting**	5–50%	50–100%	75–100%	90–100%	100%
	Time of onset	2–6 hours	1–2 hours	10–60 min	<10 min	Minutes
	Duration	<24 hours	24–48 hours	<48 hours	<48 hours	N/A (patients die in <48 hours)
	Diarrhea	None	None to mild (<10%)	Heavy (>10%)	Heavy (>95%)	Heavy (100%)
	Time of onset	N/A	3–8 hours	1–3 hours	<1 hour	<1 hour
	Headache	Slight	Mild to moderate (50%)	Moderate (80%)	Severe (80–90%)	Severe (100%)
	Time of onset	N/A	4–24 hours	3–4 hours	1–2 hours	<1 hour
	Fever	None	Moderate increase (10–100%)	Moderate to severe (100%)	Severe (100%)	Severe (100%)
	Time of onset	N/A	1–3 hours	<1 hour	<1 hour	<1 hour
	Central nervous system function	No impairment	Cognitive impairment for 6–20 hours	Cognitive impairment for >24 hours	Rapid incapacitation	Seizures, tremors, ataxia, lethargy
Latent		28–31 days	7–28 days	<7 days	None	None
Illness		Mild to moderate leukopenia, fatigue, weakness	Moderate to severe leukopenia, purpura, hemorrhage, infections, epilation (hair loss), after 300 rad (3 Gy)	Severe leukopenia, high fever, diarrhea, vomiting, dizziness, disorientation, hypotension, electrolyte disturbance	Nausea, vomiting, severe diarrhea, high fever, electrolyte disturbance, shock	N/A (patients die in <48 hours)
Mortality	Without care	0–5%	5–100%	95–100%	100%	100%
	With care	0–5%	5–50%	50–100%	100%	100%
	Death	6–8 weeks	4–6 weeks	2–4 weeks	2 days–2 weeks	1–2 days

TABLE 13.4
Federal Response Authorities (Adapted from USEPA 2023)

Incident Type, Facilities, or Materials Involved	Primary Authority for Federal Response
Nuclear facilities that are:	
Owned or operated by the Department of Defense (DOD)	DOD
Owned or operated by the Department of Energy (DOE)	DOE
Licensed by the Nuclear Regulatory Commission (NRC) or an NRC Agreement State	NRC (FEMA may coordinate the federal response for incidents with offsite consequences, but NRC coordinates the onsite response)
Not licensed, owned, or operated by a federal agency or where the owner/operator is not able to respond	USEPA
Nuclear weapons and components that are:	
In the custody of the DOD	DOD
In the custody of the DOE	DOE
Radioactive materials being transported:	
By or for the DOD	DOD
By or for the DOE	DOE
Containing NRC or NRC Agreement State-licensed materials	NRC
Within certain areas of the coastal zone that are not licensed or owned by a federal agency or an NRC Agreement State	US Coast Guard
All others	USEPA
Radioactive materials in space vehicles impacting the US that are:	
Managed by the National Aeronautics and Space Administration (NASA)	NASA
Managed by the DOD	DOD
Not managed by the DOD or NASA and impacting certain areas of the coastal zone	US Coast Guard
All others	USEPA
Disused and unwanted sealed sources with no disposition pathway:	
Offsite source recovery	DOE
Unknown or unlicensed materials and domestic response to foreign materials and international incidents:	
Certain areas of the coastal zone	US Coast Guard
Outside certain areas of the coastal zone	USEPA
Imported contaminated consumer products that are distributed before detection	USEPA
Inadvertently imported radioactive materials	US Customs and Border Protection
Other inadvertent US incidents:	
Incidents involving lost/found/orphaned radioactive material	DOE/National Nuclear Security Administration
US assistance to foreign governments for incidents with international impacts:	
US government assistance to foreign government response and recovery efforts	Department of State/US Agency for International Development
Deliberate attacks in the US:	
All deliberate attacks involving nuclear/radiological facilities or materials	Department of Homeland Security

Department of Energy, may be called upon by the Department of Homeland Security to respond to nuclear and radiological incidents (Nevada National Security Site 2024). The Department of Energy also operates the Radiation Emergency Assistance Center/Training Site (REAC/TS), which provides emergency response guidance on medical management during radiological and nuclear incidents (Oak Ridge Institute for Science and Education 2024).

13.3 EQUIP

13.3.1 Controls

13.3.1.1 Workers

Organizations may anticipate the possibility of radiation releases by developing response plans before such events occur. These plans should include selection and procurement of appropriate control measures, such as personal protective equipment (PPE), for the full range of potential hazards.

The first task in selecting controls is to conduct a hazard assessment to determine potential safety and health hazards for workers. Employers should follow the often-referenced hierarchy of controls (Figure 13.1), which ought to consider elimination/substitution, engineering, and administrative controls before relying on PPE.

Ideally, the least hazardous materials and processes should be used to reduce risk to personnel and the environment; when hazards cannot be eliminated, they should be substituted with less hazardous options. If hazards cannot be removed, engineering controls are the next best approach, such as physical barriers, ventilation, or other measures to prevent hazards from coming into contact with workers or the public. For example, gamma radiation is predominantly an external exposure pathway and best controlled with engineering controls such as dense materials (e.g., lead, concrete, or brick) placed between the radiation source and people (USEPA 2017b).

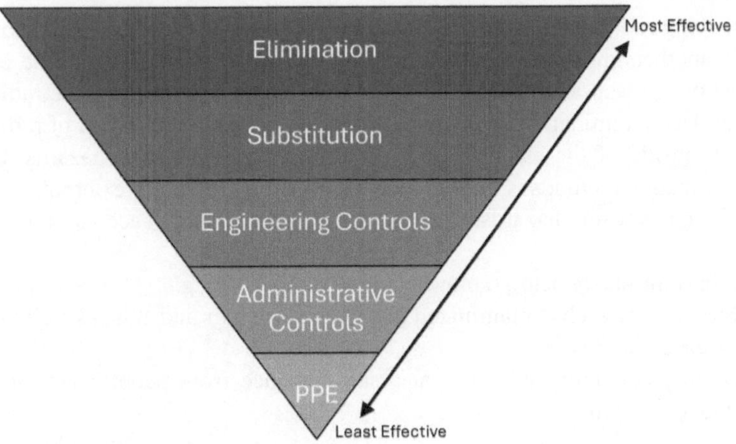

FIGURE 13.1 Hierarchy of controls

Administrative controls, such as job rotation, rest breaks, and access limitations, reduce the duration, frequency, or intensity of exposure.

Consistent with the ALARA principle, radiation doses from each of these pathways can be minimized by:

- Minimizing the time spent near radiation sources.
- Maximizing the distance between a person and radiation sources.
- Shielding a person from radiation sources (OSHA 2024b).

Minimizing the time spent near radiation sources is best achieved by planning emergency response missions such that personnel are exposed to or become contaminated with radiation as little as practicable. Sending personnel into an area with radiation contamination should be done with deliberate and careful thought to be as efficient as possible, even in an emergency.

External exposure to gamma/x-ray radiation from a "point source" follows the inverse square law, in which the intensity is inversely proportional to the square of the distance (Equation 13.1). For example, as the distance doubles, the radiation intensity is reduced to one-quarter of the initial intensity. Therefore, maximizing the distance between a person and radiation sources is another effective measure for reducing dose.

$$\frac{I_1}{I_2} = \frac{(D_2)^2}{(D_1)^2} \qquad \text{Equation 13.1}$$

where

I_1 = radiation intensity at an initial distance
I_2 = radiation intensity at a second distance
D_1 = initial distance from a radiation source
D_2 = second distance from a radiation source.

Removing radiological contamination from personnel, their clothing, and equipment is another important way to minimize the time a person would be exposed to radiation, as well as increase the distance between a person and the radioactive material. Decontamination limits radiation dose, prevents the spread of radioactive material outside of the response area, and minimizes ingestion hazards. Care in decontamination methods is needed to avoid creating secondary external, ingestion, or inhalation exposure hazards. Decontamination plans should account for:

- Areas for personnel to remove contaminated clothing.
- Showers for each contaminated person to wash hair and skin, as well as put on clean clothes.
- Storing contaminated waste at a safe distance from people and animals (OSHA 2024b).

Depending on the type of ionizing radiation, shielding may help to reduce the dose as well. One of the most common shielding options for alpha and beta radiation is

PPE. Although other methods, such as lead or concrete barriers, may also be effective for neutrons or x-rays/gamma radiation.

PPE is the least effective option, although it is almost certainly necessary in an emergency when other controls are not practical. PPE does not necessarily protect workers against most types of direct external radiation exposure but can help protect them from radiation contamination or intake, such as from inhalation or ingestion. PPE will not likely be effective for protecting against radiation from an RED, although PPE may help protect from contamination, ingestion, and inhalation from a release such as from an RDD. Workers who respond to larger events, such as from an IND or other nuclear weapon, will require PPE to protect from direct contamination but are still likely to be exposed to external radiation from fallout and from the detonation (OSHA 2024b). Airborne radiation poses particular hazards when inhaled, making respirators important PPE for responders. Skin surfaces should also be protected from alpha and beta radiation (USEPA 2017b).

An important consideration for employers is that workers who are required to wear respirators ought to be in a respiratory protection program. OSHA's respiratory protection standard under 29 CFR 1910 and 29 CFR 1926 includes provisions for a written program, such as procedures for selecting respirators; medical evaluations; fit testing; proper respirator use; cleaning, storing, and maintaining respirators; and training.

The most protective level of PPE is Level A, which consists of a self-contained breathing apparatus (SCBA) and a fully encapsulating chemical-resistant suit. However, where respiratory protection from radioactive particles is the goal, a NIOSH-approved full-face air-purifying respirator with a P-100 or high-efficiency particulate arrestance (HEPA) filter may be adequate, as determined by the hazard assessment (OSHA 2024b). Note that surgical or fabric masks are not designed or approved for protection against radioactive air contaminants or chemical vapors.

13.3.1.2 Population

Depending on the projected dose to the population, especially in large-scale incidents, protecting large populations from increased risk will be managed at higher levels of government. However, the incident commander may have to make localized sheltering or evacuation decisions to mitigate immediate suffering and loss of life.

Figure 13.2 (adapted from US Department of Homeland Security 2023) lists potential exposure pathways and associated protective actions by the three response

Potential Exposure Pathways:	External Radiation	Inhalation of Radioactivity in Plume	Skin and Clothing Contamination	External Radiation from Ground Deposition	Ingestion of Contaminated Food/Water	Inhalation of Re-suspended Radioactivity
Protective Actions:	• Sheltering • Evacuation • Access control	• Sheltering • Administration of stable iodine • Evacuation • Access control	• Sheltering • Evacuation • Decontamination of persons and animals	• Evacuation • Relocation • Decontamination of land and property	• Food and water controls	• Relocation • Decontamination of Land and Property
Protective Action Phase:	EARLY		INTERMEDIATE			LATE

FIGURE 13.2 Potential exposure pathways and protective actions by response phase (adapted from US Department of Homeland Security 2023)

phases. During the early phase, public health protective measures may include evacuations or sheltering-in-place, specifically if whole-body doses are projected to exceed 1 to 5 rem (10 to 50 mSv) over four days (USEPA 2017b). These kinds of decisions are also meant to minimize the time spent near the radiation source, maximize the distance from the source, and offer shielding. However, the decision to evacuate must consider the anticipated radiation dose during an evacuation, as well as the feasibility of an evacuation. Therefore, sheltering-in-place may be a preferred course of action when it provides at least as much protection as evacuation.

Administration of a stable iodine, namely potassium iodide (KI), will partially block thyroid uptake of radioactive iodine, which is produced by certain types of nuclear reactions (OSHA 2024b). However, medical officials should be consulted prior to making plans for its use (USEPA 2017b).

The intermediate phase occurs after the radiation release no longer poses a significant threat to human health, and the extent of radioactive contamination and exposures has been determined. Intermediate phase protective actions are aimed at reducing radiation exposure to the public, controlling worker exposures, and mitigating the spread of contamination (FEMA 2023).

Late-phase response actions reduce radiation levels in the environment to acceptable levels. This phase includes making final cleanup decisions and implementing remediation strategies. However, this phase could last for years, especially following incidents with widespread radiation contamination (FEMA 2023).

13.3.2 Radiation Measurement Equipment

Given that response decisions are made based on the level of radiation present above background, there must be a way to measure radiation at any given time following an incident. Low-cost equipment includes hand-held survey meters, particularly those that measure gamma radiation. Such meters can be used to help establish hazard zone perimeters according to the level of radioactivity. They can also be used to help determine contamination levels on personnel and equipment. However, different technologies are used to measure different types of radiation (i.e., alpha, beta, gamma/x-rays, and neutrons), and local resources may not have the necessary equipment to detect or measure the radiation of a particular incident. Conservative risk management may need to be used until further expertise and equipment arrive on scene, and more informed decisions can be made.

Another important resource is personal dosimeters that can record an individual's radiation dose. Ideally, a dosimeter or a personal radiation detector will also emit an audible alarm when the radiation levels exceed a certain threshold (FEMA 2023). Although smaller communities may not have access to such dosimeters, especially during the early phase of a response, federal and state organizations are likely to be equipped with them and should have plans for how to deploy them.

13.4 TRAIN

13.4.1 Hazardous Waste Operations and Emergency Response (HAZWOPER) Training Standard

OSHA requires responders who enter a hazardous area, such as an area with radiological material, to be trained in accordance with the HAZWOPER standard. This standard is outlined in 29 CFR 1910.120 for general industry and 29 CFR 1926.65 for the construction industry. OSHA-approved state plans or the USEPA's HAZWOPER standard (40 CFR Part 311, which adopts OSHA's HAZWOPER standard by reference) cover state and local government workers (OSHA 2024b).

HAZWOPER training must include hands-on experience that familiarizes personnel with equipment and safe practices in a non-hazardous setting. The level of training is commensurate with the type of work a person may be expected to perform. Table 13.5 lists the initial HAZWOPER training requirements for emergency response workers. All training levels also require annual refresher training (29 CFR 1910.120(q)(8)). Note that cleanup workers with a real or potential exposure to hazardous materials are required to take an initial 40 hours of instruction, 24 hours of field instruction, and an 8-hour annual refresher course (29 CFR 1910.120(e)(3)). Given the availability of additional training, many responders, especially incident

TABLE 13.5
HAZWOPER Training Requirements for Emergency Response Workers (Adapted from OSHA 2024a)

Worker Category	Initial Training
First Responder Awareness Level: Witnesses or discovers a release of hazardous substances and is trained to notify the proper authorities (29 CFR 1910.120(q)(6)(i))	Sufficient training to identify emergencies and initiate the response process and additional competencies
First Responder Operations Level: Responds to the release of hazardous substances in a defensive manner without trying to stop the release (29 CFR 1910.120(q)(6)(ii))	8-hour instruction that includes First Responder Awareness or the equivalent relevant experience and additional competencies
Hazardous Materials (HAZMAT) Technician: Responds aggressively to stop the release of hazardous substances (29 CFR 1910.120(q)(6)(iii))	24-hour First Responder Operations level training and additional competencies
HAZMAT Specialist: Responds with and in support of HAZMAT technicians and has specific knowledge of various hazardous substances (29 CFR 1910.120(q)(6)(iv))	24-hour HAZMAT Technician level training and additional competencies
Incident Commander: Assumes full control of the scene beyond the first responder awareness level (29 CFR 1910.120(q)(6)(v))	24-hour First Responder Operations level and additional competencies

commanders, choose to take a 40-hour course, which is beyond the minimum 24 hours of instruction.

13.4.2 National Fire Protection Association (NFPA) Training Standards

The Department of Homeland Security has adopted NFPA standards for personnel responding to hazardous materials and weapons of mass destruction (WMDs). NFPA 470, Hazardous Materials/Weapons of Mass Destruction (WMD) Standard for Responders, consolidated NFPA standards 1072, 472, and 473. These NFPA standards identify:

- Emergency response personnel professional qualifications.
- The minimum levels of competence for emergency responders at the awareness, operations, technician, incident commander, and other specialist levels.
- The levels of competence required of emergency medical services personnel who respond to HAZMAT or WMD incidents.

13.4.3 Training for Hospital and Triage Medical Personnel

First receivers are medical personnel who encounter contaminated patients. First receivers typically work at a site separated from where patients became contaminated, making exposures to medical personnel limited to the substances on the patients. OSHA (2005) published a best-practices guide for hospital-based first receivers of patients contaminated with hazardous substances. This guide describes training requirements, in addition to PPE and other healthcare worker needs.

Table 13.6 lists the training levels required for first receivers according to their expected duties during an emergency response. These mandatory trainings are outlined in Table 13.5. In addition, other hospital personnel who are not expected

TABLE 13.6
Mandatory Training for First Receivers (Adapted from OSHA 2005)

Mandatory Training	First Receiver Duties	Reference
Incident briefing	Employees who were not previously anticipated to work in the decontamination zone but were called in incidentally.	OSHA (1997)
HAZWOPER First Responder Awareness Level	Security personnel, set-up crew, and patient tracking clerks where they are not expected to have contact with contaminated patients, their belongings, equipment, or waste.	OSHA (1991a, 1991b)
HAZWOPER First Responder Operations Level	Workers who decontaminate patients or handle contaminated patients.	OSHA (1992, 1999, 2003)

to encounter unannounced contaminated patients, their belongings, equipment, or waste are recommended to receive training similar to what is outlined in the Hazard Communication Standard (29 CFR 1910.1200(h)). In each case, the training must be provided in a manner that the employee is capable of understanding in order to be effective (OSHA 2005).

13.5 EXERCISE

Although exercising, or testing, emergency response plans might be considered part of training, its importance warrants its own consideration. Plans have little relevance or use when personnel do not understand them. Furthermore, limitations of plans are often revealed only after putting them into practice. Thus, it is critical to exercise the plans with as many personnel as practicable, in order to have opportunities to update and refine the plans.

Emergency response plans can be exercised in various ways. Each approach should be included in an organization's overall exercise strategy.

13.5.1 Orientations

New workers ought to be introduced to the organization's emergency response plans according to the worker's duties. Those who are not expected to have a key response role may simply be informed about shelter-in-place and evacuation plans. Emergency response workers, however, may be given extensive training on how to prepare for, respond to, and recover from an emergency (OSHA 2024b).

13.5.2 Drills

Specific workplace operations or functions can be tested during coordinated, supervised drills. These activities are used as part of initial training with new equipment, in developing new policies or procedures, or to practice and maintain certain skills. Shelter-in-place or evacuation drills are common examples of workplace emergency response drills (OSHA 2024b).

13.5.3 Tabletop Exercises

During tabletop exercises, leaders in various response functions gather and discuss hypothetical emergency response actions in an informal, stress-free environment. Frequently, the participants are presented with an emergency scenario, and each person is given an opportunity to explain their respective actions. The exercise is intended to produce constructive discussion, identify problems, and find solutions as participants examine how the response actions may interact (OSHA 2024b).

13.5.4 Functional Exercises

Functional exercises are simulated and interactive events designed to validate the capability of an organization to perform a single or multiple functions of its emergency response plan. These limited-scale exercises test policies, procedures, roles, and responsibilities of one or more emergency functions. Such functions may occur before, during, or after an emergency (OSHA 2024b).

13.5.5 Full-Scale Exercises

Full-scale exercises put emergency response plans into practice with as much realism and as many personnel as practical. These exercises involve mobilizing emergency personnel, equipment, and resources to simulate actual emergency conditions (OSHA 2024b). Although full-scale exercises require the greatest amount of planning and expense, they provide organizations and personnel with the greatest amount of preparation for a real-world event. Ideally, all organizations that are likely to interact following a given scenario will help plan for and participate together in full-scale exercises.

13.6 CONCLUSIONS

Emergency incidents involving radiation can quickly become complex. Such events will likely overwhelm local governments and draw the attention of state and federal agencies. However, local governments can and should plan for their own early-phase responses. These plans must also consider what kinds of training should be provided to workers. In addition, the plans must be tested with a range of exercises in order to ensure the plans meet the needs of the organization and can be executed. Careful thought, planning, resourcing, and training can help to save lives and prevent injuries and illnesses in the event of a radiation emergency.

REFERENCES

Bushberg JT. 2022. Radiation exposure and contamination. Available at: https://www.merckmanuals.com/professional/injuries-poisoning/radiation-exposure-and-contamination/radiation-exposure-and-contamination (accessed May 1, 2024).

Calabrese EJ, Selby PB. 2023. Background radiation and cancer risks: A major intellectual confrontation within the domain of radiation genetics with multiple converging biological disciplines. *Journal of Occupational and Environmental Hygiene* 20(12): 621–632.

Federal Emergency Management Agency (FEMA). 2023. Planning guidance for responding to and recovering from Radiological Dispersal Device (RDD) incidents: After the initial response. Available at: https://www.fema.gov/sites/default/files/documents/fema_rd-planning-guidance-for-responding-to-and-recovering-from-radiological-dispersal-device-rdd-incidents.pdf (accessed April 19, 2024).

Hendee WR, Edwards M. 1986. ALARA and an integrated approach to radiation protection. *Seminars in Nuclear Medicine* XVI(2):142–150.

Nevada National Security Site. 2024. *Federal Radiological Monitoring and Assessment Center (FRMAC)*. Available at: https://nnss.gov/mission/federal-radiological-monitoring-and-assessment-center-frmac/ (accessed May 26, 2024).

Oak Ridge Institute for Science and Education. 2024. Radiation Emergency Assistance Center/Training Site. Available at: https://orise.orau.gov/reacts/index.html (accessed May 26, 2024).

Occupational Safety and Health Administration (OSHA). 1991a. Letter of Interpretation Addressed to Mr. Edward McNamara, Executive Director, Central Massachusetts Emergency Medical Systems Corporation, Re: Training requirements for emergency medical service personnel. June 14. Available at: https://www.osha.gov/laws-regs/standardinterpretations/1991-06-14-0 (accessed April 25, 2024).

Occupational Safety and Health Administration (OSHA). 1991b. Letter of Interpretation Addressed to Mr. Eugene D. McCoy, Police Department, City of Ft. Lauderdale, FL. Re: Minimum number of hours required for awareness level for police officers. June 17. Available at: https://www.osha.gov/laws-regs/standardinterpretations/1991-06-17-0 (accessed April 25, 2024).

Occupational Safety and Health Administration (OSHA). 1992. Letter of Interpretation Addressed to Howard W. Levitin, Re: Training requirements for hospital personnel involved in an emergency response of a hazardous substance. October 27. Available at: https://www.osha.gov/laws-regs/standardinterpretations/1992-10-27-1 (accessed April 25, 2024).

Occupational Safety and Health Administration (OSHA). 1997. Letter of Interpretation Addressed to Mr. Thomas Whittaker, New England Hospital Engineer's Society, Re: Emergency response training requirements for hospital staff. April 25. Available at: https://www.osha.gov/laws-regs/standardinterpretations/1997-04-25-0 (accessed April 25, 2024).

Occupational Safety and Health Administration (OSHA). 1999. Letter of Interpretation Addressed to Daniel Burke, Safety Coordinator, St. John's Medical Center, Re: Emergency response training necessary for hospital physicians/nurses that may treat contaminated patients. March 10. Available at: https://www.osha.gov/laws-regs/standardinterpretations/1999-03-10 (accessed April 25, 2024).

Occupational Safety and Health Administration (OSHA). 2003. Letter of Interpretation Addressed to Mike Bolt, Re: HAZWOPER training requirements for hospital staff whole decontaminate chemically contaminated patients. April 22. Available at: https://www.osha.gov/laws-regs/standardinterpretations/2003-04-22 (accessed April 25, 2024).

Occupational Safety and Health Administration (OSHA). 2005. OSHA best practices for hospital-based first receivers of victims from mass casualty incidents involving the release of hazardous substances. January. Available at: https://www.osha.gov/sites/default/files/firstreceivers_hospital.pdf (accessed April 25, 2024).

Occupational Safety and Health Administration (OSHA). 2024a. Hazardous Waste Operations and Emergency Response (HAZWOPER). Available at: https://www.osha.gov/emergency-preparedness/hazardous-waste-operations/preparedness (accessed April 25, 2024).

Occupational Safety and Health Administration (OSHA). 2024b. Radiation emergency preparedness and response. Available at: https://www.osha.gov/emergency-preparedness/radiation/response (accessed April 12, 2024).

US Department of Homeland Security. 2023. Nuclear/radiological incident annex to the response and recovery federal interagency operational plan. Available at: https://www.fema.gov/sites/default/files/documents/fema_incident-annex_nuclear-radiological.pdf (accessed April 15, 2024).

US Environmental Protection Agency (USEPA). 2017a. Environmental protection agency radiological emergency response plan. Available at: https://www.epa.gov/sites/default/files/2015-05/documents/rerp-1-00.pdf (accessed May 1, 2024).

US Environmental Protection Agency (USEPA). 2017b. PAG manual: Protective action guides and planning guidance for radiological incidents. EPA-400/R-17/001. Available at: https://www.epa.gov/radiation/protective-action-guides-pags (accessed April 12, 2024).

US Environmental Protection Agency (USEPA). 2023. Radiological emergency response: Authorities. Available at: https://www.epa.gov/radiation/radiological-emergency-response-authorities (accessed April 12, 2024).

Yanovskiy M, Shaki YY, Socol Y. 2019. Ethics of adoption and use of the linear no-threshold model. *Dose Response* 17(1).

14 Understanding the Impacts of Heat

Brenda Jacklitsch and W. Jon Williams

14.1 INTRODUCTION

Heat is often a major concern in response activities, due not only to environmental heat but also to the combined heat burden of metabolic heat from physical exertion during tasks and the clothing and personal protective equipment (PPE) that is worn, which can trap heat or increase physical exertion. In a study that surveyed 119 first responders (i.e., law enforcement, firefighting, explosive ordnance disposal [EOD], and hazardous materials [HAZMAT] technicians), 99% reported heat stress and heat-related illnesses (HRIs) (e.g., heat rash, heat cramps, heat exhaustion, and heat stroke) and injuries (e.g., incidents from sweaty palms or slipping on a sweat puddle on the floor, visual impairment from fogged-up safety glasses, and touching hot equipment that could result in burns) to be a risk to employee safety during occupational duties, and 47% reported having had at least one employee experience a HRI during operations in the previous year (Bach et al. 2018). For example, heat stress is an ongoing issue among responders in large-scale oil spills. The Deepwater Horizon oil spill response had 47,000 workers, including responders, at the height of the response and 978 documented heat stress incidents (Michaels and Howard 2012). During these large-scale emergencies, responders often find themselves in stressful situations where there is a great demand for tasks to be completed quickly. The tasks are physically strenuous, the shifts are long, and there is the need to wear PPE – all leading to a higher risk for HRIs and injuries (NIOSH 2016).

14.2 HEAT IMPACTS WITH OCCUPATIONAL SAFETY AND HEALTH IMPLICATIONS

14.2.1 Environmental Heat Impacts

Many workers spend their entire work shift in a variety of hot environments that may become hotter because of rising ambient temperatures, increases in extreme heat events, or shifting and expanding hot seasons (CDC 2008; Stocker 2014; Schulte et al. 2016; Dahl et al. 2019a, 2019b). Overall, occupational exposures to heat and humidity may be more hazardous than community exposures because workers generally have less control over the exposures in their response activities. Another health issue of growing concern related to rising temperatures is chronic kidney disease of

DOI: 10.1201/9781003648178-15

unknown etiology (CKDu). CKDu first started to draw attention when it was discovered in sugar cane workers in Central and South America, with over 20,000 documented deaths noted by 2013 (Chicas et al. 2019; Pundee et al. 2020). CKDu has been most often associated with chronic or repeated dehydration and heat stress from physical work in a hot environment (Chapman et al. 2021; Chicas et al. 2019; Glaser et al. 2016; Pundee et al. 2020; Shih 2023), while most cases of traditional chronic kidney disease (CKD) are caused by hypertension and diabetes (NIH 2024). Cases of chronic kidney disease have also been seen increasingly in various work populations (e.g., other agricultural workers, construction workers, and miners) and are of increasing concern as more workers labor for longer periods in higher temperatures (Glaser et al. 2016; Shih 2023; Pundee et al. 2020; Pradhan et al. 2019).

With hotter temperatures, workers may be less likely to wear appropriate clothing and PPE, reducing the protective layers over their skin that shield them from ultraviolet (UV) radiation. Overexposure to UV radiation can result in skin cancer, eye damage, and even potential immune suppression (McCarty and Taylor 2002; Jaggernath et al. 2013; Barnes et al. 2019; Parker 2021).

Extreme weather (e.g., storms, floods, droughts, and wildfires) is a hazard to many workers and results in hazardous conditions for emergency responders during and after these events (Pinkerton et al. 2019; Vaisala 2022). Many of these worker and responder populations will experience physical fatigue from long work hours, such as during post-disaster rescue or cleanup phases, as well as resulting mental health issues (Dodgen et al. 2016; Wang et al. 2016; Daghagh Yazd et al. 2019; Howard et al. 2020; Metregiste et al. 2020). As many extreme weather events occur in warmer months, these responders will also be at increased risk for HRIs and injuries (de Almeida et al. 2012).

Temperature extremes, along with precipitation and moisture levels, can affect the seasonality and distribution of vector-borne diseases, including mosquito-borne and tick-borne diseases. Vector habitats are expanding, resulting in the wider spread of ticks and mosquitoes, which may transmit diseases like Lyme disease, West Nile, and Zika (Levi et al. 2018; Caminade et al. 2019; Fouque and Reeder 2019). Poisonous plants (e.g., poison ivy, poison oak, and poison sumac) and venomous snakes may spread through expanding habitats when temperatures become more conducive to sustaining the species' populations (Klimaszyk et al. 2014; Schulte et al. 2016; Schindler et al. 2018). Increases in certain fauna and flora species may also lead to increased usage of pesticides and herbicides, resulting in the potential for additional human chemical exposures, such as particulates being spread during fires and floods of areas that were chemically treated (Gatto et al. 2016).

14.2.2 Mental Health Impacts

Responders facing post-disaster rescue and cleanup efforts from extreme weather events, including high temperatures, may face mental health disorders, as they may be more likely to suffer from new or worsened post-traumatic stress disorder (PTSD) and depression (Lowe et al. 2016; Wang et al. 2016; Orui et al. 2018). For example, during the multiday 2021 Heat Dome that affected western Canada, there was a massive increase in 911 calls for ambulance, police, and fire services to respond to hundreds of community members succumbing to the heat (Tetzlaff et al. 2024). According to the study, these responders experienced stressful job demands, consisting of work overload (e.g., the surge in call volume, firefighters responding to medical emergencies), emotional demands (e.g., severe medical emergencies, sudden deaths, unresponsive patients, distraught family members), and physical demands (e.g., resuscitation while wearing PPE, HRIs, and injuries). The study also noted that work overload is a significant factor that contributes to worker burnout (Tetzlaff et al. 2024).

14.2.3 Occupational Health Equity Impacts

Occupational health equity is an issue, particularly as increasing temperatures disproportionately impact certain workers who are already at higher risk for injury, illness, and fatality (Levy and Patz 2015; US EPA 2021a). The outdoor environments where emergencies occur may include numerous hazards, and controlling for exposures and hazards is often challenging and not always feasible due to the nature of the work (Kjellström et al. 2019; Orlov et al. 2019; NOAA NCEI 2022). As emergency response and economic situations evolve, more migrant or immigrant worker populations are participating in disaster response cleanup efforts, which may offer better pay or other incentives. A combination of factors makes these workers more susceptible to heat and other hazards, such as a lack of knowledge and safety training, poverty, seasonality of the work, extreme work conditions, cultural differences, and language barriers (Flynn et al. 2014; O'Connor et al. 2014; Spector and Sheffield 2014; Levy and Patz 2015; Kiefer et al. 2016; Fan and Qian 2017; Ellis and Stam 2018; US EPA 2021a).

When compared to larger businesses, small businesses participating in responses, including those being contracted for cleanup efforts, often face a lack of resources for safety and health practices, greater time demands on managers, and fewer employees to engage in activities such as safety committees (Lentz and Wenzl 2006; Mendeloff 2006; Buckley et al. 2008; Sinclair and Cunningham 2014). As safety and health may require additional resources, they may not always take priority. Therefore, small businesses are often burdened with higher injury and fatality rates (De Kok 2005; Hasle and Limborg 2006; Lentz and Wenzl 2006; Donato et al. 2007; Parker et al. 2007; Delp et al. 2009; Sinclair and Cunningham 2014).

14.3 BASICS OF PHYSIOLOGY AND HEAT

14.3.1 How the Body Cools

Humans have the capacity to maintain a nearly constant core (internal) body temperature. A constant core body temperature is possible because of the ability to transfer body heat (produced by the metabolism of food) to the environment (Parsons 2003). In moderate environmental temperatures (i.e., below the average skin temperature of 82.4°F–91.4°F [28°C–33.8°C]), there is a temperature difference between the environment and skin. The laws of thermodynamics dictate that energy (heat) flows from a hotter region to a cooler region to achieve thermal equilibrium (Taylor et al. 2008). Therefore, body heat will flow from warm skin to the cooler environment. When core body temperature warms the blood, which is circulated to the skin, heat is transferred to the environment through *dry heat transfer*. Dry heat transfer occurs through three primary methods: (1) convection (movement of air across the skin, taking heat away from the body), (2) conduction (direct heat transfer from the skin to a colder surface), and (3) radiation (direct heat transfer from the body to cooler objects in the environment through infrared radiation). However, when the temperature of the objects in the environment is greater than skin temperature, heat flows from the objects in the environment to the body, increasing core body temperature. For example, firefighters are exposed to fires where the heat of the flames is transferred to the firefighter (cooler object) through radiation (electromagnetic radiation in the infrared spectrum) and the firefighter gains heat (Parsons 2003; NIOSH 2016).

14.3.2 What Happens When a Body Gets Too Hot

When core body temperature increases, the cardiovascular system responds by rerouting warm blood from the deep body tissues to the blood vessels in the skin. This warm blood heats up the skin, creating a larger temperature difference between the skin and the environment. This facilitates the transfer of body heat to the environment by dry heat mechanisms (i.e., convection, conduction, radiation) and helps the body maintain a stable core body temperature (McArdle et al. 2010; Williams 2013; NIOSH 2016; Williams 2018).

When in a hot environment or when engaging in physical exertion, the body activates the sweating mechanism. When the core body temperature increases above a certain level, water is transferred to the sweat glands and is excreted onto the skin as sweat, where it evaporates. When sweat evaporates, it can remove a significant amount of heat. Each liter (L) of sweat evaporated transfers 580 kilocalories of heat from the body to the environment. A problem with this mechanism arises when the relative humidity increases and the atmosphere can no longer accept any additional moisture. In hot and humid environments, sweat does not evaporate; it remains on the skin and does not contribute to the transfer of heat to the environment. The addition of heat to the core body temperature due to increased metabolism from physical exertion adds to the heat contribution from the environment and increases the risk of an HRI or injury (Taylor et al. 2008).

14.3.3 Heat-Related Illnesses and Injuries

Heat-related illnesses and injuries lie on a continuum ranging from mild to severe (including death). If proper intervention is initiated immediately, HRIs are treatable, and those with mild to moderate HRIs generally recover completely. However, as the severity of an HRI increases, the affected individual may progress from heat exhaustion to heat stroke in a matter of minutes (Leon and Bouchama 2011; NIOSH 2016; Kenny et al. 2018). It is therefore vitally important to identify and treat HRIs rapidly (Leon and Bouchama 2011; NIOSH 2016). Heat tolerance is widely variable and depends to a large degree on an individual's prior acclimatization, physical fitness, hydration status, cardiovascular function, prescription/recreational drug use (including diuretics, alcohol, amphetamines, others), history of heat illness, and age (Taylor, Kondo, and Kenney 2008; NIOSH 2016). The following sections describe the various types of HRI and injuries, from mild to severe.

14.3.3.1 Heat Rash

Heat rash (miliaria rubra or prickly heat) appears as red papules in areas where clothing is restrictive and where the skin is continuously wet due to unevaporated sweat. This condition is caused by the reabsorption of sweat by keratinous layers of the skin, which results in regional swelling. The regional swelling causes an obstruction of the sweat ducts, which, if untreated, may develop staphylococcal infections (NIOSH 2016; Danzig et al. 2024). Miliaria crystallina, a similar skin disorder, generally occurs during the onset of sweating in areas of damaged skin (e.g., sunburn) when the damage prevents the release of sweat. Sweat becomes trapped in clear skin bumps, which resolve when sweating stops (NIOSH 2016; Palaniappan et al. 2023). Finally, a third type of heat rash known as miliaria profunda occurs when sweat ducts are blocked below the surface of the skin, usually following damage to the skin (e.g., sunburn). However, cases of miliaria profunda have been reported in the absence of any obvious injury to the skin. In contrast to miliaria rubra (prickly heat), miliaria profunda manifests as discrete pale skin bumps like gooseflesh (NIOSH 2016; Danzig, Raunig, and Acholonu 2024).

In nearly all cases, heat rashes resolve with a return to a cooler environment and with the cessation of sweating. When exposure to heat is limited and the skin is allowed to dry, the incidence of recurrence of heat rashes diminishes. Heat rashes are not by themselves dangerous but can result in a reduction of sweating and a decrease in evaporative heat loss. Generally, the skin recovers from heat rashes within a few weeks (NIOSH 2016; Danzig, Raunig, and Acholonu 2024).

14.3.3.2 Heat Cramps

Heat cramps may be associated with a continued loss of salt in sweat, accompanied by a copious intake of water without appropriate replacement of salt (NIOSH 2016). Low salt levels in the muscles can cause these painful cramps, which often occur in the abdomen, arms, or legs. If someone is experiencing heat cramps, they need to rest in a cool area, drink water, and eat some salty snacks or drink a sports drink. A worker with heat cramps will need to wait a few hours before returning to heavy work. If they have heart problems, are on a low-sodium diet, or if cramps do not subside within one hour, then additional medical care may be necessary. Salt tablets should not be taken since they are generally not necessary and can have some unexpected effects (NIOSH 2016). Each salt tablet contains about 400 mg of sodium and, if taken without water, can result in stomach irritation. Moreover, salt tablets are poorly absorbed in the stomach, but once they are absorbed they can result in significant strain on the kidneys. The kidneys will register that the body has absorbed too much salt and will excrete the excess salt in the urine while also excreting a significant amount of fluid in the process. Therefore, consumption of salt tablets may actually result in dehydration rather than increased hydration (Coyle 2004). The average diet in the United States contains more sodium than the minimum daily requirement, and sodium lost from sweating will often be replaced from dietary sources (Montain and Cheuvront 2008).

14.3.3.3 Heat Exhaustion

Heat exhaustion is the result of excessive exposure to heat coupled with reduced fluid intake (Kenny et al. 2018; Périard et al. 2021). Without adequate fluid intake, especially during increased sweating, a reduction in blood plasma volume occurs, which results in cardiovascular strain (Taylor et al. 2008; NIOSH 2016). The reduction in plasma volume may be worsened by the vomiting that is often observed in those suffering from heat exhaustion (Leon 2007; Leon and Bouchama 2011). This leads to an inability to sustain cardiac output (the amount of blood pumped by the heart per minute). Heat-related cardiovascular strain results in an increased heart rate (greater than expected due to physical activity alone) to maintain cardiac output in the presence of a decreased stroke volume (the amount of blood pumped by the heart per beat) (Lucas et al. 2018).

A reduction in cardiac output decreases the oxygen supply to cells and organ systems, compromises muscular function, and reduces the flow of blood to the skin for heat transfer (Kenny et al. 2018). Frequently, the inability of the cardiovascular system to compensate for excessive heat leads to a drop in blood pressure (due to a decrease in peripheral vascular resistance), resulting in symptoms such as lightheadedness, dizziness, or fainting (Kenny et al. 2018). If the person experiencing early levels of heat exhaustion is removed from the source of heat to rest and consume water, they will recover completely with adequate care if they continue to rest and drink water (Gauer and Meyers 2019). However, it is important to note that heat exhaustion may progress rapidly to heat stroke unless rapid cooling is applied immediately (Leon 2007; Leon and Bouchama 2011).

14.3.3.4 Heat Stroke

Heat stroke is the most severe form of HRI and is a life-threatening emergency. There are two types of heat stroke: (1) "classical" heat stroke and (2) "exertional" heat stroke.

Classical heat stroke generally occurs most frequently in the elderly or in young children and is not generally associated with physical activity (Leon and Bouchama 2011). The incidence of classical heat stroke is usually associated with exposure to prolonged environmental heat (e.g., heat waves). *Exertional heat stroke* occurs in the young, fit population engaging in physical activity, often during periods of moderate to high environmental heat (Leon and Bouchama 2011).

In general, heat stroke is diagnosed as a core body temperature of ≥104°F (40°C) in combination with symptoms of neurological dysfunction, such as exhibited by delirium (e.g., acute, reversible state of disorientation and confusion), coma, and seizures (Leon and Bouchama 2011). Importantly, regardless of the type of heat stroke (classical or exertional), the presence of neurological symptoms (e.g., confusion, dizziness, headache, syncope, seizures) is critical to the diagnosis of heat stroke.

The physiological injuries resulting from heat stroke often progress to organ system damage and often multi-organ failure, leading to death. Long-term disability from heat stroke is well documented (Leon and Bouchama 2011). Although the use of rapid cooling may restore normal core body temperature, approximately 30% of the victims of heat stroke experience poorly controlled core temperature, alterations in the level of consciousness, disseminated intravascular coagulation (DIC), acute respiratory distress syndrome (ARDS), organ system dysfunction often leading to multi-organ failure and inflammatory effects (Leon and Bouchama 2011). Although the victim survives the acute phase of heat stroke, they may suffer multi-organ system damage (e.g., liver, kidney, muscle dysfunction), neurological damage, reduced exercise capacity, heat intolerance that may last for months to years, and death may ensue at a later date due to these ongoing issues (Leon 2007; Leon and Bouchama 2011; DeGroot et al. 2022).

14.3.3.5 First Aid

It is important to learn the symptoms of heat-related illnesses and the associated first aid. First aid is important even when help (e.g., emergency medical services) is on the way, as cooling the victim quickly may prevent long-term health effects and death. Additional information is provided in Table 14.1 (adapted from NIOSH 2016).

14.3.3.6 Heat-Related Injuries

Along with HRIs, heat can also cause physical injuries such as incidents from sweaty palms or slipping on a sweat puddle on the floor, visual impairment from fogged-up safety glasses may be a concern, and touching hot equipment, which could result in burns (NIOSH 2016). Dizziness and other symptoms may also cause workers to neglect or forget safety protocols, resulting in potential traumatic injuries to themselves or others, such as experiencing falls from elevations or mishandling heavy equipment (Spector et al. 2019). In conditions of extreme heat, workers may also be more likely to loosen or remove PPE, which may lead to additional hazardous exposures.

14.4 RISK FACTORS FOR HEAT-RELATED ILLNESS

14.4.1 Environmental versus Individual Factors

Many factors can increase the risk of HRI, including environmental and individual factors. Environmental factors may include direct sun exposure, high temperatures, humidity, lack of breeze or ventilation, and radiant heat sources (e.g., equipment generating heat) (NIOSH 2016). Individual factors may include the level of acclimatization, clothing and PPE, level of physical exertion, level of hydration, physical condition, medications, advanced age, pregnancy, and having experienced a previous HRI (NIOSH 2016).

TABLE 14.1
Heat-Related Illnesses and First Aid

Type of Heat-Related Illness	First Aid
Heat Rash *Symptoms:* • Clusters of red bumps on the skin, often appearing on the neck, upper chest, groin, under the breasts, and in elbow creases	• Try to work in a cooler, less humid environment when possible. • Keep the affected area dry. • Powder may be applied to increase comfort. • Do not use ointment or creams.
Heat Cramps *Symptoms:* • Muscle pain or spasms, usually in the abdomen, arms, or legs	• Rest in a shady, cool area. • Drink water and have snacks and/or sports drinks every 15–20 minutes. • Do not use salt tablets. • Wait a few hours before returning to heavy work. • Seek medical care if the worker has heart problems, is on a low-sodium diet, or if cramps do not subside within one hour.
Heat Exhaustion *Symptoms:* • Headache • Dizziness • Heavy sweating • Nausea • Weakness • Elevated temperature • Irritability • Thirst • Decreased urine output	• Stay with the worker until help arrives. • Move to a cool area and give liquids. • Encourage frequent sips of liquids. • Remove unnecessary clothing. • Cool body with cold compresses or wash their head, face, and neck with cold water. • If the condition continues to worsen despite hydration and cooling efforts, take to an emergency room for medical evaluation or call 911!
Heat Stroke *Symptoms:* • Confusion, altered mental status, slurred speech • Loss of consciousness • Red, hot, dry skin or profuse sweating • Seizures • Very high body temperature	• MEDICAL EMERGENCY: Call 911! • Stay the with worker until help arrives. • Remove outer clothing. • Cool quickly with a cold water or ice bath; wet the skin, or soak clothing in cool water. • Place cold, wet cloths or ice on the head, neck, armpits, and groin. • Fan air around the worker.

14.4.2 Acclimatization

Workers lacking recent exposure to heat in the work environment are considered unacclimatized. Unacclimatized workers readily show signs of heat stress and have trouble replacing all the water lost in sweat (NIOSH 2016). Published studies have shown that unacclimatized workers are at a significantly higher risk of HRI, including dying from heat stroke in the first week on a new job (Day and Grimshaw 2005;

Jackson and Rosenberg 2010; Arbury et al. 2014; Spector et al. 2014; Park et al. 2017; Tustin et al. 2018; Heinzerling et al. 2020).

When a person is acclimatized to a hot environment, their body is better prepared for the heat, and the resulting adaptations make it less likely they will experience an HRI. The physiological adaptations that occur include increased sweating efficiency (which includes earlier onset of sweating, greater sweat production, and reduced electrolyte loss in sweat), stabilization of circulation, and the ability to perform work with a lower core body temperature and heart rate (NIOSH 2016). An acclimatized worker will also experience increased skin blood flow at a given core temperature, providing additional relief as heat is released back into the environment. For proper acclimatization, a worker needs to gradually be exposed to hot conditions over 7–14 days (NIOSH 2016). While both new and returning workers (i.e., those that have been away for a week or more) will need time to acclimatize, a new worker will likely need more time to acclimatize than a worker who was away (e.g., brief illness, time off).

14.4.3 Clothing and PPE

The use of PPE occupationally represents the last line of defense against external hazards (e.g., chemical, biological, and particulate exposures). In other words, PPE is used only after other control options (substitution of hazard for non-hazard, administrative controls, or engineering controls) are deemed impractical or ineffective given the occupational setting.

While PPE is crucial for protection against external hazards (e.g., chemical, biological, and particulate exposures), its use may present another set of hazards to the wearer (McLellan et al. 2013; Williams 2013). This is particularly true when the responder is wearing completely, or nearly completely, encapsulating PPE (e.g., firefighter turnout clothing, HAZMAT gear) that is potentially able to trap body heat (Havenith 1999; McLellan et al. 2013; Williams 2013). In addition, the PPE may encumber the wearer such that body motion is limited and additional physical exertion is required to move while wearing the PPE (McLellan et al. 2013).

The degree to which PPE (or clothing) traps body heat depends on the design of the PPE, which is dependent upon the nature of the hazards to which the worker will be exposed. For example, firefighter turnout ensembles are constructed of multiple layers (including the outer shell, the moisture barrier, and the insulating thermal liner) and may have various degrees of water vapor and air permeability that contribute to the heat stress imposed by the garment (Morel et al. 2014). In addition, the multiple layers add to the weight of the garment, which results in greater effort required by the wearer. This effort is accompanied by an increased metabolic rate (heat generation) that contributes to the thermal stress imposed on the wearer (McLellan et al. 2013). Unlike firefighter turnout gear with its limited moisture and air permeability, HAZMAT gear has essentially zero permeability because it is designed to completely isolate the wearer from a hazardous external environment (McLellan et al.

2013, Williams 2013). Because of this impermeability, heat cannot be transferred to the environment through any of the body's mechanisms (e.g., sweat evaporation).

14.4.4 Physical Exertion

The level of physical exertion is also a risk factor. Even when at rest, muscles produce about 20%–25% of the body's total heat (Rowell 1993). Heat produced by muscles during physical exertion will be much higher. For those experiencing high levels of physical exertion, metabolic heat will continue to increase, contributing to overall heat stress.

14.4.5 Level of Hydration

The hydration status of the worker is a balance between fluid intake and loss. During exposure to hot environments and during exercise, sweating can easily increase to 1.5–2.0 L per hour. This can result in a significant loss of body water that causes a reduction in blood volume. This contraction reduces the ability of the cardiovascular system to provide blood to the skin for heat transfer and oxygenated blood to vital organs and muscles (Taylor et al., 2008). The sweating response is normally initiated when the core body temperature increases 0.36°F–0.9°F (0.2°C–0.5°C) above the mean body temperature (98.6°F [~37°C]) (Taylor et al. 2008). If the exercise level increases, sweating will increase proportionately.

A well-acclimatized person may produce 0.3–3 L per hour or more of sweat during hard work in a hot environment (Leon and Bouchama 2011; Périard et al. 2021). Therefore, it is imperative that the supply of fluid lost to sweating be replaced by drinking the right fluids (water in the short term and balanced electrolyte/carbohydrate fluids in the longer term) (ACSM 2018; Périard et al. 2021). A guideline for rehydration involves measuring changes in body weight. Every 0.45 kg (15 fluid oz) decrease in body weight represents 450 mL of body water lost to sweating, which must be replaced with the ingestion of the same amount of fluid. A rehydration strategy during exposure to heat and physical exertion will allow for the appropriate replenishment of body water, which will allow for the continuation of the sweating response that is crucial to thermoregulation (e.g., one cup of water every 15–20 minutes or sports drinks with balanced electrolytes when sweating for several hours) (NIOSH 2016).

In addition, sweat contains some sodium, and profuse sweating over a couple of hours may result in significant sodium loss (Sawka and Montain 2000; ACSM 2018; Périard et al. 2021). Low sodium in blood plasma results in the rapid movement of fluid into the brain, leading to the development of symptoms ranging from mild (headache, confusion, malaise, nausea) to severe (seizures, coma, pulmonary edema, cardiac arrest, and death) (McArdle et al. 2010).

Generally, a person can lose approximately 2.7 kg (2.7 liters or 91.3 fluid oz) of body weight in sweat and replenish the lost electrolytes with a small amount of salt in food (Sawka and Montain 2000; ACSM 2018). A loss of 2.7 kg of body weight is equivalent to a loss of 2.7 L of sweat. This amount of sweat could be lost by an acclimatized person in an hour of intense physical exertion (although this amount may be affected by individual body weight). However, producing a greater volume of sweat over more than two hours could result in a significant loss of sodium, which could lead to hyponatremia (Sawka and Montain 2000; ACSM 2018; Périard et al. 2021). The hyponatremia would be worsened with the continued consumption of plain drinking water during this time due to the further dilution of sodium in the blood plasma. Hyponatremia may be avoided by increasing dietary sodium intake after bouts of sweating and/or the use of balanced electrolyte/carbohydrate-containing "sports" drinks during bouts of intense sweating over a period of hours (Sawka and Montain 2000; ACSM 2018; Périard et al. 2021). Given that the daily average sodium intake in the US diet is 2-4 grams (National Research Council 1989), simply eating a normal meal contains enough sodium to adequately replenish the sodium lost during sweating.

14.4.6 Physical Condition and Health Problems

A person's physical condition may influence susceptibility or resistance to heat stress. Acute illness (vomiting, diarrhea) may cause sufficient loss of body water to leave the person significantly dehydrated. The discomfort of these illnesses may cause the victim to be disinclined to rehydrate immediately, thus leaving them more vulnerable to heat illness.

Another physical condition to consider is the responder's degree of physical fitness, as frequent physical exercise provides at least partial acclimatization to heat exposure. Physical exercise results in elevated metabolic heat production from muscle activity. This metabolically produced heat must be exchanged with the environment using the physiological mechanisms discussed previously. Regular exercise induces several physiological adaptations to transfer heat more efficiently from the body to the environment. This may involve increased sweat production, induction of sweating at a lower body temperature, increased blood flow to the skin for heat exchange, reduction of blood flow to the viscera, and conservation of body electrolytes to prevent sodium depletion. All of these adaptations (acclimatization) help increase heat transfer to the environment to prevent an increase in body core temperature and reduce the possibility of HRI or injury. Conversely, a physically unfit person will be more vulnerable to HRI because these physiological adaptations to increased metabolic heat production have not been induced (Parsons 2003; McArdle et al. 2010; NIOSH 2016).

A responder's physical condition may also affect their risk for an HRI. For an overweight or obese worker, carrying extra body weight requires greater physical exertion to perform a given task (Kenny et al. 2010). The body's surface-to-body-weight ratio is also less favorable for heat dissipation, and the increased fat layers provide insulation and slow heat loss (NIOSH 2016). There may be other conditions associated with obesity that affect risk, such as lower physical fitness, decreased maximum work capacity, and decreased cardiovascular capacity.

Other health conditions that may increase the risk for an HRI include cardiovascular disease, diabetes, or any diseases in which gastrointestinal permeability is compromised (NIOSH 2016). Even seemingly more minor health concerns, like experiencing a common cold, febrile illness, and sleep deprivation or fatigue, may increase risk (Westwood et al. 2021).

14.4.7 Medications

Medications can contribute to heat sensitivity in many ways, such as reduced thirst sensation, interference with central thermoregulation, impaired sweating, hypotension, reduced cardiac output, reduced kidney blood flow, reduced blood vessel dilation, drug toxicity from reduced clearance of medications, and electrolyte imbalance (CDC 2024). In addition, heat exposure may damage medication delivery devices and may degrade medications. For example, inhalers can burst in hot environments, and EpiPens may malfunction or deliver less epinephrine when exposed to heat. Insulin may become less effective if left in the heat instead of being stored in a refrigerator.

This list of medications in Table 14.2 (adapted from CDC 2024), which increase the vulnerability to heat, is intended to augment other existing documents that describe the physical, physiological, and general health aspects of heat stress and response to heat stress. The medications in Table 14.2 are largely prescribed for the appropriate treatment of medical conditions. Workers can consult their healthcare providers to have a medication plan in place with consideration for working in the heat and to avoid abruptly stopping any medications.

14.4.8 Advanced Age (Workers 65 Years and Older)

Older workers (within this heat stress context, older workers are defined as those ≥65 years of age) have increased vulnerabilities to HRIs and injuries not generally associated with physical exertion (Leon and Bouchama 2011). The incidence of heat injury in this group usually is associated with exposure to prolonged environmental heat (most notably during severe heat waves). The increased vulnerability that older workers have to heat is associated with a greater incidence of cardiovascular disease (Leon and Bouchama 2011); a reduced sweat gland response; decreased skin blood flow; use of medications (e.g., diuretics, β-blockers, calcium channel blockers, laxatives) which reduce tolerance to heat and may compromise a number of the physiological mechanisms needed for heat transfer from the body to the environment; chronic illness; and a sedentary lifestyle (Leon and Bouchama 2011; NIOSH 2016).

14.4.9 Pregnancy

Pregnant people may also be at higher risk when working in the heat because as the pregnancy progresses, heat tolerance decreases (NIOSH 2016; Rekha et al. 2024).

TABLE 14.2
Medications That May Increase Risk of Heat-related Illness

Medication Type	Drug Class	Examples	Mechanisms
Cardiovascular medications (Antihypertensives)	• Diuretics	• Furosemide • Hydrochlorothiazide • Acetazolamide	• Electrolyte imbalance • Volume depletion, dehydration, and increased risk of fainting and falls • Reduced thirst sensation
	• β-blockers	• Atenolol • Metoprolol • Propranolol	• Reduced superficial vasodilation • Decreased sweating • Reduced blood pressure, increased risk of fainting and falls
	• Calcium channel blocker	• Amlodipine • Felodipine • Nifedipine	• Decreased blood pressure, increased risk of fainting and falls • Electrolyte imbalance
	• Angiotensin Converting Enzyme Inhibitor (ACEi) • Angiotensin II Receptor blockers (ARBs)	• ACEi: Enalapril, Lisinopril, Ramipril	• Decreased blood pressure, increased risk of fainting and falls • Reduced thirst sensation
	• Angiotensin Receptor-Neprilysin Inhibitors (ARNIs), combination drugs including ARB	• ARB: Valsartan, Losartan • Sacubitril/Valsartan	• Decreased blood pressure, increased risk of fainting and falls • Reduced thirst sensation
Cardiovascular medications (Anti-platelet medications)		• Clopidogrel • Aspirin	• Reduced superficial vasodilation

(Continued)

TABLE 14.2 (CONTINUED)
Medications That May Increase Risk of Heat-related Illness

Medication Type	Drug Class	Examples	Mechanisms
Cardiovascular medications (Antianginals)	• Nitrates	• Glyceryl Trinitrate • Isosorbide mononitrate	• Worsened hypotension
Psychiatric medications	• Mood stabilizer	• Lithium	• Diabetes insipidus-induced water loss and risk for fainting, falls • Electrolyte imbalance • Risk for toxicity in setting of dehydration because of narrow therapeutic index
	• Antipsychotics	• Haloperidol • Olanzapine • Quetiapine • Risperidone	• Impaired sweating • Impaired temperature
	• Selective Serotonin Reuptake Inhibitors (SSRI) • Serotonin and Norepinephrine Reuptake Inhibitors (SNRI) • Tricyclic antidepressants (TCAs)	• SSRI: Fluoxetine, Sertraline • SNRI: Duloxatine, Venlafaxine • Amitriptyline • Clomipramine	• Increased sweating • Decreased sweating
Antiseizure medications		• Topiramate • Oxcarbazepine • Carbamazepine	• Decreased sweating • Increased sweating • Increased urination • Dizziness and weakness, especially after an increased dose
Antihistamines with anticholinergic properties		• Promethazine • Doxylamine • Diphenhydramine	• Decreased sweating • Impaired thermoregulation

(Continued)

TABLE 14.2 (CONTINUED)
Medications That May Increase Risk of Heat-related Illness

Medication Type	Drug Class	Examples	Mechanisms
Analgesics	• Nonsteroidal anti-inflammatory drugs (NSAIDs) • Aspirin • Acetaminophen	• Ibuprofen • Naproxen	• Kidney injury with dehydration • Increased heat production with overdose • Kidney injury with dehydration • Heat-related liver injury, increased risk for acetaminophen hepatoxicity
Antibiotics	• Sulfonamides	• Sulfamethoxazole/ trimethoprim	• Kidney injury risk with dehydration
Antiretrovirals	• Protease inhibitors	• Indinavir	• Kidney injury risk with dehydration
Thyroid replacement		• Levothyroxine	• Excessive sweating
Stimulants		• Cocaine	• Reduced sweating • Reduced dilation of skin blood vessels • Impaired heat perception
		• Amphetamine • Methylphenidate	• Increased body temperature
Hallucinogens		• Methylenedioxy-methamphetamine (MDMA) (and alternatives)	• Reduced sweating • Reduced skin blood vessel dilation • Impaired heat perception
Alcohol			• Increased sweating • Increased urination • Impaired heat perception

Those who are pregnant will also need to take additional time to cool down and rehydrate more often. Normally, a pregnant person's circulation helps protect the fetus. In very hot work environments, however, a pregnant person's core body temperature may rise, and in some cases, this has been linked to birth defects and other reproductive problems (Ravanelli et al. 2019; Syed et al. 2022).

14.4.10 Previous Heat-Related Illness

Responders who have experienced a previous HRI are more likely to experience one again as they may be less tolerant to the heat (Armstrong et al. 1990; Day and Grimshaw 2005). For responders returning to hot activities after an HRI, additional precautions are needed, such as time to acclimatize and adjusting their schedule to reduce time in the heat or physical exertion. These responders may also need additional monitoring throughout the shift to ensure they are not showing symptoms of an HRI.

14.5 HEAT STRESS AND TOXICOLOGY

Exposure to heat can affect how chemicals are absorbed into the body. Previously published animal studies have shown that exposure to heat exacerbates chemical absorption and toxicity (Leon 2008). Changes to the body's core temperature can alter the absorption, distribution, metabolism, and excretion of toxicants (Leon 2008). Additionally, increases in respiration can lead to further toxicant exposure through inhalation, whereas increases in sweat and skin blood flow can lead to more efficient transcutaneous absorption of some toxicants (Gordon 2003; Leon 2008).

Studies have suggested that heat stress, with or without physical exertion, will activate skin blood flow, sweating, and respiration, which may then accelerate chemical absorption (Gordon and Leon 2005). The hazard associated with some pesticides or other chemicals increases with increased temperatures. High temperatures accelerate the dispersion of the chemicals and increase the density of airborne particles. Additionally, some workers may remove or loosen their PPE due to discomfort in the heat, and this may increase their exposure to these hazards (Gordon 2003).

Most of what is known about toxicants is derived from animal studies in which the animals were often kept in comfortable temperatures. Therefore, a better understanding of the mechanisms involved between heat exposure and toxicants in humans is needed (Gordon 2003; Gordon and Leon 2005; Leon 2008).

14.6 TRAINING AND EDUCATIONAL NEEDS

Worksite training programs should be implemented for all responders and supervisors when there is a likelihood of HRI (NIOSH 2016). Training should include heat hazards, risk factors, symptoms, and first aid. Heat stroke is an important topic to discuss because the characteristics of the individual, type of activity, and symptoms vary between the classic and exertional classifications, and the end result, if not treated emergently, is often death (DOD 2003; NIOSH 2016). Medications, alcohol, and caffeine that may reduce heat tolerance and increase risk should also be presented in training (NIOSH 2016). Refresher training may also be warranted, especially regarding symptoms, as some of the common public health messaging focuses on classic heat stroke, and those working in the heat are at higher risk for exertional heat stroke (DOD 2003, Armstrong et al. 2007; Navy Environmental Health Center 2007). In addition, there may need to be discussions about cultural attitudes toward heat stress. For example, some individuals might incorrectly believe that they can be "hardened" against the requirement for fluids by deliberately and regularly becoming dehydrated before work. This type of misinformation can be addressed (NIOSH 2016; Schwarz et al. 2016).

14.6.1 Controlling Heat Stress

Finally, considerations for how to reduce heat stress by implementing the hierarchy of controls, including engineering controls or work practice controls, can be shared, particularly during supervisor training.

These considerations should be written in a heat management plan and might include those that aim to increase air cooling, provide heat barriers, limit time in the heat or increase recovery time in a cool area, reduce the metabolic demands, institute a heat acclimatization plan, implement a buddy system and/or heat alert program, provide and encourage hydration breaks, and, in certain situations, require workers to conduct self-monitoring (NIOSH 2016). Also, as many responders find themselves experiencing significant heat strain from the environment, tasks, and PPE worn, consider implementing auxiliary cooling systems (e.g., water-cooled garments, air-cooled garments, cooling vests, and wetted overgarments) (NIOSH 2020). Auxiliary cooling may be used before (pre-cooling), during (concurrent cooling), or between operations (recovery cooling during breaks or after shift completion). Additional considerations include barriers to the use of auxiliary cooling, such as availability, cost, logistics, and knowledge (Bach et al. 2018).

14.6.2 Delivering Training and Education

Consider the most effective mechanisms for delivering heat stress education and training with the responder audience in mind. A heat-related training needs assessment on oil spill cleanup responders found that the most common training delivery methods and education received included just-in-time training and printed materials (Jacklitsch et al. 2018). However, this study also reported that the most desirable future training delivery methods and education products were smartphone or tablet applications, printed materials, and online training. Taking time to seek out various options may help identify the best tools available that will resonate with responders and provide accurate and timely information.

Disclaimer

The findings and conclusions in this report are those of the authors and do not necessarily represent the official position of the National Institute for Occupational Safety and Health, Centers for Disease Control and Prevention.

REFERENCES

ACSM. 2018. "Environmental considerations for exercise prescription." In *IACSM's Guidelines for Exercise Testing and Prescription*, 10th ed., edited by D. Riebe, J. E. Ehrman, G. Liguori, and M. Magal, 217–9. Philadelphia, PA: Wolters Kluwer.

Arbury, S., B. Jacklitsch, O. Farquah, M. Hodgson, G. Lamson, H. Martin, and A. Profitt. 2014. "Heat illness and death among workers—United States, 2012–2013." *Morbidity and Mortality Weekly Report* 63, no. 31: 661–5.

Armstrong, L. E., D. J. Casa, M. Millard-Stafford, D. S. Moran, S. W. Pyne, and W. O. Roberts. 2007. "American College of Sports Medicine Position Stand. Exertional heat illness during training and competition." *Medicine and Science in Sports and Exercise* 39, no. 3: 556–72.

Armstrong, L. E., J. P. De Luca, and R. W. Hubbard. 1990. "Time course of recovery and heat acclimation ability of prior exertional heatstroke patients." *Medicine and Science in Sports and Exercise* 22, no. 1: 36–48.

Bach, A. J. E., M. J. Maley, G. M. Minett, and I. B. Stewart. 2018. Occupational cooling practices of emergency first responders in the United States: A survey. *Temperature* 5, no. 4: 348–58. https://doi.org/10.1080/23328940.2018.1493907.

Barnes, P. W., C. E. Williamson, R. M. Lucas, S. A. Robinson, S. Madronich, N. D. Paul, J. F. Bornman, A. F. Bais, B. Sulzberger, and S. R. Wilson. 2019. "Ozone depletion, ultraviolet radiation, climate change and prospects for a sustainable future." *Nature Sustainability* 2, no. 7: 569–79.

Buckley, J. P., J. P. Sestito, and K. L. Hunting. 2008. "Fatalities in the landscape and horticultural services industry, 1992–2001." *American Journal of Industrial Medicine* 51, no. 9: 701–13.

Caminade, C., K. M. McIntyre, and A. E. Jones. 2019. "Impact of recent and future climate change on vector-borne diseases." *Annals of the New York Academy of Sciences* 1436, no. 1: 157–73.

CDC. 2008. "Heat-related deaths among crop workers—United States, 1992–2006." *Morbidity and Mortality Weekly Report* 57, no. 24: 649–53.

CDC. 2024. "Heat and medications—Guidance for clinicians." https://www.cdc.gov/heat-health/hcp/heat-and-medications-guidance-for-clinicians.html.

Chapman, C. L., H. W. Hess, R. A. Lucas, J. Glaser, R. Saran, J. Bragg-Gresham, ... & Z. J. Schlader. 2021. Occupational heat exposure and the risk of chronic kidney disease of nontraditional origin in the United States. *American Journal of Physiology-Regulatory, Integrative and Comparative Physiology* 321, no. 2: R141–51.

Chicas, R., J. Mix, V. Mac, J. Flocks, N. E. Dickman, V. Hertzberg, and L. McCauley. 2019. Chronic kidney disease among workers: A review of the literature. *Workplace Health & Safety* 67, no. 9: 481–90.

Coyle, E. F. 2004. Fluid and fuel intake during exercise. *Journal of Sports Sciences* 22: 39–55.

Daghagh Yazd, S., S. A. Wheeler, and A. Zuo. 2019. "Key risk factors affecting farmers' mental health: A systematic review." *International Journal of Environmental Research and Public Health* 16, no. 23: 4849.

Dahl, K., R. Licker, J. T. Abatzoglou, and J. Declet-Barreto. 2019a. "Increased frequency of and population exposure to extreme heat index days in the United States during the 21st century." *Environmental Research Communications* 1, no. 7: 075002.

Dahl, K., E. Spanger-Siegfried, R. Licker, A. Caldas, J. Abatzoglou, N. Mailloux, R. Cleetus, S. Udvardy, J. Declet-Barreto, and P. Worth. 2019b. *Killer Heat in the United States: Climate Choices and the Future of Dangerously Hot Days.* Union of Concerned Scientists. https://www.jstor.org/stable/resrep24062.

Danzig, R. M., J. M. Raunig, and C. J. Acholonu. 2024. "Exertional heat illness—From identifying heat rash to treating heat stroke." *Pediatric Annals* 53, no. 1: e17–21.

Day, T. K. and D. Grimshaw. 2005. "An observational study on the spectrum of heat-related illness, with a proposal on classification." *Journal of the Royal Army Medical Corps* 151, no. 1: 11–8.

DeGroot, D. W., F. G. O'Connor, and W. O. Roberts. 2022. "Exertional heat stroke: an evidence based approach to clinical assessment and management." *Experimental Physiology* 107, no. 10: 1172–83.

de Almeida, R. A. C. D. S., M. M. Veiga, F. J. de Castro Moura Duarte, L. A. Meirelles, and L. B. E. Veiga. 2012. Thermal comfort and personal protective equipment (PPE). *Work* 41(Supplement 1): 4979–82.

De Kok, J. M. 2005. "Precautionary actions within small and medium-sized enterprises." *Journal of Small Business Management* 43, no. 4: 498–516.

Delp, L., L. Podolsky, and T. Aguilar. 2009. "Risk amid recovery: occupational health and safety of Latino day laborers in the aftermath of the Gulf Coast hurricanes." *Organization & Environment* 22, no. 4: 479–90.

DOD. 2003. *Technical Bulletin: Heat Stress Control and Heat Casualty Management (TBMED 507/AFPAM 48-152 (I)).* Washington, DC: Department of Defense. https://apps.dtic.mil/sti/tr/pdf/ADA433236.pdf.

Dodgen, D., D. Donato, N. Kelly, A. La Greca, J. Morganstein, J. Reser, J. Ruzek, S. Schweitzer, M. Shimamoto, and K. T. Tart. 2016. "Mental health and well-being." In *The Impacts of Climate Change on Human Health in the United States: A Scientific Assessment*, 217–46. Washington, DC: U.S. Global Change Research Program. https://health2016.globalchange.gov/low/ClimateHealth2016_08_Mental_Health_small.pdf.

Donato, K. M., N. Trujillo-Pagan, C. L. Bankston III, and A. Singer. 2007. "Reconstructing New Orleans after Katrina: the emergence of an immigrant labor market." In *The Sociology of Katrina: Perspectives on a Modern Catastrophe*, edited by D. L. Brunsma, D. Overfelt, and J. S. Picou, 217–34. Lanham, MD: Rowman & Littlefield Publishers.

Ellis, B. D. and H. J. Stam. 2018. "Cycles of deportability: Threats, fears, and the agency of 'irregular' migrants in Canada." *Migration Studies* 6, no. 3: 321–44.

Fan, W. and Y. Qian. 2017. "Native-immigrant occupational segregation and worker health in the United States, 2004–2014." *Social Science & Medicine* 183: 130–41.

Flynn, M. A., T. Carreón, D. E. Eggerth, and A. I. Johnson. 2014. "Immigration, work, and health: A literature review of immigration between Mexico and the United States." *Revista de trabajo social* 6: 129.

Fouque, F. and J. C. Reeder. 2019. "Impact of past and on-going changes on climate and weather on vector-borne diseases transmission: A look at the evidence." *Infectious Diseases of Poverty* 8, no. 3: 1–9.

Gatto, M. P., R. Cabella, and M. Gherardi. 2016. "Climate change: the potential impact on occupational exposure to pesticides." *Annali dell'Istituto superiore di sanita* 52, no. 3: 374–85.

Gauer, R. and B. K. Meyers. 2019. "Heat-related illnesses." *American Family Physician* 99, no. 8: 482–9.

Glaser, J., J. Lemery, B. Rajagopalan, H. F. Diaz, R. García-Trabanino, G. Taduri, M. Madero, M. Amarasinghe, G. Abraham, and S. Anutrakulchai. 2016. "Climate change and the emergent epidemic of CKD from heat stress in rural communities: The case for heat stress nephropathy." *Clinical Journal of the American Society of Nephrology* 11, no. 8: 1472–83.

Gordon, C. J. 2003. "Role of environmental stress in the physiological response to chemical toxicants." *Environmental Research* 92, no. 1: 1–7.

Gordon, C. J. and L. R. Leon. 2005. "Thermal stress and the physiological response to environmental toxicants." *Reviews on Environmental Health* 20, no. 4: 235–64.

Hasle, P. and H. J. Limborg. 2006. "A Review of the literature on preventive occupational health and safety activities in small enterprises." *Industrial Health* 44, no. 1: 6–12.

Havenith, G. 1999. "Heat balance when wearing protective clothing." *Annals of Occupational Hygiene* 43, no. 5: 289–96.

Heinzerling, A., R. L. Laws, M. Frederick, R. Jackson, G. Windham, B. Materna, and R. Harrison. 2020. "Risk factors for occupational heat-related illness among California workers, 2000–2017." *American Journal of Industrial Medicine* 63, no. 12: 1145–54.

Howard, M., S. Ahmed, P. Lachapelle, and M. B. Schure. 2020. "Farmer and rancher perceptions of climate change and their relationships with mental health." *Journal of Rural Mental Health* 44, no. 2: 87.

Jacklitsch, B. L., K. A. King, R. A. Vidourek and A. L. Merianos. 2018. "Heat-related training and educational material needs among oil spill cleanup responders." *Environmental Health Insights* 12:1178630218802295.

Jackson, L. L. and H. R. Rosenberg. 2010. "Preventing heat-related illness among agricultural workers." *Journal of Agromedicine* 15, no. 3: 200–15.

Jaggernath, J., D. Haslam, and K. S. Naidoo. 2013. "Climate change: Impact of increased ultraviolet radiation and water changes on eye health." *Health* 5: 921–30.

Kenny, G. P., T. E. Wilson, A. D. Flouris, and N. Fujii. 2018. "Heat exhaustion." *Handbook of Clinical Neurology* 157: 505–29.

Kenny, G. P., J. Yardley, C. Brown, R. J. Sigal, and O. Jay. 2010. "Heat stress in older individuals and patients with common chronic diseases." *CMAJ* 182, no. 10: 1053–60.

Kiefer, M., J. Rodríguez-Guzmán, J. Watson, B. van Wendel de Joode, D. Mergler, and A. S. da Silva. 2016. "Worker health and safety and climate change in the Americas: issues and research needs." *Revista Panamericana de Salud Pública* 40: 192–7.

Kjellström, T., N. Maître, C. Saget, M. Otto, and T. Karimova. 2019. *Working on a Warmer Planet: The Impact of Heat Stress on Labour Productivity and Decent Work.* International Labour Organization, Geneva.

Klimaszyk, P., D. Klimaszyk, M. Piotrowiak, and A. Popiołek. 2014. "Unusual complications after occupational exposure to giant hogweed (Heracleum mantegazzianum): A case report." *International Journal of Occupational Medicine and Environmental Health* 27: 141–4.

Lentz, T. and T. Wenzl. 2006. "Surveillance: small businesses with high fatality rates: assessment of hazards and their prevention." *Journal of Occupational and Environmental Hygiene* 3, no. 2: D8–14.

Leon, L. R. 2007. "Heat stroke and cytokines." *Progress in Brain Research* 162: 481–524.

Leon, L. R. 2008. "Thermoregulatory responses to environmental toxicants: The interaction of thermal stress and toxicant exposure." *Toxicology and Applied Pharmacology* 233, no. 1: 146–61.

Leon, L. R. and A. Bouchama. 2011. "Heat stroke." *Comprehensive Physiology* 5, no. 2: 611–47.

Levi, M., T. Kjellstrom, and A. Baldasseroni. 2018. "Impact of climate change on occupational health and productivity: a systematic literature review focusing on workplace heat." *La Medicina del lavoro* 109, no. 3: 163.

Levy, B. S. and J. A. Patz. 2015. "Climate change, human rights, and social justice." *Annals of Global Health* 81, no. 3: 310–22.

Lowe, S. R., R. K. Kwok, J. Payne, L. S. Engel, S. Galea, and D. P. Sandler. 2016. "Why does disaster recovery work influence mental health?: Pathways through physical health and household income." *American Journal of Community Psychology* 58, no. 3–4: 354–64.

Lucas, R. A., L. C. Wilson, P. N. Ainslie, J.-L. Fan, K. N. Thomas, and J. D. Cotter. 2018. "Independent and interactive effects of incremental heat strain, orthostatic stress, and mild hypohydration on cerebral perfusion." *American Journal of Physiology-Regulatory, Integrative and Comparative Physiology* 314, no. 3: R415–26.

McArdle, W., F. Katch, and V. Katch. 2010. *Exercise Physiology: Nutrition, Energy, and Human Performance.* Philadelphia, PA: Wolters Kluwer Lippincott Williams & Wilkins. .

McCarty, C. A. and H. R. Taylor. 2002. "A review of the epidemiologic evidence linking ultraviolet radiation and cataracts." *Developments in Ophthalmology* 35: 21–31.

McLellan, T. M., H. A. Daanen, and S. S. Cheung. 2013. "Encapsulated environment." *Comprehensive Physiology* 3, no. 3: 1363–91.

Mendeloff, J. M. 2006. *Small Businesses and Workplace Fatality Risk: An Exploratory Analysis.* RAND Corporation.

Metregiste, D., D. Boucaud-Maitre, L. Aubert, L. Noubou, and L. Jehel. 2020. "Explanatory factors of post-traumatic distress and burnout among hospital staff 6 months after Hurricane Irma in Saint-Martin and Saint-Barthelemy." *PLoS One* 15, no. 3: e0229246.

Michaels, D. and J. Howard. 2012. "Review of the OSHA-NIOSH response to the Deepwater Horizon oil spill: protecting the health and safety of cleanup workers." *PLoS Currents* 18(4):e4fa83b7576b6e.

Morel, A., G. Bedek, F. Salaün, and D. Dupont. 2014. "A review of heat transfer phenomena and the impact of moisture on firefighters' clothing and protection." *Ergonomics* 57, no. 7: 1078–89.

Montain, S. J. and S. N. Cheuvront. 2008. Fluid, electrolyte and carbohydrate requirements for exercise. In *Physiological Basis of Human Performance during Work and Exercise*, edited by N. A. S. Taylor and H. Groeller, 563–73. Churchill: Livingstone; Edinburgh: Elsevier.

National Research Council. 1989. *Recommended Daily Allowances*, 10th ed. Washington, DC: National Academies Press .

Navy Environmental Health Center. 2007. Prevention and treatment of heat and cold stress injuries. https://www.med.navy.mil/sites/nmcphc/Documents/policy-and-instruction/oem-prevention-and-treatment-of-heat-and-cold-stressinjuries.pdf.

National Institutes of Health (NIH). 2024. Causes of chronic kidney disease. https://www.niddk.nih.gov/health-information/kidney-disease/chronic-kidney-disease-ckd/causes.

NIOSH. 2016. *Criteria for a Recommended Standard: Occupational Exposure to Heat and Hot Environments.* B. Jacklitsch, W. J. Williams, K. Musolin, A. Coca, J.-H. Kim, and N. Turner, eds. Cincinnati, OH: US Department of Health and Human Services, Centers for Disease Control and Prevention, National Institute for Occupational Safety and Health. https://www.cdc.gov/niosh/docs/2016-106/pdfs/2016-106.pdf?id=10.26616/NIOSHPUB2016106.

NIOSH. 2020. *Limiting Heat Burden While Wearing Personal Protective Equipment (PPE).* https://www.cdc.gov/niosh/topics/heatstress/heat_burden.html.

NOAA, NCEI. 2022. "Billion-dollar weather and climate disasters." https://www.ncdc.noaa.gov/billions/overview.

O'Connor, T., M. Flynn, D. Weinstock, and J. Zanoni. 2014. "Occupational safety and health education and training for underserved populations." *New Solutions: A Journal of Environmental and Occupational Health Policy* 24, no. 1: 83–106.

Orlov, A., J. Sillmann, A. Aaheim, K. Aunan, and K. De Bruin. 2019. "Economic losses of heat-induced reductions in outdoor worker productivity: A case study of Europe." *Economics of Disasters and Climate Change* 3, no. 3: 191–211.

Orui, M., Y. Suzuki, A. Goto and S. Yasumura. 2018. "Factors associated with maintaining the mental health of employees after the Fukushima Nuclear Disaster: Findings from companies located in the evacuation area." *International Journal of Environmental Research and Public Health* 15, no. 1: 53.

Palaniappan, V., A. Sadhasivamohan, J. Sankarapandian, and K. Karthikeyan. 2023. "Miliaria crystallina." *Clinical and Experimental Dermatology* 48, no. 5: 462–67.

Park, J., Y. Kim, and I. Oh. 2017. "Factors affecting heat-related diseases in outdoor workers exposed to extreme heat." *Annals of Occupational and Environmental Medicine* 29, no. 1: 30.

Parker, D., L. Brosseau, Y. Samant, P. Pan, Wei, M. Xi, and D. Haugan. 2007. "A comparison of the perceptions and beliefs of workers and owners with regard to workplace safety in small metal fabrication businesses." *American Journal of Industrial Medicine* 50, no. 12: 999–1009.

Parker, E. R. 2021. "The influence of climate change on skin cancer incidence – A review of the evidence." *International Journal of Women's Dermatology* 7, no. 1: 17–27.

Parsons, K. 2003. *Human Thermal Environments: The Effects of Hot, Moderate, and Cold Environments on Human Health, Comfort and Performance.* London: Taylor & Francis.

Périard, J. D., T. M. Eijsvogels, and H. A. Daanen. 2021. "Exercise under heat stress: Thermoregulation, hydration, performance implications, and mitigation strategies." *Physiological Reviews* 101, no. 4: 1873–79. https://doi.org/10.1152/physrev.00038.2020.

Pinkerton, K. E., E. Felt, and H. E. Riden. 2019. "Extreme weather resulting from global warming is an emerging threat to farmworker health and safety." *Journal of Agricultural Safety and Health* 25, no. 4: 189–90.

Pradhan, B., T. Kjellstrom, D. Atar, P. Sharma, B. Kayastha, G. Bhandari, and P. K. Pradhan. 2019. Heat stress impacts on cardiac mortality in Nepali migrant workers in Qatar. *Cardiology* 143, no. 1–2: 37–48.

Pundee, R., P. Kongtip, N. Nankongnab, S. Anutrakulchai, M. G. Robson, and S. Woskie. 2020. "Cross-shift change of acute kidney injury biomarkers in sugarcane farmers and cutters." *Human and Ecological Risk Assessment: An International Journal* 27, no. 5: 1170–87.

Ravanelli, N., W. Casasola, T. English, K. M. Edwards, and O. Jay. 2019. "Heat stress and fetal risk. Environmental limits for exercise and passive heat stress during pregnancy: A systematic review with best evidence synthesis." *British Journal of Sports Medicine* 53, no. 13: 799–805.

Rekha, S., S. J. Nalini, S. Bhuvana, S. Kanmani, J. E. Hirst, and V. Venugopal. 2024. "Heat stress and adverse pregnancy outcome: Prospective cohort study." *BJOG: An International Journal of Obstetrics & Gynaecology* 131, no. 5: 612–22.

Rowell, L. R. 1993. *Human Cardiovascular Control.* New York: Oxford University Press.

Sawka, M. N. and S. J. Montain. 2000. "Fluid and electrolyte supplementation for exercise heat stress." *The American Journal of Clinical Nutrition* 72, no. 2: 564S–72S.

Schindler, S., W. Rabitsch, F. Essl, P. Wallner, K. Lemmerer, S. Follak, and H.-P. Hutter. 2018. "Alien species and human health: Austrian stakeholder perspective on challenges and solutions." *International Journal of Environmental Research and Public Health* 15, no. 11: 2527.

Schulte, P., A. Bhattacharya, C. Butler, H. Chun, B. Jacklitsch, T. Jacobs, M. Kiefer, J. Lincoln, S. Pendergrass, and J. Shire. 2016. "Advancing the framework for considering the effects of climate change on worker safety and health." *Journal of Occupational and Environmental Hygiene* 13, no. 11: 847–65.

Schwarz, N., E. Newman and W. Leach. 2016. "Making the truth stick & the myths fade: Lessons from cognitive psychology." *Behavioral Science & Policy* 2, no. 1: 85–95.

Shih, G. 2023. "The world's torrid future is etched in the crippled kidneys of Nepali workers." *The Washington Post.*

Sinclair, R. C. and T. R. Cunningham. 2014. "Safety activities in small businesses." *Safety Science* 64: 32–8.

Spector, J. T., J. Krenz, E. Rauser, and D. K. Bonauto. 2014. "Heat-related illness in Washington State agriculture and forestry sectors." *American Journal of Industrial Medicine* 57, no. 8: 881–95.

Spector, J. T., Y. J. Masuda, N. H. Wolff, et al. 2019. "Heat exposure and occupational injuries: Review of the literature and implications." *Current Environmental Health Reports* 6: 286–96.

Spector, J. T. and P. E. Sheffield. 2014. "Re-evaluating occupational heat stress in a changing climate." *Annals of Occupational Hygiene* 58, no. 8: 936–42.

Stocker, T. 2014. *Climate Change 2013: The Physical Science Basis: Working Group I Contribution to the Fifth Assessment Report of the Intergovernmental Panel on Climate Change.* Cambridge: Cambridge University Press.

Syed, S., T. L. O'Sullivan, and K. P. Phillips. 2022. "Extreme heat and pregnancy outcomes: A scoping review of the epidemiological evidence." *International Journal of Environmental Research and Public Health* 19, no. 4: 2412.

Taylor, N., N. Kondo, and W. L. Kenney. 2008. "The physiology of acute heat exposure, with implications for human performance in the heat." In *Physiological Bases of Human Performance during Work and Exercise*, edited by N. A. Taylor and H. Groeller, 341–58. Edinburgh: Elsevier.

Tetzlaff, E. J., C. Cassan, N. Goulet, M. Gorman, B. Hogya, and G. P. Kenny. "Breaking down in tears, soaked in sweat, and sick from the heat": Media-based composite narratives of first responders working during the 2021 Heat Dome. *American Journal of Industrial Medicine* 67: 442–52. https://doi.org/10.1002/ajim.23576.

Tustin, A. W., D. L. Cannon, S. B. Arbury, R. J. Thomas, and M. J. Hodgson. 2018. "Risk factors for heat-related illness in U.S. workers: An OSHA case series." *Journal of Occupational and Environmental Medicine* 60, no. 8: e383–9.

US EPA. 2021a. *Climate Change and Social Vulnerability in the United States: A Focus on Six Impacts.* EPA 430-R-21-003. Washington, DC: U.S. Environmental Protection Agency.

Vaisala. 2022. "Total lightning statistics: 2021 annual lightning report." Vantaa. https://www.vaisala.com/sites/default/files/documents/WEA-MET-2021-Annual-Lightning-Report-B212465EN-A.pdf.

Wang, X. L., P. S. Yip, and C. L. Chan. 2016. "Suicide prevention for local public and volunteer relief workers in disaster-affected areas." *Journal of Public Health Management and Practice* 22, no. 3: E39–46.

Westwood, C. S., J. L. Fallowfield, S. K. Delves, M. Nunns, H. B. Ogden, and J. D. Layden. 2021. Individual risk factors associated with exertional heat illness: A systematic review. *Experimental Physiology* 106, no. 1: 191–9.

Williams, W. 2013. "Physiological impact of flame resistant clothing: managing heat stress." In *Handbook of Fire Resistant Textiles*, edited by F. S. Kilinc, 434–55. Amsterdam: Elsevier.

Williams, W. 2018. "Behavioral and technological adaptation." In *Human Health and Physical Activity During Heat Exposure*, edited by Y. Hosokawa, 85–9. Springer Briefs in Medical Earth Sciences. Cham: Springer.

Part II

Human Factors and Management Considerations

15 Coordinated Project Management for Emergency Response

Adedeji B. Badiru

15.1 INTRODUCTION

Every human endeavor can be modeled as a conventional project, which deserves to be managed with the usual tools and techniques of project management. This chapter presents a concise outline of what needs to be accomplished to manage any emergency response project effectively through all its steps. The usual steps of project management go through project identification, definition, initiation, planning, organizing, resource allocation, scheduling, control, and closing. The steps in the midrange constitute project execution.

According to Hanfling et al. (2012), catastrophic disasters occurring in 2011 in the United States and worldwide have demonstrated that even prepared communities can be overwhelmed. Those disasters range from the tornado in Joplin, Missouri, and the earthquake and tsunami in Japan to the earthquake in New Zealand. Successful disaster response depends on coordination and integration across the full system of key stakeholder groups: state and local governments, EMS, public health, emergency management, hospital facilities, and the outpatient sector. Vertical integration among agencies at the federal, state, and local levels also is crucial. At the cornerstone of this coordination and integration is a foundation of ethical obligations and the legal authorities and regulatory environment that allow for shifts in expectations of the best possible response based on the context of the disaster in which that response is being executed.

The contents of the chapter suggest a proactive approach to emergency response. Col. Cassie Barlow, 88th Air Base Wing Commander at Wright-Patterson Air Force Base (Dayton, Ohio) commented that "we can't wait for emergencies to happen before we respond." She also advocates for a closer relationship between business, industry, the military, and the community in executing emergency response programs. Such a wide collaborative effort is made possible by using proactive systems-based project management approaches. As a demonstration of integrating human aspects with technology assets in emergency response, in 2012, Greene County, Ohio initiated a multi-million dollar program to install communication technology hardware and six strategically placed radio towers that would link the county's first responders. The

DOI: 10.1201/9781003648178-17

goal is to link the first responders to all of the community emergency agencies in the county as well as providing a linkage to Ohio's Multi-Agency Radio Communication System (MARCS). All across the nation and in many international locations, efforts are being made to enhance emergency response. The premise of this chapter is that those efforts can yield better and more positive results through the application of project management tools and techniques. A comprehensive set of metrics offers valuable insights into a program or project, aiding in the prediction of its success. Organizations require information throughout the lifecycle of a program or project to assess its current status and forecast its success. Metrics play a crucial role in facilitating effective communication and reinforcing the project or program's purpose among stakeholders. These metrics vary by industry and the specific nature of projects. Successful organizations typically use multiple key performance indicators (KPIs) to evaluate a project from various perspectives throughout its lifecycle. Some organizations establish KPIs before the project begins, monitor multiple perspectives during implementation, and measure success after completion. They also include portfolio-level KPIs to assess performance across various programs and projects. In addition to project-specific metrics, organizations may consider broader business drivers such as resource retention and utilization. These metrics help evaluate the success of individual programs and projects, as well as the overall portfolio. Metrics can be categorized into several performance areas, including but not limited to:

- Schedule
- Financial
- Earned value
- Scope
- Quality
- Changes
- Customer satisfaction
- Process
- Risk
- Resources
- Procurement

15.2 OCCURRENCE OF DISASTERS

It is a fact of life that disasters occur every now and then, regardless of whatever preemptive preparation is made. We can take preemptive and cautionary steps to mitigate the occurrence or gravity of disasters, but they cannot be completely eliminated, due to the interplay of human factors and technical imperfection. Catastrophic disasters come in every form and shape, from a range of different causes, such as the following:

1. Accidental incidents (e.g., mechanical failure)
   Random events
   Assignable causes (e.g., design flaw)
   Unassignable causes (system wear-out)

2. Natural causes (e.g., weather-related)
3. Deliberate human acts (e.g., evil acts)
   Terrorism
   Sabotage
   Vandalism
4. Inadvertent mismanagement (e.g., error in judgment, improper work process, incompetence)
   Operator error
   Carelessness
   Incompetence
   Faulty work process
   Negligence

The risk of disasters cannot be totally eliminated. All that can be done is to mitigate the risk. As a result, it is essential to have a standing guide for emergency response. Conceptual preparedness is one thing; the reality of execution is another. A lack of communication or the occurrence of miscommunication can spell doom for the response effort. The importance of communication and coordination provides the basis for the current exposition of the human systems issues in emergency response. Disasters lead to traumatic incidents that may hamper relief project efforts. Typical results of a disaster include, but are not limited to, the following:

- Infrastructure damage
- Destruction of roads, bridges, and access ways
- Deaths
- Injuries
- Displacement of people
- Asset destruction
- Property damage
- Looting and pillaging
- Lawlessness
- Social unrest

Disasters lead to traumatic incidents that may hamper relief efforts. With the occurrence of disaster outcomes and the accompanying confusion, there will be incidents of communication breakdown, cooperation failure, and lack of coordination. To get everything back in order, a systems-oriented model is needed. Disasters will occur every now and then, regardless of whatever preemptive preparations are made. The importance of communication and coordination provides the basis for the recommendation to use the Triple C model of project management (Badiru 2012) in this chapter. The origin of the Triple C model is a successful application to an emergency response at Tinker Air Force Base in 1985 (Badiru et al. 1993).

15.3 COORDINATED RESPONSE TO EMERGENCY

It is obvious that coordination is the most crucial requirement for effective emergency response. Such coordination is predicated on human factors and managerial processes during the emergency situation. The foundation for coordination is cooperation, which depends on prior communication. This is why a collaborative structure is needed. Based on the diversity of events and issues that can develop during a disaster and the ensuing emergency response, a coordinated plan of action must be put in place and executed on the fly. Prior planning, practice, and reinforcement exercises are essential and must recognize the tools and techniques available from the following topics:

- Project systems analysis
- Systems engineering framework
- Human factors considerations

A coordinated response to an emergency will often involve the military, which brings a diversity of transportation assets, manpower resources, command and control processes, and well-honed skill sets to bear on the emergency situation. The expedited response of the military can bring efficiency and effectiveness into the overall emergency response. If a coordinated and systematic response program is not in place, citizens will run helter-skelter. In all cases, emergency response must be fast, effective, and uncompromised. Mobility, configurability, and modularity are desired elements in a coordinated response effort involving military and civilian entities. Using a systems approach, as suggested by NRC (2007) and Kossiakoff and Sweet (2003), increases the potential for a successful coordinated response.

15.4 USING A PROJECT SYSTEMS FRAMEWORK

Like any other resource-constrained and time-sensitive endeavor, emergency response programs require conventional planning, organization, scheduling, control, and phase-out. These are standard management functions for which project management tools and techniques have proven very effective. Badiru (2012) defines project management as follows:

> Project management is the process of managing, allocating, and timing resources to achieve a specific goal in an efficient and expedient manner.

The above definition suggests a systematic integration of technical, human, and other resources to achieve goals and objectives. This is precisely what is needed in a coordinated emergency response, where a multitude of goals and objectives interact in a fast-paced environment. In this chapter, emergency response challenges are seen as being amenable to a rigorous project management approach. Far too many response projects are initiated without a careful project management framework.

From a project management perspective, there are several questions to consider when executing emergency response. Some pertinent questions include the following:

1. How should emergency response be planned and executed in the presence of time-sensitive relief requirements?
2. What impact will response technology changes have on the emergency response infrastructure and facilities?
3. How agile, adaptive, and resilient is the response infrastructure to shifts in community needs?
4. What resource allocation strategies are in place to ensure sustainability of the response operation?
5. How adaptive is the project plan in the presence of demands and requests from the shareholders, city administrators, and local governments?

Emergency response is very complex, with many stakeholders, diverse inputs to the system, constraints on the work processes, and changes in resource availability. As in any project, an emergency response is executed to achieve one or more of three basic objectives:

1. Physical product (e.g., configure a rescue tool).
2. Service (e.g., provide public assistance).
3. Result (e.g., accomplish a successful rescue).

Of importance across these basic objectives is the recognition of the interrelationships between the components of the disaster event, which touch on the following categories of involvement:

1. People (first responders, victims, etc.).
2. Technology (communication hardware, transportation vehicle, medical device, etc.).
3. Process (search and rescue processes, policies, procedures, permissions, etc.).

15.5 USING A PARTICIPATIVE AND INCLUSIVE MODEL

Based on the systems view and the human factors issues discussed above, it is essential to use a participative and inclusive model. Everyone has a coordinated role to play, from the federal level to the personal level, where individual actions and reactions are paramount for a successful coordinated emergency response. The role of the federal government is to provide assurance and resources to execute the emergency response. If possible, business and industry must continue to operate to provide basic amenities, goods, and services that may be needed for the emergency response. This is particularly important for cases where the impact of the emergency situation or disaster may be protracted, stretching over several days or weeks. Medical facilities must remain open and accessible to cater to the needs of victims. First responders must be ready, agile, and adaptive as situations on the ground evolve. Schools and higher education facilities are often used as shelters in emergency situations. As such, they must be robust and resilient. Relief organizations, working in consonance with victims, must be visible but not constitute an impediment to the movement of first responders. Individuals, homes, and neighborhoods must be cooperative in following response instructions, announcements, and alerts. Utility companies must be swift in creating a safe pathway for rescue and evacuation teams to have access to emergency response structures. Finally, local and state governments must cooperate to work within the response decision hierarchy. All units must be involved in a collaborative, inclusive, and participatory systems framework. A single point of obstinance can prove to be the cog in the wheel of the response system.

15.6 EXECUTING THE STEPS OF PROJECT MANAGEMENT

Figure 15.1 illustrates the steps of a project framework, starting with the identification of a need and ending with a phase-out after the need has been met. The steps provide a structured framework for executing an emergency response endeavor, ranging from identifying the need for a response, establishing response objectives, rescue planning, personnel organization, resource allocation, task scheduling, progress tracking, process control, and termination of response. Response termination, in this case, does not imply conclusion of the overall effort, but rather, the completion of a particular phase, which may then serve as the initiating point for other follow-on efforts, such as rebuilding. Further explanations of the elements in the steps are provided below.

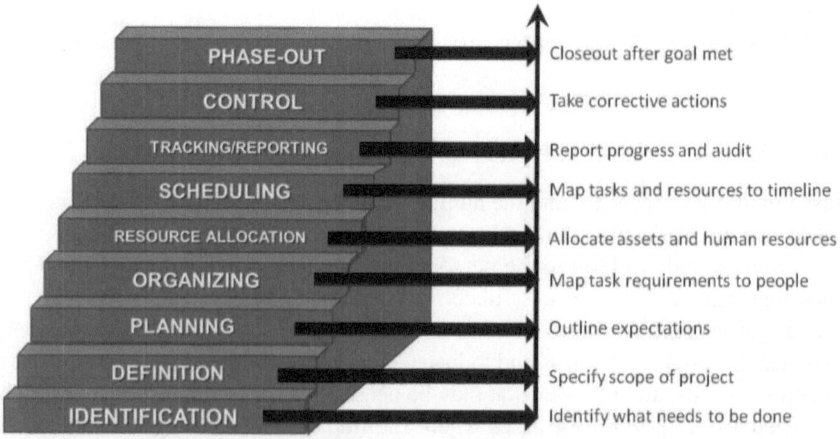

FIGURE 15.1 Steps of project management applied to emergency response

15.6.1 Identification

Identification is the process of recognizing the need for an emergency response. This recognition may be initiated by the announcement of the occurrence of a disaster.

15.6.2 Definition

Project definition requires an explicit articulation of what exactly should be accomplished by the response effort, identifying goals and strategies to meet them. This step outlines a clear understanding regarding what the final accomplishment is expected to look like. Questions that can be asked during this step, that can preempt or mitigate problems later on, include the following:

1. Who is in charge of the emergency response program?
2. When will the response be initiated?
3. How will the response contribute to the overall welfare of the community?
4. How will the emergency response affect different groups of people within the community?
5. What organizations within the community will be involved?
6. What will happen after the emergency response is implemented?
7. How do the emergency response objectives fit the overall priority of the community?

15.6.3 Planning

Expectations of the emergency response, quality control techniques, communication hierarchy, technology selection, and transportation modes are established at this step. Planning should not commence until a clear definition of the project objectives from the previous step has been developed. Quality control techniques include expert reviews to detect logic errors and logistical impediments. Stakeholders can benchmark other successful response programs when designing and outlining the structure and activities of the response. Also during this step, methods that will be used to assess the performance of the program should be outlined.

15.6.4 Organization

Organization requires a mapping of tasks and responsibilities to specific individuals involved in the emergency response. Individuals and organizations that will contribute to the response are identified. If possible, a responsibility matrix can be used as an effective tool for organizing projects. Simple codes may be used to outline responsibilities. Examples are **R** (Responsible), **I** (Inform), **S** (Support), and **C** (Consult), while the task tracking codes could be **D** (Done), **O** (On Track), and **L** (Late).

15.6.5 Resource Allocation

Resource allocation is a critical part of executing a project effectively. One common complaint about emergency response infrastructure is the inadequate allocation of resources (i.e., human assets, technology, and service support). The needs of first responders and victims should dictate the type of technology, or combination of technology, used to deliver emergency response services. Without dependable technology, emergency responders are likely to become frustrated, disappointed, and detached, which can be detrimental to the overall goal. When resource allocation is addressed as an explicit step, the process of communicating resource requirements to decision makers is better structured and more effective.

15.6.6 Task Scheduling

Task scheduling is often the most visible part of project management, but it is not the first step, as most people often falsely assume. If the preceding steps of project management are executed properly, they will pave the way for a more effective task-scheduling process. This will prevent scheduling conflicts between first responders, rescuers, facility managers, and law enforcement officers.

15.6.7 Tracking

Tracking the response project once it has been launched is important. Tracking entails reporting and auditing the performance of those involved in the operations to ensure that actions are aligned with plans, goals, and standards.

15.6.8 Control

At the control step, corrective actions are taken to determine if operations meet expectations. Corrective actions must be taken in a timely manner before minor incidents become major events.

15.6.9 Phase-out

A phase-out denotes that a specific goal has been accomplished and efforts can proceed to the next contiguous undertaking in the overall emergency response project.

15.7 USING SYSTEMS ENGINEERING FRAMEWORK

The George Washington University Institute for Crisis, in a guide entitled "Disaster and Risk Management," provides a definition of a systems approach to emergency response as a "management strategy that recognizes that disparate components must be viewed as interrelated components of a single system, and so employs specific methods to achieve and maintain the overarching system. These methods include the use of standardized structure and processes and foundational knowledge and concepts in the conduct of all related activities." This aligns directly with the project management and systems approach theme presented in this chapter as a recommended approach.

Any project is ultimately a component of a larger system. As such, a systems view facilitates a complete look at all factors involved in emergency response. Systems engineering efficiency and effectiveness are of interest across the spectrum of project management for the purpose of improving organizational performance. Emergency responders should be interested in having systems engineering serve as the umbrella for a coordinated approach to emergency response. This will get everyone properly connected with the prevailing organizational goals, as well as create collaborative avenues among the responders. Systems application applies across the spectrum of any organization and encompasses the following elements:

- Technological systems (e.g., engineering control systems and mechanical systems).
- Organizational systems (e.g., work process design and operating structures).
- Human systems (e.g., interpersonal relationships and human-machine interfaces).

A systems view of emergency response will make everything work better and projects more likely to succeed. A systems view provides a disciplined process for the design, development, and execution of complex projects, both in engineering and non-engineering organizations. One of the major advantages of a systems approach is the win-win benefit for everyone. A systems view also allows full involvement of all stakeholders in a response effort. Every emergency response environment is very complex because of the diversity of factors involved. There are differing human personalities. There are differing technical requirements. There are differing expectations. There are differing environmental factors. Each specific context and the prevailing circumstances will determine the specific structure of what can and cannot be done in the effort. The best approach for effective project management is to adapt to what each project needs. This requires taking a systems view of the project. Project management represents an excellent platform for the implementation of a systems approach. Project management integrates various technical and management requirements. Project management requires control techniques, such as operations research, operations management, forecasting, quality control, and simulation, to deliver goals. In systems-based project management, it is essential that related techniques be employed in an integrated fashion so as to maximize the total project output. There should not be an over-reliance on technology, nor should there be an over-dependence on human processes. Similarly, there should not be too much emphasis on analytical models to the detriment of common-sense human-based decisions. The comprehensive systems engineering definition below illustrates the importance of a systems framework in emergency response:

Systems engineering is the application of engineering to solutions of a multifaceted problem through a systematic collection and integration of parts of the problem with respect to the lifecycle of the problem. It is the branch of engineering concerned with the development, implementation, and use of large or complex systems. It focuses on specific goals of a system, considering the specifications, prevailing constraints, expected services, possible behaviors, and structure of the system. It also involves a consideration of the activities required to ensure that the system's performance matches the stated goals. Systems engineering addresses the integration of tools, people, and processes required to achieve a cost-effective and timely operation of the system.

Logistics can be defined as the planning and implementation of a complex task, the planning and control of the flow of goods and materials through an organization or manufacturing process, or the planning and organization of the movement of personnel, equipment, and supplies. Just as it is in the corporate world, logistics plays a direct role in emergency response activities. Complex projects represent a hierarchical system of operations. Thus, we can view an emergency response as a collection of interrelated projects, all serving a common end goal. Consequently, the following definition is applicable to the diversity of needs in an emergency response situation:

Project systems logistics is the planning, implementation, movement, scheduling, and control of people, equipment, goods, materials, and supplies across the interfacing boundaries of several related projects.

Conventional project management must be modified and expanded to address the unique logistics of emergency response.

15.8 HUMAN FACTORS CONSIDERATIONS

Human attitude is a big part of emergency response. Some of the human issues that can impede a smooth emergency response include the following:

- Bureaucracy
- Complacency
- Incompetence
- Indifference
- Arrogance
- Inaccessibility
- Personal rigidity
- Obstinate
- Stubbornness
- Administrative inflexibility

Human behavior in emergency situations is subject to the "cry wolf syndrome," whereby repeated warnings become so persistent that the warnings lose effectiveness, validity, and impact. Citizens may then become complacent and indifferent to warnings by giving emergency announcements a cold shoulder. These adverse behaviors can be mitigated by reemphasizing the structure of top-down and bottom-up communication in emergency response scenarios. This suggests that each interface within the communication structure should be managed to maximize the perception of the gravity of what is communicated.

15.9 TRIPLE C MODEL FOR EMERGENCY RESPONSE

Managing a project in the wake of a tragedy is complicated and involves various emotional, sentimental, reactive, and chaotic responses. This makes it difficult to clearly pursue the traditional methods of planning and execution. This is the time when a structured communication model is most needed. Unfortunately, practical models are often not readily available. Conventional wisdom and assumptions, in lieu of direct communication, portend failure for a project. At a time of disaster, reactive rhetoric may not coincide with action or reality. Having a guiding model can help put things in proper focus.

Using the basis of the communication, cooperation, and coordination presented earlier, we now present a Triple C-based model for disaster rapid response. The Triple C model presented by Badiru (2012) is an effective tool for emergency response project planning. The model states that project management can be enhanced by implementing it within the integrated functions of

- Communication
- Cooperation
- Coordination

The Triple C model provides a specification of what, why, who, how, where, and when parameters as they relate to managing emergency response. The model facilitates a systematic approach to project planning, organizing, scheduling, and control. The Triple C model complements the usual military command, control, and communication processes as may be applied to emergency response. The Triple C suggests communication as the first and foremost function in any coordinated endeavor. It highlights what must be done and when. It can also help to identify the resources (personnel, equipment, facilities, etc.) required for each effort. It points out important questions, such as

- Does each project participant know what the objective is?
- Does each participant know his or her role in achieving the objective?
- What obstacles may prevent a participant from playing his or her role effectively?

An adaptive version of the Triple C model for disaster response uses an integrative and inclusive process so that communication, cooperation, and coordination points are identified throughout the stages of implementing the model. The Triple C approach leverages level-to-level interfaces for communication, cooperation, and coordination within the top-down and bottom-up response hierarchy.

15.10 COMMUNICATION FOR EMERGENCY RESPONSE

Communication makes working together possible. The communication function of project management involves making all those concerned become aware of project requirements and progress. Those who will be affected by the project, directly or indirectly, as direct participants or as beneficiaries, should be informed as appropriate regarding the following:

- The scope of the project.
- Personnel contribution required.
- Expected cost, schedule, performance requirements, and merits of the project.
- Project organization and implementation plan.
- Potential adverse effects if the project should fail.
- Alternatives, if any, for achieving the project goal.
- Potential direct and indirect benefits of the project.

The communication channel must be kept open throughout the project life cycle. In addition to internal communication, appropriate external sources should also be consulted. The project manager must:

- Exude commitment to the project.
- Utilize a communication responsibility matrix.
- Facilitate multichannel communication interfaces.
- Identify internal and external communication needs.
- Resolve organizational and communication hierarchies.
- Encourage both formal and informal communication links.

When clear communication is maintained between management and employees and among peers, many project problems can be averted. Project communication may be carried out in one or more of the following formats:

- One-to-many
- One-to-one
- Many-to-one
- Written and formal
- Written and informal
- Oral and formal
- Oral and informal
- Nonverbal gestures

Good communication is achieved when what is implied is perceived as intended. Effective communication is vital to the success of any project. Despite the awareness that proper communication forms the blueprint for project success, many organizations still fail in their communications functions. The study of communication is complex. Factors that influence the effectiveness of communication within a project organization structure include the following:

1. **Personal perception**. Each person perceives events on the basis of personal psychological, social, cultural, and experimental background. As a result, no two people can interpret a given event the same way. The nature of events is not always the critical aspect of a problem situation. Rather, the problem is often the different perceptions of the different people involved.
2. **Psychological profile**. The psychological makeup of each person determines personal reactions to events or words. Thus, individual needs and levels of thinking will dictate how a message is interpreted.
3. **Social Environment**. Communication problems sometimes arise because people have been conditioned by their prevailing social environment to interpret certain things in unique ways. Vocabulary, idioms, organizational status, social stereotypes, and economic situation are among the social factors that can thwart effective communication.
4. **Cultural background**. Cultural differences are among the most pervasive barriers to project communications, especially in today's multinational organizations. Language and cultural idiosyncrasies often determine how communication is approached and interpreted.
5. **Semantic and syntactic factors**. Semantic and syntactic barriers to communication usually occur in written documents. Semantic factors are those that relate to the intrinsic knowledge of the subject of the communication. Syntactic factors are those that relate to the form in which the communication is presented. The problems created by these factors become acute in situations where response, feedback, or reaction to the communication cannot be observed.
6. **Organizational structure**. Frequently, the organizational structure in which a project is conducted has a direct influence on the flow of information and, consequently, on the effectiveness of communication. Organizational hierarchy may determine how different personnel levels perceive a given communication.
7. **Communication media**. The method of transmitting a message may also affect the value ascribed to the message and, consequently, how it is interpreted or used. The common barriers to project communication are:
   - Inattentiveness
   - Lack of organization
   - Outstanding grudges
   - Preconceived notions
   - Ambiguous presentation
   - Emotions and sentiments

- Lack of communication feedback
- Sloppy and unprofessional presentation
- Lack of confidence in the communicator
- Lack of confidence by the communicator
- Low credibility of the communicator
- Unnecessary technical jargon
- Too many people involved
- Untimely communication
- Arrogance or imposition
- Lack of focus

Some suggestions on improving the effectiveness of communication are presented next. The recommendations may be implemented as appropriate for any of the forms of communication listed earlier. The recommendations are for both the communicator and the audience.

1. Never assume that the integrity of the information sent will be preserved as the information passes through several communication channels. Information is generally filtered, condensed, or expanded by the receivers before being relayed to the next destination. When preparing a communication that needs to pass through several organizational structures, one safeguard is to compose the original information in a concise form to minimize the need for recomposition.
2. Give the audience a central role in the discussion. A leading role can help make a person feel a part of the project effort and responsible for the project's success. He or she can then have a more constructive view of project communication.
3. Do homework and think through the intended accomplishment of the communication. This helps eliminate trivial and inconsequential communication efforts.
4. Carefully plan the organization of the ideas embodied in the communication. Use indexing or points of reference whenever possible. Grouping ideas into related chunks of information can be particularly effective. Present the short messages first. Short messages help create focus, maintain interest, and prepare the mind for the longer messages to follow.
5. Highlight why the communication is of interest and how it is intended to be used. Full attention should be given to the content of the message with regard to the prevailing project situation.
6. Elicit the support of those around you by integrating their ideas into the communication. The more people feel they have contributed to the issue, the more expeditious they are in soliciting the cooperation of others. The effect of the multiplicative rule can quickly garner support for the communication's purpose.
7. Be responsive to the feelings of others. It takes two to communicate. Anticipate and appreciate the reactions of members of the audience.

Recognize their operational circumstances and present your message in a form they can relate to.
8. Accept constructive criticism. Nobody is infallible. Use criticism as a springboard to higher communication performance.
9. Exhibit interest in the issue in order to arouse the interest of your audience. Avoid delivering your messages as a routine organizational requirement.
10. Obtain and furnish feedback promptly. Clarify vague points with examples.
11. Communicate at the appropriate time, at the right place, to the right people.
12. Reinforce words with positive action. Never promise what cannot be delivered. Value your credibility.
13. Maintain eye contact in oral communication and read the facial expressions of your audience to obtain real-time feedback.
14. Concentrate on listening as much as speaking. Evaluate both the implicit and explicit meanings of statements.
15. Document communication transactions for future reference.
16. Avoid asking questions that can be answered yes or no. Use relevant questions to focus the attention of the audience. Use questions that make people reflect upon their words, such as, "How do you think this will work?" compared to, "Do you think this will work?"
17. Avoid patronizing the audience. Respect their judgment and knowledge.
18. Speak and write in a controlled tempo. Avoid emotionally charged voice inflections.
19. Create an atmosphere for formal and informal exchange of ideas.
20. Summarize the objectives of the communication and how they will be achieved.

A communication responsibility matrix can be used to show the linking of sources of communication and targets of communication. Cells within the matrix would indicate the subject of the desired communication. With a communication responsibility matrix, a clear understanding of what needs to be communicated to whom can be developed. Communication in a project environment can take any of several forms. The specific needs of a project may dictate the most appropriate mode. Three popular computer communication modes are discussed next in the context of communicating data and information for emergency response.

15.10.1 Simplex Communication

Simplex communication is a unidirectional arrangement in which one project entity initiates communication to another entity or individual within the project environment. The entity addressed in the communication does not have a mechanism or capability for responding to the communication. An extreme example of this is a one-way, top-down communication from top management to the project personnel. In this case, the personnel have no communication access or input to top management. A budget-related example is a case where top management allocates a budget to a project without requesting and reviewing the actual needs of the project. Simplex communication is common in authoritarian organizations.

15.10.2 Half-Duplex Communication

Half-duplex communication is a bi-directional arrangement whereby one project entity can communicate with another entity and receive a response within a certain time lag. Both entities can communicate with each other, but not at the same time. An example of half-duplex communication is a project organization that permits communication with top management without a direct meeting. Each communicator must wait for a response from the target of the communication. Request and allocation without a budget meeting is another example of half-duplex data communication in project management.

15.10.3 Full-Duplex Communication

Full-duplex communication involves an arrangement that permits a dialogue between the communicating entities. Both individuals and entities can communicate with each other at the same time or face-to-face. As long as there is no clash of words, this appears to be the most receptive communication mode. It allows participative project planning in which each member of the project team has an opportunity to contribute to the planning process.

Each member of a response team needs to recognize the nature of the prevailing communication mode in the response environment. An evaluation of who is to communicate with whom about what may help improve the project data/information communication process. A communication matrix may include notations about the desired modes of communication between individuals and groups in the project environment.

15.11 COOPERATION FOR EMERGENCY RESPONSE

The cooperation of project personnel must be explicitly elicited. Merely voicing consent for a project is not enough assurance of full cooperation. The participants and beneficiaries of the project must be convinced of the merits of the project. Some of the factors that influence cooperation in a project environment include personnel requirements, resource requirements, budget limitations, past experiences, conflicting priorities, and lack of uniform organizational support. A structured approach to seeking cooperation should clarify the following:

- Cooperative efforts required
- Precedents for future projects
- Implications of lack of cooperation
- Criticality of cooperation to project success
- Organizational impact of cooperation
- Time frame involved in the project
- Rewards of good cooperation

Cooperation is a basic virtue of human interaction. More projects fail due to a lack of cooperation and commitment than for any other reason. To secure and retain the cooperation of project participants, you must elicit a positive first reaction to the project. The most positive aspects of a project should be the first items of project communication. For project management, there are different types of cooperation that should be understood.

15.11.1 Functional Cooperation

Functional cooperation is induced by the nature of the functional relationship between two groups. The two groups may be required to perform related functions that can only be accomplished through mutual cooperation.

15.11.2 Social Cooperation

Social cooperation is driven by the social relationship between two groups. The prevailing social relationship motivates cooperation that may be useful in getting project work done.

15.11.3 Legal Cooperation

Legal cooperation is imposed through some authoritative requirement. In this case, the participants may have no choice other than to cooperate.

15.11.4 Administrative Cooperation

Administrative cooperation is brought on by administrative requirements that make it imperative that two groups work together on a common goal.

15.11.5 Associative Cooperation

Associative cooperation may also be referred to as collegiality. The level of cooperation is determined by the association that exists between two groups.

15.11.6 Proximity Cooperation

Proximity cooperation may result when groups are geographically close. Being close makes it imperative that the two groups work together.

15.11.7 Dependency Cooperation

Dependency cooperation is caused when one group depends on another group for some important aspect. Such dependency is usually of a mutual, two-way nature. One group depends on the other for one thing, while the latter group depends on the former for some other thing.

15.11.8 Imposed Cooperation

In imposed cooperation, external agents must be employed to induce cooperation between two groups. This is applicable for cases where the two groups have no natural reason to cooperate. This is where the approaches presented earlier for seeking cooperation can become very useful.

15.11.9 Lateral Cooperation

Lateral cooperation involves cooperation with peers and immediate associates. Lateral cooperation is often easy to achieve because existing lateral relationships create a conducive environment for project cooperation.

15.11.10 Vertical Cooperation

Vertical or hierarchical cooperation refers to cooperation that is implied by the hierarchical structure of the project. For example, subordinates are expected to cooperate with their vertical superiors.

Whichever type of cooperation is available in a project environment, the cooperative forces should be channeled toward achieving project goals. Documentation of the prevailing level of cooperation is useful for winning further support for a project. Clarification of project priorities will facilitate personnel cooperation. Relative priorities of multiple projects should be specified and communicated broadly so that all groups within the organization understand the relative importance of work. Some guidelines for securing cooperation for most projects are:

- Establish achievable goals for the project.
- Clearly outline the individual commitments required.
- Integrate project priorities with existing priorities.
- Eliminate the fear of job loss due to industrialization.
- Anticipate and eliminate potential sources of conflict.
- Use an open-door policy to address project grievances.
- Remove skepticism by documenting the merits of the project.

15.11.11 Commitment

Cooperation must be supported with commitment. To cooperate is to support the ideas of a project. To commit is to willingly and actively participate in project efforts again and again through the thick and thin of the project. Provision of resources is one way that management can express commitment to a project.

15.12 TRIPLE C + COMMITMENT = PROJECT SUCCESS

15.12.1 Coordination in Emergency Response

After the communication and cooperation functions have successfully been initiated, the efforts of the project personnel must be coordinated. Coordination facilitates the harmonious organization of project efforts. The construction of a responsibility chart can be very helpful at this stage. A responsibility chart is a matrix consisting of columns of individual or functional departments and rows of required actions. Cells within the matrix are filled with relationship codes that indicate who is responsible for what. The matrix helps avoid neglecting crucial communication requirements and obligations. It can help resolve questions such as:

- Who is to do what?
- How long will it take?
- Who is to inform whom of what?
- Whose approval is needed for what?
- Who is responsible for which results?
- What personnel interfaces are required?
- What support is needed from whom and when?

15.12.2 Resolving Conflicts in Emergency Response

When implemented as an integrated process, the Triple C model can help avoid conflicts in emergency response. When conflicts do develop, Triple C can help in resolving the conflicts. Several sources of conflicts can exist in large emergency response scenarios. Some of these are discussed below.

15.12.2.1 Schedule Conflict

Conflicts can develop because of improper timing or sequencing of project tasks. This is particularly common in large, multiple projects. Procrastination can lead to having too much to do at once, thereby creating a clash of project functions and discord among project team members. Inaccurate estimates of time requirements may lead to infeasible activity schedules. Project coordination can help avoid schedule conflicts.

15.12.2.2 Cost Conflict

Project cost may not be generally acceptable to the clients of a project. This can lead to project conflict. Even if the initial cost of the project is acceptable, a lack of cost control during implementation can lead to conflicts. Poor budget allocation approaches and the lack of a financial feasibility study will cause cost conflicts later on in a project. Communication and coordination can help prevent most of the adverse effects of cost conflicts.

15.12.2.3 Performance Conflict

If clear performance requirements are not established, performance conflicts will develop. A lack of clearly defined performance standards can lead each person to evaluate his or her own performance based on personal value judgments. In order to uniformly evaluate the quality of work and monitor project progress, performance standards should be established by using the Triple C approach.

15.12.2.4 Management Conflict

There must be a two-way alliance between management and the project team. The views of management should be understood by the team. The views of the team should be appreciated by management. If this does not happen, management conflicts will develop. A lack of a two-way interaction can lead to strikes and industrial actions, which can be detrimental to project objectives. The Triple C approach can help create a conducive dialogue environment between management and the project team.

15.12.2.5 Technical Conflict

If the technical basis of a project is not sound, technical conflicts may develop. New industrial projects are particularly prone to technical conflicts because of their significant dependence on technology. A lack of comprehensive technical feasibility study will lead to technical conflicts. Performance requirements and systems specifications can be integrated through the Triple C approach to avoid technical conflicts.

15.12.2.6 Priority Conflict

Priority conflicts can develop if project objectives are not defined properly and applied uniformly across a project. Without a clear project definition, each project member may define his or her own goals, which may be in conflict with the intended goals of the project. Lack of consistency of the project mission is another potential source of priority conflicts. Over-assignment of responsibilities with no guidelines for relative significance levels can also lead to priority conflicts. Communication can help defuse priority conflict.

15.12.2.7 Resource Conflict

Resource allocation problems are a major source of conflict in project management. Competition for resources, including personnel, tools, hardware, software, and so on, can lead to disruptive clashes among project members. The Triple C approach can help secure resource cooperation.

15.12.2.8 Power Conflict

Project politics lead to a power play that can adversely affect the progress of a project. This can manifest itself in terms of power play between the various groups involved in emergency response programs. Project authority and project power should be clearly delineated. Project authority is the control that a person has by virtue of his or her functional post. Project power relates to the clout and influence that a person can exercise due to connections within the administrative structure. People with popular personalities can often wield a lot of project power in spite of low or nonexistent project authority. The Triple C model can facilitate a positive marriage of project authority and power to the benefit of project goals. This will help establish clear leadership for a project.

15.12.2.9 Personality Conflict

Personality conflict is a common problem in projects involving a large group of people. The larger the project, the larger the size of the management team needed to keep things running. Unfortunately, the larger management team creates an opportunity for personality conflicts. Communication and cooperation can help defuse personality conflicts.

In summary, conflict resolution through Triple C can be achieved by observing the following guidelines:

1. Confront the conflict and identify the underlying causes.
2. Be cooperative and receptive to negotiation as a mechanism for resolving conflicts.
3. Distinguish between proactive, inactive, and reactive behaviors in a conflict situation.
4. Use communication to defuse internal strife and competition.
5. Recognize that short-term compromise can lead to long-term gains.
6. Use coordination to work toward a unified goal.
7. Use communication and cooperation to turn a competitor into a collaborator.

The application of the Triple C model is in direct alignment with contingency planning strategies for emergency response, as summarized in Table 15.1.

TABLE 15.1
Emergency Contingency Planning Compared to Conventional Planning

Characteristics	Preparedness Planning	Contingency Planning	Operations Planning
When (contingency)	Planning phase	Before the emergency	During emergency
What (scope of plan)	General	Time-frame specific	More specific
Who (involved partners)	Everybody within system	People knowledgeable	People actually involved
How (focus)	All types	Specific/Projected	Actual
How (planning style)	Long-term, global	Specific time frame	Actual
What (allocation)	Estimated	Quantified	Precise
Where (planning level)	All levels	Managerial level	Actual/field level
When (time frame)	Annual (one year)	Specific (but uncertain)	Executed right time, fixed
Who (relationships)	Long-term	Developing	Utilizing

15.13 CONCLUSIONS

Education is an important part of any coordinated emergency response. Using a systems approach will foster collaborative, interdisciplinary alliances among schools, higher education academic programs, and community groups through research and development and service programs. Graduate students can plan direct research roles through studies dealing with not only technical systems but also social sciences and behavioral studies. Information technology and cyber infrastructure can also impinge upon how a response program is executed. New academic specialization tracks can evolve to address specific issues and unique issues of emergency response. These could include the following:

- Systems integration, systems management, and resilience engineering.
- Computational statistics, simulation, and risk analysis to assess emergency-related data sets.
- Optimization and control for emergency medical response.
- Organizational processes and human behavioral tendencies.
- Information technology research and product development for emergency response.

REFERENCES

Badiru, A. B. (2012). *Project Management: Systems, Principles, and Applications.* Boca Raton, FL: CRC Press/Taylor & Francis.

Badiru, A. B., Foote, B. L., Leemis, L., Ravindran, A., & Williams, L. (1993). Recovering from a crisis at tinker air force base. *PM Network*, Vol. 7, No. 2, pp. 10–23.

Hanfling, D., et al. (2012). *Crisis Standards of Care: A Systems Framework for Catastrophic Disaster Response.* Washington, DC: The National Academies Press. http://www.nap.edu/catalog.php?record_id=13351.

Kossiakoff, A., & Sweet, W. N. (2003). *Systems Engineering: Principles and Practice.* Hoboken, NJ: Wiley InterScience.

National Research Council (NRC) (2007). *Improving Disaster Management: The Role of IT in Mitigation, Preparedness, Response, and Recovery.* Washington, DC: The National Academies Press.

16 DEJI Systems Model
Factors and Elements for Emergency Response

Adedeji B. Badiru

16.1 ELEMENTS OF THE DEJI SYSTEMS MODEL

This chapter presents the application of the Design, Evaluate, Justify, and Integrate (DEJI) systems model to the management of emergency response processes, with particular emphasis on the issues of activity management and coordination, especially with respect to using innovative approaches. The model provides a generic pathway for process design, evaluation, justification, and integration. The pursuit of innovative ideas, actions, and processes is essential to how we respond to the challenges of emergency response. Although there are many components of emergency response, innovation is a viable factor to focus on. Thus, we use the framework of innovation to introduce the DEJI systems model in this chapter. The theme and focus of innovation run throughout this chapter. With its capstone of "systems integration," the DEJI systems model is applicable to both the qualitative and quantitative aspects of emergency response.

"A new way of doing things" is one of the definitions of innovation. Emergency response requires new ways of doing things. Whether it is this definition or any other definition, emergency response must have buy-in from stakeholders and be integrated into the operating environment. The DEJI systems model (Badiru, 2012, 2019) is a good tool for ensuring that the proposed innovation fits the operating environment of the organization, the community, or the nation. The DEJI systems model is applicable for innovation design, evaluation, justification, and integration. Figure 16.1 illustrates the overall framework of the DEJI systems model. More details on the model can be obtained from www.DEJImodel.com.

The elements and factors of the model are summarized below, with specific sub-considerations.

- Design
- Evaluation
- Justification
- Integration
- Integrate

DOI: 10.1201/9781003648178-18

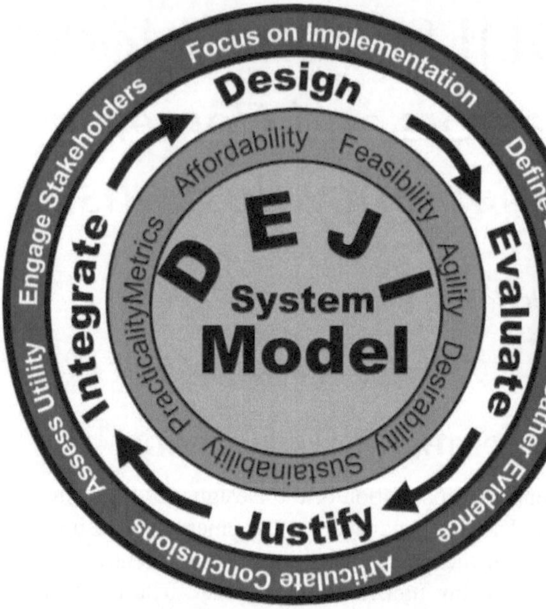

FIGURE 16.1 Elements and factors within the DEJI systems model

- Feasibility
- Agility
- Desirability
- Sustainability
- Practicality
- Metrics
- Affordability
- Focus on implementation
- Definition of end goal
- Gathering of operational evidence
- Articulation of conclusions
- Assessment of utility
- Engagement of stakeholders

Figure 16.2 illustrates the coalescence of many of the applicable considerations in the application of the DEJI systems model.

16.2 WHY THE DEJI SYSTEMS MODEL?

Driven by analytical tools, technical professionals tend to want to jump to the coordination and implementation stage of a project. That is, jumping to the design functionality stage while dispensing with intermediate steps, where non-technical and

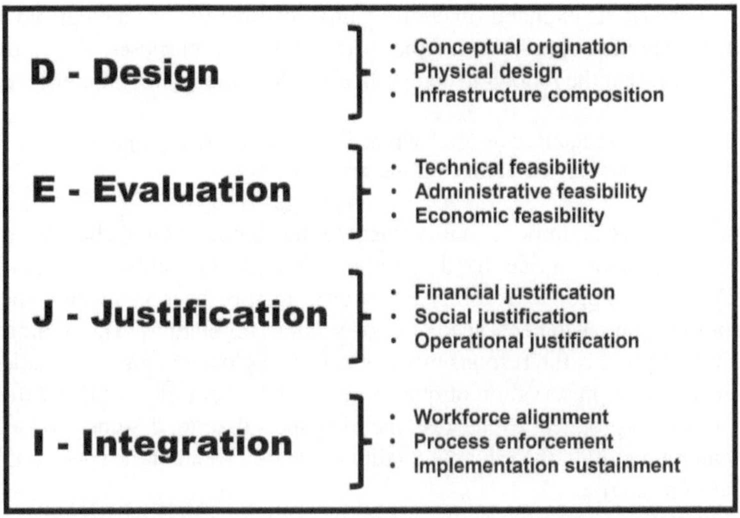

FIGURE 16.2 Operational considerations within the DEJI systems model

"soft" issues might exist. However, those intermediate stages are often more critical for system success than the pure analytical foundation. Items such as needs analysis, gap analysis, user involvement, communication, cooperation, resource requirement analysis, budget flow, leadership support, workforce acceptance, project desirability, and so on, are essential before getting to the end point of the project. This is the essential narrative that highlights the efficacy of the approach of the DEJI systems model, which takes a project sequentially through the stages of design, evaluation, justification, and, finally, integration. These step-by-step stages allow important considerations, technical or otherwise, to be addressed in the project. It is of utmost importance to understand how the proposed product of the project will integrate with and align with the existing organizational framework. The DEJI model makes it imperative to do an a priori evaluation of the potential impact that the project output might have on the prevailing environment.

In implementation, the model can be customized for specific needs related to sustainability. Explanations and examples for design, evaluation, justification, and integration are provided throughout the chapter. Several factors related to sustainability innovation are amenable to the application of the DEJI systems model. Some of these are discussed in the sections that follow. Wherever innovation is mentioned in this chapter, the specific focus is on sustainability innovation.

16.3 QUALITY MANAGEMENT IN EMERGENCY RESPONSE

Sustainable "sustainability" requires innovation, which can come in various modes and flavors, technical or non-technical, each requiring a measure of quality management. Quality is a measure of customer satisfaction and a product's "fit-for-use" status. To perform its intended functions, a product must provide a balanced level of satisfaction to both the producer and the customer. For the purposes of sustainability pursuits, we present the following comprehensive definition of sustainability quality:

> Quality refers to an equilibrium level of functionality possessed by a product or service based on the producer's capability and the customer's needs.

Based on the above definition, quality refers to the combination of characteristics of a product, process, or service that determines the product's ability to satisfy specific needs. Quality is a product's ability to conform to specifications, where specifications represent the customer's needs or government regulations. The attainment of quality in a product is the responsibility of every employee in an organization, and the production and preservation of quality should be a commitment that extends all the way from the producer to the customer. Products that are designed to have high quality cannot maintain the inherent quality at the user's end of the spectrum if they are not used properly.

The functional use of a product should match the functional specifications for the product within the prevailing usage environment. The ultimate judge of the quality of a product, however, is the perception of the user, and differing circumstances may alter that perception. A product that is perceived as being of high quality for one purpose at a given time may not be seen as having acceptable quality for another purpose at another time. Industrial quality standards provide a common basis for global commerce. Customer satisfaction or production efficiency cannot be achieved without product standards. Regulatory, consensus, and contractual requirements should be taken into account when developing product standards driven by innovation. These are described below:

16.3.1 Regulatory Standards

Regulatory standards are imposed by a governing body, such as a government agency. All firms within the jurisdiction of the agency are required to comply with the prevailing regulatory standards.

16.3.2 Consensus Standards

Consensus standards refer to a general and mutual agreement between companies to abide by a set of self-imposed standards.

16.3.3 Contractual Standards

Contractual standards are imposed by the customer based on case-by-case or order-by-order needs. Most international standards fall into the category of consensus standards, simply because a lack of an international agreement often leads to trade barriers.

16.3.4 Industry and Legal Standards

Along with the aforementioned standards, there are also self-coordinated standards, such as industry standards and legal standards.

16.4 ROLE OF PRODUCT DESIGN AND MANUFACTURING

The initial step in any effort is the development of a manufacturable and marketable product suitable for emergency response applications. An analysis of what is required for a design and what is available should be conducted in the planning phase of a design project. The development process must cover analyses of the product configuration, the raw materials required, production costs, and potential profits. Design engineers must select appropriate materials; the product must be expected to operate efficiently for a reasonable length of time (reliability and durability), and it must be possible to manufacture the product at a competitive cost. The design process will be influenced by the required labor skills, production technology, and raw materials. Product planning is substantially influenced by the level of customer sophistication, enhanced technology, and competition pressures. These are all project-related issues that can be addressed by project management. The designer must recognize changes in all these factors and incorporate them into the design process. Design project management provides guidelines for the initiation, implementation, and termination of a design effort. It sets guidelines for specific design objectives, structure, tasks, milestones, personnel, cost, equipment, performance, and problem resolution. The steps involved include planning, organizing, scheduling, and control. The availability of technical expertise within an organization and outside of it should be reviewed. The primary question of whether or not a design is needed at all should be addressed. The "make" or "buy," "lease" or "rent," and "do nothing" alternatives to a proposed design should be among the considerations.

In the initial stage of design planning, the internal and external factors that may influence the design should be determined and given relative weights according to priority. Examples of such influential factors include organizational goals, labor situations, market profile, expected return on design investment, technical manpower availability, time constraints, state of the technology, and design liabilities. The desired components of a design plan include a summary of the design plan, design objectives, design approach, implementation requirements, design schedule, required resources, available resources, design performance measures, and contingency plans.

16.4.1 Design Feasibility

The feasibility of a proposed design can be ascertained in terms of technical factors, economic factors, or both. A feasibility study is documented with a report showing all the ramifications of the design. A report of the design's feasibility should cover statements about the need, the design process, the cost feasibility, and the design effectiveness. The need for a design may originate from within the organization, from another organization, from the public, or from the customer. Pertinent questions for design feasibility review include: Is the need significant enough to warrant the proposed design? Will the need still exist by the time the design is finished? What are alternative means of satisfying the need? What technical interfaces are required for the design? What is the economic impact of the need? What is the return, financially, on the design change?

A design breakdown structure (DBS) is a flowchart of design tasks required to accomplish design objectives. Tasks that are contained in the DBS collectively describe the overall design. The tasks may involve hardware products, software products, services, and information. The DBS helps to describe the link between the end objective and its components. It shows design elements in the conceptual framework for the purposes of planning and control. The objective of developing a DBS is to study the elemental components of a design project in detail, thus permitting a "divide and conquer" approach. Overall design planning and control can be significantly improved by using DBS. A large design may be decomposed into smaller sub-designs, which may, in turn, be decomposed into task groups. Definable sub-goals of a design problem may be used to determine appropriate points at which to decompose the design.

Individual components in a DBS are referred to as "DBS elements," and the hierarchy of each is designated by a level identifier. Elements at the same level of subdivision are said to be of the same DBS level. Descending levels provide increasingly detailed definition of design tasks. The complexity of a design and the degree of control desired are used to determine the number of levels to have in a DBS. Level I of a DBS contains only the final design purpose. This item should be identifiable directly as an organizational goal. Level II contains the major subsections of the design. These subsections are usually identified by their contiguous location or by their related purpose. Level III contains definable components of the Level II subsections. Subsequent levels are constructed in more specific details depending on the level of control desired. If a complete DBS becomes too crowded, separate DBSs may be drawn for the Level II components, for example. A specification of design (SOD) should accompany the DBS. A statement of design is a narrative of the design to be generated. It should include the objectives of the design, its nature, the resource requirements, and a tentative schedule. Each DBS element is assigned a code (usually numeric) that is used for the element's identification throughout the design life cycle.

16.4.2 Design Stages

The guidelines for the various stages in the life cycle of a design can be summarized in the following way:

1. **Definition of design problem**: Define the problem and specify the importance of the problem, emphasize the need for a focused design problem, identify designers willing to contribute expertise to the design process, and disseminate the design plan.

2. **Personnel assignment**: The design group and the respective tasks should be announced, and a design manager should be appointed to oversee the design effort.
3. **Design initiation**: Arrange an organizational meeting, discuss the general approach to the design problem, announce the specific design plan, and arrange for the use of required hardware and tools.
4. **Design prototype**: Develop a prototype design, test an initial implementation, and learn more about the design problem from test results.
5. **Full design development**: Expand the prototype design and incorporate user requirements.
6. **Design verification**: Get designers and potential users involved, ensure that the design performs as designed, and modify the design as needed.
7. **Design validation**: Ensure that the design yields the expected outputs. Validation can address design performance level, deviation from expected outputs, and the effectiveness of the solution to the problem.
8. **Design integration**: Implement the full design, ensure the design is compatible with existing designs and manufacturing processes, and arrange for design transfer to other processes.
9. **Design feedback analysis**: What are the key lessons from the design effort? Were enough resources assigned? Was the design completed on time? Why or why not?
10. **Design maintenance**: Arrange for continuing technical support of the design and update the design as new information or technology becomes available.
11. **Design documentation**: Prepare full documentation of the design and document the administrative process used in generating the design.

16.4.3 Cultural and Social Compatibility Issues

Cultural infeasibility is one of the major impediments to outsourcing sustainability innovation in a wide-open market. The business climate can be very volatile. This volatility, coupled with cultural limitations, creates problematic operations, particularly in emerging technologies. The pervasiveness of online transactions overwhelms the strict cultural norms in many markets. The cultural feasibility of information-based outsourcing needs to be evaluated from the standpoint of where information originates, where it is intended to go, and who comes into contact with the information. For example, the revelation of personal information is frowned upon in many developing countries, where there may be an interest in outsourced innovation engagements. Consequently, this impedes the collection, storage, and distribution of workforce information that may be vital to the success of outsourcing. For outsourcing to be successfully implemented in such settings, assurances must be incorporated into the hardware and software implementations so as to conciliate the workforce. Accidental or deliberate mismanagement of information is a more worrisome aspect of IT than it is in the Western world, where enhanced techniques are available to correct information errors. What is socially acceptable in the outsourcing culture may not be acceptable in the receiving culture, and vice versa.

16.4.4 Administrative Compatibility

Administrative or managerial feasibility involves the ability to create and sustain an infrastructure to support an operational goal. Should such an infrastructure not be in existence or be unstable, then we have a case of administrative infeasibility. In developing countries, a lack of trained manpower precludes a stable infrastructure for some types of industrial outsourcing. Even where trained individuals are available, the lack of coordination makes it almost impossible to achieve a collective and dependable workforce. Systems that are designed abroad for implementation in a different setting frequently get bogged down when imported into a developing environment that is not conducive to such systems. Differences in the perception of ethics are also an issue of concern in an outsource location. A lack of administrative vision and limited managerial capabilities limit the ability of outsource managers in developing countries. Both the physical and conceptual limitations on technical staff lead to administrative infeasibility that must be reckoned with. Overzealous entrepreneurs are apt to jump on opportunities to outsource production without a proper assessment of the capabilities of the receiving organization. More often than not, outsourcing organizations don't fully understand the local limitations. Some organizations take the risk of learning as they go, without adequate prior preparation.

16.4.5 Technical Compatibility

Hardware maintenance and software upgrades are, perhaps, the two most noticeable aspects of the technical infeasibility for information technology in a developing country. The mistake is often made that once you install IT and all its initial components, you have the system for life. This is very far from the truth. The lack of proximity to the source of hardware and software enhancement makes this situation particularly distressing in a developing country. The technical capability of the personnel, as well as the technical status of the hardware, must be assessed in view of the local needs. Overdoing the infusion of IT just for the sake of keeping up is as detrimental as doing nothing at all.

16.4.6 Workforce Integration Strategies

Any outsourcing enterprise requires adapting from one form of culture to another. The implementation of a new technology to replace an existing (or nonexistent) technology can be approached through one of several cultural adaptation options. Below are some suggestions:

16.4.6.1 Parallel Interface

The host culture and the guest culture operate concurrently (side by side), with mutual respect on either side.

16.4.6.2 Adaptation Interface

This is the case where either the host culture or the guest culture makes a conscious effort to adapt to each other's ways. The adaptation often leads to new (but not necessarily enhanced) ways of thinking and acting.

16.4.6.3 Superimposition Interface

The host culture is replaced (annihilated or relegated) by the guest culture. This implies cultural imposition on local practices and customs. Cultural incompatibility, for the purpose of business goals, is one reason to adopt this type of interface.

16.4.6.4 Phased Interface

Modules of the guest culture are gradually introduced to the host culture over a period of time.

16.4.6.5 Segregated Interface

The host and guest cultures are separated both conceptually and geographically. This used to work well in colonial days, but it has become more difficult with modern flexibility of movement and communication facilities.

16.4.6.6 Pilot Interface

The guest culture is fully implemented on a pilot basis in a selected cultural setting in the host country. If the pilot implementation works with good results, it is then used to leverage further introduction to other localities.

16.4.7 Cultural Differences

The increased interface of cultures through industrial outsourcing is gradually leading to the emergence of hybrid cultures in many developing countries. A hybrid culture derives its influences from diverse factors, where there are differences in how the local population views education, professional loyalty, social alliances, leisure pursuits, and information management. A hybrid culture is, consequently, not fully embraced by either side of the cultural divide. This creates a big challenge for managing outsourcing projects.

Sustainability quality is at the intersection of efficiency, effectiveness, and productivity. Efficiency provides the framework for quality in terms of resources and inputs required to achieve the desired level of quality. Effectiveness comes into play with respect to the application of product quality to meet specific needs and requirements of an organization. Productivity is an essential factor in the pursuit of quality as it relates to the throughput of a production system. To achieve the desired levels of quality, efficiency, effectiveness, and productivity, a new research framework must be adopted for sustainability to take hold across national and cultural boundaries.

Several aspects of quality must undergo rigorous research along the realms of both quantitative and qualitative characteristics. Many times, quality is taken for granted, and the flaws only come out during the implementation stage, which may be too late to rectify. The growing trend in product recalls is a symptom of insufficient a priori analysis of the sources and implications of quality at the product conception stage. This chapter advocates the use of the DEJI model for enhancing quality design, quality evaluation, quality justification, and quality integration through hierarchical and stage-by-stage processes.

Better quality is achievable, and there is always room for improvement in the quality of products and services. But we must commit greater effort to research at the outset of the product development cycle. Even the human elements of the perception of quality can benefit from more directed research from a social and behavioral sciences point of view.

16.5 FUNCTIONAL ACCOUNTABILITY

Throughout history, engineering has answered the call of society to address specific challenges. With such answers comes a greater expectation of professional accountability. Consider the level of social responsibility that existed during the time of the Code of Hammurabi. Two of the laws are echoed below:

Hammurabi's Law 229:

> If a builder builds a house for someone, and does not construct it properly, and the house which he built falls in and kill its owner, then that builder shall be put to death.

Hammurabi's Law 230:

> If it kills the son of the owner, the son of that builder shall be put to death.

These are drastic measures designed to curb professional dereliction of duty and enforce social responsibility with particular focus on product quality. Research and education must play bigger and more direct roles in the design, practice, and management of quality. Modern aspects of social responsibility should be presented in the context of day-to-day personal and professional activities. The global responsibility of the greater society is essential with respect to world development challenges covering the global economy, human development, global governance, and social relationships. Quality is the common theme in the development challenges. Focusing on the emerging field of Big Data, we should advocate engineering education collaboration, which aligns well with data-intensive product development. With the above principles as possible tenets for better research, education, and practice of quality in engineering and technology, this chapter suggests the DEJI model as a potential methodology. The model encourages the practice of building sustainability into a product right from the beginning so that the product integration stage can be more successful.

The design of quality in product development should be structured to follow point-to-point transformations. A good technique to accomplish this is the use of state-space transformation, with which we can track the evolution of a product from the concept stage to the final product stage. For the purpose of product quality design, the following definitions are applicable:

Product state: A state is a set of conditions that describe the product at a specified point in time. The *state* of a product refers to a performance characteristic of the product, which relates input to output, such that knowledge of the input function over time and the state of the product at time $t = t_0$ determines the expected output for $t \geq t_0$. This is particularly important for assessing where the product stands in the context of new technological developments and the prevailing operating environment.

Product state-space: A product *state-space* is the set of all possible states of the product lifecycle. State-space representation can solve product design problems by moving from an initial state to another state, and eventually to the desired end-goal state. The movement from state to state is achieved by means of actions. A goal is a description of an intended state that has not yet been achieved. The process of solving a product problem involves finding a sequence of actions that represents a solution path from the initial state to the goal state. A state-space model consists of state variables that describe the prevailing condition of the product. The state variables are related to inputs by mathematical relationships. Examples of potential product state variables include schedule, output quality, cost, due date, resources, resource utilization, operational efficiency, productivity throughput, and technology alignment. For a product described by a system of components, the state-space representation can use state-by-state transfer of product characteristics. Each intermediate state may represent a significant milestone in the product. Thus, a descriptive state-space model facilitates the analysis of what actions to apply in order to achieve the next desired product state. A graphical representation can be developed for a product transformation from one state to another through the application of human or machine actions. This simple representation can be expanded to cover several components within the product information framework. Hierarchical linking of product elements provides an expanded transformation structure. The product state can be expanded in accordance with implicit requirements. These requirements might include grouping of design elements, linking precedence requirements (both technical and procedural), adapting to new technology developments, following required communication links, and accomplishing reporting requirements. The actions to be taken at each state depend on the prevailing product conditions. The nature of subsequent alternate states depends on what actions are implemented. Sometimes there are multiple paths that can lead to the desired end result. At other times, there exists only one unique path to the desired objective. In conventional practice, the characteristics of the future states can only be recognized after the fact, thus, making it impossible to develop adaptive plans. In the implementation of the DEJI model, adaptive plans can be achieved because the events occurring within and outside the product state boundaries can be taken into account.

If we describe a product by P state variables s_i, then the composite state of the product at any given time can be represented by a vector **S** containing P elements. The components of the state vector could represent either quantitative or qualitative variables (e.g., cost, energy, color, time). We can visualize every state vector as a point in the state-space of the product. The representation is unique since every state vector corresponds to one and only one point in the state-space. Suppose we have a set of actions (transformation agents) that we can apply to the product information so as to change it from one state to another within the project state-space. The transformation will change a state vector into another state vector. A transformation may be a change in raw material or a change in design approach. The number of transformations available for a product characteristic may be finite or unlimited. We can construct trajectories that describe the potential states of a product evolution as we apply successive transformations with respect to technology forecasts. Each transformation may be repeated as many times as needed. Given an initial state $\mathbf{S}_0$, the sequence of state vectors can be represented by successive state transitions.

16.6 EVALUATION OF QUALITY OF WORK

A product can be evaluated on the basis of cost, quality, schedule, and its ability to meet requirements. There are many quantitative metrics that can be used in evaluating a product at this stage. Learning curve productivity is one relevant technique that can be used, because it offers an evaluation basis for a product with respect to the concept of growth and decay. The half-life extension (Badiru, 2012) of the basic learning curve is directly applicable because the half-life of the technologies going into a product can be considered. In today's technology-based operations, retention of learning may be threatened by fast-paced shifts in operating requirements. Thus, it is of interest to evaluate the half-life properties of new technologies as they impact the overall product quality. Information about the half-life can tell us something about the sustainability of learning-induced technology performance. This is particularly useful for designing products whose life cycles stretch into the future in a high-tech environment.

16.7 JUSTIFICATION OF WORK PLAN

We need to justify an innovation program on the basis of quantitative value assessment. The systems value model (SVM) is a good quantitative technique that can be used for innovation justification on the basis of value. The model provides a heuristic decision aid for comparing project alternatives. It is presented here again for the present context. Value is represented as a deterministic vector function that indicates the value of tangible and intangible attributes that characterize the product. It can be represented as V – the assessed value based on the contributing attributes of the components making up the product. Examples of product attributes are quality, throughput, manufacturability, capability, modularity, reliability, interchangeability, efficiency, and cost performance. Attributes are considered to be a combined function of factors. Examples of product factors are market share, flexibility, user acceptance, capacity utilization, safety, and design functionality. Factors are themselves considered to be composed of indicators. Examples of indicators are debt ratio, acquisition volume, product responsiveness, substitutability, lead time, learning curve, and scrap volume. By combining the above definitions, a composite measure of the operational value of a product can be quantitatively assessed. In addition to the quantifiable factors, attributes, and indicators that impinge upon overall project value, human-based, subtle factors should also be included in assessing overall project value.

16.8 INTEGRATION OF WORK QUALITY

Without integration, a system will be in isolation, and it may be worthless. We must integrate all the elements of a system on the basis of alignment of functional goals. The overlap of systems for integration purposes can conceptually be viewed as projection integrals by considering areas bounded by the common elements of subsystems. Quantitative metrics can be applied at this stage for effective assessment of the product state. Trade-off analysis is essential in quality integration. Pertinent questions include the following:

- What level of trade-offs on the level of quality are tolerable?
- What is the incremental cost of higher quality?
- What is the marginal value of higher quality?
- What is the adverse impact of a decrease in quality?
- What is the integration of quality of time?

Presented below are guidelines and important questions relevant for quality integration.

- What are the unique characteristics of each component in the integrated system?
- How do the characteristics complement one another?
- What physical interfaces exist among the components?
- What data/information interfaces exist among the components?
- What ideological differences exist among the components?
- What are the data flow requirements for the components?
- What internal and external factors are expected to influence the integrated system?
- What are the relative priorities assigned to each component of the integrated system?
- What are the strengths and weaknesses of the integrated system?
- What resources are needed to keep the integrated system operating satisfactorily?
- Which organizational unit has primary responsibility for the integrated system?

The proposed approach of the DEJI model will facilitate a better alignment of product technology with future development and needs. The stages of the model require research for each new product with respect to design, evaluation, justification, and integration. Existing analytical tools and techniques can be used at each stage of the model.

An extensive review of the literature concludes that an overarching theory was lacking to guide the process of innovation. The key to a successful actualization of innovation centers on how people work and behave in team collaborations. Hence, the proposed methodology of "umbrella theory for innovation" takes into account the interplay between people, tools, and processes. The umbrella theory for innovation capitalizes on the trifecta of human factors, process design, and technology tool availability within the innovation environment. The theory harnesses the proven efficacies of existing tools and principles of systems engineering and management. Two specific techniques in this regard are the Triple C model and the DEJI systems model.

A semantic network, also called a frame network, is a knowledge base that represents semantic relationships between elements in an operational network or system. It is often used for knowledge representation purposes in software systems. In innovation, a semantic network can be used to represent the relationships among elements (people, technology, and process) in the innovation system. This representation can give a visual cue of the critical paths in the innovation network. The requirements for the success of an innovation effort include the following:

1) **Relative advantage**: This is the degree to which an innovation is perceived as better than the idea it supersedes by a particular group of users, measured in terms that matter to those users, like economic advantage, social prestige, convenience, or satisfaction. The greater the perceived relative advantage of an innovation, the more rapid its rate of adoption is likely to be. There are no absolute rules for what constitutes "relative advantage." It depends on the particular perceptions and needs of the user group.
2) **Compatibility with existing values and practices**: This is the degree to which an innovation is perceived as being consistent with the values, past experiences, and needs of potential adopters. An idea that is incompatible with their values, norms, or practices will not be adopted as rapidly as an innovation that is compatible.
3) **Simplicity and ease of use**: This is the degree to which an innovation is perceived as difficult to understand and use. New ideas that are simpler to understand are adopted more rapidly than innovations that require the adopter to develop new skills and understandings.
4) **Trialability**: This is the degree to which an innovation can be experimented with on a limited basis. An innovation that is triable represents less uncertainty to the individual who is considering it.
5) **Observable results**: The easier it is for individuals to see the results of an innovation, the more likely they are to adopt it. Visible results lower uncertainty and also stimulate peer discussion of a new idea, as friends and neighbors of an adopter often request information about it.

16.8.1 Response Risk Management

Risk is an essential element in any pursuit. No risk means no accomplishment. The important thing is to manage risk constructively. Risk management is an integral part of innovation. For innovation, particularly for those dealing with new ventures, risk management can be carried out effectively by investigating and identifying the sources of risks associated with each activity. These risks can be assessed or measured in terms of likelihood and impact. Because of the exploratory basis of new technology, a different and diverse set of risk concerns will be involved. So, as risks are assessed for managerial processes, technical and managerial risks must also be assessed. The major activities in innovation analysis consist of feasibility studies, design, transportation, utility, survey work, construction, permanent structure work, mechanical and electrical installations, maintenance, and so on.

Risk is often ambiguously defined as a measure of the probability, level of severity, and exposure to all hazards for a project activity. Practitioners and researchers often debate the exact definition, meaning, and implications of risk. Two alternate definitions of risk are presented below:

1) Risk is an uncertain event or condition that, if it occurs, has a positive or negative effect on a project objective.
2) Risk is an uncertain event or set of circumstances that, should it occur, will have an effect on the achievement of the project's objectives.

In this book, we present the following definition of risk management:

> Risk management is the state of having a contingency ready to respond to the impact (good or bad) of occurrence of risk, such that risk mitigation or risk exploitation becomes an intrinsic part of the project plan.

For any innovation undertaking, there is always a chance that things will not turn out exactly as planned. Thus, project risk pertains to the probability of uncertainties in the technical, schedule, and cost outcomes of the project. All technology-based projects are complex and involve risks in all the phases of the project, starting from the feasibility phase to the operational phase. These risks have a direct impact on the project schedule, cost, and performance. These projects are inherently complex and volatile, with many variables. A proper risk-mitigation plan, if developed for identified risks, will ensure better and smoother achievement of project goals within the specified time, cost, and technical requirements. Conventional project management techniques, without a risk management component, are not sufficient to ensure time, cost, and quality achievement of a large-scale project, which may be mainly due to changes in scope and design, changes in government policies and regulations, changes in industry agreement, unforeseen inflation, underestimation, and improper estimation. Projects that are exposed to such risks and uncertainty can be effectively managed with the incorporation of risk management throughout their life cycle.

16.8.2 Impacts of Regulations

Risks can be mitigated, not eliminated. In fact, risk is the essence of any enterprise. In spite of government regulations designed to reduce accident risks, accidents will occasionally happen. Government regulators can work with organizations to monitor data and operations. This will only preempt a fraction of potential risks of incidents. For this reason, government agencies must work with organizations to ensure that adequate precautions are taken in all operating scenarios. Government and industry must work together in a risk-mitigation partnership, rather than in an adversarial and dictatorial relationship. There is no risk-free activity in business and industry today. For example, many of the safety and security incidents observed over the years involved human elements – errors, incompetence, negligence, and so on. How do you prevent negligence? You can encourage non-negligent operation or incentivize a perfect record, but humans will still be human when bad things happen. Effective risk management requires a reliable risk analysis technique. Below is how to deal with risk management:

- Avoid
- Assign
- Assume
- Mitigate
- Manage

Below is a four-step process for managing risk:

STEP ONE: Identify the Risks.
STEP TWO: Assess the Risks.
STEP THREE: Plan Risk Mitigation.
STEP FOUR: Communicate the Risk.

We must venture out on the risk limb in order to benefit from what the innovation offers. Many leaders profess the call of "taking risk," but guidance is often lacking on to what extent risks can be taken. A quote that typifies the benefit of taking risk is echoed below:

Consider the quote below:

Behold the lowly Turtle – he only makes progress when he sticks his neck out.

James Conan Bryan, 1954

Let us take another look at the basic definition of risk:

Risk – "Potential Realization of an Unwanted Negative Consequence."

Reward – "Potential Realization of a Desired Positive Consequence."

A master list of risk management involves the following:

- New technology
- Functional complexity
- New vs. replacement
- Leverage on company
- Intensity of business need
- Interface with existing applications
- Staff availability
- Commitment of team
- Team morale

- Applications knowledge
- Client information system (IS) knowledge
- Technical skills availability
- Staff conflicts
- Quality of information available
- Dependability on other projects
- Conversion difficulty
- End-date dictate
- Conflict resolution mechanism
- Continued budget availability
- Project standards used
- Large/small project
- Size of team
- Geographic dispersion
- Reliability of personnel
- Availability of support organization
- Availability of champion
- Vulnerability to change
- Stability of business area
- Organizational impact
- Tight time frame
- Turnover of key people
- Change budget accepted
- Change process accepted
- Level of client commitment
- Client attitude toward IS
- Readiness for takeover
- Client design participation
- Client participation in acceptance test
- Client proximity to IS
- Acceptance process

Possible risk response planning can follow the following options:

- Accept – Do nothing because the cost to fix is more expensive than the expected loss.
- Avoid – Elect not to do part of the project associated with the risk.
- Contingency planning – Frame plans to deal with risk consequences and monitor risk regularly (identify trigger points).
- Mitigate – Reduce either the probability of occurrence, the loss, or both.
- Transfer – Outsource.

The perspectives and guidance offered by the umbrella model for innovation management can create an avenue for managing, controlling, or mitigating risk in innovation pursuits.

16.9 CONCLUSIONS

It is expected that the methodology of the umbrella theory of innovation will inspire new research inquiries into the human factors of driving innovation in organizations. The theory has the benefit of providing coverage for all the typical nuances (qualitative and quantitative) that may be encountered in the innovation environment. Of particular importance is the consideration of the people factors of innovation. The common flawed view of innovation is that it is predicated on the acquisition of technological items. While technology may be the underpinning of a specific innovation project, more often than not, the human factors will determine the success or failure of innovation. The umbrella theory explicitly calls out the people aspects of the pursuit of innovation. The quantitative measure of innovation readiness can be adapted and expanded to fit specific research, development, and implementation themes related to the pursuit of innovation. Quality is an integrative process that must be evaluated on a stage-by-stage approach. This requires research, education, and implementation strategies that consider several pertinent factors. This chapter suggests the DEJI systems model, which has been used successfully for product development applications, as a viable methodology for quality design, quality evaluation, quality justification, and quality integration. This chapter is intended as a source to spark the interest of researchers to apply this tool in new product development efforts. Further details and examples of the diverse applications of the DEJI systems model can be found in Badiru (2012, 2014, 2015, 2016, 2019, 2023), Badiru and Maloney (2016), and Badiru et al. (2015).

REFERENCES

Badiru, A. B. (2012), "Application of the DEJI Model for Aerospace Product Integration," *Journal of Aviation and Aerospace Perspectives (JAAP)*, Vol. 2, No. 2, pp. 20–34.

Badiru, A. B. (2014), "Quality Insights: The DEJI Model for Quality Design, Evaluation, Justification, and Integration," *International Journal of Quality Engineering and Technology*, Vol. 4, No. 4, pp. 369–378.

Badiru, A. B. (2015), "A Systems Model for Global Engineering Education: The 15 Grand Challenges," *Engineering Education Letters*, Vol. 1, No. 1, pp. 1–14. http://dx.doi.org/10.5339/eel.2015.3.

Badiru, A. B. (2019), *Systems Engineering Models: Theory, Methods, and Applications*, Taylor & Francis/CRC Press, Boca Raton, FL.

Badiru, A. B. (2023), *Systems Engineering Using DEJI Systems Model: Design, Evaluation, Justification, and Integration with Case Studies and Applications*, Taylor & Francis CRC Press, Boca Raton, FL.

Badiru, A. B., Elshaw, J., and Badiru, I. A. (2015), "Quality Insights: Systems-based Product Quality Assessment for Customer Preferences," *International Journal of Quality Engineering and Technology* (IJQET), Vol. 5, No. 3/4, 2015, pp. 266–280.

Badiru, A. B., and Maloney, A. E. (2016), "A Conceptual Framework for the Application of Systems Approach to Intelligence Operations: Using HUMINT to Augment SIGINT," *American Intelligence Journal*, Vol. 33, No. 2, pp. 41–46.

17 Cooperation and Compliance in Emergency Response

Adedeji B. Badiru

17.1 INTRODUCTION

The human environment, whether at home, at work, or on the road, faces unimaginable vulnerabilities with respect to emergency occurrences. In each case, a cataclysmic, apocalyptic, or catastrophic event triggers an emergency response. While great and satisfactory responses have been recorded in each emergency case in the past, the premise of this chapter is to strengthen emergency response preparation before any disaster occurs. This is particularly essential in the case of forecasted natural disasters, such as hurricanes and tornadoes. The greatest risk to emergency preparation is human compliance or failure thereof. The expanded Triple C model (Badiru, 2008) highlighted in this chapter is useful for preemptive compliance actions on the part of residents in forecasted disaster zones. Cases of reluctance and refusal to evacuate disaster areas have been recorded in several incidents of flash floods, hurricanes, volcanoes, and brush fires, in spite of early-warning systems. Ignorance, obstinate attitude, stubbornness, property fixation, adamant stance, lackadaisical disposition, ego, and social resistance are all human flaws that can impede emergency preparedness and response to disasters. This is why compliance is advocated in this chapter as a recommended component of the usual communication, cooperation, and coordination principles.

This chapter explicitly emphasizes the critical issue of compliance in emergency response scenarios. A typical concern in emergency events is communication, but there are subtle factors that are rarely considered or recognized. An example of a subtle factor is compliance, which is a human factors issue. Communication may be present, cooperation may be in effect, but voluntary compliance may not happen. Consequently, emergency response efforts may be impeded or even compromised. The chapter presents integrated guidelines for communication, cooperation, compliance, and coordination for emergency response. The conventional Triple C principle of communication, cooperation, and coordination can be expanded to highlight compliance, which is an inherent characteristic of humans, based on individual hierarchies of needs. Noncompliance cases can happen in hurricanes, train derailments, flash floods, bridge collapses, and other disasters.

DOI: 10.1201/9781003648178-19

17.2 POTENTIAL SOURCES OF CALAMITY

In environmental disasters, vulnerability can quickly materialize into actual emergency developments. Sources can be in any or a combination of the following categories:

- Natural events
- Man-made events
- Operational mismanagement
- Negligence
- Mischief
- Terrorism
- Deliberate act
- Prank
- Human error
- Accident

Some possible sources include the following (not quite an exhaustive list):

1. Bridge collapse
2. Brush fires
3. Building collapse
4. Dam collapse
5. Earthquake
6. Electrical fires
7. Erosion
8. Explosion
9. Fires
10. Floods
11. Geysers
12. Glacier
13. Hailstorms
14. Hurricanes
15. Icebergs
16. Landslide
17. Lightning
18. Mountain collapse
19. Ocean creep
20. Plane crash
21. Quicksand
22. Rainstorms
23. Sabotage
24. Sandstorms
25. Sea wall
26. Ship collision

27. Sinkhole
28. Snowstorms
29. Thunderstorms
30. Tornadoes
31. Tree falls
32. Volcano
33. War invasion
34. Windstorms

This is quite an extensive list, illuminating the vulnerability that we are all subject to in our present society. To be forewarned is to be forearmed. Thus, the theme of this chapter is of great importance in changing or advancing typical human reactions to disaster warnings.

17.3 THE TRIPLE C MODEL

The Triple C model of project management with respect to communication, cooperation, and coordination was first introduced by Badiru (1987) and formally documented by Badiru (2008). It has been applied rewardingly in many practical project management communication challenges and corporate strategies. While cooperation is usually the cog in the wheel of project execution, emergency response situations necessitate highlighting compliance as a critical element. That critical element can be the platform for involvement and adherence to alerts and warnings. The following Chinese proverb is applicable:

> Tell me, and I forget;
> Show me, and I remember;
> Involve me, and I understand.
>
> **–Confucius**

To be involved is to understand and remember what needs to be done in an emergency. Another Chinese proverb says:

> The person who says it cannot be done should not interrupt the person doing it.

This implies a requirement for not only cooperation but also compliance and support.

As edified by the Chinese proverb above, the involvement of every team member is critical for the overall success of a project. The Triple C model facilitates better understanding and involvement based on foundational communication. The Triple C approach elucidates the integrated involvement of communication, cooperation, and coordination. Communication is the foundation for cooperation, which in turn is the foundation for coordination. Communication leads to cooperation, which leads to coordination, which leads to project harmony, which leads to project success. Emergency response works in this order as well. In fact, any human act can be defined as a project, thereby making it amenable to the application of project management tools and techniques. Thus, in effect, emergency response, as presented in this chapter, is akin to a project that must be executed under extreme stress, nervousness, and confusion.

The primary lesson of the Triple C model is not to take cooperation for granted. It must be pursued, solicited, and secured explicitly. The process of securing cooperation requires structured communication upfront. It is only after cooperation is in effect that all project efforts can be coordinated.

The Triple C model has been used effectively in practice to enhance project performance because most project problems can be traced to initial communication problems. The Triple C approach works because it is very simple – simple to understand and simple to implement. The simplicity comes from the fact that most of the required elements of the approach are already being done within every organization, albeit in a nonstructured manner. The Triple C model puts the existing processes into a structured approach to communication, cooperation, and coordination. Embedding a requirement for compliance into the process increases the potential for the success of emergency response activities.

The idea for the Triple C model originated from a complex facility redesign project (Badiru et al., 1993) conducted for Tinker Air Force Base (TAFB) in Oklahoma City by the School of Industrial Engineering, University of Oklahoma from 1985 to 1989. The project was part of a reconstruction project following a disastrous fire that occurred in the base's repair/production facility in November 1984. The urgency, complexity, scope ambiguity, confusion, and disjointed directions that existed in the early days of the reconstruction effort led to the need to develop a structured approach to communication, cooperation, and coordination of the various work elements. Despite the high-pressure timing of the project, the author called a Time-Out-Of-time (TOOT) so that a process could be developed for project communication, leading to personnel cooperation and eventually facilitating task coordination. The investment of TOOT time resulted in a remarkable resurgence of cooperation where none existed at the beginning of the project. Encouraged by the intrinsic occurrence of cooperation, the process was further enhanced and formalized as the Triple C approach to the project's success. The approach was credited with the overall success of the project. The qualitative approach of Triple C complemented the technical approaches used in the project to facilitate harmonious execution of tasks. Many projects fail when the stakeholders get too wrapped up in the technical requirements at the expense of qualitative requirements. The importance of Triple C can be summarized by the sequential relationship below:

Triple C ➔ Communication ➔ Cooperation ➔ Coordination ➔ Success

Embedding compliance leads to the expanded relationship below:

Triple C ➔ Communication ➔ Cooperation ➔ Compliance ➔ Coordination ➔ Safety

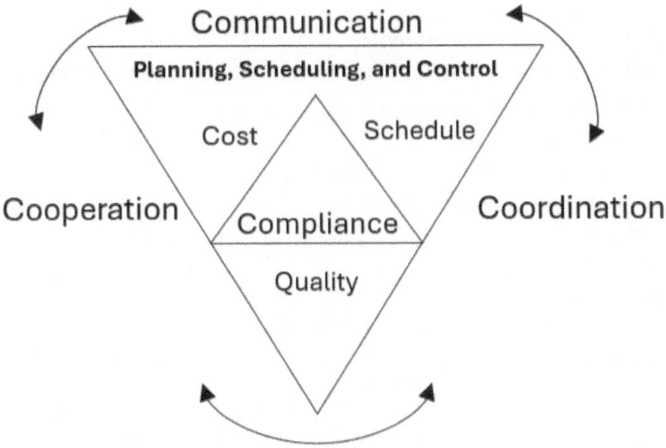

FIGURE 17.1 Triple C model in emergency response

Other elements of "C," such as collaboration, commitment, and correlation, are implicitly embedded in the Triple C structure. Of course, the constraints of time, cost, and performance must be overcome all along the way.

Organizations thrive by investing in three primary resources: the people who do the work, the tools that the people use to do the work, and the process that governs the work that the people do. Of the three, investing in people is the easiest thing an organization can do, and we should do it whenever we have an opportunity. The Triple C approach incorporates the qualitative (human) aspects of a project into the overall project requirements. Again, human compliance takes center stage for emergency response. Figure 17.1 illustrates the execution of the Triple C model for emergency response.

The expanded Triple C model answers the questions of what, who, why, how, where, and when in emergency response. It highlights what must be done and when. It can also help to identify the resources (personnel, equipment, facilities, etc.) required for each effort. It points out important questions such as the following:

- Does each project participant know what the objective is?
- Does each participant know his or her role in achieving the objective?
- What obstacles may prevent a participant from playing his or her role effectively?

Triple C can mitigate the disparity between idea and practice because it explicitly solicits information about the critical aspects of an emergency response.

Types of communication:

- Verbal
- Written

- Body language
- Visual tools (e.g., graphical tools)
- Sensual (Use of all five senses: sight, smell, touch, taste, hearing: olfactory, tactile, auditory)
- Simplex (unidirectional)
- Half-duplex (bi-directional with time lag)
- Full-duplex (real-time dialogue)
- One-on-one
- One-to-many
- Many-to-one

Types of cooperation:

- Proximity
- Functional
- Professional
- Social
- Romantic
- Power influence
- Authority influence
- Hierarchical
- Lateral
- Cooperation by intimidation
- Cooperation by enticement

Types of coordination:

- Teaming
- Delegation
- Supervision
- Partnership
- Token-passing
- Baton hand-off

Questioning is the best approach to getting information for effective project management. Everything should be questioned. By upfront questions, we can preempt and avert project problems later on. Typical questions to ask under the Triple C approach are:

- What is the purpose of the project?
- Who is in charge of the project?
- Why is the project needed?
- Where is the project located?
- When will the project be carried out?

- How will the project contribute to increased opportunities for the organization?
- What is the project designed to achieve?
- How will the project affect different groups of people within the organization?
- What will the project approach or methodology be?
- What other groups or organizations will be involved (if any)?
- What will happen at the end of the project?
- How will the project be tracked, monitored, evaluated, and reported?
- What resources are required?
- What are the associated costs of the required resources?
- How do the project objectives fit within the goals of the organization?
- What respective contribution is expected from each participant?
- What level of cooperation is expected from each group?
- Where is the coordinating point for the project?

The key to getting everyone on board with a project is to ensure that task objectives are clear and comply with the principle of SMART, as outlined below:

Specific: The task objective must be specific.
Measurable: The task objective must be measurable.
Aligned: The task objective must be achievable and aligned with the overall project goal.
Realistic: The task objective must be realistic and relevant to the organization.
Timed: The task objective must have a time basis.

If a task has the above intrinsic characteristics, then communicating the task will more likely lead to personnel cooperation.

Communication makes working together possible. The communication function of project management involves making all those concerned aware of project requirements and progress. Those who will be affected by the project directly or indirectly, as direct participants or as beneficiaries, should be informed as appropriate regarding the following:

- Scope of the project.
- Personnel contribution required.
- Expected cost and merits of the project.
- Project organization and implementation plan.
- Potential adverse effects if the project should fail.
- Alternatives, if any, for achieving the project goal.
- Potential direct and indirect benefits of the project.

The communication channel must be kept open throughout the project life cycle. In addition to internal communication, appropriate external sources should also be consulted. The project manager must

- Exude commitment to the project.
- Utilize the communication responsibility matrix.
- Facilitate multi-channel communication interfaces.
- Identify internal and external communication needs.
- Resolve organizational and communication hierarchies.
- Encourage both formal and informal communication links.

When clear communication is maintained between management and employees and among peers, many project problems can be averted. Project communication may be carried out in one or more of the following formats:

- One-to-many
- One-to-one
- Many-to-one
- Written and formal
- Written and informal
- Oral and formal
- Oral and informal
- Nonverbal gestures

Good communication is achieved when what is implied is perceived as intended. Effective communication is vital to the success of any project. Despite the awareness that proper communication forms the blueprint for project success, many organizations still fail in their communication functions. The study of communication is complex. Factors that influence the effectiveness of communication within a project organizational structure include the following.

1. **Personal perception and past experiences**. Each person perceives events on the basis of personal psychological, social, cultural, and experiential background. As a result, no two people can interpret a given event the same way. The nature of events is not always the critical aspect of a problem situation. Rather, the problem is often the different perceptions of the people involved.
2. **Psychological profile**. The psychological makeup of each person determines personal reactions to events or words. Thus, individual needs and levels of thinking will dictate how a message is interpreted.
3. **Social environment**. Communication problems sometimes arise because people have been conditioned by their prevailing social environment to interpret certain things in unique ways. Vocabulary, idioms, organizational status, social stereotypes, and economic situation are among the social factors that can thwart effective communication.
4. **Cultural background**. Cultural differences are among the most pervasive barriers to project communication, especially in today's multinational organizations. Language and cultural idiosyncrasies often determine how communication is approached and interpreted.

5. **Semantic and syntactic factors**. Semantic and syntactic barriers to communications usually occur in written documents. Semantic factors are those that relate to the intrinsic knowledge of the subject of the communication. Syntactic factors are those that relate to the form in which the communication is presented. The problems created by these factors become acute in situations where response, feedback, or reaction to the communication cannot be observed.
6. **Organizational structure**. Frequently, the organizational structure in which a project is conducted has a direct influence on the flow of information and, consequently, on the effectiveness of communication. Organization hierarchy may determine how different personnel levels perceive a given communication.
7. **Communication media**. The method of transmitting a message may also affect the value ascribed to the message and consequently, how it is interpreted or used. Common barriers to project communications are

1. Inattentiveness
2. Lack of organization
3. Outstanding grudges
4. Preconceived notions
5. Ambiguous presentation
6. Emotions and sentiments
7. Lack of communication feedback
8. Sloppy and unprofessional presentation
9. Lack of confidence in the communicator
10. Lack of confidence by the communicator
11. Low credibility of communicator
12. Unnecessary technical jargon
13. Too many people involved
14. Untimely communication
15. Arrogance or imposition
16. Lack of focus.

Some suggestions on improving the effectiveness of communication are presented next. The recommendations may be implemented as appropriate for any of the forms of communication listed earlier. The recommendations are for both the communicator and the audience.

1. Never assume that the integrity of the information sent will be preserved as the information passes through several communication channels. Information is generally filtered, condensed, or expanded by the receivers before relaying it to the next destination. When preparing a communication that needs to pass through several organizational structures, one safeguard is to compose the original information in a concise form to minimize the need for re-composition of the project structure.

2. Give the audience a central role in the discussion. A leading role can help make a person feel a part of the project effort and responsible for the project's success. He or she can then have a more constructive view of project communication.
3. Do homework and think through the intended outcome of the communication. This helps eliminate trivial and inconsequential communication efforts.
4. Carefully plan the organization of the ideas embodied in the communication. Use indexing or points of reference whenever possible. Grouping ideas into related chunks of information can be particularly effective. Present the short messages first. Short messages help create focus, maintain interest, and prepare the mind for the longer messages to follow.
5. Highlight why the communication is of interest and how it is intended to be used. Full attention should be given to the content of the message with regard to the prevailing project situation.
6. Elicit the support of those around you by integrating their ideas into the communication. The more people feel they have contributed to the issue, the more expeditious they are in soliciting the cooperation of others. The effect of the multiplicative rule can quickly garner support for the communication purpose.
7. Be responsive to the feelings of others. It takes two to communicate. Anticipate and appreciate the reactions of members of the audience. Recognize their operational circumstances and present your message in a form they can relate to.
8. Accept constructive criticism. Nobody is infallible. Use criticism as a springboard to higher communication performance.
9. Exhibit interest in the issue in order to arouse the interest of your audience. Avoid delivering your messages as a matter of a routine organizational requirement.
10. Obtain and furnish feedback promptly. Clarify vague points with examples.
11. Communicate at the appropriate time, at the right place, to the right people.
12. Reinforce words with positive action. Never promise what cannot be delivered. Value your credibility.
13. Maintain eye contact in oral communication and read the facial expressions of your audience to obtain real-time feedback.
14. Concentrate on listening as much as speaking. Evaluate both the implicit and explicit meanings of statements.
15. Document communication transactions for future reference.
16. Avoid asking questions that can be answered yes or no. Use relevant questions to focus the attention of the audience. Use questions that make people reflect upon their words, such as, "How do you think this will work?" rather than "Do you this will work?"
17. Avoid patronizing the audience. Respect their judgment and knowledge.
18. Speak and write in a controlled tempo. Avoid emotionally charged voice inflections.

19. Create an atmosphere for formal and informal exchange of ideas.
20. Summarize the objectives of the communication and how they will be achieved.

17.4 USING A COMMUNICATION MATRIX

Figure 17.2 shows an example of a communication responsibility matrix. A communication responsibility matrix shows the linking of sources of communication and targets of communication. Cells within the matrix indicate the subject of the desired communication. There should be at least one filled cell in each row and each column of the matrix. This assures that each individual of a department has at least one communication source or target associated with him or her. With a communication responsibility matrix, a clear understanding of what needs to be communicated to whom can be developed. Communication in a project environment can take any of several forms. The specific needs of a project may dictate the most appropriate mode. Three popular computer communication modes are discussed next in the context of communicating data and information for project management.

Simplex communication is a unidirectional communication arrangement in which one project entity initiates communication to another entity or individual within the project environment. The entity addressed in the communication does not have a mechanism or capability for responding to the communication. An extreme example of this is a one-way, top-down communication from top management to project personnel. In this case, the personnel have no communication access or input to top management. A budget-related example is when top management allocates the

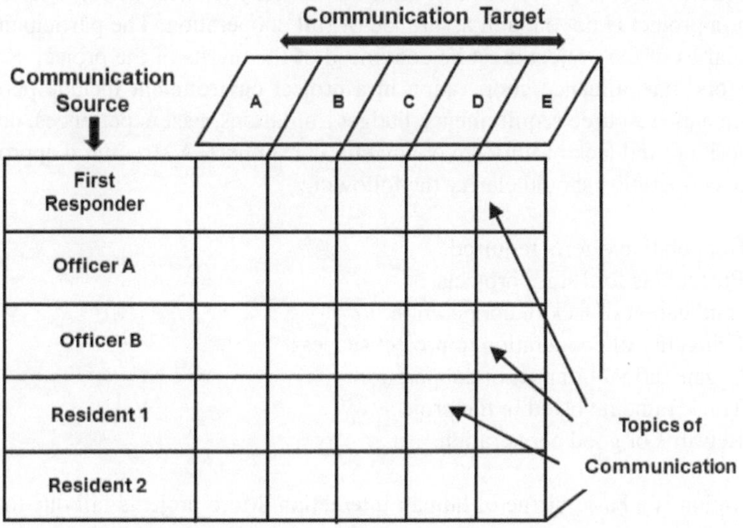

FIGURE 17.2 Triple C communication matrix for emergency response

budget to a project without requesting and reviewing the actual needs of the project. Simplex communication is common in authoritarian organizations.

Half-duplex communication is a bi-directional communication arrangement whereby one project entity can communicate with another entity and receive a response within a certain time lag. Both entities can communicate with each other but not at the same time. An example of half-duplex communication is a project organization that permits communication with top management without a direct meeting. Each communicator must wait for a response from the target of the communication. Request and allocation without a budget meeting is another example of half-duplex data communication in project management.

Full-duplex communication is a communication arrangement that permits a dialogue between the communicating entities. Both individuals and entities can communicate with each other at the same time or face-to-face. As long as there is no clash of words, this appears to be the most receptive communication mode. It allows participative project planning in which each project member has an opportunity to contribute to the planning process.

Each member of a project team needs to recognize the nature of the prevailing communication mode in the project. Management must evaluate the prevailing communication structure and attempt to modify it if necessary to enhance project functions. An evaluation of who is to communicate with whom about what may help improve the project data/information communication process. A communication matrix may include notations about the desired modes of communication between individuals and groups in the project environment.

17.5 COOPERATION

The cooperation of project personnel must be explicitly elicited. Merely voicing consent for a project is not enough assurance of full cooperation. The participants and beneficiaries of the project must be convinced of the merits of the project. Some of the factors that influence cooperation in a project environment include personnel requirements, resource requirements, budget limitations, past experiences, conflicting priorities, and lack of uniform organizational support. A structured approach to seeking cooperation should clarify the following:

- Cooperative efforts required.
- Precedents for future projects.
- Implication of lack of cooperation.
- Criticality of cooperation to project success.
- Organizational impact of cooperation.
- Time frame involved in the project.
- Rewards of good cooperation.

Cooperation is a basic virtue of human interaction. More projects fail due to a lack of cooperation and commitment than any other factor. To secure and retain the cooperation of project participants, you must elicit a positive first reaction to the project.

The most positive aspects of a project should be the first items of project communication. For project management, there are different types of cooperation that should be understood.

Functional cooperation. This is cooperation induced by the nature of the functional relationship between two groups. The two groups may be required to perform related functions that can only be accomplished through mutual cooperation.

Social cooperation. This is the type of cooperation created by the social relationship between two groups. The prevailing social relationship motivates cooperation that may be useful in getting project work done.

Legal cooperation. Legal cooperation is imposed by some authoritative requirement. In this case, the participants may have no choice but to cooperate.

Administrative cooperation. This is cooperation brought on by administrative requirements that make it imperative that two groups work together on a common goal.

Associative cooperation. This type of cooperation may also be referred to as collegiality. The level of cooperation is determined by the association that exists between two groups.

Proximity cooperation. Cooperation due to the fact that two groups are geographically close is referred to as proximity cooperation. Being close makes it imperative that the two groups work together.

Dependency cooperation. This is cooperation caused by the fact that one group depends on another group for some important aspect. Such dependency is usually of a mutual two-way nature. One group depends on the other for one thing while the latter group depends on the former for some other thing.

Imposed cooperation. In this type of cooperation, external agents must be employed to induce cooperation between two groups. This is applicable in cases in which the two groups have no natural reason to cooperate. This is where the approaches presented earlier for seeking cooperation can become very useful.

Lateral cooperation. Lateral cooperation involves cooperation with peers and immediate associates. Lateral cooperation is often easy to achieve because existing lateral relationships create an environment that is conducive to project cooperation.

Vertical cooperation. Vertical or hierarchical cooperation refers to cooperation that is implied by the hierarchical structure of the project. For example, subordinates are expected to cooperate with their vertical superiors.

Whichever type of cooperation is available in a project environment, the cooperative forces should be channeled toward achieving project goals. Documentation of the prevailing level of cooperation is useful for winning further support for a project. Clarification of project priorities will facilitate personnel cooperation. Relative priorities of multiple projects should be specified so that a priority is clear to all groups within the organization. Some guidelines for securing cooperation for most projects are:

- Establish achievable goals for the project.
- Clearly outline the individual commitments required.
- Integrate project priorities with existing priorities.
- Eliminate the fear of job loss due to industrialization.
- Anticipate and eliminate potential sources of conflict.
- Use an open-door policy to address project grievances.
- Remove skepticism by documenting the merits of the project.

17.6 COMPLIANCE

Compliance must be supported with commitment. To cooperate is to support the ideas of a project. To commit is to willingly and actively participate in project efforts again and again through the thick and thin of the project. Provision of resources is one way that management can express commitment to a project. Compliance can be enforced through several means, including the following:

- Legislative
- Punitive
- Threat of harm
- Peer pressure
- Enticement
- Encouragement
- Reasoning and logic
- Compensation

17.7 COORDINATION

After the communication and cooperation functions have been successfully initiated, the efforts of the project personnel must be coordinated. Coordination facilitates harmonious organization of project efforts. The construction of a responsibility chart (See Figure 17.3) can be very helpful at this stage. A responsibility chart is a matrix consisting of columns of individual or functional departments and rows of required actions. Cells within the matrix are filled with relationship codes that indicate who is responsible for what.

- Who is to do what?
- How long will it take?
- Who is to inform whom of what?
- Whose approval is needed for what?
- Who is responsible for which results?
- What personnel interfaces are required?
- What support is needed from whom and when?

Tasks	Person Responsible				Status of Task			
	Staff A	Staff B	Staff C	Staff D	Date 1	Date 2	Date 3	Date 4
Task 1	R	R	R	R	D			
Task 2				R		O		
Task 3	I	R	R			O		
Task 4	R	R				D		
Task 5		C	R	I	O	O	D	
....		C	R					D
Task N			R			L	L	

R = Responsible; D = Done; I = Inform; O = On Track; S = Support; L = Late; C = Consult

FIGURE 17.3 Responsibility matrix for emergency response

Conflicts can and do develop in any work environment. Conflicts, whether intended or inadvertent, prevent an organization from getting the most out of the workforce. When implemented as an integrated process, the Triple C model can help avoid conflicts in a project. When conflicts do develop, it can help in resolving them. The key to conflict resolution is open and direct communication, mutual cooperation, and sustainable coordination. Several sources of conflicts can exist in projects. Some of these are discussed below.

Schedule conflict. Conflicts can develop because of improper timing or sequencing of project tasks. This is particularly common in large or multiple projects. Procrastination can lead to having too much to do at once, thereby creating a clash of project functions and discord among project team members. Inaccurate estimates of time requirements may lead to infeasible activity schedules. Project coordination can help avoid schedule conflicts.

Cost conflict. Project costs may not be generally acceptable to the clients of a project. This will lead to project conflict. Even if the initial cost of the project is acceptable, a lack of cost control during implementation can lead to conflicts. Poor budget allocation approaches or lack of a financial feasibility study can cause cost conflicts later in a project. Communication and coordination can help prevent most of the adverse effects of cost conflicts.

Performance conflict. If clear performance requirements are not established, performance conflicts will develop. Lack of clearly defined performance standards can lead each person to evaluate his or her own performance based on personal value judgments. In order to uniformly evaluate the quality of work and monitor project progress, performance standards should be established using the Triple C approach.

Management conflict. There must be a two-way alliance between management and the project team. The views of management should be understood by the team. The views of the team should be appreciated by management.

If this does not happen, management conflicts will develop. A lack of two-way interaction can lead to strikes and industrial actions, which can be detrimental to project objectives. The Triple C approach can help create a conducive dialogue environment between management and the project team.

Technical conflict. If the technical basis of a project is not sound, technical conflict will develop. New industrial projects are particularly prone to technical conflicts because of their significant dependence on technology. Lack of a comprehensive technical feasibility study will lead to technical conflicts. Performance requirements and systems specifications can be integrated through the Triple C approach to avoid technical conflicts.

Priority conflict. Priority conflicts can develop if project objectives are not defined properly and applied uniformly across a project. Lack of a direct project definition can lead each project member to define his or her own goals which may be in conflict with the intended goal of a project. Lack of consistency in the project mission is another potential source of priority conflicts. Over-assignment of responsibilities with no guidelines for relative significance levels can also lead to priority conflicts. Communication can help defuse priority conflict.

Resource conflict. Resource allocation problems are a major source of conflict in project management. Competition for resources, including personnel, tools, hardware, software, and so on, can lead to disruptive clashes among project members. The Triple C approach can help secure resource cooperation.

Power conflict. Project politics lead to a power play that can adversely affect the progress of a project. Project authority and project power should be clearly delineated. Project authority is the control that a person has by virtue of his or her functional post. Project power relates to the clout and influence a person can exercise due to connections within the administrative structure. People with popular personalities can often wield a lot of project power in spite of low or nonexistent project authority. The Triple C model can facilitate a positive marriage of project authority and power to the benefit of project goals. This will help define clear leadership for a project.

Personality conflict. Personality conflict is a common problem in projects involving a large group of people. The larger the project, the larger the size of the management team needed to keep things running. Unfortunately, the larger management team creates an opportunity for personality conflicts. Communication and cooperation can help defuse personality conflicts.

In summary, conflict resolution through Triple C can be achieved by observing the following guidelines:

1. Confront the conflict and identify the underlying causes.
2. Be cooperative and receptive to negotiation as a mechanism for resolving conflicts.

3. Distinguish between proactive, inactive, and reactive behaviors in a conflict situation.
4. Use communication to defuse internal strife and competition.
5. Recognize that short-term compromise can lead to long-term gains.
6. Use coordination to work toward a unified goal.

Use communication and cooperation to turn a competitor (or naysayer) into a collaborator. It is the little and often neglected aspects of a project that lead to project failures. Several factors may constrain project implementation. All the relevant factors can be evaluated under the Triple C model from the project-initiation stage. The adaptation of the nursery rhyme below illustrates the importance of the little "things" in a project.

17.8 THINGS FALLING THROUGH THE CRACKS

The adaptation of the nursery rhyme below illustrates the importance of the little "things" that can fall through the cracks in emergency response situations. This is particularly a great concern in high-pressure and high-intensity response environments. The nursery rhyme is as follows:

For the want of a nail, the horse shoe was lost;
For the loss of the horse shoe, the horse was lost;
For the loss of the horse, the rider was lost;
For the loss of the rider, the message was lost;
For the loss of the message, the battle was lost;
For the loss of the battle, the war was lost;
For the loss of the war, the Kingdom was lost.
All for the want of a nail!

An analogy to the rhyme is the failure of the little things in emergency response. The narrative goes as follows:

For the want of communication, the data was lost;
For the lack of the data, the information was lost;
For the lack of the information, the decision was lost;
For the lack of the decision, the cooperation was lost;
For the lack of compliance, the coordination was lost;
For the lack of the coordination, the emergency response failed.
All for the want of simple communication!

A summary of lessons to be inferred from a Triple C approach is:

- Use proactive planning to initiate project functions.
- Use preemptive planning to avoid project pitfalls.

- Use meetings strategically. A meeting is not a *work element.* A meeting should be convened to facilitate work.
- Use project assessment to properly frame the problem, adequately define the requirements, continually ask the right questions, cautiously analyze risks, and effectively scope the project.
- Be bold about terminating a project when it is the right course of action. Every project needs an exit plan. In some cases, there is victory in capitulation.

The sustainability of the Triple C model for emergency response is summarized below:

1. For effective communication, create good communication channels.
2. For enduring cooperation, establish partnership arrangements.
3. For steady coordination, use a workable organization structure.

17.9 UPSTREAM AND DOWNSTREAM COMMUNICATION

Time is of the essence in emergency response. Good organizational skills and time consciousness are essential for a successful emergency response. Figure 17.4 illustrates upstream and downstream communication channels for upward and downward communication flows. Depending on the type of emergency response needed, communication can flow upward (from individual residents) or downward (from

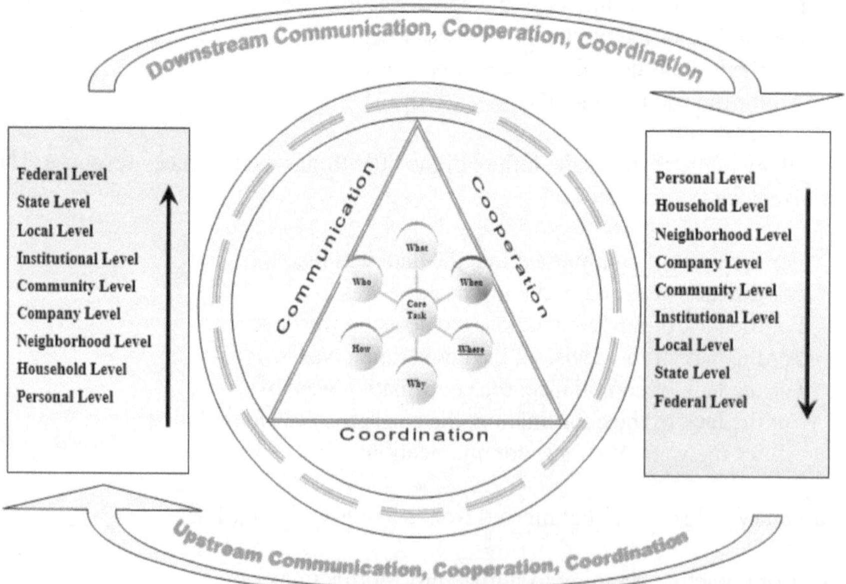

FIGURE 17.4 Upward and downward communication flows for emergency response

government authorities to residents). Compliance through the stages of the communication flow is essential for an overall positive result in emergency response. Barriers that typically develop in layers of communication can be resolved or mitigated by the Triple C model.

17.10 THE EFFECT OF HIERARCHY OF NEEDS

There could be an unrecognized effect of the respective hierarchies of needs in emergency response situations. In today's social-media-influenced society, just because we are all communicating more on our mobile phones does not mean that we are engaged in meaningful and constructive exchanges of relevant content. This chapter suggests that reception of and reaction to communication may be influenced by the respective hierarchies of needs of the communication sources and the communication targets. If an emergency response situation is modeled as a project (which it is), we can see a common basis for applying the project management tool of the hierarchy of needs to emergency response activities. The needs of project participants must be taken into consideration in any project-planning task in accordance with the prevailing personal and behavioral landscape of the project. A common tool for accomplishing this is Maslow's hierarchy of needs (Maslow, 1943). With this framework, the following considerations are proposed:

1. **Physiological needs**: The needs for the basic things of life, such as food, water, housing, and clothing. *This is the level where access to money is most critical.*
2. **Safety needs**: The needs for security, stability, and freedom from the threat of physical harm. *The fear of adverse environmental impact may inhibit project efforts.*
3. **Social needs**: The needs for social approval, friends, love, affection, and association. *For example, public service projects may bring about a better economic outlook that may enable individuals to be in a better position to meet their social needs.*
4. **Esteem needs**: The needs for accomplishment, respect, recognition, attention, and appreciation. *These needs are important not only at the individual level but also at the national level.*
5. **Self-actualization needs**: These are the needs for self-fulfillment and self-improvement. They also involve the availability of opportunities to grow professionally. *Work improvement projects may lead to self-actualization opportunities for individuals to assert themselves socially and economically. Job achievement and professional recognition are two of the most important factors that lead to employee satisfaction and better motivation.*

17.11 INCORPORATING THE DEJI SYSTEMS MODEL

Along with the Triple C approach, the DEJI systems model (Badiru, 2019) can enhance the overall systems-thinking approach to emergency response. The DEJI model of systems engineering provides one additional option for systems engineering development applications. Although the model is generally applicable in all types of systems modeling, it is particularly effective for emergency response scenarios. The core stages of the DEJI systems model are:

- Design
- Evaluation
- Justification
- Integration

Design encompasses any system initiative providing a starting point for a project. Thus, design can include technical product design, process initiation, and concept development. In essence, we can say that "design" represents requirements and specifications. Evaluation can use a variety of metrics, both qualitative and quantitative, depending on the organization's needs. Justification can be done on the basis of monetary, technical, or social reasons. Integration needs to be done with respect to the normal or standard operations of the organization. In other words, it can be implemented within the context of the people, community, and locality affected by the emergency response. Figure 17.5 illustrates the full profile of the DEJI model. In this context, a system is defined as:

> A collection (or partnership) of interrelated elements, whose collective output together (in unison) is higher than the mere sum of the individual outputs of the elements.

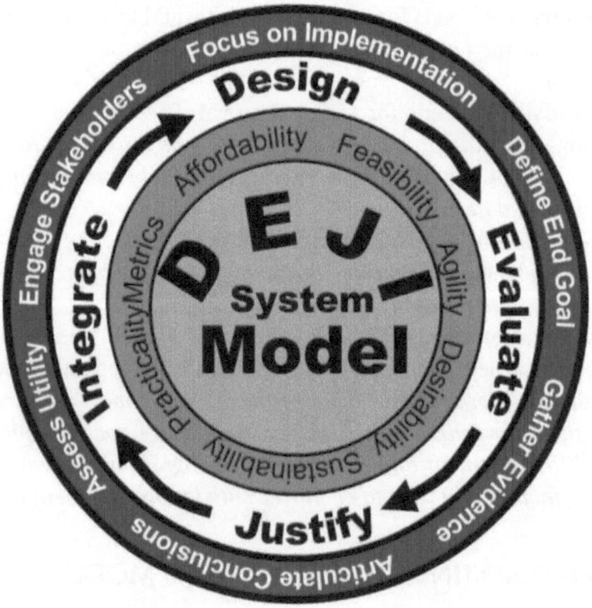

FIGURE 17.5 The DEJI systems model

This highlights the fact that emergency response requires partnerships across many platforms of emergency response groups. Working together, from a systems-thinking approach maximizes the benefits of positive outputs.

17.12 CONCLUSIONS

Having now understood the intrinsic elements of the Triple C model, we can see how and where it could be applicable to the steps of project management in emergency response. Communication explains project scope and requirements through the stages of planning, organizing, scheduling, and control. Cooperation is required to get human resource buy-in and stakeholder endorsement across all facets of planning, organizing, scheduling, and control. Coordination facilitates adaptive interfaces over all the elements of planning, organizing, scheduling, and control. If compliance is embedded within the Triple C model, it can enhance the implementation of the model. The Triple C model should be implemented as an iterative loop process that moves an effort through the communication, cooperation, and coordination functions in any emergency response situation.

REFERENCES

Badiru, A. B. (1987), "Communication, Cooperation, Coordination: The Triple C of Project Management," in *Proceedings of 1987 IIE Spring Conference*, Washington, DC, May, pp. 401–4.

Badiru, A. B. (2008), *Triple C Model of Project Management: Communication, Cooperation, and Coordination*, Taylor & Francis CRC Press, Boca Raton, FL.

Badiru, A. B. (2019), *Systems Engineering Models: Theory, Methods, and Applications*, Taylor & Francis/CRC Press, Boca Raton, FL.

Badiru, A. B., B. L. Foote, L. Leemis, A. Ravindran, and L. Williams (1993), "Recovering from a Crisis at Tinker Air Force Base," *PM Network* 7(2):10–23.

Maslow, A. (1943), "A theory of human motivation." *Psychological Review* 50(4): 370–96.

18 Emergency Response
Systems-based Use of Finland's Concept of Sisu

Adedeji B. Badiru

18.1 INTRODUCTION

The world is becoming more and more unstable and unpredictable due to environmental, economic, social, and political developments. Weather phenomena bring about more extreme and more frequent stress on the population. Economic, social, and political developments can create unstable pressures on the delicate balance in our human relationships and physical infrastructure. These are unplanned or unexpected developments that often necessitate some form of emergency response. In each case, extreme dedication is the cornerstone of an effective response. The methodology advocated in this chapter is to leverage Finland's concept of "Sisu." Sisu is a Finnish concept that describes stoic determination, tenacity of purpose, grit, bravery, resilience, and hardiness, particularly in the face of extreme hardship. Hardship is a precursor for instituting an emergency response in a community.

18.2 SOFT AND HARD SCIENCE

Because of people's involvement in emergency response, we must employ a hybrid method that includes both soft and hard science. In this regard, a systems thinking approach is necessary. We recommend the DEJI systems model, which provides a structured approach to design, evaluation, justification, and integration. A precursor to using the DEJI systems model is the Triple C model, which uses a step-wise approach to communication, cooperation, and coordination. The response surface for emergency response is not smooth. There must always be a compromise region weighing time, quality, and performance against expectations. Only a systems approach can give each measure its due within the scheme of an emergency response. Lahmidi et al. (2013) emphasize the necessity of focusing on social transformations in solving complex technological problems. The Finnish concept of Sisu fits the socially centric approach.

 DOI: 10.1201/9781003648178-20

18.3 DEJI SYSTEMS MODEL

The iconic representation of the DEJI systems model is shown in Figure 18.1. Design is not necessarily the physical design of a product. Rather, it could be a concept of operation or action that must be evaluated, justified, and integrated into the prevailing work environment. Design can also be a specification of requirements, which must be executed under pressure, albeit effectively, within the emergency response framework. Without a well-designed, well-defined, and well-articulated set of requirements, all emergency response efforts will be misguided and ineffective. Many organizations are now inserting the highly functional DEJI systems framework into nearly every aspect of their operations. Everything is connected and very interdependent in our present digital-oriented world. So, everything now requires a systems engineering approach. The DEJI systems model is a flagship framework for planning contemporary projects, systems, teams, and ventures.

With the structured framework of the DEJI systems model, emergency response can be executed faster, more efficiently, effectively, and economically. Moreover, the approach ensures that systems integration is done within the local context and the prevailing work environment. Based on the preceding emergency response

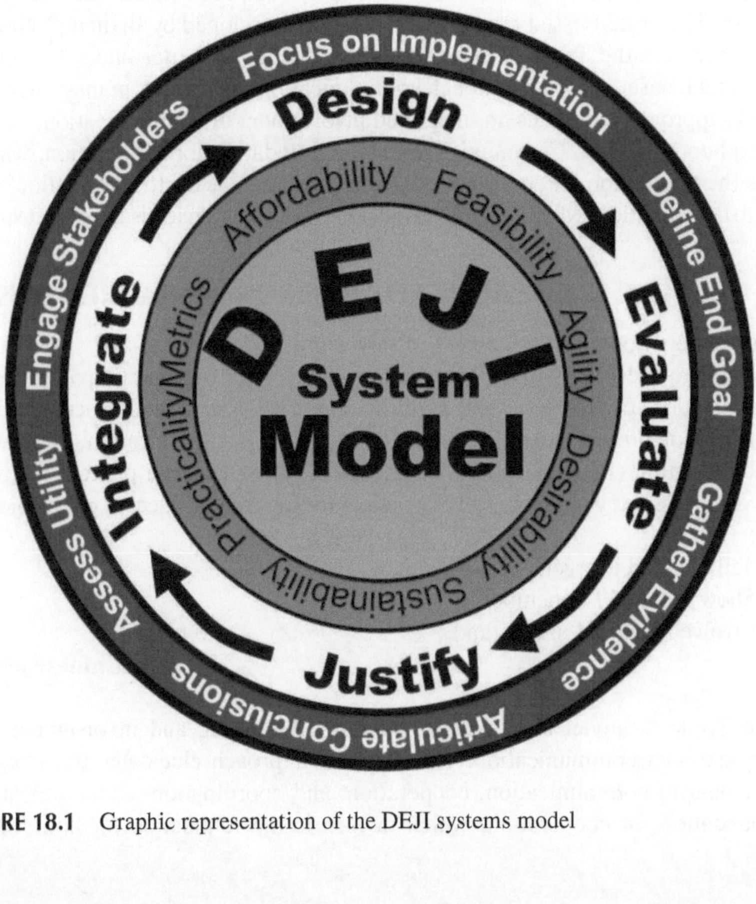

FIGURE 18.1 Graphic representation of the DEJI systems model

considerations, it is recommended that we look at some of the systems engineering tools and techniques available in the literature (see Badiru, 2019). Of particular importance is systems integration to link the technical elements of emergency response to the social human elements through the application of the DEJI systems model. A condensed summary of the essential application of the model to a power-supply scenario is described below:

- **Design**: Design of the technical aspects of power plants (whether renewable or nonrenewable).
- **Evaluation**: An assessment of power supply needs vis-à-vis the power plant capabilities.
- **Justification:** A hybrid review of power-supply flow to areas of need (home, business, and industry).
- **Integration**: Mapping of power-supply realities to human behavior in consumption and conservation.

A total systems-based approach facilitates a consideration of all the nuances of human involvement in emergency response. Of particular importance is the system of communication, cooperation, and coordination required in complex emergency response. This is addressed by the Triple C model developed by Badiru (2008). This chapter presents the Triple C principle, which facilitates better understanding and involvement based on foundational communication in project management. The Triple C approach facilitates an integrated involvement of communication, cooperation, and coordination. Communication is the foundation for cooperation, which in turn is the foundation for coordination. Communication leads to cooperation, which leads to coordination, which leads to project harmony, which leads to project success.

18.4 TRIPLE C FRAMEWORK FOR ENVIRONMENTAL RESPONSE

Getting things done, in the context of environmental response and sustainability, ultimately requires the involvement of many participants. Such participation requires communication, cooperation, and coordination. This chapter introduces the Triple C principle of project execution based on stages of communication, cooperation, and coordination (Badiru, 2008). As presented by the Chinese proverb below, the involvement of every team member is critical for the overall success of a project.

> Tell me, and I forget;
> Show me, and I remember;
> Involve me, and I understand.
>
> **– Chinese proverb**

The Triple C model facilitates a better understanding and involvement based on foundational communication. The Triple C approach elucidates the integrated involvement of communication, cooperation, and coordination. Communication is the foundation for cooperation, which in turn is the foundation for coordination.

Communication leads to cooperation, which leads to coordination, which leads to project harmony, which leads to project success.

The primary lesson of the Triple C model is not to take cooperation for granted. It must be pursued, solicited, and secured explicitly. The process of securing cooperation requires structured communication upfront. It is only after cooperation is in effect that all project efforts can be coordinated.

The Triple C model has been used effectively in practice to enhance project performance because most project problems can be traced to initial communication problems. The Triple C approach works because it is very simple – simple to understand and simple to implement. The simplicity comes from the fact that most of the required elements of the approach are already being done within every organization, albeit in a nonstructured manner. The Triple C model puts the existing processes into a structural approach to communication, cooperation, and coordination.

The idea for the Triple C model originated from a complex facility redesign project (Badiru et al., 1993) conducted for Tinker Air Force Base (TAFB) in Oklahoma City by the School of Industrial Engineering, University of Oklahoma, from 1985 to 1989. The project was part of a reconstruction project following a disastrous fire that occurred in the base's repair/production facility in November 1984. The urgency, complexity, scope ambiguity, confusion, and disjointed directions that existed in the early days of the reconstruction effort led to the need to develop a structured approach to communication, cooperation, and coordination of the various work elements. Despite the high-pressure timing of the project, the author called a Time-Out-of-Time (TOOT) so that a process could be developed for project communication, leading to personnel cooperation and eventually facilitating task coordination. The time invested in TOOT resulted in a remarkable resurgence of cooperation where none existed at the beginning of the project. Encouraged by the intrinsic occurrence of cooperation, the process was further enhanced and formalized as the Triple C approach to the project's success. The approach was credited with the overall success of the project. The qualitative approach of Triple C complemented the technical approaches used on the project to facilitate the harmonious execution of tasks. Many projects fail when the stakeholders get too wrapped up in the technical requirements at the expense of qualitative requirements. Other elements of "C," such as collaboration, commitment, and correlation, are embedded in the Triple C structure. Of course, the constraints of time, cost, and performance must be overcome all along the way.

Organizations thrive by investing in three primary resources: the people who do the work, the tools that the people use to do the work, and the process that governs the work that the people do. Of the three, investing in people is the easiest thing an organization can do, and we should do it whenever we have an opportunity. The Triple C approach incorporates the qualitative (human) aspects of a project into overall project requirements.

The Triple C model was first used in 1985 and subsequently introduced in print in 1987 (Badiru 1987). The project scenario that led to the development of the Triple C model was later documented in Badiru et al. (1993). The model is an effective project planning and control tool. The model states that project management can be enhanced by implementing it within the integrated functions summarized below:

- Communication
- Cooperation
- Coordination

The model facilitates a systematic approach to project planning, organizing, scheduling, and control. The Triple C model is distinct from the 3C approach commonly used in military operations. The military approach emphasizes personnel management in the hierarchy of command, control, and communication. This places communication as the last function. The Triple C, by contrast, suggests communication as the first and foremost function. The Triple C model can be implemented for project planning, scheduling, and control purposes.

Figure 18.2 shows the application of Triple C for project planning, scheduling, and control within the confines of the Triple Constraints of cost, schedule, and performance. Each of these three primary functions of project management requires effective communication, sustainable cooperation, and adaptive coordination.

Triple C illustrates the basic questions of what, who, why, how, where, and when. It highlights what must be done and when. It can also help to identify the resources (personnel, equipment, facilities, etc.) required for each effort. It points out important questions such as:

- Does each project participant know what the objective is?
- Does each participant know his or her role in achieving the objective?
- What obstacles may prevent a participant from playing his or her role effectively?

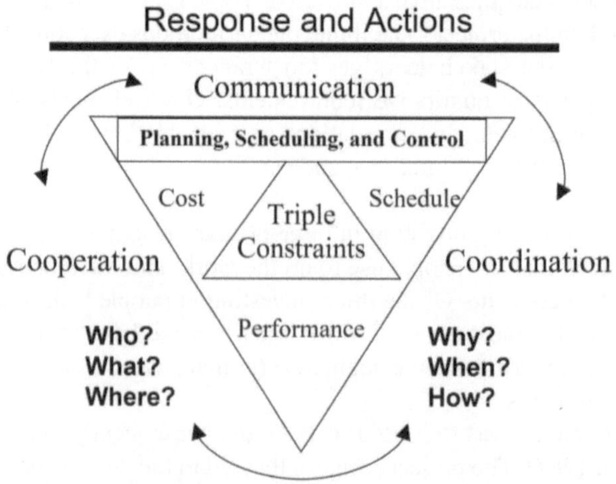

FIGURE 18.2 Triple C for communication, cooperation, and coordination

Triple C can mitigate the disparity between idea and practice because it explicitly solicits information about the critical aspects of a project in terms of the following queries.

18.4.1 Types of Emergency Communication

- Verbal
- Written
- Body language
- Visual tools (e.g., graphical tools)
- Sensual (the use of all five senses: sight, smell, touch, taste, hearing – olfactory, tactile, auditory)
- Simplex (unidirectional)
- Half-duplex (bi-directional with time lag)
- Full-duplex (real-time dialogue)
- One-on-one
- One-to-many
- Many-to-one

18.4.2 Types of Emergency Cooperation

- Proximity
- Functional
- Professional
- Social
- Romantic
- Power influence
- Authority influence
- Hierarchical
- Lateral
- Cooperation by intimidation
- Cooperation by enticement

18.4.3 Types of Emergency Coordination

- Teaming
- Delegation
- Supervision
- Partnership
- Token-passing
- Baton hand-off

18.4.4 Triple C Questions for Emergency Response

Questioning is the best approach to gathering information for effective project management. Everything should be questioned. Questions up front can preempt and avert project problems later on. Typical questions to ask under the Triple C approach are:

- What is the purpose of the project?
- Who is in charge of the project?
- Why is the project needed?
- Where is the project located?
- When will the project be carried out?
- How will the project contribute to increased opportunities for the organization?
- What is the project designed to achieve?
- How will the project affect different groups of people within the organization?
- What will be the project approach or methodology?
- What other groups or organizations will be involved (if any)?
- What will happen at the end of the project?
- How will the project be tracked, monitored, evaluated, and reported?
- What resources are required?
- What are the associated costs of the required resources?
- How do the project objectives fit into the goals of the organization?
- What respective contribution is expected from each participant?
- What level of cooperation is expected from each group?
- Where is the coordinating point for the project?

The key to getting everyone on board with a project is to ensure that task objectives are clear and comply with the principle of SMART as outlined below:

- **Specific**: The task objective must be specific.
- **Measurable**: The task objective must be measurable.
- **Aligned**: The task objective must be achievable and aligned with the overall project goal.
- **Realistic**: The task objective must be realistic and relevant to the organization.
- **Timed**: The task objective must have a time basis.

If a task has the above intrinsic characteristics, then the function of communicating the task will more likely lead to personnel cooperation.

18.5 SISU-BASED COMMUNICATION

Communication makes working together possible. The communication function of project management involves keeping stakeholders aware of project requirements and progress. Those who will be affected by the project directly or indirectly, as direct participants or as beneficiaries, should be informed as appropriate regarding the following:

- Scope of the project.
- Personnel contribution required.
- Expected cost and merits of the project.
- Project organization and implementation plan.
- Potential adverse effects if the project should fail.
- Alternatives, if any, for achieving the project goal.
- Potential direct and indirect benefits of the project.

The communication channel must be kept open throughout the project life cycle. In addition to internal communication, appropriate external sources should also be consulted. The project manager must

- Exude commitment to the project.
- Utilize the communication responsibility matrix.
- Facilitate multi-channel communication interfaces.
- Identify internal and external communication needs.
- Resolve organizational and communication hierarchies.
- Encourage both formal and informal communication links.

When clear communication is maintained between management and employees and among peers, many project problems can be averted. Project communication may be carried out in one or more of the following formats:

- One-to-many
- One-to-one
- Many-to-one
- Written and formal
- Written and informal
- Oral and formal
- Oral and informal
- Nonverbal gestures

Good communication is affected when what is implied is perceived as intended. Effective communication is vital to the success of any project. Despite the awareness that proper communication form the blueprint for project success, many organizations still fail in their communication functions. The study of communication is complex. Factors that influence the effectiveness of communication within a project organization structure include the following.

1. Personal perception. Each person perceives events on the basis of personal psychological, social, cultural, and experiential background. As a result, no two people can interpret a given event the same way. The nature of events is not always the critical aspect of a problem situation. Rather, the problem is often the different perceptions of the different people involved.
2. Psychological profile. The psychological makeup of each person determines personal reactions to events or words. Thus, individual needs and levels of thinking will dictate how a message is interpreted.
3. Social Environment. Communication problems sometimes arise because people have been conditioned by their prevailing social environment to interpret certain things in unique ways. Vocabulary, idioms, organizational status, social stereotypes, and economic situation are among the social factors that can thwart effective communication.
4. Cultural background. Cultural differences are among the most pervasive barriers to project communication, especially in today's multinational organizations. Language and cultural idiosyncrasies often determine how communication is approached and interpreted.
5. Semantic and syntactic factors. Semantic and syntactic barriers to communication usually occur in written documents. Semantic factors are those that relate to the intrinsic knowledge of the subject of the communication. Syntactic factors are those that relate to the form in which the communication is presented. The problems created by these factors become acute in situations where response, feedback, or reaction to the communication cannot be observed.
6. Organizational structure. Frequently, the organizational structure in which a project is conducted has a direct influence on the flow of information and, consequently, on the effectiveness of communication. Organizational hierarchy may determine how different personnel levels perceive a given communication.
7. Communication media. The method of transmitting a message may also affect the value ascribed to the message and, consequently, how it is interpreted or used. The common barriers to project communication are
   - Inattentiveness
   - Lack of organization
   - Outstanding grudges
   - Preconceived notions
   - Ambiguous presentation
   - Emotions and sentiments
   - Lack of communication feedback
   - Sloppy and unprofessional presentation
   - Lack of confidence in the communicator
   - Lack of confidence by the communicator
   - Low credibility of the communicator
   - Unnecessary technical jargon
   - Too many people involved

- Untimely communication
- Arrogance or imposition
- Lack of focus

Some suggestions on improving the effectiveness of communication are presented next. The recommendations may be implemented as appropriate for any of the forms of communication listed earlier. The recommendations are for both the communicator and the audience.

1. Never assume that the integrity of the information sent will be preserved as the information passes through several communication channels. Information is generally filtered, condensed, or expanded by the receivers before relaying it to the next destination. When preparing a communication that needs to pass through several organization structures, one safeguard is to compose the original information in a concise form to minimize the need for re-composition of the project structure.
2. Give the audience a central role in the discussion. A leading role can help make a person feel a part of the project effort and responsible for the project's success. He or she can then have a more constructive view of project communication.
3. Do homework and think through the intended accomplishment of the communication. This helps eliminate trivial and inconsequential communication efforts.
4. Carefully plan the organization of the ideas embodied in the communication. Use indexing or points of reference whenever possible. Grouping ideas into related chunks of information can be particularly effective. Present the short messages first. Short messages help create focus, maintain interest, and prepare the mind for the longer messages to follow.
5. Highlight why the communication is of interest and how it is intended to be used. Full attention should be given to the content of the message with regard to the prevailing project situation.
6. Elicit the support of those around you by integrating their ideas into the communication. The more people feel they have contributed to the issue, the more expeditious they are in soliciting the cooperation of others. The effect of the multiplicative rule can quickly garner support for the communication purpose.
7. Be responsive to the feelings of others. It takes two to communicate. Anticipate and appreciate the reactions of members of the audience. Recognize their operational circumstances and present your message in a form they can relate to.
8. Accept constructive criticism. Nobody is infallible. Use criticism as a springboard to higher communication performance.
9. Exhibit interest in the issue in order to arouse the interest of your audience. Avoid delivering your messages as a matter of a routine organizational requirement.

10. Obtain and furnish feedback promptly. Clarify vague points with examples.
11. Communicate at the appropriate time, at the right place, to the right people.
12. Reinforce words with positive action. Never promise what cannot be delivered. Value your credibility.
13. Maintain eye contact in oral communication and read the facial expressions of your audience to obtain real-time feedback.
14. Concentrate on listening as much as speaking. Evaluate both the implicit and explicit meanings of statements.
15. Document communication transactions for future reference.
16. Avoid asking questions that can be answered with a "yes" or "no." Use relevant questions to focus the attention of the audience. Use questions that make people reflect upon their words, such as, "How do you think this will work?" compared to, "Do you this will work?"
17. Avoid patronizing the audience. Respect their judgment and knowledge.
18. Speak and write in a controlled tempo. Avoid emotionally charged voice inflections.
19. Create an atmosphere that encourages formal and informal exchange of ideas.
20. Summarize the objectives of the communication and how they will be achieved.

Within the framework of Triple C, a communication responsibility matrix links sources of communication to targets of communication. Cells within the matrix indicate the subject of the desired communication. There should be at least one filled cell in each row and each column of the matrix. This ensures that each individual in a department is associated with at least one communication source or target. With a communication responsibility matrix, a clear understanding of what needs to be communicated to whom can be developed. Communication in a project environment can take several forms. The specific needs of a project may dictate the most appropriate mode. Three popular computer communication modes are discussed next in the context of communicating data and information for project management.

18.5.1 Simplex Communication

Simplex communication is a unidirectional communication arrangement in which one project entity initiates communication with another entity or individual within the project environment. The entity addressed in the communication does not have a mechanism or capability for responding to the communication. An extreme example of this is a one-way, top-down communication from top management to the project personnel. In this case, the personnel have no communication access or input to top management. A budget-related example is a case where top management allocates a budget to a project without requesting and reviewing the actual needs of the project. Simplex communication is common in authoritarian organizations.

18.5.2 Half-Duplex Communication

Half-duplex communication is a bi-directional arrangement whereby one project entity can communicate with another entity and receive a response within a certain time lag. Both entities can communicate with each other, but not at the same time. An example of half-duplex communication is a project organization that permits communication with top management without a direct meeting. Each communicator must wait for a response from the target of the communication. Request and allocation without a budget meeting is another example of half-duplex data communication in project management.

18.5.3 Full-Duplex Communication

Full-duplex communication involves an arrangement that permits a dialogue between the communicating entities. Both individuals and entities can communicate with each other at the same time or face-to-face. As long as there is no clash of words, this appears to be the most receptive communication mode. It allows participative project planning in which each project personnel has an opportunity to contribute to the planning process.

Each member of a project team needs to recognize the nature of the prevailing communication mode in the project. Management must evaluate the prevailing communication structure and attempt to modify it if necessary to enhance project functions. An evaluation of who is to communicate with whom about what may help improve the project data/information communication process. A communication matrix may include notations about the desired modes of communication between individuals and groups in the project environment.

18.6 SISU-FOCUSED COOPERATION

The cooperation of the project personnel must be explicitly elicited. Merely voicing consent for a project is not enough assurance of full cooperation. The participants and beneficiaries of the project must be convinced of the merits of the project. Some of the factors that influence cooperation in a project environment include personnel requirements, resource requirements, budget limitations, past experiences, conflicting priorities, and lack of uniform organizational support. A structured approach to seeking cooperation should clarify the following:

- Cooperative efforts required.
- Precedents for future projects.
- Implication of lack of cooperation.
- Criticality of cooperation to project success.
- Organizational impact of cooperation.
- Time frame involved in the project.
- Rewards of good cooperation.

Cooperation is a basic virtue of human interaction. More projects fail due to a lack of cooperation and commitment than any other factors. To secure and retain the cooperation of project participants, you must elicit a positive first reaction to the project. The most positive aspects of a project should be the first items of project communication. For project management, there are different types of cooperation that should be understood.

18.6.1 Functional Cooperation

Functional cooperation is induced by the nature of the functional relationship between two groups. The two groups may be required to perform related functions that can only be accomplished through cooperation.

18.6.2 Social Cooperation

Social cooperation is influenced by the social relationship between two groups. The prevailing social relationship motivates cooperation that may be useful in getting project work done.

18.6.3 Legal Cooperation

Legal cooperation is the type of cooperation that is imposed through some authoritative requirement. In this case, the participants may have no choice other than to cooperate.

18.6.4 Administrative Cooperation

Administrative cooperation is brought on by administrative requirements that make it imperative that two groups work together on a common goal.

18.6.5 Associative Cooperation

Associative cooperation may also be referred to as collegiality. The level of cooperation is determined by the association that exists between two groups.

18.6.6 Proximity Cooperation

Proximity cooperation results when two groups are geographically close. Being close makes it imperative that the two groups work together.

18.6.7 Dependency Cooperation

Dependency cooperation occurs when one group depends on another group for some important aspect. Such dependency is usually of a mutual, two-way nature. One group depends on the other for one thing, while the latter group depends on the former for some other thing.

18.6.8 Imposed Cooperation

In imposed cooperation, external agents must be employed to induce cooperation between two groups. This is applicable in cases where the two groups have no natural reason to cooperate. This is where the approaches presented earlier for seeking cooperation can become very useful.

18.6.9 Lateral Cooperation

Lateral cooperation involves cooperation with peers and immediate associates. Lateral cooperation is often easy to achieve because existing lateral relationships create an environment that is conducive to project cooperation.

18.6.10 Vertical Cooperation

Vertical or hierarchical cooperation refers to cooperation that is implied by the hierarchical structure of the project. For example, subordinates are expected to cooperate with their vertical superiors.

Regardless of the type of cooperation available in a project environment, the cooperative forces should be channeled toward achieving project goals. Documentation of the prevailing level of cooperation is useful for winning further support for a project. Clarification of project priorities will facilitate personnel cooperation. Relative priorities of multiple projects should be specified so that a priority is established for all groups within the organization. Some guidelines for securing cooperation in emergency responses are provided below. Sisu can facilitate a positive outcome out of these expectations.

- Establish achievable goals for the project.
- Clearly outline the individual commitments required.
- Integrate project priorities with existing priorities.
- Eliminate the fear of job loss due to industrialization.
- Anticipate and eliminate potential sources of conflict.
- Use an open-door policy to address project grievances.
- Remove skepticism by documenting the project's merits.

18.6.11 Commitment

Cooperation must be supported with commitment. To cooperate is to support the ideas of a project. To commit is to willingly and actively participate in project efforts again and again through the thick and thin of the project. Providing resources is one way management can demonstrate its commitment to a project.

18.7 SISU-ORIENTED COORDINATION

After the communication and cooperation functions have been successfully initiated, the efforts of the project personnel must be coordinated. Coordination facilitates the harmonious organization of project efforts. Creating a responsibility chart can be very helpful at this stage. A responsibility chart is a matrix consisting of columns of individual or functional departments and rows of required actions. Cells within the matrix are filled with relationship codes that indicate who is responsible for what. The matrix helps avoid neglecting crucial communication requirements and obligations. It can help resolve questions such as:

- Who is to do what?
- How long will it take?
- Who is to inform whom of what?
- Whose approval is needed for what?
- Who is responsible for which results?
- What personnel interfaces are required?
- What support is needed from whom and when?

18.8 CONFLICT RESOLUTION IN EMERGENCY RESPONSE

Conflicts can and do develop in any work environment. Conflicts, whether intended or inadvertent, prevent an organization from getting the most out of the workforce. When implemented as an integrated process, the Triple C model can help avoid conflicts in a project. When conflicts do develop, it can help resolve them. The key to conflict resolution is open and direct communication, cooperation, and sustainable coordination. Several sources of conflicts can exist in a project. Some of these are discussed below.

18.8.1 Schedule Conflict

Conflicts can develop because of improper timing or sequencing of project tasks. This is particularly common in large, multi-project settings. Procrastination can lead to having too much to do at once, thereby creating a clash of project functions and discord among project team members. Inaccurate estimates of time requirements may lead to infeasible activity schedules. Project coordination can help avoid schedule conflicts.

18.8.2 Cost Conflict

The project cost may not be generally acceptable to the project's clients. This will lead to project conflict. Even if the initial cost of the project is acceptable, a lack of cost control during implementation can lead to conflicts. Poor budget allocation approaches and the lack of a financial feasibility study may cause cost conflicts later in a project. Communication and coordination can help prevent most of the adverse effects of cost conflicts.

18.8.3 Performance Conflict

If clear performance requirements are not established, performance conflicts will develop. A lack of clearly defined performance standards can lead each person to evaluate his or her own performance based on personal value judgments. In order to uniformly evaluate the quality of work and monitor project progress, performance standards should be established using the Triple C approach.

18.8.4 Management Conflict

There must be a two-way alliance between management and the project team. The views of management should be understood by the team. The views of the team should be appreciated by management. If this does not happen, management conflicts will develop. A lack of a two-way interaction can lead to strikes and industrial actions, which can be detrimental to project objectives. The Triple C approach can help create a conducive dialogue environment between management and the project team.

18.8.5 Technical Conflict

If the technical basis of a project is not sound, technical conflict will develop. New industrial projects are particularly prone to technical conflicts because of their significant dependence on technology. The lack of a comprehensive technical feasibility study will lead to technical conflicts. Performance requirements and systems specifications can be integrated through the Triple C approach to avoid technical conflicts.

18.8.6 Priority Conflict

Priority conflicts can develop if project objectives are not defined properly and applied uniformly across a project. The lack of a direct project definition can lead each project member to define his or her own goals, which may be in conflict with the intended goal of a project. A lack of consistency in the project mission is another potential source of priority conflicts. Over-assignment of responsibilities with no guidelines for relative significance levels can also lead to priority conflicts. Communication can help defuse priority conflict.

18.8.7 Resource Conflict

Resource allocation problems are a major source of conflict in project management. Competition for resources, including personnel, tools, hardware, software, and so on, can lead to disruptive clashes among project members. The Triple C approach can help secure resource cooperation.

18.8.8 Power Conflict

Project politics lead to a power play, which can adversely affect the progress of a project. Project authority and project power should be clearly delineated. Project authority is the control that a person has by virtue of his or her functional post. Project power relates to clout and influence, which a person can exercise due to connections within the administrative structure. People with popular personalities can often wield a lot of project power despite low or nonexistent project authority. The Triple C model can facilitate a positive marriage of project authority and power to the benefit of project goals. This will help define clear leadership for a project.

18.8.9 Personality Conflict

Personality conflict is a common problem in projects involving a large group of people. The larger the project, the larger the size of the management team needed to keep things running. Unfortunately, the larger management team creates an opportunity for personality conflicts. Communication and cooperation can help defuse personality conflicts. In summary, conflict resolution through Triple C can be achieved by observing the following guidelines:

1. Confront the conflict and identify the underlying causes.
2. Be cooperative and receptive to negotiation as a mechanism for resolving conflicts.
3. Distinguish between proactive, inactive, and reactive behaviors in a conflict situation.
4. Use communication to defuse internal strife and competition.
5. Recognize that short-term compromise can lead to long-term gains.
6. Use coordination to work toward a unified goal.
7. Use communication and cooperation to turn a competitor into a collaborator.

It is the little and often neglected aspects of a project that lead to project failures. Several factors may constrain the project implementation. All the relevant factors can be evaluated under the Triple C model right from the project initiation stage.

18.9 SISU AND TRIPLE C

Having now understood the intrinsic elements of Triple C, we can see how and where it could be applicable to emergency response project management. Communication explains project scope and requirements through the stages of planning, organizing, scheduling, and control. Cooperation is required to get human resource buy-in and stakeholder acceptance across all facets of planning, organizing, scheduling, and control. Coordination facilitates adaptive interfaces over all the elements of planning, organizing, scheduling, and control in high-stakes emergency response. The Triple C model should be implemented as an iterative loop process that moves emergency response through the communication, cooperation, and coordination functions. This chapter has presented a general introduction to the Triple C approach, focusing on Communication, Cooperation, and Coordination within the context of Finland's Sisu. A summary of lessons to be inferred from a Triple C approach is presented below. Further details on Triple C can be found in Badiru (2008).

- Use proactive planning to initiate project functions.
- Use preemptive planning to avoid project pitfalls.
- Use meetings strategically. A meeting is not *work*. Meetings should be done to facilitate work.
- Use project assessment to properly frame the problem, adequately define the requirements, continually ask the right questions, cautiously analyze risks, and effectively scope the project.
- Be bold to terminate a project when termination is the right course of action. Every project needs an exit plan. In some cases, there is victory in capitulation.

The applicability and sustainability of the Triple C approach within the context of Sisu is summarized below:

1. For effective communication, create good communication channels, using the dedicated seriousness of Sisu.
2. For enduring cooperation, establish partnership arrangements, based on Sisu's spirit of collaboration.
3. For steady coordination, use a workable organization structure, based on Sisu's stoic determination.

REFERENCES

Badiru, A. B. (1987), "Communication, Cooperation, Coordination: The Triple C of Project Management," in *Proceedings of 1987 IIE Spring Conference*, Washington, DC, May, pp. 401–4.

Badiru, A. B. (2008), *Triple C Model of Project Management: Communication, Cooperation, and Coordination*, Taylor & Francis/CRC Press, Boca Raton, FL.

Badiru, A. B. (2019), *Systems Engineering Models: Theory, Methods, and Applications*, CRC Press/Taylor & Francis, Boca Raton, FL.

Badiru, A. B., B. L. Foote, L. Leemis, A. Ravindran, and L. Williams (1993), "Recovering from a Crisis at Tinker Air Force Base," *PM Network*, Vol. 7, No. 2, pp. 10–23.

Lahmidi, W., Z. Lahmidi, and S. El-Boujnouni (2013), "Social Transformation through Social Innovation: The Case Study of a Moroccan Waste Recycling Cooperative," *International Journal of Engineering, Business and Management (IJEBM)*, Vol. 7, No. 4. https://dx.doi.org/10.22161/ijebm.7.4.5.

19 Emergency Response Process Improvement Using Lean Six Sigma Techniques

Charlie A. Marquez and Damirson A. Co

19.1 APPLICABILITY OF LEAN SIX SIGMA

Emergency response is like any coordinated human endeavor to which Lean Six Sigma techniques can be applied to improve operations. If we define the activities embodied in an emergency response as human production activities, then the production management concept of Lean Six Sigma can be applied. The end result of a successful emergency response depends on process improvement, which is the bastion of Lean Six Sigma techniques. If we can improve how we do emergency response, we can increase the likelihood of success.

The history of Lean traces back to the start of modern manufacturing. Henry Ford created what is known as "flow production," which involves the continuous movement of elements through the production process. Ford used mass production to fabricate and assemble the components of his vehicles in few minutes rather than hours or days. This process was very successful and allowed the Ford Motor Company to produce over 15 million Model T cars between 1908 and 1927. During World War II, the US military adopted Ford's mass production system (Skhmot 2017).

After World War II, Kiichiro Toyoda, son of Toyoda Automatic Loom Works founder Sakichi Toyoda, and his nephew Eiji Toyoda collaborated with Taiichi Ohno to develop a new means of production which they called the Toyota Production System. Compared to Ford's mass production system, this system enabled faster, cheaper production, improved quality, and, most importantly, greater product variety (Lean Enterprise Institute 2024).

The concept of Six Sigma was introduced in 1986 by Bill Smith, a senior engineer and scientist at Motorola, to standardize the way defects are counted. He is considered the father of Six Sigma (Skhmot 2017). Bill, along with Mikel Harry, convinced Robert "Bob" W. Galvin, Motorola's CEO at that time, of the benefits of using statistical analysis to improve quality, resulting in Motorola's Six Sigma Quality Program in 1987. This helped Motorola become the first company to receive the Malcolm

 DOI: 10.1201/9781003648178-21

Baldridge National Quality Award in 1988, just a year after initiating the Six Sigma concept. Because of the success of Six Sigma at Motorola, many companies, such as General Electric, Dow Chemical, DuPont, Honeywell, and Whirlpool, became early adopters. Inspired by their success, numerous other companies also adopted Six Sigma to improve their processes, reduce their defects, and increase customer satisfaction (RP News Wires 2024).

Lean Six Sigma, or LSS, is a combination of two disciplines that complement each other. Lean focuses on *waste* reduction, while Six Sigma focuses on *variation* reduction. Lean uses less technical tools such as *kaizen* (continuous improvement), workplace organization (commonly called *5S*), and visual controls, whereas Six Sigma uses statistical data analysis, design of experiments, and hypothesis testing (ASQ 2024). Tom Ehrenfeld noted that both Six Sigma and Lean programs had significant gaps, causing them to fall short of the Toyota Production System. As a result, many organizations combined Lean and Six Sigma to address the shortcomings inherent in each approach (Ehrenfeld 2010).

19.2 THE FIVE LEAN PRINCIPLES

In 1991, James P. Womack, Daniel T. Jones, and Daniel Roos wrote a book called *The Machine That Changed the World*, in which they introduced the principles of Lean. Together, they studied several manufacturing systems and documented their observations of Toyota's system (Skhmot 2017). Figure 19.1 shows the five Lean principles (Lean Enterprise Institute 2024).

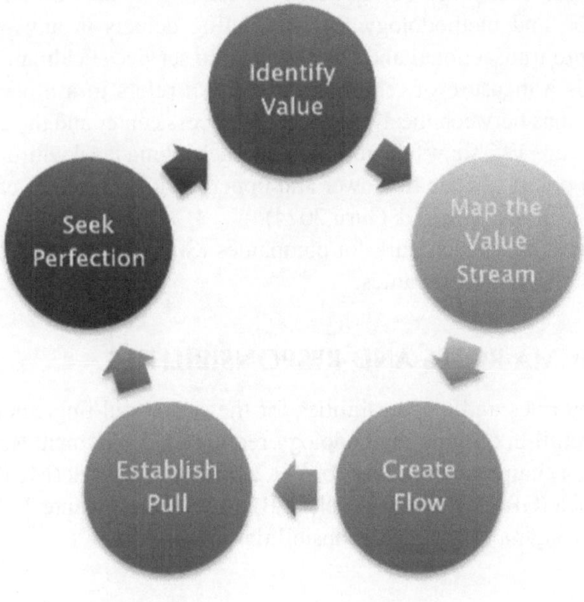

FIGURE 19.1 The Five Lean principles

The Lean Enterprise Institute summarized these principles as follows:

1. Specify value from the standpoint of the end customer by product family.
2. Identify all the steps in the value stream for each product family, eliminating whenever possible those steps that do not create value.
3. Make the value-creating steps occur in a tight sequence so the product can flow smoothly towards the customer.
4. As flow is introduced, let customers pull value from the next upstream activity.
5. As value is specified, value streams are identified, wasted steps are removed, and flow and pull are introduced, repeat the process continuously until a state of perfection is reached, in which perfect value is created with no waste.

19.3 THE EIGHT FORMS OF WASTE

For easy recall, the eight forms of waste, or *muda*, can be written as DOWNTIME (Six Sigma BELT Guru 2024). This acronym and its meaning are shown in Table 19.1.

19.4 SIX SIGMA DEFINED

According to Jack Welch, CEO of General Electric (2018–present), "Six Sigma is a quality program that, when all is said and done, improves your customer's experience, lowers your costs, and builds better leaders." It is also a disciplined, data-driven approach and methodology for eliminating defects in any process—from manufacturing to transactional and from product to service (Feldman 2022).

Six Sigma is a measure of "sigma level," which refers to a process having six standard deviations between the average of the process center and the closest specification limit. Figure 19.2 shows the total area of each sigma level within a normal distribution. Data points outside the lower and upper limits are said to cause customer dissatisfaction (Six Sigma BELT Guru 2024).

Six Sigma is also a benchmark for companies (SixLeanSigma 2021). Table 19.2 shows the sigma level of companies.

19.5 SIX SIGMA ROLES AND RESPONSIBILITIES

There are many roles and responsibilities for the successful implementation of Six Sigma. The overall Six Sigma methodology requires a deployment leader or executive leadership, a champion or process owner, a master black belt (MBB), a black belt (BB), a green belt (GB), and a yellow belt (YB) (Six Sigma Institute 2024). Table 19.3 outlines the Six Sigma roles and responsibilities.

TABLE 19.1
Eight Forms of Waste and Their Meanings

Type of Waste	Meaning	Examples
Defects	Anything that does not meet customer spssecification or is incomplete.	- Wrong vendor number. - Incorrect traveler detail.
Overproduction	Producing more, better, or sooner than required by the customer.	- Parts produced beyond the production plan and forecast. - Printing paperwork (that might change) before it is needed.
Waiting	Any delay throughout the value stream.	- Waiting for parts to be delivered from the vendor. - Waiting for qualification testing results from the engineering team.
Non-utilization of Skills	Not using employees' full intellectual contribution.	- Supervisors doing admin tasks. - Having highly paid staff do routine tasks that don't require their unique expertise.
Transportation	Too many hand-offs or extra movement of work across the value stream.	- Excessive movement of parts from one area to another. - Manual transport of production parts from front line to end of line.
Inventory	Work waiting in a queue to be processed.	- Overstock of nonmoving raw materials in storage.
Motion	Movement of body or mind to perform work.	- Dragging too many data fields that could be auto-uploaded with a macro. - Walking to copier, printer, fax.
Extra-processing	Exerting more effort than needed.	- Unnecessary approvers/reviewers. - Duplicate processes.

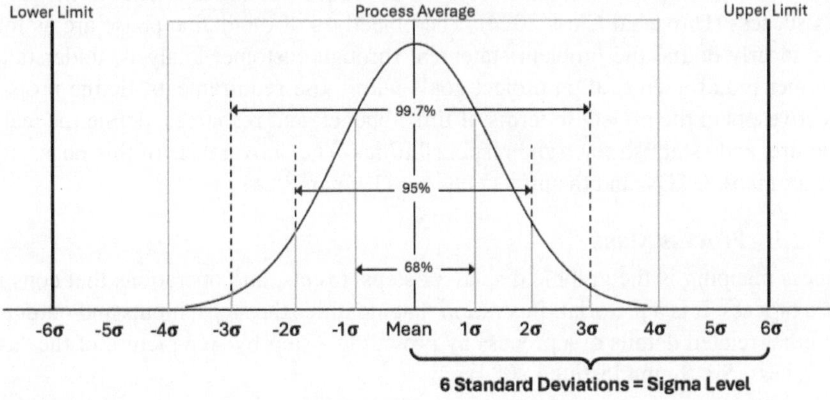

FIGURE 19.2 Six standard deviations

TABLE 19.2
Sigma Level of Companies

Yield	Defects per Million Opportunities	Cost of Poor Quality	Sigma	Company Classification
99.9997%	3.4	<10%	6	World Class Benchmarks
	233	10–15%	5	
	6,210	16–20%	4	Industry Average
	66,807	21–30%	3	
	308,537	31–40%	2	Non-competitive
	500,000	>40%	1	

19.5.1 The Phase Approach of Six Sigma

Six Sigma created a realistic and quantifiable goal of 3.4 defects per million opportunities, along with a methodology to attain that goal. This methodology, introduced by Motorola, was a problem-solving strategy made up of four steps, namely: measure, analyze, improve, and control. But when General Electric launched Six Sigma, they improved the methodology to include the define phase (Six Sigma BELT Guru 2024). Today, the define phase is an important aspect of the methodology and is now called DMAIC (define, measure, analyze, improve, control). Figure 19.3 shows the roadmap for the DMAIC approach.

19.5.2 Define Phase

The define phase is the first phase in all Six Sigma projects, whether the goals of the project are process improvement or better-designed products (6σ Certification Course 2024). It lays the foundation for the entire project and is crucial to the project's success (Universal Class 2024). The objectives of the define phase are as follows: clearly define the problem statement through customer analysis, understand customer requirements, align project goals with those requirements, define project objectives, plan the project in terms of time, budget, and resources, define the team structure, and establish roles and responsibilities. The deliverables of this phase are process maps, CTQs, and the project charter (Kumar 2024).

19.5.2.1 Process Maps

Process mapping is the graphic display of steps, events, and operations that constitute a process. It is a pictorial illustration that identifies the steps, inputs and outputs, and other related details of a process by providing a step-by-step picture of the "as-is" process (Six Sigma Institute 2024).

Process maps are very important because they help all process members understand their role and how their work fits into the big picture. They show you where you can take measurements that will help you run the process better, help you understand

TABLE 19.3
Six Sigma Roles and Responsibilities

Six Sigma Role	Responsibilities
Six Sigma Deployment Leader or executive—owns the vision for the business, they provide sponsorship and set expectations for the results from Six Sigma. They enable the organization to apply Six Sigma and then monitor the progress against expectations.	- Establishes business objectives and the role of Six Sigma to achieve those goals.- Creates an environment which enables success including goals, measures, coaching, and communication, among others.- Actively participates in Six Sigma activities and projects.
Six Sigma Champion/Sponsor—Project Champions or sponsors are the managers of the business, function, or value stream which has been identified as high priority.	- Identifies and selects the most meaningful projects to work on.- Provides guidance to the Six Sigma belters.- Obtains needed project resources.- Eliminates roadblocks and must ensure process improvements are captured and sustained.- Participates in all project reviews.
Six Sigma Master Black Belts (MBB)—Are technical expert, a go-to person for Six Sigma methodology. Responsible for translating the high-level business goals into a Six Sigma strategy for the division and the supporting tactics. Works with the Deployment Leader to achieve business goals.	- Provides advice and counsel to executive leadership.- Leads the development of Six Sigma skills in the organization through providing training (in class and onsite mentoring) and support for Black Belts, Green Belts, and the general associate base.- Develops sustainability for the business.- Facilitates cultural change.- Coordinates and lead activity on key cross-functional value streams.
Six Sigma Black Belts (BB)—Are application experts and work projects within the business. A BB is a project team leader, working full time to solve problems under the direction of a Champion, and with technical support from the MBB. BB's work on projects that are relatively complex and requires significant focus to resolve. Most BB's conduct an average of four to six projects a year—with a high financial return to the company.	- Acts a project team leader.- Facilitates DMAIC teams in applying Six Sigma methods to solve problems.- Works cross-functionally.- Contributes to the accomplishment of organizational goals.- Provides technical support to improvement efforts.
Six Sigma Green Belts (GB)—Are practitioners of Six Sigma methodology and typically work within their functional areas or support larger black belt projects. They usually address less-complex problems than black belts and perform at least two projects per year.	- - Supports projects with process knowledge and data collection.- Helps in the definition and measurement of critical processes.
Six Sigma Yellow Belts (YB)—They fully understand the principles of six sigma and are capable of characterizing processes, solving problems associated with their work responsibilities, and implementing and maintaining the gains from improvements.	- Provides support to GB's and BB's in developing process maps, helping with data capture, facilitating simulation, and improvements.

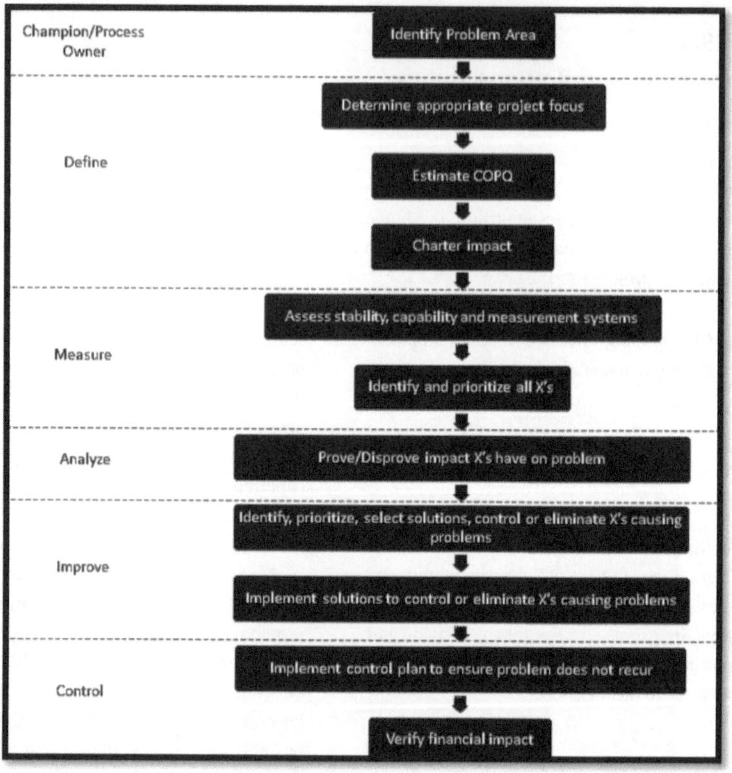

FIGURE 19.3 DMAIC phases roadmap

where problems like bottlenecks or delays occur, identify some of the causes, and can be used as aids in training people (Six Sigma BELT Guru 2024).

Some of the process maps commonly used are:

1. SIPOC or Supplier-Input-Process-Output-Customer: A high-level SIPOC chart helps identify the process outputs and their customers so that the voice of the customer (VoC) can be captured.
2. Cross-Functional Chart or Swim-lane Chart: Best used in transactional processes where multiple departments or functional groups are involved in a complex process. It can be drawn in a horizontal or vertical manner. In using this chart, one can see how the various departments are interdependent in this process.
3. Value Stream Map: A flowchart used to illustrate, analyze, and improve the steps required to deliver a product or service. It is used to review the flow of process steps and information from origin to delivery to the customer. This is especially useful for finding and eliminating waste.

If you want to drill down into a process, you can also try using process flow charts and process flow diagrams.

19.5.2.2 Project CTQs

Critical to Quality or CTQs are measures we use to capture the VoC properly. CTQs are sometimes difficult to understand, especially when they are vague and difficult to measure. The steps in developing CTQs include identifying the customer, capturing the voice of the customer, and validating the CTQ. To fully understand customer needs, CTQ Trees are created. CTQ Trees are diagram-based tools that help organizations develop and deliver high-quality products and services. They are used to translate broad customer needs into specific, actionable, and measurable performance requirements (MindTools 2024).

19.5.2.3 The Project Charter

A Lean Six Sigma project charter outlines key details, goals, intentions, and many other essential components of your project, serving as a roadmap. It is also used as a contract between the team implementing the project and the person funding it, who is known as the sponsor. This project charter helps lay out expectations, including milestones and expected deliverables, to keep everyone on schedule and in the loop, including both stakeholders and team members (Ciccarelli 2024).

There is no standard way of presenting a project charter. Each organization has its own standardized way to present a Six Sigma project charter. Therefore, the Six Sigma project charter can take many forms (Master of Project Academy 2024). However, it must have these common elements, which are found in every Six Sigma project charter.

19.5.2.3.1 Business Case

The business case is a high-level articulation of the area of concern. This case answers two primary questions: (1) What is the business motivation for considering the project? (2) What is the general area of focus for the improvement effort? It communicates the need for the project in terms of meeting business objectives. The components are: (a) output unit (product/service) for the external customer; (b) primary business measure of output unit for the project; (c) baseline performance of primary business measure; and (d) gap in baseline performance of primary business measure from the business objective (Six Sigma BELT Guru 2024).

Business Case Example: From *Academic Year 2012–2016* (period of time for baseline performance), *the average annual expenditure deviation* (primary business measure) for *office, school, and other supplies* (key business process) was *17.20%* (baseline performance). This gap of *12.2%* (business objective target vs. baseline) from *5%* (business objective) represents an annualized average cost impact of *USD195,000* (cost impact of gap).

19.5.2.3.2 Problem/Opportunity Statement

The problem statement may describe a business problem or pain point, while an opportunity statement identifies to an improvement opportunity (Master of Project Academy 2024, Six Sigma BELT Guru 2024).

Problem and Opportunity Statement Example: The inventory levels at the storage facility of ABC Company are consuming space, taking up asset management time and creating cash flow issues. The average inventory levels are 20 days, with a high of 33 days. These levels have exceeded the target of 14 days 77% of the time since March 2020 (problem statement). If inventory levels meet the target of 14 days, we could save an annualized average of USD450,000 (opportunity statement).

19.5.2.3.3 Objective Statement

The objective statement defines the expected improvement the team is seeking to achieve in clear, concise, and measurable terms. A good objective statement is SMART (specific, measurable, attainable, relevant, and time-bound), does not assign blame, presume cause, or prescribe a solution, and starts with a verb (reduce, achieve, control, increase, and so on) (SSDSI 2024).

Objective Statement Example: Increase the fill in rate of parts ordered by dealers in the ABC region from 84.80% to 90% starting February of 2020 and onward. This will result in an additional revenue of USD338,815.96 per month.

19.5.2.3.4 Project Scope

Project scope focuses on the boundaries and resources of the improvement efforts. The scope statement should include what is *in scope* (this could be departments, personnel, sites, equipment, and so on within the scope of the investigation and controllable) and what is *out of scope* (departments, personnel, sites, equipment, etc., outside the project's scope or control). If the scope has not been clearly defined, projects are subject to scope creep, which can result in projects that stall indefinitely. Scope creep can include a change request, update, or addition that was not in the initial scope. These changes can alter the intended outcome of the project and cause alterations or delays to the scope (SSDSI 2024).

Scope Statement Example:

- **In Scope:** Spare parts ordering and delivery process, inventory process, and accounting process for the ABC Region.
- **Out of Scope:** Production and marketing process.

19.5.2.3.5 Project Plan

The project plan contains a chart with the major milestones of the project. Often, the chart will contain the steps of DMAIC as a start (Master of Project Academy 2024). Figure 19.4 shows an example of a high-level project plan/timeline. Of course, the project team must follow this chart with a more detailed project plan.

Team structure refers to project resources like project managers, leaders, and project team members who are involved in the project (Master of Project Academy 2024). Figure 19.5 shows an example of a project team composition.

HIGH-LEVEL PROJECT TIMELINE				
	TARGET START	ACTUAL START	TARGET COMPLETION DATE	ACTUAL COMPLETION DATE
DEFINE	08/01/2019	08/15/2019	08/30/2019	
MEASURE	09/01/2019			
ANALYZE	10/01/2019			
IMPROVE	11/01/2019			
CONTROL	12/01/2019			

FIGURE 19.4 High-level project timeline

PROJECT TEAM COMPOSITION	
NAME	ROLE
	PROJECT CHAMPION / SPONSOR
	BLACK BELT / TEAM LEADER
	GREEN BELT / TEAM MEMBER
	YB / TEAM MEMBER
	TEAM MEMBER

FIGURE 19.5 Project team composition

Remember though that the project charter is a "living document," meaning the charter will be revised as you gain more knowledge about the project. Your problem statement, goal statement, and scope may change as you progress in your project (SSDSI 2024). Figure 19.6 shows a sample project charter template.

PROJECT CHARTER					
PROJECT NAME:					
BUSINESS CASE					PROBLEM/OPPORTUNITY STATEMENT
GOAL STATEMENT					PROJECT SCOPE
HIGH-LEVEL TIMELINE					PROJECT TEAM
	TARGET START	ACTUAL START	TARGET COMPLETE	ACTUAL COMPLETE	
DEFINE					
MEASURE					
ANALYZE					
IMPROVE					
CONTROL					
Prepared by:					Approved by:

FIGURE 19.6 Sample project charter template

19.5.3 Measure Phase

The measure phase focuses on identifying the problem by collecting data and conducting extensive analysis, including numerical and statistical studies. In this phase, you will identify which metric has the greatest impact on the problem so that it can be prioritized. The objective of this phase is to determine the significant measures that are essential to assess success, meet significant customer requirements, and start developing procedures to effectively gather data for quantifying performance (What Is Six Sigma 2024).

Deliverables in the measure phase include: (1) a robust description of the process workflow; (2) a quantitative assessment of how well the process is actually working; (3) an assessment of any measurement systems used to gather data for making decisions or to describe the performance of the process; and (4) a shortlist of potential causes of our problem—these are the X's that are most likely related to the problem (Six Sigma BELT Guru 2024).

The first deliverable refers to the tools used to facilitate process discovery, such as detailed process maps. In the define phase we enumerated different process mapping tools such as SIPOC, cross-functional charts, and value stream maps. Mapping the process identifies many important characteristics and develops information for other analytical tools. These tools will provide information about process inputs (X's), supplier requirements, process outputs (Y's), actual customer needs, value-adding and nonvalue-adding tasks and steps, data-collection points (such as cycle time, defects, COPQ, and so on), decision points, problems that have immediate fixes, and process control needs.

Many people think that process mapping is just drawing some shapes on a diagram, but it means much more than that. There are three levels of process mapping that are commonly accepted among the Six Sigma crowd (Six Sigma BELT Guru 2024, SPC Business Consulting 2020).

19.5.3.1 Level 1 Process Map

The Level 1 process map is typically how management views the processes of the organization. It is a big-picture, future-strategy kind of view. It also enables management to position the organization or resources in a way that complements the product/service being created. This is a high-level map that generally includes:

- Activities that relate to one major process step.
- How the process fits into the big picture.
- Little specific detail.
- Visualizes only major process steps.
- Can be used with only a general understanding of the purpose of the process and its steps.

19.5.3.2 Level 2 Process Map

The Level 2 process map is the "worker bee" process map, where the people who have specific knowledge of the process come in. This is the map that is used to identify all the major steps a worker takes to complete a process. Within Level 2, there are four types of process maps (Six Sigma BELT Guru 2024; SPC Business Consulting 2020):

- **Linear Flow:** A straight line from beginning to end.
- **Swim Lane:** Shows you who is responsible for each task.
- **SIPOC:** A little more complicated. It covers five areas: suppliers, inputs, process, outputs, and customers.
- **Value Stream:** A map that helps to visualize and understand performance metrics for major steps.

19.5.3.3 Level 3 Process Flow Chart and Process Flow Diagram or Micro Process Map

Level 3 process maps, also called improvement-level or viewpoint maps, similar to Level 2, show more steps and tasks and present performance data such as yield, cycle time, value-added and nonvalue-added time, defects, and so on (Six Sigma BELT Guru 2024). They focus on specific areas and the steps in the process that are causing whatever challenges you are having. It is a lot of information, but mapping a process is a fundamental step in your improvement project. It is absolutely critical that you get it right (SPC Business Consulting 2020).

19.5.3.4 Six Sigma Statistics

Peter Drucker once said, "What cannot be measured, cannot be improved." Therefore, we need to learn to communicate with processes in the language of data. Statistics provide tools and techniques to analyze data and turn it into useful information that you can use to make your decisions and manage your processes. Statistics is the science that deals with the collection, classification, analysis, and interpretation of numerical facts and data. It also provides a basis for making inferences about the future and provides the foundation for assessing process capability (Six Sigma BELT Guru 2024, GreyCampus 2024).

19.5.3.5 Types of Data

Using data to measure, analyze, improve, and control processes forms the foundation of Six Sigma methodology. Data turned into information, then transformed into knowledge, lowers the risks of poor decisions. The goal is to make decisions based on data and not on opinion or gut feel. One of the first steps for a Six Sigma practitioner is to understand the types of data they will be using and needing. There are two types of data:

- **Attribute Data:** Also called qualitative data, attribute data is binary in nature, for example, good or bad, yes or no. You cannot make much analysis based on this data. It must be converted to a form of variable data called discrete in order to make it useful (Six Sigma BELT Guru 2024).
- **Variable Data:** There are two types of variable data, namely discrete and continuous. Discrete data cannot be broken down into smaller units to add

meaning. It typically consists of whole numbers or integers. For example, there is no such thing as half a defect. Examples include number of chairs produced, population of college students, and so on. On the other hand, continuous data can be meaningfully divided into finer levels. It can be measured on a scale or continuum and can have almost any numeric value. For example, you can measure your height precisely in meters, centimeters, millimeters, and so on. You can record continuous data at so many different measurements—width, temperature, time, and so on. This is the key difference from discrete data (Valcheva 2024).

19.5.3.5 Process Capability

Process capability is the inherent reproducibility of a process's output. It measures how well the process is currently performing with respect to the output specifications. It refers to the uniformity of the process. Capability is often thought of in terms of the proportion of output that will be within product specification tolerances. The frequency of defectives produced may be measured in percentage (%), parts per million (ppm), and parts per billion (ppb) (Six Sigma BELT Guru 2024).

Cp and Cpk are process capability indices (Hessing 2024). Pp and Ppk are process performance indices. Both aim to verify if the process meets customer CTQs (requirements). Use Cp when the process is in statistical control and centered; use Cpk when in statistical control but not centered. This often happens with mature processes. Process capability uses sigma values determined from either the moving range, range, or sigma control charts. Pp and Ppk are used for process performance. Generally, you use these when a process is too new to determine if it is under statistical control. For example, during short preproduction runs or pilot processes. Because there is not a lot of historical data, we take large samples from the process to account for variation. Process performance generally uses sample sigma in its calculation.

19.5.4 Analyze Phase

The analyze phase focuses on brainstorming possible causes and validating root causes. Two of the most common tools used in this phase are root cause analysis (RCA) and the failure mode and effect analysis (FMEA). Later, we will enumerate the questions to ask and answer before proceeding to the next phase.

19.5.4.1 Root Cause Analysis

There are a lot of tools being used to brainstorm and validate root causes. The most widely used tools for root cause analysis are the Pareto chart and fishbone diagram.

19.5.4.2 Pareto Chart

A Pareto chart is a series of bars whose heights reflect the frequency or impact of categories under study. The bars are arranged in descending order of height from left to right. The categories represented by the tall bars on the left are relatively more significant than those of the right.

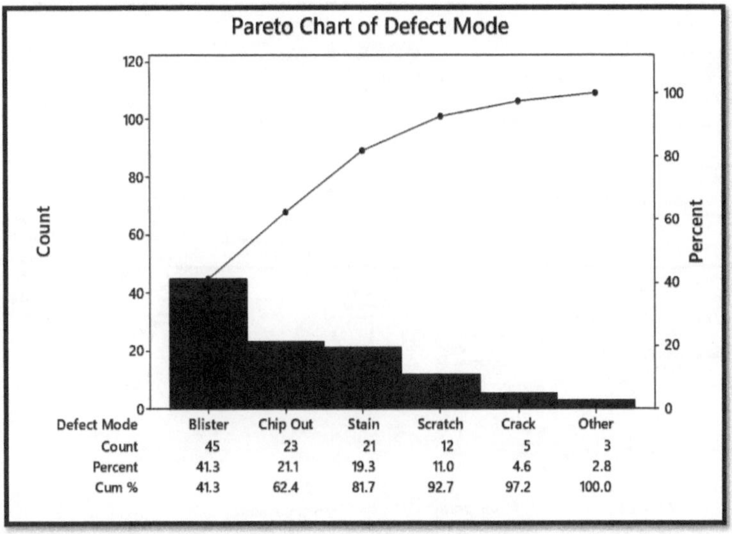

FIGURE 19.7 Sample Pareto chart of defect mode

The Pareto chart was based on the principle of "vital few and trivial many." For example, 80% of the total process output variability comes from 20% of the causes in the process. The Pareto chart can be an effective tool for problem identification as it can help separate the vital few from the trivial many. In addition to problem identification, the Pareto chart can also be used for problem analysis. For example, Figure 19.7 shows the same set of data plotted in two different ways using a Pareto chart.

19.5.4.3 Fishbone Diagram

The fishbone diagram, also known as a cause-and-effect diagram or Ishikawa diagram, is a graphical display of potential causes of a problem and their relationship to the effect (Figure 19.8). It is a visual tool used to identify, explore, and graphically display all the possible causes related to a problem to discover root causes. It was formalized by Dr. Kaoru Ishikawa, a quality statistician and one of the pioneers of Japan's quality revolution in the 1940s.

As the name implies, the fishbone diagram resembles a fishbone. The head of the fish is the effect being examined. The ribs that are connected to the backbone usually represent the categories from which potential causes of the problem would come. From the ribs, there are medium-sized bones that are connected. These represent the secondary causes. Lastly, the small bones are the root cause(s).

In constructing the fishbone diagram, you first need to decide which quality characteristic, outcome, or effect you want to examine. You may use the Pareto chart for this. Write the problem or effect on the head of the fish. Identify possible causes through brainstorming. Sort possible causes into categories and assign labels. The most common categories are man, machine, material, method, and environment (Mother Nature). Develop the main bones for each category. Afterward, develop

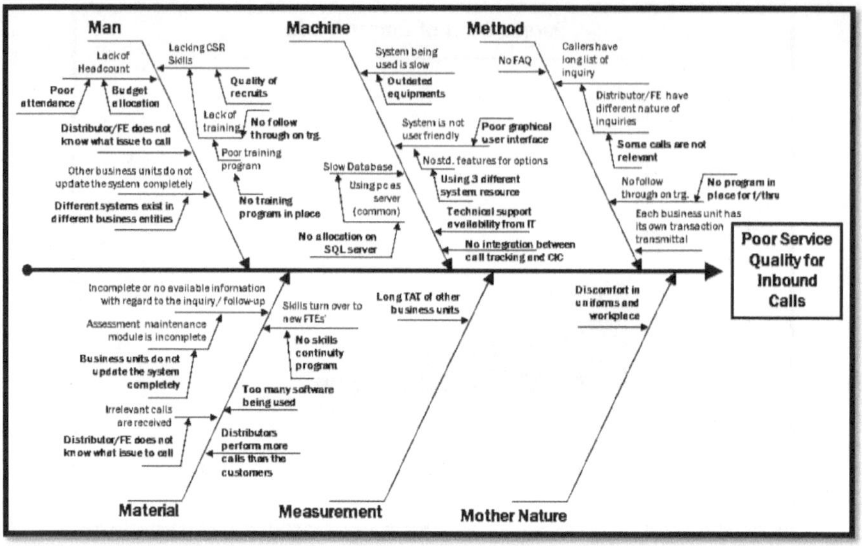

FIGURE 19.8 Sample fishbone diagram for poor service quality of inbound calls

the secondary bones of each category and ask, "Why did it happen?" until you have obtained the root cause.

When the fishbone diagram is completed, label every root cause as either a "C," "N," or "X," where:

"C": Variables that must be held as constant and require standard operating procedures to ensure consistency. Also known as controllable potential key performance input variables (KPIVs) or quick wins.

"N": Uncontrolled variables or noise that cannot be cheaply or easily held constant.

"X": Variables considered to be critical KPIVs that need to be experimented on to determine their influence on the output and what their optimal settings should be to achieve customer-desired performance. These usually need long-term or high-level interventions to be eliminated.

After labeling every root cause with "C," "N," or "X," the team shall analyze and zoom in on those "most likely causes." A helpful hint is to look out for causes that appear in more than one category, as they may be the "most likely causes." Prioritize these causes and perform further investigation or verification.

19.5.4.4 Failure Mode and Effect Analysis

FMEA is a systematic evaluation procedure whose purpose is to recognize and evaluate potential failure modes and causes associated with designing and manufacturing a new product or a change to an existing product. This tool includes identifying actions to eliminate or reduce the chance of potential failures and documenting the process.

FMEA is function-driven; it begins with a definition of the functions an item is supposed to perform. The inputs must come from several resources to be effective.

FMEA works on the principle of single-point failure, where failure of a specific item causes system failure. A failure mode is any design flaw, out-of-specification condition, or change in a product that prevents the product from functioning properly. By defining and eliminating failure modes, FMEA serves as a reliability tool by improving product reliability and focusing on potential failure modes early in the design process.

Types of failure modes include:

1. Failure to perform a defined function.
2. Unexpected or undesired occurrences.
3. Wrong application.

Types of FMEA include:

1. System FMEA is used to analyze systems and subsystems in the early concept and design stages.
2. Design FMEA is used to analyze products before they are released to production.
3. Process FMEA is used to analyze manufacturing, assembly, and administrative processes.

When to start conducting FMEA:

1. When new systems, products, and processes are being designed.
2. When the existing designs and processes are being changed.
3. When carryover designs or processes are used in new applications or environments.
4. After completing a problem-solving study to prevent recurrence of a problem.

Elements of FMEA:

1. **Failure Mode:** The manner in which the process could fail to perform its intended function. It could be a cause in a subsequent (downstream) operation or an effect associated with a potential failure in a previous (upstream) operation.
2. **Failure Effect:** The effect on both downstream operations and the end user if a failure occurs.
3. **Severity:** Rate the seriousness of the effect on a scale from 1 (least severe) to 10 (most severe).
4. **Causes:** The potential causes/root causes of the failure modes.
5. **Occurrence:** The likelihood of the failure to occur, rated from 1 (rare) to 10 (almost certain).

6. **Current Controls:** Methods for detecting the failure mode before it reaches downstream processes or the customer.
7. **Effectiveness:** How effective each current control method is; 10 implies no control/detection, and 1 suggests detection is nearly certain.

Three typical items that are scored to measure the FMEA:

1. **Severity:** Magnitude of the impact of the failure mode on either the customer or downstream process.
2. **Occurrence:** Frequency of the failure mode or cause occurring, based on actual performance data or historical references.
3. **Detection:** Capability of the process to detect and prevent defects from being shipped out.

The product of the scores derived from severity, occurrence, and detection is called the risk priority number. Figure 19.9 provides a template for a typical FMEA.

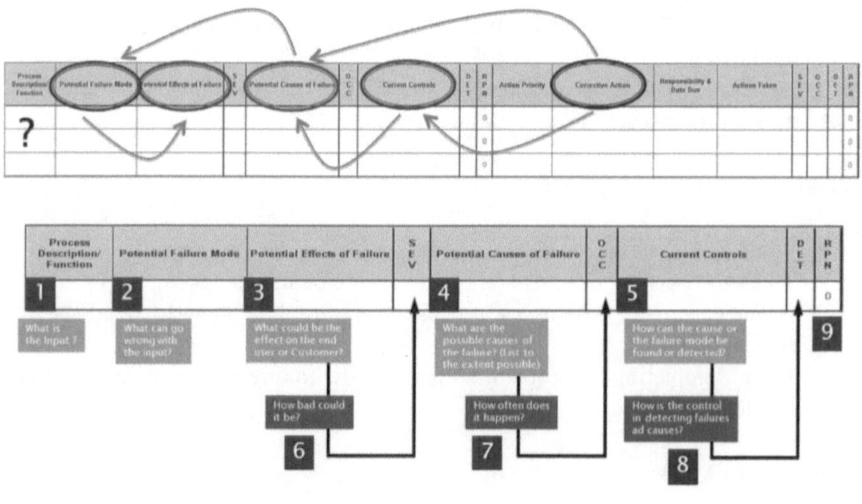

FIGURE 19.9 Typical FMEA template

Here are the questions that the team needs to ask and answer before proceeding to the next DMAIC phases:

1. What are the significant inputs (X's) affecting the output of concern (also known as Y's or critical-to-quality characteristics)?
2. Have you asked "why" enough times to move upstream and identify the root cause(s)?
3. Have you considered the relationships among multiple variables?

19.5.5 Improve Phase

The improve phase focuses on identifying improvement measures. This phase involves discussing commonly used improvement tools, error proofing, and validating improvement. Later, we will list the questions to ask and answer before proceeding to the next phase.

The key steps in the improve phase are:

1. Brainstorm potential solutions.
2. Evaluate and select the best solution.
3. Develop an action plan.
4. Perform potential risks assessment and stakeholder analysis.
5. Pilot solutions and check effectiveness.

19.5.5.1 Improvement Tools

19.5.5.1.1 Brainstorming

How to brainstorm?

a. Generate a long list of possibilities. This requires a maximum level of creativity.
b. Being creative means identifying ideas that might sound farfetched at the beginning. This improves the chances of exploring more innovative and out-of-the-box solutions.
c. Do not be restricted by boundaries, rules, constraints, policies, procedures, and norms.
d. Go for quantity—target at least 20 or so potential solutions.

Keep the following in mind:

a. Consider many possible solutions; do not assume the first solution is the best.
b. Look outside standard practice. Do not be constrained by the current system.
c. Challenge inbuilt rules and assumptions.
d. Logic can sometimes be helpful and sometimes inhibiting. At times, impractical and silly thoughts can lead to new ideas.
e. Do not be afraid of being laughed at.

19.5.5.1.2 Creativity Techniques

These methods help generate a long list of ideas:

a. **Analogy:** Identify another but similar (analogous) situation and generate ideas from there first.
b. **Antisolution:** Brainstorm the opposite of what you want to accomplish.

c. **Chain Letter:** Instead of a meeting, generate and pass ideas around via memo or email.
d. **Billboard:** Instead of meeting, gather ideas from the public.

19.5.5.1.3 Effectiveness and Practicality Matrix (Figure 19.10)

How to prepare an effectiveness and practicality matrix:

a. Copy the ideas on Post-it notes.
b. Place the ideas in the appropriate locations on the matrix.
c. Focus on the idea that is effective. If it is not practical, see what can be done to make it workable by asking questions such as:
   1. What is this idea trying to accomplish? Are there other means to accomplish the same thing?
   2. Is there a new technology that can make it work?
   3. Capture the refined ideas and add them to the list.

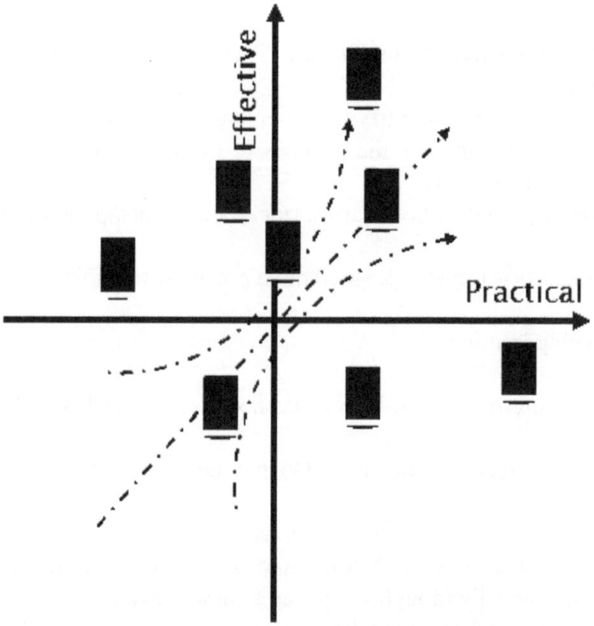

FIGURE 19.10 Effectiveness and practicality matrix

19.5.5.1.4 Solutions Evaluation Checklist

How to prepare a solutions evaluation matrix:

a. Generate a list of criteria.
b. Clearly define each criterion so that everyone has the same definition in mind.
c. Discuss and rate the solutions using the criteria.
d. Be open to new perspectives.
e. Look for the possibility to combine parts of different solutions.

Evaluation criteria:

a. Effectiveness of solution: How effective is the solution in addressing the root cause?
b. Impact on the organization: Which employees will be affected and how? How much resistance might there be?
c. Ease of implementation: How easy would it be to implement the solution?
d. Cost: Dollars, time, additional investments needed (e.g., equipment, training).
e. Time: How long will it take to implement the solution?

19.5.5.1.5 Paired-Choice Matrix

How to prepare a solution evaluation matrix:

a. Assign a letter to each solution. Set up a paired-choice matrix as shown previously.
b. Begin with the first row and decide which is the better solution between each pair.
c. Write in the box the choice between the two.
d. Skip the box with the same solutions.
e. Repeat the process for each row.
f. Tally up the number of A's, B's, and so on. The solutions chosen most frequently become the short list.

19.5.5.1.6 Potential Risk Assessment

Implementing improvement solutions usually involves making changes to the process. These changes may result in unexpected problems or side effects for the process involved or related processes. It is necessary to identify these potential risks and take preventive measures using the risk assessment tool.

How to prepare a risk assessment:

a. Brainstorm potential risk items:
    1. Possible adverse effects from introducing new methods.
    2. New factors that could cause the process to deteriorate from its improved state.

b. Quantify the risk level of each risk item.
c. For high-risk items, identify the appropriate preventive measures.

Quantifying risk level:

a. Rate the probability of the risk item occurring as high (H), medium (M), or low (L).
b. Rate the impact or severity of the risk item if it does occur. Again, use high (H), medium (M), or low (L).
c. Quantify the risk level of each risk item by multiplying its ratings of probability and impact. H is assigned a score of 3, M is 2, and L is 1.
d. The product is the risk level of the item.

19.5.5.1.7 Piloting Solution

The purposes of pilot testing are:

a. To further improve the solution.
b. To validate the expected results.
c. To facilitate buy-in.
d. To reduce the risk of failure.
e. To identify unknown performance problems.

Here are situations requiring pilot testing:

a. There are a lot of unknown factors involved, causing high risk of failure.
b. Implementing the change is costly, so effectiveness should be checked before full implementation.
c. The scope of change is large, and reversing the change would be difficult.
d. The change would have far-reaching, unforeseen consequences.

The pilot test and full implementation differ in terms of:

a. Scope/scale
b. Complexity
c. Duration/quantity
d. Both involve:
   1. Understanding the objective.
   2. Planning and executing of tasks that are necessary to achieve the objective.

19.5.5.1.8 Improvement Action Plan

After the best solutions have been selected comes the critical part: turning the solutions into reality. This takes much work, involves many people, and requires investment. It requires planning and follow through. Most importantly, the solutions must be able to solve the problem and result in the expected improvement. The improvement action plan outlines how to implement the selected solutions.

19.5.5.1.9 Contingency Planning

An implementation plan may be stalled due to unexpected problems that happen along the way. Prepare for potential problems by having a contingency plan. With a contingency plan in place, the team can keep the implementation plan going when these problems occur.

How to prepare contingency plans:

a. For each solution implementation plan, review the tasks and subtasks involved.
b. Identify the threats or potential problems may occur along the way.
c. Find out:
   1. What can be done to prevent those potential problems from occurring.
   2. How to deal with them if they occur.

In addition to effective use of tools, an innovative mindset and subject matter knowledge are also important for achieving effective solutions.

19.5.5.2 Error Proofing—Poke-Yoke

Poka-yoke (poh-kah yoh-keh) was coined in Japan during the 1960s by Shigeo Shingo, an industrial engineer at Toyota. Shingo is also credited with creating and formalizing zero quality control, combining poka-yoke techniques to correct possible defects with source inspection to prevent defects.

Poka-yoke helps people and processes work right the first time. Poka-yoke refers to techniques that make it impossible to make mistakes. These techniques can drive defects out of products and processes and substantially improve quality and reliability. Poka-yoke can be thought of as an extension of FMEA and can be used to fine-tune improvements and process designs from Six Sigma DMAIC projects. Simple poka-yoke ideas and methods in product and process design can eliminate both human and mechanical errors.

Poka-yoke can be used wherever something can go wrong or an error can be made. It is a technique that can be applied to any type of process, whether in manufacturing or the service industry. Error types include:

1. Processing Error: Process operation was missed or not performed according to the standard operating procedure.
2. Set-up Error: Using the wrong tooling or setting machine adjustments incorrectly.
3. Missing Part: Not all parts were included in the assembly, welding, or other processes.
4. Improper Part: Wrong part was used in the process.

Three Levels of Error Proofing:

1. Level 1: Prevent errors from happening.
2. Level 2: Detect the error after it has occurred.
3. Level 3: Detect the defect as soon as it is made.

Error Proofing Steps:

1. Create a process map.
2. If procedures are available, check if they are being followed.
3. List the defects that are usually found. Use a Pareto diagram to identify major defects.
4. Identify red flags that may cause the defects at each process step.
5. Identify appropriate prevention and detection measures.
6. Test the measures.
7. Check the effectiveness of measures.

19.5.5.3 Validating Improvements

We can validate the effectiveness of the solutions implemented by:

1. Comparing the variation of the process before and after improvement.
2. Comparing the process capability (Cpk and Ppk) before and after improvement.
3. Checking the variation of the process using a run chart to confirm improvement on spread.

Here are the questions that the team needs to ask and answer first before proceeding to the next DMAIC phases:

1. What actions can be taken to eliminate each root cause?
2. What benefits are expected?
3. Were the actions successful in addressing the root cause?
4. What is the new process capability?
5. What actions are in place to mitigate the risk of the changes to the process?

19.5.6 Control Phase

The control phase focuses on establishing a control system and disseminating lessons learned. This includes considerations for control phase, standardized work, process monitoring, and process dashboards. Finally, we will list questions that we need to ask and answer to determine the completeness of this phase.

19.5.6.1 Considerations for Control Phase

1. Create a process control plan.
2. Finalize documentation for the new or improved process.

3. Implement solution.
4. Regularly evaluate process performance utilizing a combination of leading and lagging indicators.
5. Make appropriate process adjustments where necessary.
6. Document learning.
7. Identify other areas in the organization where improvements and learning may be leveraged and create a transfer plan.

19.5.6.2 Standardized Work

Standardized work is used in project and process documentation, training of process owners, and monitoring and feedback systems. It can also be used as a control mechanism, including:

1. Policy Statements: Contain policy statements that prescribe the way an organization intends to carry out its business within its various functions.
2. Operating Procedures: Describe the established methods for performing and administering tasks.
3. Other Supporting Documents: Detail how the various tasks are to be carried out.

19.5.6.3 Process Monitoring

Process monitoring is critical to ensure that process improvements are sustained. It is most effective when applied to the Xs (leading indicators), but can also be applied to the process Y. A process control plan supports the process monitoring strategy. This is a documented method for how the process owners should respond to any out-of-control conditions that may occur in the process. It specifies required actions, timing, and owner.

19.5.6.4 Process-Monitoring Methods

1. Checklist: Listing of critical process activities needed to complete the process or operation successfully. Used as real-time verification that critical process steps have been completed. Used for standardized, low-throughput processes.
2. Statistical Process Control: Used for highly standardized process (X or Y with a high throughput).
3. Graphical Analysis: Keep statistical data on the output of the process and analyzes it to decide where adjustments are needed. This reactive, "after the fact" approach is used for nonstandardized, high-throughput processes.
4. Periodic Status Reports: Establish key milestones and deliverables. Review status and issues at defined frequency. Used for nonstandardized, low-throughput processes.

19.5.6.5 Process Dashboards

Process dashboards are visual trend charts that display the performance of the process. The two types of process dashboards are:

1. Time series dashboards: Show trends over time, as well as current performance.
2. Control charts: Identify the presence of special cause variation in the process and provide a trigger for action.

Here are the questions that the team needs to ask and answer in the control phase:

1. Did the actions in the large-scale implementation successfully accomplish the goal?
2. Is the process stable and in control?
3. Are plans in place to ensure that control will be maintained? Who is responsible?
4. What benefits were realized?
5. Where can the learning from this project be applied?

REFERENCES

6σ Certification Course. 2024. Define Phase of Lean Six Sigma Project – A Beginner's Guide. Available at: http://www.sixsigmacertificationcourse.com/define-phase-of-lean-six-sigma-project-a-beginners-guide/.

ASQ. 2024. What Is Six Sigma? Available at: https://asq.org/quality-resources/six-sigma.

Ciccarelli D. 2024. How to Write a Lean Six Sigma Project Charter in 7 Steps. Available at: https://www.goskills.com/Lean-Six-Sigma/Resources/Lean-six-sigma-project-charter.

Ehrenfeld T. 2010. The Lean and Six Sigma Marriage. Available at: http://artoflean.com/index.php/2011/01/05/the-lean-and-six-sigma-marriage/.

Feldman K. 2022. What Is Six Sigma? Available at: https://www.isixsigma.com/new-to-six-sigma/getting-started/what-six-sigma/.

GreyCampus. 2024. Introduction on Six Sigma Statistics. Available at: https://www.greycampus.com/opencampus/lean-six-sigma-green-belt/introduction-on-six-sigma-statistics.

Hessing T. 2024. Process Capability (Cp & Cpk). Available at: https://sixsigmastudyguide.com/process-capability-cp-cpk/.

Kumar P. 2024. What is Six Sigma: Everything You Need to Know About It. Available at: https://www.simplilearn.com/define-phase-of-lean-six-sigma-tutorial.

Lean Enterprise Institute. 2024. A Brief History of Lean. Available at: https://www.lean.org/whatslean/history.cfm.

MindTools. 2024. Available at: https://www.mindtools.com/pages/article/ctq-trees.

Master of Project Academy. 2024. 7 Elements of the Six Sigma Project Charter. Available at: https://blog.masterofproject.com/six-sigma-project-charter/.

RP News Wires. 2024. Robert W. Galvin Inducted into Six Sigma Hall of Fame. Available at: https://www.reliableplant.com/Read/22762/Galvin-Six-Sigma-Hall-of-Fame.

SixLeanSigma. 2021. Is Your Company Six Sigma? Available at: https://www.sixleansigma.com/index.php/2015/08/01/is-your-company-6-sigma-5-sigma-4-sigma-confuse-what-is-5-4-sigma/.

Six Sigma BELT Guru. 2024. Available at: https://www.6sigmabelt.com.

Six Sigma Institute. 2024. Six Sigma Roles and Responsibilities. https://www.sixsigma-institute.org/Six_Sigma_Roles_And_Responsibilities.php.

Skhmot N. 2017. What Is Lean? Available at: https://theleanway.net/what-is-lean.

SPC Business Consulting. 2020. 6 Sigma Tools: Process Mapping Levels. Available at: https://www.spcconsulting.org/2012/08/6sigma-tools-process-mapping-levels/.

SSDSI. 2024. How to Complete a Lean Six Sigma Project Charter. Available at: https://sixsigmadsi.com/how-to-complete-a-six-sigma-project-charter/.

Universal Class. 2024. The Define Phase in Six Sigma Projects. Available at: https://www.universalclass.com/articles/business/the-define-phase-in-six-sigma-projects.htm.

Valcheva S. 2024. Discrete vs Continuous Data: with Comparison Chart. Available at:: http://www.intellspot.com/discrete-vs-continuous-data/.

What Is Six Sigma. 2024. Six Sigma DMAIC – Measure Phase. Available at: https://www.whatissixsigma.net/six-sigma-dmaic-measure-phase/.

20 Learning Curve Application for Emergency Response

Adedeji B. Badiru

20.1 INTRODUCTION

Many manufacturing firms today operate in a fiscally constrained and financially conscious environment, where the level of improvement based on the number of repetitions is very important. Managers throughout these organizations are expected to maximize the utility of every dollar as budgets and profit margins shrink. Increased financial scrutiny has added greater emphasis on the accuracy of program and project management cost estimates to ensure production programs are sufficiently funded. Cost-estimating models and tools organizations use must be evaluated for their relevance and accuracy for reliable cost estimates. Many of the cost-estimating procedures for learning curves appeared following Wright's (1936) work and are still used today as a primary method for modeling learning. As automation and robotics increasingly replace human manual labor in many manufacturing processes, the current decades-old learning curve model may no longer provide the most accurate approach to productivity estimates.

It is necessary, therefore, to develop new learning curve models to capture the performance of automated production, and other technological factors that lead to reduced learning should be examined.

Since Wright's (1936) learning curve, researchers have found other functions to model learning within the manufacturing process (Badiru 2012; Boone et al. 2021; Carr 1946; Chalmers and DeCarteret 1949; Crawford 1944; De Jong 1957; Towill 1990; Towill and Cherrington 1994).

This chapter presents an application of the techniques and modeling of learning curves in emergency response activities. Typically applied in industrial production activities, learning curves have far broader applications in a variety of human pursuits. Wherever humans can learn and improve, learning curves can be applied to track levels of improvement based on the number of repetitions. In the case of emergency response, learning curves mirror the case of learning-and-forgetting models because repetitions occur infrequently. Because the same types of emergencies requiring the same types of responses do not occur frequently enough to facilitate continuous learning, the learning-and-forgetting models of learning curves

 DOI: 10.1201/9781003648178-22

are important to examine from a practical application perspective. Badiru's half-life curve model is applicable, and it is the primary basis for this chapter.

20.2 LITERATURE REVIEW

Learning curve research dates back to 1936 when Theodore Paul Wright published the original learning curve equation, which predicted the production effects of learning. Wright (1936) modeled the relationship between the time it takes for a worker to complete a single task and the number of times that worker has performed that task. The mathematical relationship developed from this hypothesis is that as workers complete the same process repeatedly, they get better at it. Specifically, Wright realized that the rate at which they improve at that task is constant. The relationship between these two variables is as follows: as the number of units produced doubles, the worker will do it faster at a constant rate. He proposed the following relationship:

$$F = N^x \text{ or } x = \frac{Log\, F}{Log\, N} \qquad \text{Equation 20.1}$$

where F is a cost variation factor proportional to the quantity N. The reciprocal of F then represents a direct percent variation of cost vs. quantity (Wright 1936). The relationship between these variables can be modified to predict the expected cost of a given unit number in production by multiplying F by the theoretical cost of the first unit produced—this relationship was stated in the fundamental equation of learning curves. It is a log-linear relationship, as demonstrated through algebraic manipulation. The logarithmic form of this equation (taking the natural log of both sides of the equation) allows practitioners to run linear regression analysis on the data to find the slope that best fits the data using a straight line (Martin 2019).

The goal of using learning curves is to increase the accuracy of cost estimates and production output. Accurate cost estimates allow an organization to efficiently budget while providing as much operational capability as possible, allowing resources to be allocated to higher priorities. While learning curves focus on creating accurate cost estimates, they often use the labor hours it takes to perform a task. When Wright originated the theory, he proposed the output in terms of time to produce, not production cost. However, many organizations perform learning curve analysis on production cost and production time per unit, depending on the available data. Nevertheless, labor hour cost is relevant because it is based on factors such as labor rates and other associated values. Using labor hours in learning curve development allows a common comparison over time without the effects of inflation convoluting the results. However, the same goal can be achieved by using inflation-adjusted cost values.

Wright's model has been compared to some of the more contemporary models that have surfaced in recent years since the original learning curve theory was established (Moore et al. 2015). Moore compared the Stanford-B, DeJong, and S-curve models to Wright's model to see if any of these functions could provide a more accurate estimate of the learning phenomenon. The DeJong and S-curve models both use an incompressibility factor in their calculations. Incompressibility is a factor used to account for the percentage of automation in the production process. Values of the incompressibility factor can range from 0 to 1, where 0 is all touch labor and 1 is complete automation. Moore found that when using an incompressibility factor between 0 and 0.1, the DeJong and S-curve models were more accurate than that of Wright (Moore et al. 2015). In other words, when a production process had very little automation and high amounts of touch labor, the newer learning curve models tended to be more accurate. Wright's model was more accurate for incompressibility values larger than 0.1 but less than 1.

More recently, Johnson (2016) proposed that a flattening effect is evident at the end of the production process, where learning does not continue at a constant rate near the end of a production cycle. Using the same models as Moore, Johnson explored the difference in accuracy between Wright's model and contemporary models at earlier versus later stages in the production process. He had similar findings to Moore in that Wright's model was most accurate except when the incompressibility factor values were close to zero. When the incompressibility factor is low, more touch labor is involved in the process, allowing for the possibility of additional learning to occur. He also found that Wright's learning curve was more accurate early in the production process, whereas the DeJong and S-curve models were more accurate later in the production process (Johnson 2016).

Another key concept in learning curve estimation and modeling is the idea of a forgetting curve (Honious et al. 2016). A forgetting curve explains how configuration changes in the production process can cause a break in learning, which diminishes the efficiency that had previously been gained. When a configuration change occurs, the production process changes. Changes may include factors such as using different materials, different tooling, adding steps to a process, or might even be attributed to workforce turnover. The new process affects how workers complete their tasks and causes previously learned efficiencies to be lost. If manufacturers fail to take these breaks into account, they may underestimate the total effort needed to produce a product. Honious et al. (2016) found that configuration changes significantly changed the learning curve and that the new learning curve slope was steeper than the previous steady slope prior to a configuration change. The distinction between pre- and post-configuration changes is important to ensure both types of effects are taken into account.

The International Cost Estimating and Analysis Association (ICEAA) published learning curve training material in 2013. While presenting the basics of learning curve theory, it also presented some rules of thumb for learning. The first rule is that learning curves are steepest when the production process is touch-labor intensive. Conversely, learning curves are the flattest when the production process is highly automated (ICEAA 2013). Another key piece of information is that adding new work to the process can affect the overall cost. ICEAA states that this essentially adds a new curve for the added work, which increases the original curve by the amount of the new curve (ICEAA 2013). Equation 20.2 is as follows:

$$Cost(x) = A_1 x^{b_1} + A_2 (x - L)^{b_2} \qquad \text{Equation 20.2}$$

where:

$Cost(x)$ = cumulative average cost per unit.
A_1 = theoretical cost to produce the first unit prior to the addition of new work.
A_2 = theoretical cost to produce the first unit after the addition of new work.
x = cumulative number of units produced.
L = last unit produced before addition of new work.
ϕ_1 = learning rate ($0 < \phi_1 < 1$), before additional work.
ϕ_2 = learning rate ($0 < \phi_2 < 1$), after additional work.
$b_i = \phi_i / \ln(2)$, learning exponent where i = 1, 2.

Equation 20.2 is important to consider when generating an estimate after a major configuration change or engineering change proposal (ECP). For example, while producing the eighth unit of an aircraft, the customer realizes they need to drastically change the aircraft's radar. Learning has already taken place on the first eight aircraft; the new radar has not yet been installed, and therefore, no learning has taken place. To accurately take into account the new learning, the radar would be treated as a second part of the equation, ensuring we account for the learning on the eight aircraft while also accounting for no learning on the new radar.

Lastly, Anderlohr (1969) and Mislick and Nussbaum (2015) write about production breaks and the effects they have on the learning curve. These production breaks can cause a direct loss of learning, which can fully or partially reset the learning curve. For example, a 50% loss of learning would result in a loss of half of the cost reduction that has occurred (ICEAA 2013). This information is important when analyzing past data to ensure that breaks in production are accounted for.

Thus far, we have laid out the fundamental building blocks of learning curve theory and how they might be applied in a production environment. Wright's learning curve formula established the method by which many organizations account for learning during the procurement process. Following Wright's findings, other methods have emerged that account for breaks in production, the natural loss of learning over time, incompressibility factors, and half-life analysis (Benkard 2000). This chapter adds to the discussion by examining the flattening effect and how various models predict learning at different points in the production process.

When examining learning curve theory and the effects learning has on production, it is critical to understand the production process being estimated. Since Wright established the learning curve theory in 1936, factory automation and technology have grown tremendously and continue to grow. Contemporary learning curve methods try to account for this automation. To get the best understanding, we examine the aircraft industry, specifically how it operatees in relation to the rest of the manufacturing industry.

The aircraft industry has relatively low automation compared to other industries (Kronemer and Henneberger 1993). Kronemer and Henneberger (1993) state that the aircraft industry is a fairly labor-intensive process with relatively little reliance on automated production techniques, despite it being a high-tech industry. Specifically, they list three main reasons why manufacturing aircraft is so labor-intensive. First, aircraft manufacturers usually build multiple models of the same aircraft, typically for the commercial sector alone. These different aircraft models mean different tooling and configurations are needed to meet the customer's demand. Second, aircraft manufacturers deal with a very low unit volume compared to other manufacturing industries. The final reason for low levels of automation is the fact that aircraft are highly complex and have very tight tolerances. To attain these specifications, manufacturers must continue to use highly skilled touch laborers or spend extremely large amounts of money on machinery to replace them (Kronemer and Henneberer 1993). For these reasons, we typically use low incompressibility factors in learning curve models when estimating within the aircraft industry.

Although the aircraft industry remains largely unaffected by the shift from human labor to machine production, many industries are seeing a rise in the percentage of manufacturing processes that are automated. In a 2012 *Wall Street Journal* article, the author showed how companies have been increasing the amount of money spent on machines and software while spending less on manpower. They proposed that part of the reason behind this shift was a temporary tax break "that allowed companies in 2011 to write off 100% of investments in the first year" (Aeppel 2012). Tax breaks combined with extremely low interest rates provide the industry with incentives to invest in future production. Investment in production technology increases the incompressibility factor that should be used when estimating the effects of learning. In a separate article for *The Wall Street Journal*, Madigan (2011) also pointed out the increase in spending on capital investments in labor. Madigan stated that "businesses had increased their real spending on equipment and software by a strong 26%, while they have added almost nothing to their payrolls."

20.3 IMPLICATIONS FOR EMERGENCY SUPPLY CHAINS

Although the methodology of this research centers on general production systems using US Air Force data, it is directly applicable to the case of general relationships between a production system and supply chain networks. The half-life learning curve model presented by Badiru (2012) is particularly relevant for dynamic technology-sensitive supply chains where learning and relearning can change over a short period. An appreciation and incorporation of learning curves can help mitigate supply chain risks.

20.3.1 Learning Curves and Innovations for Emergency Response

Learning curves, also known as performance progress functions, are used extensively in business, science, technology, engineering, and industry to predict system performance over time. Learning curves have a direct application in the quantitative analysis of innovation, particularly because of the dynamism of technology driving innovation. The innovation of today may be outdated tomorrow. Innovation of the future may not yet be conceived. Although most of the early development and applications of learning curves were in the area of production engineering, contemporary applications can be found in all areas of applications. Technology, in particular, offers a fertile area for the application of learning curves. This chapter applies the concept of the half-life of learning curves to innovation management. This is useful for predictive measures of technology system performance. In the parlance of radioactive elements in physical science, half-life is the amount of time it takes for a quantity to diminish to half of its original size through natural processes. The approach of half-life computation provides an additional decision tool for researchers and practitioners in technological innovation management. The derivation of the half-life equations for learning curves can reveal more about the properties of these curves, particularly with respect to the unique lifecycle properties of new and old technologies. The half-life theory of learning curves introduced by Badiru and Ijaduola (2009) offers a good technique for an accurate assessment.

Innovation has several unique characteristics that make its management challenging. Some of these characteristics include frequent lifecycle changes in technology and uncertainty in the operating environment. Learning curve analysis offers a viable approach for evaluating innovation systems that involve human learning and forgetting. With an effective learning curve evaluation, an assessment can be made of how the pursuit of innovation meets organizational objectives and maximizes its benefits to the organization. Figure 20.1 illustrates a conventional curve of the lifecycle of innovation as a function of resource infusion. In reality, there will be dips in the curve due to the effects of learning and forgetting phenomena. It is essential to be able to predict the locations of such dips so that an accurate assessment of the overall technology performance can be performed.

The fact is that the fast pace of technology affects learning curves, and frequent changes in technology can degrade them. Thus, a specialized analytical assessment of learning curves is needed for innovation management. The degradation of learning curves is often depicted analytically by incorporating forgetting components into conventional learning curves, as has been shown in the literature over the past few decades (Badiru 1994, 1995a; Jaber and Sikström 2004; Jaber et al. 2003; Jaber and Bonney 1996; Jaber and Bonney 2007; Nembhard and Osothsilp 2001; Nembhard and Uzumeri 2000; Sule 1978; Globerson et al. 1998).

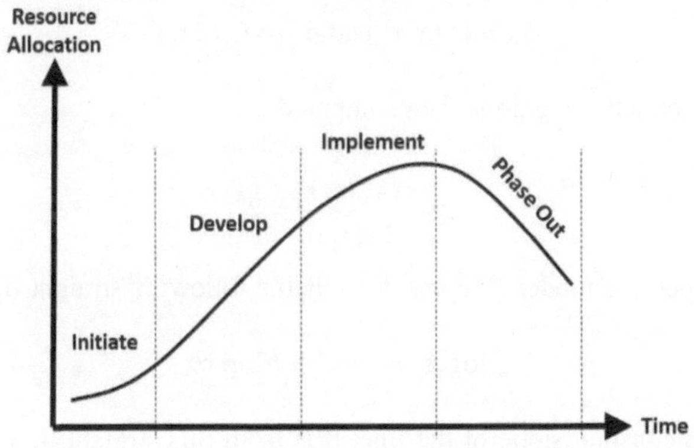

FIGURE 20.1 Innovation lifecycle

20.3.2 Basic Learning Curve Calculations

There are several models of learning curves in use in business and industry. The log-linear model is perhaps the most extensively used. The log-linear model states that productivity improvement is constant (i.e., it has a constant slope) as output increases. There are two basic forms of the log-linear model: the average cost function and the unit cost function.

The average cost model is used more than the unit cost model. It specifies the relationship between the cumulative average cost per unit and cumulative production. The relationship indicates that the cumulative cost per unit will decrease by a constant percentage as the cumulative production volume doubles. The *average cost* model is expressed as:

$$A_x = C_1 x^b \qquad \text{Equation 20.3}$$

where:

A_x = cumulative average cost of producing x units.
C_1 = cost of the first unit.
x = cumulative production count.
b = the learning curve exponent (i.e., a constant slope on log-log paper).

The relationship between the learning curve exponent, b, and the learning rate percentage, p, is given by:

$$b = \frac{\log p}{\log 2} \text{ or } p = 2^b \qquad \text{Equation 20.4}$$

The derivation of the above relationship can be seen by considering two production levels where one level is double the other, as shown below. Let Level I = x_1 and Level II = $x_2 = 2x_1$. Then,

$$A_{x_1} = C_1(x_1)^b \text{ and } A_{x_2} = C_1(2x_1)^b \qquad \text{Equation 20.5}$$

The percent productivity gain is then computed as:

$$p = \frac{C_1(2x_1)^b}{C_1(x_1)^b} = 2^b \qquad \text{Equation 20.6}$$

On log-log paper, the model is represented by the following straight-line equation:

$$\log A_x = \log C_1 + b \log x \qquad \text{Equation 20.7}$$

where b is the constant slope of the line. It is from this straight line that the name log-linear was derived.

20.3.2.1 Computational Example 1

Assume that 50 units of an item are produced at a cumulative average cost of \$20 per unit. Suppose we want to compute the learning percentage when 100 units are produced at a cumulative average cost of \$15 per unit. The learning curve analysis would proceed as follows:

(i) Initial production level = 50 units; average Cost = \$20.
(ii) Double production level = 100 units; cumulative average cost = \$15.
(iii) Using the log relationship, we obtain the following equations:

$$\log(20) = \log C_1 + b\log(50) \qquad \text{Equation 20.8 and 20.9}$$

$$\log(15) = \log C_1 + b\log(100)$$

(iv) Solving the equations simultaneously yields

$$b = \frac{\log(20) - \log(15)}{\log(50) - \log(100)} = -0.415$$

Thus, $p = (2)^{-0.415} = 0.75$, i.e., a 75% learning rate. In general, the learning curve exponent, *b*, may be calculated directly from actual data or computed analytically. That is:

$$b = \frac{\log A_{x_1} - \log A_{x_2}}{\log x_1 - \log x_2} \qquad \text{Equation 20.10}$$

or

$$\text{b} = \frac{\ln(\text{p})}{\ln(2)} \qquad \text{Equation 20.11}$$

where

x_1 = first production level.
x_2 = second production level.
A_{x_1} = cumulative average cost per unit at the first production level.
A_{x_2} = cumulative average cost per unit at the second production level.
p = learning rate percentage.

Using the basic cumulative average cost function, the total cost of producing *x* units is computed as:

$$TC_x = (x)A_x = (x)C_1x^b = C_1x^{(b+1)}$$ Equation 20.12

The unit cost of producing the *x*th unit is given by:

$$U_x = C_1\left[x^{1+b} - (x-1)^{1+b}\right]$$ Equation 20.13

The marginal cost of producing the *x*th unit is given by:

$$MC_x = \frac{d[TC_x]}{dx} = (b+1)C_1x^b$$ Equation 20.14

20.3.2.2 Computational Example 2

Suppose in a production run of a certain product, it is observed that the cumulative hours required to produce 100 units is 100,000 hours with an 85% learning curve. For project planning purposes, an analyst needs to calculate the number of hours spent producing the 50th unit. Following the notation used previously, we have the following information: $p = 0.85$, $x = 100$ units, $A_x = 100{,}000$ hours/100 units = 1,000 hours/unit. Now, $0.85 = 2^b$ corresponding to $b = -0.2345$, with $C_1 = (1{,}000)100^{0.2345}$ = 2,944.42 hours. Thus, the cumulative average hours for 50 units is $C_{50} = (2{,}944.42)(50)^{-0.2345}$ = 1,176.50 hours, and the cumulative total hours for 50 units is 58,824.91 hours. Similarly, $C_{49} = (2{,}944.42)(50)^{-0.2345}$ = 1,182.09 hours, and the cumulative total hours for 49 units is 57,922.17 hours. Consequently, the number of hours for the fiftieth unit is $C_{50} - C_{49}$ = 902.74 hours.

The unit cost model is expressed in terms of the specific cost of producing the *x*th unit. The unit cost formula specifies that the individual cost per unit will decrease by a constant percentage with the doubling of cumulative production. The formulation of the unit cost model is presented below. Define the average cost as:

$$A_x = C_1x^b$$ Equation 20.15

The total cost is defined as:

$$TC_x = (x)A_x = (x)C_1x^b = C_1x^{(b+1)}$$ Equation 20.16

The marginal cost is given by:

$$MC_x = \frac{d[TC_x]}{dx} = (b+1)C_1x^b$$ Equation 20.17

This is the cost of one specific unit. Therefore, define the unit cost model as:

$$U_x = (1+b)C_1x^b$$ Equation 20.18

where U_x is the cost of producing the xth unit. To derive the relationship between A_x and U_x

$$U_x = (1+b)C_1 x^b \qquad \text{Equation 20.19}$$

$$\frac{U_x}{(1+b)} = C_1 x^b = A_x \qquad \text{Equation 20.20}$$

$$A_x = \frac{U_x}{(1+b)} \qquad \text{Equation 20.21}$$

$$U_x = (1+b)A_x \qquad \text{Equation 20.22}$$

To derive an expression for finding the cost of the first unit, C_1, we will proceed as follows. Since $A_x = C_1 x^b$, we have:

$$C_1 x^b = \frac{U_x}{(1+b)} \qquad \text{Equation 20.23}$$

$$\therefore C_1 = \frac{U_x x^{-b}}{(1+b)} \qquad \text{Equation 20.24}$$

For the case of continuous product volume (e.g., chemical processes), we have the following corresponding expressions:

$$TC_x = \int_0^x U(z)\,dz = C_1 \int_0^x z^b\,dz = \frac{C_1 x^{(b+1)}}{b+1} \qquad \text{Equation 20.25}$$

$$Y_x = \left(\frac{1}{x}\right)\frac{C_1 x^{(b+1)}}{b+1} \qquad \text{Equation 20.26}$$

$$MC_x = \frac{d[\mathrm{TC}_x]}{dx} = \frac{d\left[\dfrac{C_1 x^{(b+1)}}{b+1}\right]}{dx} = C_1 x^b \qquad \text{Equation 20.27}$$

20.3.3 Half-lives

As another approach to capturing the essence of performance degradation in learning curves, Badiru and Ijaduola (2009) introduced the half-life theory of learning curves.

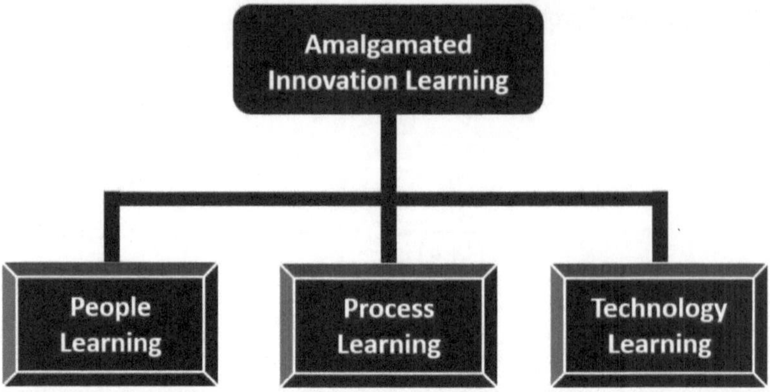

FIGURE 20.2 Learning in the innovation environment

Traditionally, the standard time has been used as an indication of when learning should cease or when resources need to be transferred to another job. It is possible that half-life theory can supplement standard time analysis. The half-life approach will encourage researchers and practitioners to reexamine conventional applications of existing learning curve models. Organizations invest in people, work processes, and technology to achieve performance improvement. The systematic nature of such an investment strategy requires that the investment be strategically planned over multiple years. Thus, changes in learning curve profiles over those years become very crucial. Forgetting analysis and half-life computations can provide additional insights into learning curve changes. Through the application of robust learning curve analysis, system innovation can be achieved in terms of cost, time, and performance, with respect to the strategic investment of funds and other organizational assets in people, processes, and technology, as shown in Figure 20.2. The predictive capability of learning curves helps plan for integrated system performance improvement that can drive innovation.

Formal analysis of learning curves first emerged in the mid-1930s in connection with the analysis of the production of airplanes (Wright 1936). Learning refers to the improved operational efficiency and cost reduction obtained from the repetition of a task. This directly impacts training purposes and the design of work. Workers learn and improve by repeating operations. But they also regress due to the impact of forgetting, prolonged breaks, work interruptions, and the natural degradation of performance. Half-life computations can provide a better understanding of actual performance levels over time. Half-life is the amount of time it takes for a quantity to diminish to half of its original size through natural processes. Duality is of natural interest in many real-world processes. We often speak of "twice as much" and "half as much" as benchmarks for process analysis. In economic and financial principles, the "rule of 72" refers to the length of time required for an investment to double in value. These common "double" or "half" concepts provide the motivation for half-life analysis.

The usual application of half-life is in natural sciences. For example, in physics, the half-life is a measure of the stability of a radioactive substance. In practical terms, the half-life attribute of a substance is the time it takes for one-half of the atoms in an initial magnitude to disintegrate. The longer the half-life of a substance, the more stable it is. This provides a good analogy for modeling learning curves with the recognition of increasing performance or decreasing cost with respect to the passage of time. The approach provides another perspective on the large body of literature on learning curves. Badiru and Ijaduola (2009) present the following formal definitions:

For learning curves: *Half-life* is the production level required to reduce the cumulative average cost per unit to half of its original size.

For forgetting curves: *Half-life* is the amount of time it takes for performance to decline to half its original magnitude.

20.3.4 Degradation over Time

Although there is an extensive collection of classical studies of *improvement* due to learning curves, only very limited attention has been paid to performance *degradation* due to the impact of forgetting. Some of the classical works on process improvement due to learning include Belkaoui (1976), Camm et al. (1987), Liao (1979), Mazur and Hastie (1978), McIntyre (1977), Nanda (1979), Pegels (1976), Richardson (1978), Smith (1989), Smunt (1986), Sule (1978), Womer (1979, 1981, 1984), Womer and Gulledge (1983), and Yelle (1976, 1979, 1983). It is only in recent years that the recognition of "forgetting" curves has begun to emerge, as can be seen in more recent literature (Badiru 1995b; Jaber and Sikström 2004; Jaber et al. 2003; Jaber and Bonney 2003, 2007; Jaber and Guiffrida 2008). The new and emerging research on the forgetting components of learning curves motivated studying the half-life properties of learning curves. Performance decay can occur due to several factors, including a lack of training, reduced retention of skills, lapses in performance, extended breaks in practice, and natural forgetting. The conventional learning curve equation introduced by Wright (1936) has a drawback whereby the cost or time per unit approaches zero as the cumulative output approaches infinity. That is:

$$\lim_{x\to\infty} C(x) = C_1 \lim_{x\to\infty} x^{-b} \to 0 \qquad \text{Equation 20.28}$$

Researchers who initially embraced Wright's learning curve (WLC) assumed a lower bound for the equation such that WLC could be represented as:

$$C(x) = \begin{cases} C_1 x^{-b}, & \text{if } x < x_s \\ C_s \;, & \text{otherwise} \end{cases} \qquad \text{Equation 20.29}$$

where x_s is the number of units required to reach standard cost C_s. A half-life analysis can reveal more information about the properties of WLC, particularly when we consider the operating range of $x_0 < x_s$.

20.3.5 Half-Life of Learning Curves

Learning curves present the relationship between cost (or time) and the level of activity on the basis of the effect of learning. An early study by Wright (1936) disclosed the "80% learning" effect, which indicates that a given operation is subject to a 20% productivity improvement each time the activity level or production volume *doubles*. The proposed half-life approach is the antithesis of the double-level milestone. A learning curve can serve as a predictive tool for obtaining time estimates for tasks that are repeated within a project lifecycle. A new learning curve does not necessarily commence each time a new operation is started, since workers can sometimes transfer previous skills to new operations. The point at which the learning curve begins to flatten depends on the degree of similarity of the new operation to previously performed operations. Typical learning rates that have been encountered in practice range from 70% to 95%. Several alternate models of learning curves have been presented in the literature, including the *log-linear model, S-curve model, Stanford-B model, DeJong's learning formula, Levy's adaptation function, Glover's learning formula, Pegels' exponential function, Knecht's upturn model,* and *Yelle's product model.* The basic log-linear model is the most popular learning curve model. It expresses a dependent variable (e.g., production cost) in terms of some independent variable (e.g., cumulative production). The model states that the improvement in productivity is constant (i.e., it has a constant slope) as output increases and is given as:

$$C(x) = C_1 x^{-b} \qquad \text{Equation 20.30}$$

where:

$C(x)$ = cumulative average cost of producing x units.
C_1 = cost of the first unit.
x = cumulative production unit.
b = learning curve exponent.

The expression for $C(x)$ is practical only for $x > 0$. This makes sense because the learning effect cannot realistically kick in until at least one unit ($x \geq 1$) has been produced. For the standard log-linear model, the expression for the learning rate, p, is derived by considering two production levels where one level is double the other. The performance curve, $P(x)$, can be defined as the reciprocal of the average cost curve, $C(x)$. Thus, we have:

$$P(x) = \frac{1}{C(x)} \qquad \text{Equation 20.31}$$

which will have an increasing profile compared to the asymptotically declining cost curve. In terms of practical application, learning to drive is one example where maximum performance can be achieved in a relatively short time compared to the half-life of performance. That is, learning is steep, but the performance curve is relatively

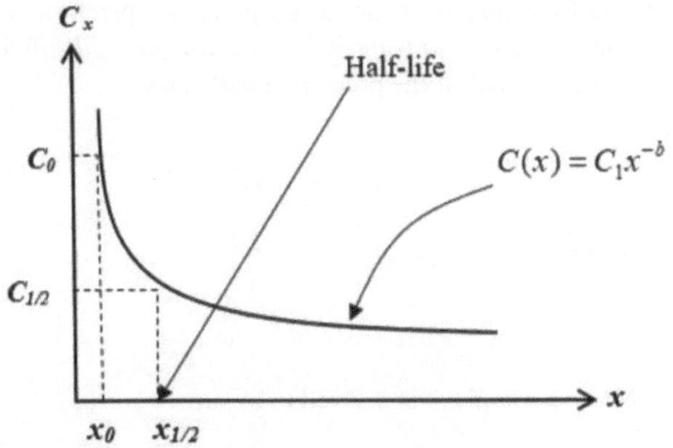

FIGURE 20.3 Profile of basic learning curve with half-life point

flat after a steady state is achieved. The application of half-life analysis to learning curves can help address questions such as the ones below:

- How fast and how far can system performance be improved?
- What are the limitations to system performance improvement?
- How resilient is a system to shocks and interruptions to its operation?
- Are the performance goals that are set for the system achievable?

20.3.6 Half-Life of the Log-Linear Model

Figure 20.3 shows the basic log-linear model, with the half-life point indicated as $x_{1/2}$. The half-life of the log-linear model is computed as follows: Let:

C_0 = Initial performance level.

$C_{1/2}$ = Performance level at half-life.

$$C_0 = C_1 x_0^{-b} \text{ and } C_{1/2} = C_1 x_{1/2}^{-b} \qquad \text{Equation 20.32}$$

But $C_{1/2} = \frac{1}{2} C_0$

Therefore, $C_1 x_{1/2}^{-b} = \frac{1}{2} C_1 x_0^{-b}$, which leads to $x_{1/2}^{-b} = \frac{1}{2} x_0^{-b}$, which, by taking the (–1/b)th exponent of both sides, simplifies to yield the following expression as the general expression for the standard log-linear learning curve model,

$$x_{1/2} = \left(\frac{1}{2}\right)^{-\frac{1}{b}} x_0, \quad x_0 \geq 1 \qquad \text{Equation 20.33}$$

where $x_{1/2}$ is the half-life and x_0 is the initial point of operation. We refer to $x_{1/2}$ (Figure 20.3) as the *first-order half-life*. The *Second-order half-life* is computed as the time corresponding to half of the preceding half. That is:

$$C_1 x_{1/2(2)}^{-b} = \frac{1}{4} C_1 x_0^{-b}, \quad \text{Equation 20.34}$$

which simplifies to yield:

$$x_{1/2(2)} = (1/2)^{-2/b} x_0, \quad \text{Equation 20.35}$$

Similarly, the *third-order half-life* is derived to obtain:

$$x_{1/2(3)} = (1/2)^{-3/b} x_0, \quad \text{Equation 20.36}$$

In general, the ***kth**-order half-life* for the log-linear model is represented as:

$$x_{1/2(k)} = (1/2)^{-k/b} x_0, \quad \text{Equation 20.37}$$

20.3.7 Computational Examples of Half-Life

This section uses examples of log-linear learning curves with $b = 0.75$ and $b = 0.3032$, respectively, to illustrate the characteristics of learning, which can dictate the half-life behavior of the overall learning process. Knowing the point where the half-life of each curve occurs can be very useful in assessing learning retention when designing training programs. For $C(x) = 250x^{-0.75}$, the first-order half-life is computed as:

$$x_{1/2} = (1/2)^{-1/0.75} x_0, \quad x_0 \geq 1 \quad \text{Equation 20.38}$$

If the above expression is evaluated for $x_0 = 2$, the first-order half-life yields $x_{1/2} =$ 5.0397, which indicates a fast drop in the value of $C(x)$, where $C(2) = 148.6509$ corresponding to a half-life of 5.0397. Note that C(5.0397) = 74.7674, which is about half of 148.6509. The conclusion from this analysis is that if we operate at the point $x = 2$, we can expect the curve to reach its half-life decline point at $x = 5$. For $C(x) =$ $240.03x^{-0.3032}$, the first-order half-life is computed as:

$$x_{1/2} = (1/2)^{-1/0.3032} x_0, \quad x_0 \geq 1 \quad \text{Equation 20.39}$$

If we evaluate the above function for $x_0 = 2$, the first-order half-life is $x_{1/2} = 19.6731$. Several models and variations of learning curves are used in practice. Models are developed through one of the following approaches:

1. Conceptual models
2. Theoretical models

3. Observational models
4. Experimental models
5. Empirical models

20.3.7.1 The S-Curve Model

The S-curve (Towill and Kaloo 1978) is based on an assumption of a gradual start-up. The function has the shape of the cumulative normal distribution function for the start-up curve and the shape of an operating characteristics function for the learning curve. The gradual start-up is based on the fact that the early stages of production are typically in a transient state with changes in tooling, methods, materials, design, and even changes in the workforce. The basic form of the S-curve function is:

$$C(x) = C_1 + M(x+B)^{-b} \quad \text{Equation 20.40}$$

$$MC(x) = C_1\left[M + (1-M)(x+B)^{-b}\right] \quad \text{Equation 20.41}$$

where:

$C(x)$ = learning curve expression.
b = learning curve exponent.
M(x) = marginal cost expression.
C_1 = cost of first unit.
M = incompressibility factor (a constant).
B = equivalent experience in units (a constant).

Assumptions about at least three out of the four parameters (M, B, C1, and b) are needed to solve for the fourth one. Using the $C(x)$ expression and derivation procedure outlined earlier for the log-linear model, the half-life equation for the S-curve learning model is derived to be:

$$x_{1/2} = (1/2)^{-1/b}\left[\frac{M(x_0+B)^{-b} - C_1}{M}\right]^{-1/b} - B \quad \text{Equation 20.42}$$

where:

$x_{1/2}$ = half-life expression for the S-curve learning model.
x_0 = initial point of evaluation of performance on the learning curve.

In terms of practical application of the S-curve, consider when a worker begins learning a new task. The individual is slow initially at the tail end of the S-curve. However, the rate of learning increases as time goes on, with additional repetitions. This helps the worker to climb the steep-slope segment of the S-curve very rapidly. At the top of the slope, the worker is classified as being proficient with the learned task. From then on, even if the worker puts much effort into improving upon the task, the resultant learning will not be proportional to the effort expended. The top end of the S-curve is often called the slope of *diminishing returns*. At the top of the S-curve, workers succumb to the effects of *forgetting* and other performance-impeding factors. As the work environment continues to change, a worker's level of skill and expertise can become obsolete. This is an excellent reason for the application of half-life computations.

20.3.7.2 The Stanford-B Model

The Stanford-B model is represented as:

$$UC(x) = C_1 (x + B)^{-b} \qquad \text{Equation 20.43}$$

where:

$UC(x)$ = direct cost of producing the xth unit.
b = learning curve exponent.
C_1 = cost of the first unit when $B = 0$.
B = slope of the asymptote for the curve, where $1 < B < 10$.

This is equivalent units of previous experience at the start of the process, which represents the number of units produced prior to first unit acceptance. It is noted that when $B = 0$, the Stanford-B model reduces to the conventional log-linear model. The general expression for the half-life of the Stanford-B model is derived to be:

$$x_{1/2} = (1/2)^{-1/b} (x_0 + B) - B \qquad \text{Equation 20.44}$$

where:

$x_{1/2}$ = half-life expression for the Stanford-B Learning Model
x_0 = initial point of evaluation of performance on the learning curve

20.3.7.3 Badiru's Multi-Factor Model

Badiru (1994) presents applications of learning and forgetting curves to productivity and performance analysis. One example presented used production data to develop a predictive model of production throughput. Two data replicates are used for each of the ten selected combinations of cost and time values. Observations were recorded for the number of units representing double production levels. The resulting model has the following functional form.

$$C(x) = 298.88 x_1^{-0.31} x_2^{-0.13} \qquad \text{Equation 20.45}$$

where:

$C(x)$ = cumulative production volume.
x_1 = cumulative units of Factor 1.

x_2 = cumulative units of Factor 2.
$b_1 = -0.31$ (first learning curve exponent)
$b_1 = -0.13$ (second learning curve exponent).

A general form of the modeled multi-factor learning curve model is:

$$C(x) = C_1 x_1^{-b_1} x_2^{-b_2} \quad \text{Equation 20.46}$$

The half-life expression for the multi-factor learning curve was derived to be:

$$x_{1(1/2)} = (1/2)^{-1/b_1} \left[\frac{x_{1(0)} x_{2(0)}^{b_2/b_1}}{x_{2(1/2)}^{b_2/b_1}} \right]^{-1/b_1} \quad \text{Equation 20.47}$$

$$x_{2(1/2)} = (1/2)^{-1/b_2} \left[\frac{x_{2(0)} x_{1(0)}^{b_1/b_2}}{x_{1(1/2)}^{b_2/b_1}} \right]^{-1/b_2} \quad \text{Equation 20.48}$$

where:

$x_{i(1/2)}$ = half-life component due to Factor *i* (*i* = 1, 2).
$x_{i(0)}$ = initial point of Factor *i* (*i* = 1, 2) along the multi-factor learning curve.

Knowledge of the value of one factor is needed to evaluate the other factor. Just as in the case of single-factor models, the half-life analysis of the multi-factor model can be used to predict when the performance metric will reach half of a starting value.

20.3.7.4 DeJong's Learning Formula

DeJong's learning formula is a power function that incorporates parameters for the proportion of manual activity in a task. When operations are controlled by manual tasks, the time will be compressible as successive units are completed. If, by contrast, machine cycle times control operations, then the time will be less compressible as the number of units increases. DeJong's formula introduces an incompressible factor, *M*, into the log-linear model to account for the man-machine ratio. The model is expressed as:

$$C(x) = C_1 + Mx^{-b} \quad \text{Equation 20.49}$$

$$MC(x) = C_1\left[M + (1-M)x^{-b}\right] \quad \text{Equation 20.50}$$

where:

$C(x)$ = learning curve expression.
$M(x)$ = marginal cost expression.
b = learning curve exponent.
$_1$ = cost of first unit.
M = incompressibility factor (a constant).

When $M = 0$, the model is reduced to the log-linear model, which implies a completely manual operation. In completely machine-dominated operations, $M = 1$. In that case, the unit cost reduces to a constant equal to C_1, which suggests that no learning-based cost improvement is possible in machine-controlled operations. This represents a condition of high incompressibility. This profile suggests impracticality at higher values of production. Learning is very steep, and average cumulative production cost drops rapidly. The horizontal asymptote for the profile is below the lower bound on the average cost axis, suggesting an infeasible operating region as production volume increases. The analysis above agrees with the fact that no significant published data is available on whether or not DeJong's learning formula has been successfully used to account for the degree of automation in any given operation. Using the expression *MC(x)*, the marginal cost half-life of DeJong's learning model is derived to be:

$$x_{1/2} = (1/2)^{-1/b}\left[\frac{(1-M)x_0^{-b} - M}{2(1-M)}\right]^{-1/b} \quad \text{Equation 20.51}$$

where:

$x_{1/2}$ = half-life expression for the DeJong's learning curve marginal cost model.
x_0 = initial point of evaluation of performance on the marginal cost curve.

If the $C(x)$ model is used to derive the half-life, then we obtain the following derivation:

$$x_{1/2} = (1/2)^{-1/b}\left[\frac{Mx_0^{-b} - C_1}{M}\right]^{-1/b} \quad \text{Equation 20.52}$$

where:

$x_{1/2}$ = half-life expression for the DeJong's learning curve model.
x_0 = initial point of evaluation of performance on the DeJong's learning curve.

20.3.7.5 Levy's Technology Adaptation Function

Recognizing that the log-linear model does not account for the leveling off of the production rate and the factors that may influence learning, Levy (1965) presented the following learning cost function:

$$MC(x) = \left[\frac{1}{\beta} - \left(\frac{1}{\beta} - \frac{x^{-b}}{C_1}\right)k^{-kx}\right]^{-1} \quad \text{Equation 20.53}$$

where:

β = production index for the first unit.
k = constant used to flatten the learning curve for large values of x.

The flattening constant, k, forces the curve to reach a plateau instead of continuing to decrease or turning upward. The half-life expression for Levy's learning model is a complex nonlinear expression derived as shown below:

$$\left(1/\beta - x_{1/2}^{-b}/C_1\right)k^{-kx_{1/2}} = 1/\beta - 2\left[1/\beta - \left(1/\beta - x_0^{-b}/C_1\right)k^{-kx_0}\right]$$

Equation 20.54

where:

$x_{1/2}$ = half-life expression for Levy's learning curve model.
x_0 = initial point of evaluation of performance on Levy's learning curve.

Knowledge of some of the parameters of the model is needed to solve for the half-life as a closed-form expression.

20.3.7.6 Glover's Learning Model

Glover's learning formula (Glover 1966) is a learning curve model that incorporates a work commencement factor. The model is based on a bottom-up approach that uses individual worker learning results as the basis for plant-wide learning curve standards. The functional form of the model is expressed as:

$$\sum_{i=1}^{n} y_i + a = C_1\left(\sum_{i=1}^{n} x_i\right)^m \qquad \text{Equation 20.55}$$

where:

y_i = elapsed time or cumulative quantity.
x_i = cumulative quantity or elapsed time.
a = commencement factor.
n = index of the curve (usually $1+b$).
m = model parameter.

This is a complex expression for which half-life expression is not easily computable. We defer the half-life analysis of Levy's learning curve model for further research by interested readers.

20.3.7.7 Pegels' Exponential Function

Pegels (1976) presented an alternate algebraic function for the learning curve. His model, a form of an exponential function of marginal cost, is represented as:

$$MC(x) = \alpha a^{x-1} + \beta \qquad \text{Equation 20.56}$$

where α, β , and a are parameters based on empirical data analysis. The total cost of producing x units is derived from the marginal cost as follows:

$$TC(x) = \int \left(\alpha a^{x-1} + \beta \right) dx = \frac{\alpha a^{x-1}}{\ln(a)} + \beta x + c \qquad \text{Equation 20.57}$$

where c is a constant to be derived after the other parameters are found. The constant can be found by letting the marginal cost, total cost, and average cost of the first unit be all equal. That is, $MC_1 = TC_1 = AC_1$, which yields:

$$c = \alpha - \frac{\alpha}{\ln(a)} \qquad \text{Equation 20.58}$$

The model assumes that the marginal cost of the first unit is known. Thus,

$$MC_1 = \alpha + \beta = y_0 \qquad \text{Equation 20.59}$$

The mathematical expression for the total labor cost in Pegels' start-up curves is expressed as:

$$TC(x) = \frac{a}{1-b} x^{1-b} \qquad \text{Equation 20.60}$$

where:

x = cumulative number of units produced,
a, b = empirically determined parameters.

The expressions for marginal cost, average cost, and unit cost can be derived as shown earlier for other models. Using the total cost expression, $TC(x)$, we derive the expression for the half-life of Pegels' learning curve model to be as shown below:

$$x_{1/2} = \left(\frac{1}{2} \right)^{-1/(1-b)} x_0 \qquad \text{Equation 20.61}$$

20.3.7.8 Knecht's Upturn Model

Knecht (1974) presents a modification to the functional form of the learning curve to analytically express the observed divergence of actual costs from those predicted by learning curve theory when the number of units produced exceeds 200. This permits the consideration of nonconstant slopes for the learning curve model. If UC_x is defined as the unit cost of the xth unit, then it approaches zero asymptotically as x increases. To avoid a zero-limit unit cost, the basic functional form is modified. In the continuous case, the formula for cumulative average costs is derived as:

$$C(x) = \int_0^x C_1 z^b dz = \frac{C_1 x^{b+1}}{(1+b)} \qquad \text{Equation 20.62}$$

This cumulative cost also approaches zero as x goes to infinity. Knecht alters the expression for the cumulative curve to allow for an upturn in the learning curve at large cumulative production levels. He suggested the functional form below:

$$C(x) = C_1 x^{-b} e^{cx} \qquad \text{Equation 20.63}$$

where c is a second constant. Differentiating the modified cumulative average cost expression gives the unit cost of the xth unit, as shown below.

$$UC(x) = \frac{d}{dx}\left[C_1 x^{-b} e^{cx}\right] = C_1 x^{-b} e^{cx}\left(c + \frac{-b}{x}\right) \qquad \text{Equation 20.64}$$

The half-life expression for Knecht's learning model turns out to be a nonlinear complex function as shown below:

$$x_{1/2} e^{-cx_{1/2}/b} = \left(\frac{1}{2}\right)^{-1/b} e^{-cx_0/b} x_0 \qquad \text{Equation 20.65}$$

where:

$x_{1/2}$ = half-life expression for the Knecht's learning curve model.
x_0 = initial point of evaluation of performance on Knecht's learning curve.

Given that x_0 is known, iterative, interpolation or numerical methods may be needed to solve for the half-life value.

20.3.7.9 Yelle's Combined Technology Learning Curve

Yelle (1979) proposed a learning curve model for products by aggregating and extrapolating the individual learning curve of the operations making up a product on a log-linear plot. The model is expressed as shown below:

$$C(x) = k_1 x_1^{-b_1} + k_2 x_2^{-b_2} + \cdots + k_n x_n^{-b_n} \qquad \text{Equation 20.66}$$

where:

$C(x)$ = cost of producing the xth unit of the product.
n = number of operations making up the product.
$k_i x_i^{-b_i}$ = learning curve for the ith operation.

20.3.8 Aggregated Learning Curves

In comparing the models discussed in the preceding sections, the deficiency of Knecht's model is that a product-specific learning curve seems to be a more reasonable model than an integrated product curve. For example, an aggregated learning curve with a 96.6% learning rate obtained from individual learning curves with the respective learning rates of 80%, 70%, 85%, 80%, and 85% does not appear to represent reality. If this type of composite improvement is possible, then one can always improve the learning rate for any operation by decomposing it into smaller integrated operations. The additive and multiplicative approaches of reliability functions support the conclusion of the impracticality of Knecht's integrated model. Jaber and Guiffrida (2004) presented an aggregated form of the WLC where some of the items produced are defective and require reworking. The quality learning curve that they provide is of the form:

$$t(x) = y_1 x^{-b} + 2r_1 \left(\frac{\theta}{2}\right)^{1-\varepsilon} x^{1-2\varepsilon} \qquad \text{Equation 20.67}$$

where y_1 is the time to produce the first unit, r_1 is the time to rework the first defective unit, θ is the probability of the process going out of control ($\theta < 1$), and b is the learning exponent of the reworks learning curve. The variable $t(x)$ has three behavioral patterns, for $0 < b < 1/2$(Case I), $b = 1/2$ (Case II), and $1/2 < b < 1$(Case III). Assuming no production error, we computed the half-life for $t(x)$ for case 1 as:

Case I: $x_{1/2} = \left(\frac{1}{2}\right)^{-\frac{1}{b}} x$ and $x_{1/2} = \left(\frac{1}{2}\right)^{-\frac{1}{1-2\varepsilon}} x$

Case II: $t(x) = y_1 x^{-b} + 2r_1 \left(\frac{\rho}{2}\right)^{1-\varepsilon} x^{1-2\varepsilon}$ reduces to $t(x) = +t(x) = y_1 x^{-b} + 2r_1 \sqrt{\frac{\rho}{2}}$,

where $2r_1 \sqrt{\frac{\rho}{2}}$ is the lower bound, or the plateau of the learning curve, when $\epsilon = 0.5$.

Case III: The behavior of $t(x)$ follows that of the WLC: monotonically decreasing as cumulative output increases. It is noted that Jaber and Guiffrida (2008) assumed that the percentage defective reduces as the number of interruptions to restore the process increases. They found that $t(x)$ could converge to the WLC when learning in reworking (quality learning curve) is fast $\epsilon = 0.5$.

20.3.9 Half-Life of Decline Curves

Over the years, the decline curve technique has been extensively used by the oil and gas industry to evaluate future oil and gas predictions. These predictions are used as the basis for economic analysis to support development, property sale or purchase, industrial loan provisions, and also to determine if a secondary recovery project should be carried out. It is expected that the profile of the hyperbolic decline curve can be adapted for application to learning curve analysis. The graphical solution of the hyperbolic equation is through the use of a log-log paper, which sometimes provides a straight line that can be extrapolated for a useful length of time to predict future production levels. This technique, however, sometimes fails to produce the straight line needed for extrapolation for some production scenarios. Furthermore, the graphical method usually involves some manipulation of data, such as shifting, correcting, and/or adjusting scales, which eventually introduces bias into the actual data. To avoid the noted graphical problems of hyperbolic decline curves and to accurately predict the future performance of a producing well, a nonlinear least-squares technique is often considered. This method does not require any straight-line extrapolation for future predictions. The mathematical analysis proceeds as follows. The general hyperbolic decline equation for oil production rate (q) as a function of time (t) can be represented as:

$$q(t) = q_0 \left(1 + mD_0 t\right)^{-1/m}, \text{ where } 0 < m < 1 \qquad \text{Equation 20.68}$$

where:

$q(t)$ = oil production at time t.
q_0 = initial oil production.
D_0 = initial decline.
m = decline exponent.

Also, the cumulative oil production at time t, $Q(t)$ can be written as

$$Q(t) = \frac{q_0}{(m-1)D_0}\left[\left(1 + mD_0 t\right)^{\frac{m-1}{m}} - 1\right] \qquad \text{Equation 20.69}$$

where $Q(t)$ = Cumulative production as of time t. By combining the above equations and performing some algebraic manipulations, it can be shown that

$$q(t)^{1-m} = q_0^{\,1-m} + (m-1)D_0 q_0^{\,-m} Q(t), \qquad \text{Equation 20.70}$$

which shows that the production at time t is a nonlinear function of its cumulative production level. By rewriting the equations in terms of cumulative production, we have:

$$Q(t) = \frac{q_0}{(1-m)D_0} + q(t)^{1-m} \frac{q_0^{\,m}}{(m-1)D_0} \qquad \text{Equation 20.71}$$

The model can be investigated in terms of conventional learning curve techniques, forgetting decline curve, and half-life analysis. The forgetting function has the same basic form as the standard learning curve model, except that the forgetting rate will be negative, indicating a decay process. Figure 20.4 shows some of the possible profiles of the forgetting curve. Profile (a) shows a case where forgetting occurs rapidly along a convex curve. Profile (b) shows a case where forgetting occurs more slowly along a concave curve. Profile (c) shows a case where the rate of forgetting shifts from convex to concave along an S-curve.

The profile of the forgetting curve and its mode of occurrence can influence the half-life measure. This is further evidence that the computation of half-life can help distinguish between learning curves, particularly if a forgetting component is

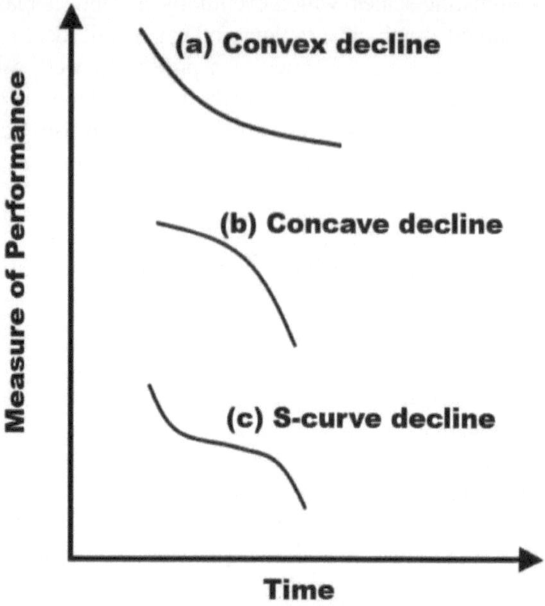

FIGURE 20.4 Shapes of innovation degradation curves

involved. The combination of the learning and forgetting functions presents a more realistic picture of what actually occurs in a learning process. The combination is not necessarily as simple as resolving two curves to obtain a resultant curve. The resolution may be particularly complex in the case of intermittent periods of forgetting. Figure 20.5 shows representations of periods where forgetting occurs and the resulting learn-forget profile.

Degradation of performance occurs naturally, either due to internal processes or externally imposed events, such as extended production breaks. For productivity assessment purposes, it may be of interest to determine the length of time it takes for a production metric to decay to half of its original magnitude. For example, for a career planning strategy, one may be interested in how long it takes for skill sets to degrade by half regarding the current technological needs of the workplace. The half-life phenomenon may be due to intrinsic factors, such as forgetting, or due to external factors, such as a shift in labor requirements. Half-life analysis can have applications in intervention programs designed to achieve reinforcement of learning. It can also have applications for assessing the sustainability of skills acquired through training programs. Further research on the theory of the half-life of learning curves should be directed to topics such as the following:

- Half-Life Interpretations
- Training and Learning Reinforcement Program
- Forgetting Intervention and Sustainability Programs

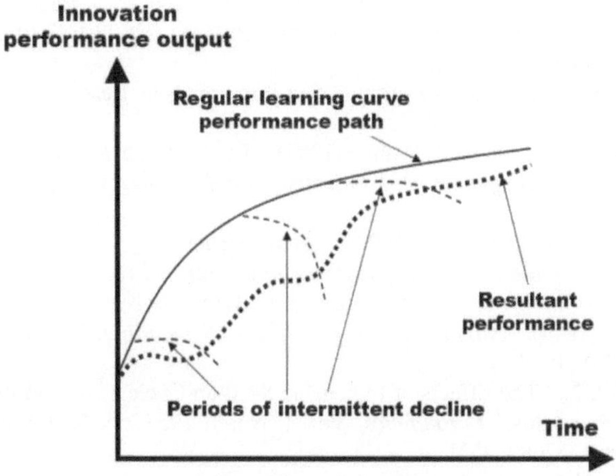

FIGURE 20.5 Resolution of learn-forget performance curves

20.4 SUMMARY

Inasmuch as emergency response activities can be modeled as repeatable production activities, learning curve models are applicable. In addition to the predictive benefits of half-life expressions, they also reveal the ad hoc nature of some of the classical learning curve models that have been presented in the literature. The case of applications to emergency response requires nonclassical modeling considerations.

REFERENCES

Aeppel, T. (2012), "Man vs. Machine: Behind the Jobless Recovery," *Wall Street Journal*, January 17. http://www.wsj.com/articles/SB10001424052970204468004577164710231081398.

Anderlohr, G. (1969), "What Production Breaks Cost," *Industrial Engineering*, Vol. 1, No. 9, 1969, pp. 34–36.

Badiru, A. B. (1994), "Multifactor Learning and Forgetting Models for Productivity and Performance Analysis," *International Journal of Human Factors in Manufacturing*, Vol. 4, No. 1, 1994, pp. 37–54.

Badiru, A. B. (1995b), "Multivariate Analysis of the Effect of Learning and Forgetting on Product Quality," *International Journal of Production Research*, Vol. 33, No. 3, 1995, pp. 777–794.

Badiru, A. B. (2012), "Half-life Learning Curves in the Defense Acquisition Life Cycle," *Defense Acquisition Research Journal*, Vol. 19, No. 3, 2012, pp. 283–308. https://www.afit.edu/BIOS/publications/HalflifeLearningCurvesinDefenseAcquisitionLifeCycleBadiruDARJ2012.pdf.

Badiru, A. B. and A. Ijaduola (2009), "Half-Life Theory of Learning Curves for System Performance Analysis," *IEEE Systems Journal*, Vol. 3, No. 2, 2009, pp. 154–165.

Belkaoui, A. (1976), "Costing through Learning," *Cost and Management*, Vol. 50, No. 3, 1976, pp. 36–40.

Boone, E., J. J. Elshaw, C. M. Koschnick, J. D. Ritschel, and A. B. Badiru (2021), *Defense Acquisition Research Journal*, Vol. 28, No. 1, 2021, pp. 72–97. https:// doi.org/10.22594/10.22594/dau.20-850.28.01.

Carr, G. W. (1946), "Peacetime Cost Estimating Requires New Learning Curves," *Aviation*, Vol. 45, No. 4, 1946, pp. 220–228.

Camm, J. D., J. R. Evans, and N. K. Womer (1987), "The Unit Learning Curve Approximation of Total Cost," *Computers and Industrial Engineering*, Vol. 12, No. 3, 1987, pp. 205–213.

Chalmers, G. and N. DeCarteret (1949), *Relationship for Determining the Optimum Expansibility of the Elements of a Peacetime Aircraft Procurement Program*, USAF Air Materiel Command, Wright-Patterson AFB, OH, 1949.

Crawford, J. R. (1944), *Estimating, Budgeting and Scheduling*, Lockheed Aircraft Co, Burbank, CA, 1944.

De Jong, J. R. (1957), "The Effects of Increasing Skill on Cycle Time and Its Consequences for Time Standards," *Ergonomics*, Vol. 1, No. 1, 1957, pp. 51–60. https://doi.org/10.1080/00140135708964571.

Globerson, S., A. Nahumi, and S. Ellis (1998), "Rate of Forgetting for Motor and Cognitive Tasks," *International Journal of Cognitive Ergonomics*, Vol. 2, 1998, pp. 181–191.

Glover, J. H. (1966), "Manufacturing Progress Functions: An Alternative Model and Its Comparison with Existing Functions," *International Journal of Production Research*, Vol. 4, No. 4, 1966, pp. 279–300.

Honious, C., B. Johnson, J. Elshaw, and A. Badiru (2016), "The Impact of Learning Curve Model Selection and Criteria for Cost Estimation Accuracy in the DoD," in Maj Gen C. Blake, USAF (Chair), *Proceedings of the 13th Annual Acquisition Research Symposium,* Monterey, CA , May 4–5. https://apps.dtic.mil/dtic/tr/fulltext/u2/1016823.pdf.

International Cost Estimating and Analysis Association (2013), *Cost Estimating Body of Knowledge,* ICEAA. https://www.iceaaonline.com/cebok/.

Jaber, M. Y. and M. Bonney (1996), "Production Breaks and the Learning Curve: The Forgetting Phenomena," *Applied Mathematical Modelling*, Vol. 20, 1996, pp. 162–169.

Jaber, M. Y. and M. Bonney (2003), "Lot Sizing With Learning and Forgetting in Setups and in Product Quality," *International Journal of Production Economics*, Vol. 83, No. 1, 2003, pp. 95–111.

Jaber, M. Y. and M. Bonney (2007), "Economic Manufacture Quantity (EMQ) Model With Lot Size Dependent Learning and Forgetting Rates," *International Journal of Production Economics*, Vol. 108, Nos. 1–2, 2007, pp. 359–367.

Jaber, M. Y. and A. L. Guiffrida (2004), "Learning Curves for Processes Generating Defects Requiring Reworks," *European Journal of Operational Research*, Vol. 159, No. 3, 2004, pp. 663–672.

Jaber, M. Y. and A. L. Guiffrida (2008), "Learning Curves for Imperfect Production Processes with Reworks and Process Restoration Interruptions," *European Journal of Operational Research*, Vol. 189, No. 1, 2008, pp. 93–104.

Jaber, M. Y., H. V. Kher, and D. Davis (2003), "Countering Forgetting through Training and Deployment," *International Journal of Production Economics*, Vol. 85, No. 1, 2003, pp. 33–46.

Jaber, M. Y. and S. Sikström (2004), "A Numerical Comparison of Three Potential Learning and Forgetting Models," *International Journal of Production Economics*, Vol. 92, No. 3, 2004, pp. 281–294.

Johnson, B. J. (2016), *A Comparative Study of Learning Curve Models and Factors in Defense Cost Estimating Based on Program Integration, Assembly, and Checkout* [Master's thesis], Air Force Institute of Technology. https://apps.dtic.mil/dtic/tr/fulltext/u2/1056447.pdf.

Knecht, G. R. (1974), "Costing, Technological Growth, and Generalized Learning Curves," *Operations Research Quarterly*, Vol. 25, No. 3, 1974, pp. 487–491.

Kronemer, A. and J. E. Henneberger (1993), "Productivity in Aircraft Manufacturing," *Monthly Labor Review*, Vol. 16, No. 6, 1993, pp. 24–33. http://www.bls.gov/mfp/mprkh93.pdf.

Levy, F. K. (1965), "Adaptation in the Production Process," *Management Science*, Vol. 11, No. 6, 1965, pp. B136–B154.

Liao, W. M. (1979), "Effects of Learning on Resource Allocation Decisions," *Decision Sciences*, Vol. 10, 1979, pp. 116–125.

Madigan, K. (2011), "It's Man vs. Machine and Man is Losing," *Wall Street Journal*, September 28. https://blogs.wsj.com/economics/2011/09/28/its-man-vs-machine-and-man-is-losing/.

Martin, J. R. (2019), *What is a Learning Curve?* Management and Accounting Web. http://maaw.info/LearningCurveSummary.htm.

Mazur, J. E. and R. Hastie (1978), "Learning as Accumulation: A Reexamination of the Learning Curve," *Psychological Bulletin*, Vol. 85, 1978, pp. 1256–1274.

McIntyre, E. V. *(1977), "Cost-Volume-Profit Analysis Adjusted for Learning," *Management Science*, Vol. 24, No. 2, 1977, pp. 149–160.

Mislick, G. K. and D. A. Nussbaum (2015). *Cost Estimation: Methods and Tools*, Wiley. https://www.academia.edu/24430098/Cost_Estimation_Methods_and_Tools_by_Gregory_K_Mislick_and_Daniel_A_Nussbaum_1st_Edition.

Moore, J. R., J. Elshaw, A. B. Badiru, and J. D. Ritschel (2015), "Acquisition Challenge: The Importance of Incompressibility in Comparing Learning Curve Models," *Defense Acquisition Research Journal*, Vol. 22, No. 4, 2015, pp. 416–449. https://www.dau.edu/library/arj/ARJ/ARJ75/ARJ75-ONLINE-FULL.pdf.

Nanda, R. (1979), "Using Learning Curves in Integration of Production Resources," *Proceedings of 1979 IIE Fall Conference*, 1979, pp. 376–380.

Nembhard, D. A. and N. Osothsilp (2001), "An Empirical Comparison of Forgetting Models," *IEEE Transactions on Engineering Management*, Vol. 48, 2001, pp. 283–291.

Nembhard, D. A. and M. V. Uzumeri (2000), "Experiential Learning and Forgetting for Manual and Cognitive Tasks," *International Journal of Industrial Ergonomics*, Vol. 25, 2000, pp. 315–326.

Pegels, C. C. (1976), "Start Up or Learning Curves - Some New Approaches," *Decision Sciences*, Vol. 7, No. 4, 1976, pp. 705–713.

Richardson, W. J. (1978), "Use of Learning Curves to Set Goals and Monitor Progress in Cost Reduction Programs," *Proceedings of 1978 IIE Spring Conference*, 1978, pp. 235–239.

Smith, J. (1989), *Learning Curve for Cost Control*, Industrial Engineering and Management Press, Norcross, GA, 1989.

Smunt, Timothy L. (1986), "A Comparison of Learning Curve Analysis and Moving Average Ratio Analysis for Detailed Operational Planning," *Decision Sciences*, Vol. 17, No. 4, pp. 475-495.

Sule, D. R. (1978), "The Effect of Alternate Periods of Learning and Forgetting on Economic Manufacturing Quantity," *AIIE Transactions*, Vol. 10, No. 3, 1978, pp. 338–343.

Towill, D. R. (1990), "Forecasting Learning Curves," *International Journal of Forecasting*, Vol. 6, No. 1, 1990, pp. 25–38.

Towill, D. R. and J. E. Cherrington (1994), "Learning Curve Models for Predicting the Performance of Advanced Manufacturing Technology," *International Journal of Advanced Manufacturing Technology*, Vol. 9, No. 3, 1994, pp. 195–203.

Towill, D. R. and U. Kaloo (1978), "Productivity Drift in Extended Learning Curves," *Omega*, Vol. 6, No. 4, 1978, pp. 295–304.

Womer, N. K. (1984), "Estimating Learning Curves from Aggregate Monthly Data," *Management Science*, Vol. 30, No. 8, 1984, pp. 982–992.

Womer, N. K. (1979), "Learning Curves, Production Rate, and Program Costs," *Management Science*, Vol. 25, No. 4, 1979, pp. 312–219.

Womer, N. K. (1981), "Some Propositions on Cost Functions," *Southern Economic Journal*, Vol. 47, 1981, pp. 1111–1119.

Womer, N. K. and T. R. Gulledge, Jr., (1983), "A Dynamic Cost Function for an Airframe Production Program," *Engineering Costs and Production Economics*, Vol. 7, 1983, pp. 213–227.

Wright, T. P. (1936), "Factors Affecting the Cost of Airplanes," *Journal of Aeronautical Science*, Vol. 3, No. 2, 1936, pp. 122–128.

Yelle, Louis E. (1976), "Estimating Learning Curves for Potential Products," *Industrial Marketing Management*, Vol. 5, No. 2/3, 1976, pp. 147–154.

Yelle, Louis E. (1979), "The Learning Curve: Historical Review and Comprehensive Survey," *Decision Sciences*, Vol. 10, No. 2, 1979, pp. 302–328.

Yelle, Louis E. (1983), "Adding Life Cycles to Learning Curves," *Long Range Planning*, Vol. 16, No. 6, 1983, pp. 82–87.

21 Systems Engineering Framework for Environmental Conservation and Restoration Management

Aisha Tarfa and Adedeji B. Badiru

21.1 INTRODUCTION TO ENVIRONMENTAL EMERGENCY

An emergency is defined as a sudden, urgent, and unexpected situation that requires an immediate response. An emergency, in our common understanding, can develop from catastrophic events due to a variety of factors, including human negligence, human error, impacts of nature, accidental occurrences, deliberate acts, technical failures, and other unintended developments. This conventional interpretation of "suddenness" in an emergency draws us away from the more subtle and gradual developments that later may necessitate an "emergency" response. The focus of this chapter is to highlight the impacts of the gradual degradation of the environment due to some biological incursions, such as soil contaminants. Sooner or later, such adverse occurrences require urgent remediation actions, thus fitting the emergency response backdrop of this handbook of emergency response. In the context of this chapter, environmental emergencies are not necessarily sudden occurrences. With this broadened viewpoint, we can address many environmental considerations of an emergency response, including environmental cleanup, regulatory issues, community priorities, budgetary limitations, safety risks, health impacts, and so on. In particular, the Comprehensive Environmental Response, Compensation, and Liability Act (CERCLA) is of great interest.

This type of emergency response is best addressed from a systems engineering framework. For this purpose, a system is defined as a collection of interrelated elements, whose outcome (in unison) is higher than the summation of the individual outcomes of the sub-elements.

DOI: 10.1201/9781003648178-23

21.2 ENVIRONMENTAL SYSTEMS

It's all in the system. Based on the concept of systems thinking, an environmental system encompasses many aspects of what is addressed in this chapter. This is in consonance with the theme of this handbook, which focuses on identifying and highlighting the tools and techniques of systems engineering that can be brought to bear on global environmental challenges. The US National Academy of Engineering (NAE), in 2008, released a list of the 14 grand challenges for engineering. Each area of the challenges constitutes a complex emergency response that must be planned and executed strategically. The 14 challenges, which can be viewed as science, technology, engineering, and mathematics (STEM) areas, are listed as follows:

1. Make solar energy affordable.
2. Provide energy from fusion.
3. **Develop carbon sequestration methods.**
4. Manage the nitrogen cycle.
5. **Provide access to clean water.**
6. Restore and improve urban infrastructure.
7. Advance health informatics.
8. Engineer better medicines.
9. Reverse-engineer the brain.
10. Prevent nuclear terror.
11. Secure cyberspace.
12. Enhance virtual reality.
13. Advance personalized learning.
14. Engineer the tools for scientific discovery.

Items 3 and 5, highlighted in the list above, represent the environmental emergency response focus of this chapter, with respect to biological impacts on the environment, albeit through gradual processes.

21.3 CERCLA AND EMERGENCY RESPONSE

Consistent efforts have been made over the years to provide legislative and industry guidelines for responding to environmental degradation. One such effort is CERCLA, commonly known as Superfund, which was enacted by the US Congress on December 11, 1980. This law created a tax on the chemical and petroleum industries and provided broad Federal authority to respond directly to releases or threatened releases of hazardous substances that may endanger public health or the environment. Over five years, $1.6 billion was collected, and the tax went into a trust fund for cleaning up abandoned or uncontrolled hazardous waste sites. CERCLA provides for the following:

- Established prohibitions and requirements concerning closed and abandoned hazardous waste sites.

- Provided for the liability of persons responsible for releases of hazardous waste at these sites.
- Established a trust fund to provide for cleanup when no responsible party could be identified.

The law authorizes two kinds of response actions:

- Short-term removals, where actions may be taken to address releases or threatened releases requiring a prompt response.
- Long-term remedial response actions that permanently and significantly reduce the dangers associated with releases or threats of releases of hazardous substances that are serious but not immediately life-threatening. These actions can be conducted only at sites listed on the national priorities list of the US Environmental Protection Agency (EPA).

CERCLA also enabled the revision of the National Contingency Plan (NCP). The NCP provided the guidelines and procedures needed to respond to releases and threatened releases of hazardous substances, pollutants, or contaminants from a comprehensive project management perspective (Badiru, 2019).

21.3.1 Gradual Biological Degradation of the Environment

This section presents details of the biological degradation of the environment that may necessitate an emergency response in alignment with two of the 14 grand challenges outlined by the US NAE in 2008. According to Tarfa (2021), the key task of the 21st century will be to satisfy the fundamental needs of human beings while maintaining the integrity of the agroecosystem by sustaining global biodiversity and promoting social-ecological development through understanding that all species living on Earth are dependent on carbon molecules. Soil organic carbon (SOC) is an essential component of carbon solids, including relative plant and animal tissues, in the form of microbial biomass at different levels of decomposition. Two cross-border cropping systems with the ability to investigate carbon 13 (13C) isotopic composition through the net ecosystem production (NEP) components (also known as the vertical inputs) were chosen. In contrast to perennial plants, annual plants use water and nutrients inefficiently, which can cause soil degradation and deterioration of water quality. Cropping schemes have been perennial and periodic. Collectively, the design of the relative carbon budget is commonly estimated by computing the difference between vertical inputs and outputs of C while ignoring any lateral component. The litter content and certain phenological properties can allow the 13C to deviate from its source. The NEP component collected consists of plant-relative tissue from shoots, litter, roots, soil, earthworms, and earthworm casts. Studies suggest that earthworm casts constitute hotspots for carbon turnover and the development of biogeochemical interfaces in soils, and an isotopic study of the carbon (C) flow across different reservoirs of the global C cycle will provide vital information on neighboring farming systems. Earthworm cast material can play a direct role in key areas of soil rehabilitation by SOC biosequestration. The paper explores the possibilities of different 13C ratios across different herbs, litter content, earthworms, and soil material, as it applies to the biosequestration of organic carbon in the ecosystem. C to N Ratio Isotopic Composition considers the scientific context to better examine the observational data on which the theories are based by incorporating predictive simulation into environmental research interactions.

21.3.2 Terrestrial Ecosystems

Comprehensive data on carbon flow in terrestrial ecosystems is a requirement for understanding agroecosystem services and managing agricultural systems in a sustainable way. Relevant data is available on total amounts, individual fractions, and residence time of C in soil (Marhan et al., 2011). The reason is that carbon is not just another nutrient but an essential component of soil organic matter (SOM). This is because SOM controls biotic activities in soil, which is the essential core of life in soil. Measured in gigaton/C, carbon is found in three major forms in the carbon cycle: the atmosphere, aboveground biomass, and SOM. Soil microorganisms transform fresh organic matter (FOM), entering the soil into chemically stable, biologically inactive organic matter through the so-called humification process (Brookes et al., 2008).

The measurable component of SOM is SOC, found in three pools of soil, which includes the labile pool, the slow pool, and the inert pool. Tarfa (2021) provides a figure that illustrates the movement of carbon is through the pools. The model neglects important knowledge derived from slow and inert forms of soil organic matter, such as the existence of different chemical forms of carbon, i.e., carbohydrates or lignin, having different stability against decomposition. The model shows SOM has the highest share of organic carbon content compared to both aboveground biomass and the atmosphere.

Photosynthesis continuously extracts CO_2 from the atmosphere to form plant biomass mineralized by microorganisms to reform atmospheric CO_2. Some of the plant carbon formed accumulates as plant biomass in terrestrial ecosystems, and some is transformed into biodegradable matter such as microbial biomass or new molecules. The product is then synthesized to SOM. It is important to note that the model focuses on the liable pool in connection to soil fauna related to the pools. It also ignores the existence of chemical gradients in soil profiles. In addition, microorganisms typically mineralize as CO_2 40–60% of the carbon in organic matter. As a consequence, SOM is a field of organic molecules relating to the various intermediates of the FOM to the biologically inactive phase of the transfer of organic matter. Global modification in management practices leading to the increased cultivation of perennial-annual neighboring crop research has led to the secondary laboratory-based analysis for earthworm cast, leading to a direct role in key areas of soil rehabilitation. Collectively, these seemingly insignificant animals can make a significant contribution to achieving sustainable human development without affecting environmental quality (soil health). The link between perennial and annual crops entails information relating to the connection between earth resources and human activities on the agroecosystem. The findings can be a promising alternative to help mitigate the impact of global change on world ecosystems to promote the increased storage of atmospheric carbon dioxide in components of terrestrial ecosystems (Houghton et al., 2001; McCarthy et al., 2001). Cropping systems such as annual and perennial play a central role in storing organic carbon two to three times more in soil. Studies indicate that stability and time play a vital role in the accumulation of organic carbon content, however, not in composition. Studies also indicate that SOM can measure the storage of C input from the liable pool. This is because plant cells have a nonrandom isotopic distribution of 13C.

The replacement of annual crops by perennial crops has a major role to play not only in energy transition but also in key processes in the carbon cycle, such as the gross primary production (GPP), net primary production (NPP), and NEP variables in the agroecosystem. Replacing annual crops with perennial crops is, therefore, a sustainable agricultural practice that focuses not only on nutrient recovery strategies for reusing existing minerals, increasing the search for alternate supplies of nutrition that have less harmful environmental consequences, but also on estimating the input of soil carbon content build-up or losses in the agroecosystem. Since the carbon content of the relative tissue of plants is recognized as a photosynthesis-weighted carbon supply and demand integrator, and feedback mechanisms between plant and microbial communities control the richness of plant species and productivity, it is significant to integrate soil fauna such as earthworms into the perennial – annual crop research. This is because they have the ability to directly affect the decomposition of soil through gut-associated processes via the effects of ingestion, digestion, and stimulation of the organic matter (OM) breakdown and microorganisms (Monroy et al., 2011; Aira et al., 2008).

Earthworm activity can amend the beneficial microflora and nutrient recycling. This is because soil worm casts are a rich source of micronutrients, macronutrients, and microbial enzymes (Lavelle and Martin, 1992). Decomposition and nutrient recycling begin in the gut by a diverse group of microbes in a cascading network of biochemical processes that proceeds to soil. Through decomposition processes in soil, microbes release simpler carbon compounds, nitrogen, CO_2, and minerals from dead organic material, which are ultimately consumed by higher plants. The dynamic interactions involved in the process, where nutrients contained in the organic matter are partly converted to more bioavailable forms, are crucial. In contrast, the fate of belowground carbon (C) is misunderstood, particularly the flow of C through the soil food web. The transfer of C from plant roots to soil through rhizodeposition annually recycles about 10% of atmospheric CO_2, an order of magnitude greater than the current rate of fossil fuel C combustion (Marhan et al., 2011).

21.4 ISOTOPIC COMPOSITION OF ORGANIC MATERIALS

The isotopic composition of organic materials can provide extremely useful information about NPP in identifying the carbon supply and demand in plant tissue. The 13C of plant tissue is known to be a photosynthesis-weighted integrator of carbon supply and demand (Farquhar et al., 1982). Variation in 13C may be driven by changes in cropping systems, changes in photosynthetic capacity, or changes in both because 13C has been shown to be positively related to the ratio of intercellular to atmospheric CO_2 concentration (Farquhar et al., 1982). Cropping systems such as annual and perennial, as seen in the model, play a central role in storing organic carbon two to three times more in soil. The model indicates that stability and time play a vital role in the accumulation of organic carbon content, however, not for composition. Studies indicate that soil organic matter can measure the storage of C input from the labile pool because plant cells have a nonrandom isotopic distribution of 13C.

Earthworms are key organisms in organic matter decomposition because of their interactions with soil properties and microflora (Aira and Dominguez 2011). The casts produced by the earthworm represent hotspots for carbon turnover and the formation of biogeochemical interfaces in soils. Because of the complex microscale cast architecture, it remains challenging to understand the casting formation and development mechanisms at a process-relevant scale, i.e., within microaggregates and at the interface between plant residues, microorganisms, and mineral particles.

Earthworms enhance decomposition rates through the joint action of direct effects (i.e., effects due to direct earthworm activity such as digestion, burrowing, etc.) and indirect effects (i.e., effects derived from earthworm activities such as gut content and cast aging). Many studies of plant and ecosystem function use measurements of shoot material as a basic tool in understanding carbon and water fluxes. An integrative measure of the NEP component requiring little (and unskilled) labor in the field would be of great merit. However, the same cautions as outlined above for breeding applications apply to ecophysiological applications.

Carbon flow in the agroecosystem is evidence that soil organic carbon is mainly distributed among:

- Net primary production from plants.
- Decomposition rate of organic material.

21.5 CARBON FLOW IN THE AGROECOSYSTEM

Studies indicate the movement of carbon can be examined through various environmental isotopes found in the global C cycle. Tarfa (2021) provides a diagram that illustrates the carbon flow found in the plant-soil system. Readers may refer to that reference for further details. Firstly, atmospheric CO_2 in the presence of sunlight is assimilated and converted to organic carbon by plants and enters the soil through decomposition processes aided by shredder organisms and soil microbiota from root and leaf litter.

Each component in the system plays a different role in the formation of SOM through the decomposition pathway of the agroecosystem. Agroecosystems have depleted the original soil organic carbon levels by 25–75% with a loss of 10–50 tons C/ha, causing ecosystem damage, loss of soil carbon, and increased atmospheric CO_2 levels, contributing to climate change. However, isotope measurements reflect assimilated carbon and nitrogen isotopes, offering novel insights into the ecological positions of earthworms. The relationship between plants and soil is distinguished by a given zone called the "rhizosphere," where microbial behavior is affected by the root system. The effective association of soil-plant-microbial species separates this region from the rest of the soil mass (Russell, 1923; Herman et al., 2012). Contacts between microorganisms and the root system include a variety of activities in the root region within the soil community that lead to plant growth. Such activity between soils and microbes plays an important part in improving the bioavailability and utilization of plant mineral nutrients (Glick et al., 1999).

This study observes the natural abundance of carbon content between neighboring cropping systems, as well as the indirect earthworm effects of earthworms on carbon content in the substrate found in the NEP component using the plant–soil fauna–soil system. The study was reviewed by analyzing the C:N ratio required for plant-residue decomposition without N immobilization, which was determined to be approximately 25:1, a number that is still appropriate unless large amounts of poorly degradable residues are involved, as in forest litter Waksman (1932). The study focuses on the transfer of assimilated C of perennial and annual plants by analyzing the microbial decomposition rate in shoot, litter, root, earthworm casts, and earthworm in order to identify and generate an ideal microbial diet for soil microbes, relating the findings to the large stock of nutrients in the soil.

21.6 EMERGENCY RESPONSE QUESTIONS

Is the earthworm community of perennial land-use systems governed by the provided litter quality or the related soil moisture condition? Pertinent objectives include the following:

- To investigate perennial and annual neighbor plant systems related to carbon content and isotopic NEP composition.
- To investigate the explanatory variables content in C and N turnover of herbaceous plant material derived from perennial crops in soil.
- To test the indirect earthworm effects affecting microbial community functioning in the substrate, such as when earthworms are present using plant residues like perennial crops.
- To compare the effects of perennial crops and annual crops on soil microbial activities.
- To examine the response of the soil ecosystem to different plant residues as it relates to earthworm ecotypes.
- To explore possible relationships between 13C signatures of supposed sources of carbon in natural agroecosystems and consumer biota (earthworms).

21.7 SOIL DEPLETION AND CARBON SEQUESTRATION

Agricultural soil is an important component of the terrestrial ecosystem. It allows food production but also helps in reducing greenhouse gas emissions through C sequestration (Lal, 2004). The impact of human activities such as farming on the environment has led to a various decline in different ecosystems and the functionality of their components. A major component that has some undefined effects in soil due to the fact that many components are unidentified, and the need for exploration has become a necessity. Scientific research is necessary for the declaration dealing with financial and political support for reorganization. Knowledge must be more rapidly generated and translated into social and political action. This requires a focus on scientists to provide alternative solutions to global sustainability (Lal, 2004).

Maintaining both food productivity and the integrity of our natural habitats is a defining mission of the 21st century. Annual crop monocultures, presently supplying the majority of the food and fiber needs of mankind, pose a strong contrast to the complex perennial plant populations that constitute natural habitats, with few exceptions.

Soil depletion is the loss of nutrients, biodiversity, and soil quality due to improper extractive practices. This occurs when components contributing to fertility are not replaced after removal, and also when conditions supporting soil fertility are not properly maintained. This results in short-term effects, such as low crop yield, and long-term effects, such as endangered soil. According to the United Nations Global Opportunity Report 2017, soil depletion is one of the biggest challenges in soil, with approximately 40% of soil used for agriculture being degraded. Seventy percent of topsoil is gone. The United Nations (FAO) estimates that food production must increase by 70% from 2017 to 2050. Increasing food production with current practices will lead to a reduction in the decomposition rate, which will, in turn, lead to loss in soil biodiversity.

Under the Marrakech Agreements of the Kyoto Protocol, Articles 3.3 (activities limited to afforestation, reforestation, and deforestation) and 3.4 (activities limited to forest management, cropland management, grazing land management, and revegetation) allow the biospheric sinks and sources to be included to meet reduction targets of greenhouse gas emissions for the first commitment period of 2008–2012 of the Protocol. Therefore, the methods for the assessment, monitoring, and verification of soil C changes under these Articles are needed. In simple terms, soil C sequestration over a two-time period (e.g., commitment period of 2008–2012) may be defined as the difference between C addition and C loss and for known amounts of C input as:

$$\text{Soil C sequestration} = \text{C input} - \text{C loss (or turnover)} = I - kC \quad (1)$$

where:

I = C input.
k = decomposition rate or constant.

Various procedures can be used for measuring C accumulation based on mass balance measurements either by determining the net C retained (C stocks) at the end of the period or the turnover rate of C input each of the years for the period.

21.7.1 Soil Quality Indicators for C/N Turnover

Soil depletion has been shown to decrease the rate of decomposition due to loss in soil biota. (Santru et al., 2000). Knowledge of carbon and nitrogen distributions in vegetation and soil is important for understanding the carbon and nitrogen cycle on terrestrial croplands. Microorganisms play vital roles in soil processes such as substance turnover (decomposition), biogeochemical cycling, and plant growth, contributing essentially to soil ecosystem services (Wu et al., 2017). During decomposition, essential elements are converted from organic combinations to simple inorganic forms – a process called mineralization. The various interlocking processes of synthesis and decomposition by which carbon is circulated through soil, plants, animals, and air – collectively the biosphere – comprise the carbon cycle.

For the past 200 years or so, the release of CO_2 from the combustion of fossil fuels, respiration by organisms, land clearing, and burning has exceeded the sequestration of C in living and dead organisms on land and in water. This has led to a steady rise in the CO_2 concentration in the atmosphere, currently at an annual rate of 0.4%, and to what has been described as the enhanced "greenhouse effect." Globally, C in soil organic matter is a very large sink (c. 1,580 Gt or 1,580 × 109 t C, with an additional 800 Gt C in inorganic carbonates), so changes in the dynamic balance between the soil, vegetation, and the atmosphere can significantly affect the net flux of CO_2 to the atmosphere. Indeed, changing land management practices to achieve greater sequestration of C in SOM is part of the overall strategy to decrease net CO_2 emissions to the atmosphere. This makes the study of SOM – its composition, accumulation, and decomposition – a very important topic.

Soil contains a myriad of bacteria, the diversity and community structure of which are crucial to soil functional stability. Considerable efforts have been invested to address how bacteria respond to the changing environment, as terrestrial ecosystems are increasingly under the pressure of human activities (Wu et al., 2017). Cropland is such a hotspot of anthropogenic disturbance due to the lasting input of agricultural chemicals and pollutants over recent decades, resulting in significant changes in soil characteristics, as exemplified by acidification and pollution, particularly in some rapidly developed areas (Wu et al.,2017).

21.7.2 Impacts of Soil Quality on Soil Biota

The pronounced impact of anthropogenic activities on soil causes significant negative impacts on the SOM and the status of litter quality, leading to a decline in soil health and function. Soil biota, the "bio-engine of the earth," are one of the most affected properties of soil. Scientific principles of fundamental soil processes and properties should be recognized in order to assign the appropriate threshold values necessary to underline the impact of activities on SOM and prevent the extinction of soil biota species (Ritz et al. 2010). Microorganisms are key players in important ecological processes, such as carbon, nitrogen, phosphorus, and sulfur biogeochemical cycles (Garbeva et al., 2004), as seen in Table 21.1. A diverse group of microorganisms is present in the environment, including soil, and for their isolation, identification,

TABLE 21.1
Contributions of Soil Biota in the Biogeochemical Cycling

Carbon Cycle	Nitrogen Cycle
Carbon Assimilation	Nitrogen fixation
Carbon Mineralization	Nitrification
Methanogenesis	Denitrification

characterization, and culture-based microbial diversity analysis purposes, different standard culture-based techniques (Curtis et al., 2002).

Soil biota, such as bacteria, play a significant role in the cycle of a wide range of elements. However, the relative abundance of the most abundant microorganisms in a particular group is not necessarily associated with the importance of that group in the functioning of the community. The most abundant organisms may not always play the most critical role in a community, while organisms constituting only 0.1% of the community (e.g., nitrogen fixers) can have very important functions (Dinsdale et al., 2008).

21.7.3 Carbon Sequestration

The long-term absorption, sequestration, or preservation of carbon dioxide from the atmosphere to delay or reverse CO_2 emissions and to mitigate or reverse global warming are referred to as carbon sequestration or carbon dioxide removal. Readers are referred to Bregliani et al. (2010) for a figure showing the said relationships. The figure shows a diagrammatic interplay of atmospheric carbon dioxide and combustion from human activities, combustion from fossil fuels, assimilation by plants and animals, plant respiration, animal respiration, assimilation into soil, assimilation by phytoplankton, organic decomposition (animal waste, dead animals, and plants), formation of fossil fuels, and marine deposits of $CaCO_3$. The dynamic relationships and feedback in terrestrial ecosystems between the carbon cycles. Carbon is stored in soil organic matter. SOM is a diverse carbon mixture composed of plant and animal tissue splitting, microbial (protozoa, nematodes, fungi, and bacteria) and soil mineral carbon. Soil organisms require food for two different purposes: to provide nutrition for their basic and vital processes and to construct their body tissues. For these two reasons, though, the origins of food for various species can be different. In order to transform carbon from inorganic sources, all autotrophic species need much more energy for growth than many heterotrophs, because greater energy is required than for organic substances such as sugar (Russell, 1973). Autotrophic species may also fulfill their nitrogen needs from ammonium or nitrate salts. Heterotrophic species, however, are characterized by their dietary requirements or the metabolic modifications they offer. Most heterotrophs may use glucose as their primary source and, if necessary, generate an enzyme to turn a large variety of carbohydrates into sugar

(Herman et al., 2021). For the transformation of soil organic carbon for plant nutrient provision, the relationship between soil, plants, and microorganisms is important (Bregliani et al., 2010).

21.7.4 Biosequestration

Terrestrial biosequestration requires the net removal of CO_2 and storage of vegetative biomass and soils from the environment by plants and microorganisms. The sequestration of agricultural carbon will greatly alleviate the effects of global warming. At the same time, it would also increase soil quality using technologies to boost carbon sequestration in soil. Procedures that dramatically increase soil carbon sequestration include:

- Conservation of tillage (low-till/no-till farming) – A planting system that reduces or removes soil for crop production. It involves tilling that leaves crop residues on the soil surface, which in turn improves soil structure. These processes typically decrease soil degradation, enhance water quality, and increase carbon concentrations in the topsoil. Conservation tillage can also decrease the amount of fossil fuel used by farm operations.
- Cover crop – The usage of plants and small grains to sustain and stimulate soil between regular crop production. They boost carbon sequestration by altering the composition of the surface by increasing organic matter in the soil.
- Crop rotation – Growing multiple crops in a revolving schedule of years (e.g., maize-oats-clover) decreases the carbon loss from the soil and, with certain additions (e.g., manure, lime, phosphorous), contributes carbon to the soil.

Many of the above techniques are used more widely in organic farming than in conventional farming. Carbon stored in soils oxidizes rapidly. Management of the soil and the adoption of conservation practices provide a positive impact on the ability of soil to supply water for crop demands, and practices that enhance soil C provide a means of reducing yield variation under a changing climate (Huyet al., 2025). The use of a range of climate change models with environmental models to provide a clear projection of soil C rises (Yurova et al., 2010). The difference in soil C shifts depends on temperature, precipitation, evaporation, and original soil properties. Recent studies test a number of climate change scenarios with the possible change in soil C (Jan et al., 2011). Adoption of farming activities like neighbor cropping systems to improve soil C will benefit crop production and serve as an atmospheric CO_2 sink. Increasing soil C will depend upon the cropping system placed on the landscape (Brown et al., 2014). In order to establish a plan to modify soil C, the identified land-use shifts must be related to climate change scenarios.

The variations between soil types and their reactions to management systems make things more difficult (Brown and Castellazzi, 2014). The dominant factors that influence soil C shift and land transfer with tillage to annual cultivation systems were found by the rangeland method (Byrd et al., 2015), which merged patterns of land use and precipitation patterns. They proposed that input should be understood from land use to climate change, with the goal of designing efficient systems for soil management to improve soil. Understanding this dynamic provides a framework to determine the C-sequestration capacity in various environments and the predicted soil changes.

21.7.5 Cropping System

The cropping method refers to the form and sequence of plants grown and the techniques used to grow plants. This covers all crop sequences practiced over time and space depending on available crop processing technologies (Haramoto and Gallandt, 2004). Species and variety selection are based on the content of vegetative plant relative tissues and higher soil fertility status, along with seed termination coverage. Traditionally, it has also been structured to optimize crop yields in herbaceous plants. There is also a clear need to design cropping systems that take into account evolving social, economic, and environmental or environmental issues. When tillage activities are limited, organic farming systems that integrate crop rotations, cover crops, and crop diversification increase soil organic C concentration.

Crop diversification has the capacity to break the pest cycle in organic farming, suppress weed reproduction and decrease unnecessary labor. Rotations have been used for a long since pesticides and herbicides were introduced to combat weeds. These methods are effective in decreasing and eradicating particular weed species. Planting legumes, grasses, perennials, or winter plants disrupts weed cycles while maximizing organic C soil storage. The conservation of soil and water and the preservation of long-term soil fertility depends to a large extent on the management of crop systems, which affect the extent of soil erosion and the dynamics of soil organic matter. Although extremely degraded land may require conversion to nonagricultural systems (e.g., woodland, perennial grass) for regeneration, prudently selected and carefully maintained crop systems may sustain or even increase soil fertility and restore moderately degraded land by improving soil resilience. Crop diversification is an important choice for sustainable agricultural systems.

21.7.6 Herbaceous Plant

This (herb) is nonwoody vascular plant comprised of grasses and grass-like plants clustered together as graminoids, forbs, and ferns. It is used to classify plants by the number of growing seasons required to complete their life cycle. Generally, these groups are annuals, biennials, and perennials (Fuller and Carothers, 1963), with no permanent woody stems but containing an array of cytoplasm and cell wall components that require a complex scheme for decomposition. The use of lignin as a complex phenotypic polymer stored in the secondary cell walls of all vascular plants does not result in the perennialization of aboveground structures. Since many woody plants are perennial with a longer life cycle, they take longer to produce persistently growing significant, dry tree trunks, and because they require more time and more energy (nutrients and water), they cannot colonize as easily as herbs. During the evolution of vascular plants, lignin was formed, providing mechanical strength, rigidity, and hydrophobicity to secondary cell walls, allowing plants to grow extensively by holding water and nutrients inside the plant body for longer distances.

21.7.7 Annual Crop

An annual crop is a plant that completes its life cycle in one season, from germination to seed development, and then dies. Based on geographical location, the time and duration of the growing seasons may not correspond to the four conventional seasonal divisions of the year (Collinson, 1988). Having achieved their reproductive mission, they die when the first hard frosts of autumn arrive. With respect to the traditional seasons, annual plants are generally categorized into summer annuals and winter annuals; a good example is wheat. The roots, stems, and leaves of the plant die annually. Only the dormant seed bridges the gap between one generation and the next. Toward the end of the growing season (late summer or early fall), annual flowers yield seeds, signaling to the plants that their life cycle is complete. Even though they do not compete directly with cultivated plants, sometimes winter annuals are considered a pest in commercial agriculture because they can host insect pests or fungal diseases (ovary smut – *Microbotryum* sp.) that attack crops being cultivated. Their property of preventing the soil from drying out can also be problematic for commercial agriculture. In 2008, it was discovered that the inactivation of only two genes in one species of annual plant leads to its conversion into a perennial plant.

The summer annuals sprout, flower, produce seed, and die during the warmer months of the year. Summer annuals germinate during spring or early summer and mature by autumn of the same year. Winter annuals germinate during the autumn and mature during the spring or summer of the following calendar year. One seed-to-seed life cycle for an annual can occur in as little as a month in some species, though most last several months. In cultivation, many food plants are or are grown as, annuals, including virtually all domesticated grains (Siegbert et al. 2008).

Winter annuals develop in autumn or winter, live through the winter, and then bloom in winter or spring. The plants grow and bloom during the cool season when most other plants are dormant, or other annuals are in seed form, waiting for warmer weather to germinate. Winter annuals die after flowering and setting seed. The seeds germinate in the autumn or winter when the soil temperature is cool. Winter annuals typically grow low to the ground, where they are usually sheltered from the coldest nights by snow cover, and make use of warm periods in winter for growth when the snow melts.

Some common winter annuals include wheat, henbit, deadnettle, chickweed, and winter cress. Winter annuals are important ecologically, as they provide vegetative cover that prevents soil erosion during winter and early spring when no other cover exists, and they provide fresh vegetation for animals and birds that feed on them. Although they are often considered to be weeds in gardens, this viewpoint is not always necessary, as most of them die when the soil temperature warms up again in early to late spring, when other plants are still dormant and have not yet leafed out.

21.7.7.1 Triticum aestivum (Winter Wheat)

Triticum aestivum, or "winter wheat," is the oldest C_3 plant and the most widely produced and consumed cereal crop on earth, cultivated for more than ten thousand years. It grows in a diverse range of climates and soils. CIMMYT (1996) and Tarfa (2021) provide a plot of worldwide wheat area and production. It is one of the first food crops of domesticated origin and was the basic staple food of large European, West Asian, and North African civilizations for 8,000 years (Curtis et al., 2002). It develops in greater elevations near the equator from the Arctic cycle. In a number of nations, wheat is the largest source of carbohydrates. It contains nutrients, vitamins, and fats (lipids) and is extremely nutritious even without the inclusion of animal or legume protein (Curtis et al., 2002). In recent years, the proportion of wheat production from high-income nations dropped from around 45% at the beginning of the 1950s to around 35%. Policy adjustments in grain reserve systems for the protection of soils in high-income countries have taken up a large wheat production area.

More than 45% of global wheat has been produced by developed countries in the last five years. During the 1951–1990 period, the world wheat output increased significantly, even though the expansion of the sown wheat field was a significant source of increased wheat production for several years (CIMMYT, 1996). Output in 1990 still reached a peak of 592 million tons. Since 1986, 500 million tons or more. Output has been largely stable since 1990. It is also a common source of animal food, particularly when harvests have a negative effect on rain, and substantial amounts of grain are not suitable for food consumption (CIMMYT, 1996).

21.7.7.2 Zea mays (Maize)

Part of the grass family, *Zea mays* (maize) is one of the most diverse C_4 plants, usually called corn. The monoecious annual summer seasonal plant has thick alternating leaves, an upright stalk and its steady inflorescence consisting of a main spike (tassel) and several branches. The inflorescences of one to several pistillate and the huge fiber root system are noteworthy. The staple grain has been eaten for around 10,000 years in many parts of the world. It is one of the main food crops in the world, cultivated at nearly 370 million tons (Ranum et al., 2014) and provides more than 50% of the world's food in temperate climate countries. Maize is widely cultivated around the world and achieves higher annual yields than any other crop. Pollination is carried out by the wind, which results in self-fertilization as well as cross-fertilization. A high degree of variation has arisen from cross-fertilization, broad distribution, and human selection. Maize grows only under cultivation; no fully wild varieties are known, but wild teosinte and maize have shared genetic access where they occur (Galinat, 1971; Wilkes, 1972). While research indicates that cold temperatures cause long-term damage to maize production, it contains both male and female reproductive structures and is recorded by cross-pollination and self-pollination. Early planting due to climate change is becoming more common, although the associated risks are slowly increasing. Increasing maize toleration may increase latitude and enhance yield and productivity during the growing season (Dohleman and Long, 2009).

21.7.8 Perennial Crop

Perennial crops live for more than two years. The word is commonly used to identify plants with little or no woody development, unlike trees and shrubs, which are technically annual. Requiring no yearly cultivation, they grow back naturally after harvesting. By avoiding replanting, their yields will decrease soil losses to erosion and increase biological carbon sequestration due to decreased soil disruption. This also substantially reduces water emissions by farm runoff due to less nitrogen intake (Berry, 2009). It usually has a growing structure that enables them to survive by vegetative reproduction instead of seeding from one year to the next. These systems include flowers, tubers, woody crowns, and rhizomes. They comprise specialized stems or crowns that allow them to withstand periods of dormancy during the cold or dry seasons of the year.

Annuals, however, produce seeds to begin the species as a new generation when the growing season is sufficient, and the seeds live through the cold or dry season to resume growing when the conditions are again appropriate. Many perennials have special features that allow them to withstand severe climate and environmental conditions. Some have evolved to survive warm and dry or freezing conditions. They seem to invest a great deal of energy in adjusting and often do not flower and generate seeds until after a few years of development. Many perennials produce comparatively large seeds, which may offer a benefit, with larger seedlings produced after germination that are better able to compete with other plants. Some annuals produce far more seeds per plant in one season, while some (polycarpic) perennials are not under the same strain to produce many seeds but can produce seeds over many years. Dividing perennial plants is something that gardeners do in the months of September and October or early spring. The point of division in early autumn is to allow for sufficient root growth of approximately six weeks until the ground freezes.

Soil is properly moisturized to quickly expand due to leaves that come from crops and the amount of rain that falls in most areas during the autumn months. Perennials that are loosely or marginally hardy are better separated in the season. Each type of plant may be divided differently; for example, plants with fibrous root systems may be separated. However, some plants have a root system of rhizomes; these root systems can be planted at the top of the rhizome just above the ground floor, with the leaves showing from the following year.

21.7.8.1 Miscanthus giganteus (Miscanthus)

Miscanthus giganteus is a power plant, also called miscanthus, with key potential for renewable energy because of its fuel efficiency. It is a tall, highly active, resistant variety, a rhizomatous C_4 photosynthesis perennial grass with excellent rapid growth. It has unusually high photosynthetically active radiation at low temperatures and remains highly active in cold climates among C_4 species usually susceptible to cold weather damage (Long, 1983). it is a perennial crop that stores a large amount of biomass below ground level. About half of the biomass is lower, with rhizomes making up 65–89% under the layer (Kahle et al., 2001). The grass has been researched and used to produce heat and energy by combustion in Europe since the 1980s, but since 2005, the US government has encouraged experiments using herbaceous feedstocks to convert to ethanol for use as transport fuel, because of its potential to produce large quantities of biomass (Anderson et al., 2014).

The grass species and varieties have been primarily categorized and defined by phenotypic features. The phenolic features play a vital role in neighboring cropping because they improve the resistance of neighboring crops, inhibit the growth of weeds, and prevent shallow soil erosion. They enhance carbon content and encourage the activity and variety of microorganisms that are essential to the aggregation and rehabilitation phase of soil particles (Nsanganwimana et al., 2015). The authors say the three-fold benefit of this practice is that soil fertility is increased, biomass yields are increased, and wastewater sludge treatment and disposal costs are reduced in compliance with particular regulations in every region. It provides a wide variety of economic end goods and uses depending on the processes involved in conversion.

21.7.8.2 Silphium perfoliatum (Cup Plant)

Silphium perfoliatum, or "cup plant," is a perennial C_3 flora belonging to the Asteraceae and Heliantheae families. It is often called a cup plant because its cup-shaped leaves allow it to store moisture and avoid drought (Standford, 1990). It needs very little crop maintenance because it is understood that after the first year of development, it has enduring disease and pest-resistant forms requiring much less pesticide. The herbicide is effective enough to deal with weeds, and from the second vegetation cycle, herbicide steps are not needed as the plant responds well to the European environment. It seeks humus on deep-seated ground, usually along streams and waterways with a lot of moisture. It is grown as a medicinal plant with an intense scent of resin of the form turpentine and emitting more eco-friendly facilities than maize as both a food and ornamental plant. Current research provides promising alternatives to maize as the cup plant is an energy culture that not only has similar properties for biogas production of biogas is concerned, but also has ecological benefits such as soil preservation and providing food for pollinators. It offers food and shelter for herbivores, birds, and insects and is typically used to make maize cultivation more environmentally friendly as an alternative or neighborly cultivation method for large biogas plants. The extraction of proteins from the biomass of cup plants could lead to the replacement of soy for feeding cattle with locally produced proteins. The new European regulation on advanced biofuels, which was applied to greening acts in 2018, is compliant. The cup plant is much better than maize, as it is more resistant to marginal soil conditions such as adverse roots, wetness, and polluted soil. Cup plant farming is increasingly rising in Germany. The biomass yields are roughly 20 mg/ha in Europe and 20 mg/ha in South America, according to Frączek et al. (2011) and Pichard (2012).

Good quality planting must be produced to improve cup plant energy use. Before winter, in the first year, the plant grows leaves and roots. It steadily increases in its second spring year, and its first production is expected to take place in early autumn (Biertümpfel et al., 2013). The Karpenstein-Machan (Platen et al. 2017), which is similar to maize production, shows a higher average return. Weeds and pest control are generally only required in the first year; thus, no herbicides or pesticides are needed in the following years. There is no tillage, which raises carbon sequestration and, after the first year, encourages pollination. It is very valuable in Europe because of its sustainability characteristics, such as increased energy supplies (biomass production), weather/disease resistance, and suitability as the fundamental key to a sustainable agricultural transformation (Gansberger et al. 2015). Generally speaking, the perennial neighbor crop system, such as miscanthus, is used to increase soil physical and chemical fertility properties (Melligan et al., 2012) and to boost the yields of some crops like maize (Kwapinski et al., 2010). The choice and control of plants will have a direct effect on the soil microbial communities and their processes.

Various types of soil have no specific effect on the dry matter production of the plant, but the longer the growth location, the shorter the growing time and, thus, the lower the output. The plant is ideal for many different places in Europe owing to its low land requirements. In comparison, the cup plant has high productivity and is thus resistant to drought conditions, even though drought resistance and water efficiency are lower than for maize in the cup plant. It's because of its long roots. The minimum water needs are equivalent to 400–500 mm for corn, but in arid years, the cup plant can provide more biomass than maize.

21.7.9 C_3 Plants

The first step in the Calvin cycle is to fix carbon dioxide by rubisco, with C_3 plants forming three-carbon compounds, which only use this normal mechanism. C_3 plants, including corn, wheat, soybeans, and all trees, comprise around 85% of the plant species on earth. It is a "natural" plant with no adaptation to photosynthesize. Plants with C_3 photosynthesis have dominated the background of terrestrial vegetation, as a limited percentage of typical habitats are inhabited by Crassulacean Acid Metabolism (CAM) plants. A wide spectrum of compositions of carbon isotopes (–20 to –37 km, V-PDB) is found in C_3 plants (Koch et al., 2004).

21.7.10 C_4 Plants

C_4 plants physically distinguish the light-based reactions and the Calvin cycle, and the light-dependent reactions occur in mesophyll cells (spongy tissue in the center of the leaf). Special cells in the leaves, known as bundle-sheath cells, perform the cycle of Calvin. C_4 plants are also known. The bundling-sheath cells are these cells. Second, in mesophyll cells, atmospheric CO_2 is fixed to form a basic, organic four-carbon acid (oxaloacetate) by an enzyme that does not bind to O_2, the non-rubisco phosphoenolpyruvate carboxylase (PEP) carboxylase. Oxaloacetate is then converted into a related molecule, malate, which is malate and can be transported to the bundle-sheath cells. In the bundle sheath, malate breaks down and releases a CO_2 molecule. This CO_2 is then fixed into sugar by rubisco, in photosynthesis C_3 in the Calvin cycle. The photosynthetic C_4 cycle, which is practically unable to operate at low temperatures, would greatly reduce the probability of phenotypes and genera entirely adapted to cold temperate and cool climates compared to those in the Calvin cycle. Furthermore, the selection is likely for higher potential production, water quality, and nitrogen efficiency. This probable chosen advantage of C_4 relative to C_3 species is limited by low temperatures in terms of higher potential production, water quality, and productivity in nitrogen use (Long, 1983).

21.7.11 Plant Structure

Plant is the photosynthetic eukaryote, making up the Plantae kingdom. It needs water, carbon dioxide, and sunlight (i.e., inorganic substances) in its individual environment/habitat to synthesize sugar/nutrients functioning as food for different organisms. In addition to the synthesis of their own food, plants in diverse ecosystems (aquatic, terrestrial, etc.) play an important role in the production of oxygen, making them vital to all life on Earth. Though plant biology allows photosynthesis (a unifying feature), various types of plants have different physical and genetic characteristics. Plant structure can be subdivided into three different groups comprising shoot, litter and root.

21.7.11.1 Plant Shoot

The shoot includes the stem, leaves, and bulbs. It is often used for a young plant that grows out of the soil after the seed has germinated. It consists of stalks, flowers, lateral buds, and flower stalks attached to each other, structurally developing on a shooting frame that grows over the soil. The gravity of the shoot mechanism is recognized in the growth zone by specialized cells (Moulia et al., 2011; Morita, 2010). When the annual plant sprouts from the seed, the root grows into the soil, and the shoot grows towards the sun. As the bulb of a perennial plant becomes active in the spring, it sends out roots further into the soil and shoots into the air. The stem is the part of the shoot that carries water up the shoot and dissolves food to all other areas of the plant. It assists the remainder of the shoot.

21.7.11.2 Plant Stem

The stem is part of the shoot system found above the ground, which protects the plant, supplies water and nutrients from roots to other parts of the plant, supplies food from leaves to other parts of the plant, serves as food storage, and creates new living tissue. Normally, the stem is split into nodes and internodes. Nodes contain one or two leaves as well as buds that develop into branches (with leaves, coniferous cones, or inflorescences). Adventitious roots can also be created from the nodes; the internodes distance one node from another. The normal life cycle of a plant cell is one to three years, but stem cells, or meristems, develop new living tissue every year. The roots have the tissues xylem and phloem like two pipes. The xylem tissue holds water by pulling the sap, capillaries, and root strain. The tissues of the phloem are made up of sieve tubes and cells. All tissues are divided into xylem or phloem cells by a cambium tissue. Typically, the tissue of the stem consists of three tissues: blood, soil and vascular tissue.

The dermal tissue protects the exterior surface of the trunk and typically acts to shield, prevent water loss, and regulate the exchange of gases. The tissue in the field normally consists of parenchymal cells and fills the space surrounding the vascular tissue. It often helps in photosynthesis. The vascular tissue is responsible for the long-distance transport of vascular tissue and provides structural support. In woody stems, any or all ground tissue on the ground can be lost over time. Waterproofing in aerial stems may be absent from the dermal tissue of aquatic plants. The vascular tissue varies extensively between plant species.

21.7.11.3 Plant Leaf

The leaf is the most essential organ of most vascular plants. The leaf is usually flattened with distinct upper (adaxial) and lower (abaxial) surfaces that vary in color, hairiness, the number of stomata (pores that ingest and output gases), the volume and composition of epicuticular wax, and other characteristics. It is mostly green in color due to the presence of a compound called chlorophyll, which is essential for photosynthesis as it absorbs light energy from the sun. A leaf with white spots or edges is called a variegated leaf. Green plants are autotrophic, meaning that they produce their food with the aid of sunlight, carbon dioxide, water, and minerals. This mechanism is called photosynthesis. The mechanism of photosynthesis happens as leaves absorb the energy in sunlight and turn it into basic sugars, such as glucose and sucrose, from carbon dioxide and water. The sugars are then deposited as starch, further converted by chemical synthesis into more complex organic molecules such as proteins or cellulose, the essential structural material in plant cell walls, or metabolized by cellular respiration to provide chemical energy to run cellular processes.

Leaf extract water from the ground in the transpiration process by a vascular conducting mechanism known as xylem and receive carbon dioxide from the environment through diffusion by openings called stomata in the outer covering layer of the leaf (epidermis), while leaves are oriented to increase their exposure to sunlight. When sugar has been synthesized, it needs to be transferred to areas of active growth, such as the plant shoots and roots. Vascular plants transport sucrose in a special tissue called the phloem. The phloem and xylem are parallel to each other, but the transport of materials is ordinarily in inverse directions. Inside the leaf, these vascular structures branch to make veins that supply as much of the leaf as possible, ensuring that cells carrying out photosynthesis are near to the transportation structure.

21.7.11.4 Litter Material

Litter material is the largest source of organic matter that enters many stream ecosystems (Abelho, 2001). The decomposition of plant litter is a crucial step in nutrient recycling. Litterfall is the dominant pathway for nutrient return to the soil. In tropical rainforests, there is a thin litter layer due to rapid decomposition. In boreal forests, the rate of decomposition is slower and leads to the accumulation of a thick litter layer, also known as a mor. Latitude also has a strong effect on litterfall rates and thickness. Litterfall declines with increasing latitude. In highly weathered tropical soils, most of the plant biomass-derived carbon is mineralized in the litter layer. This is known as soil immobilization. The accumulation of these nutrients in the top layer of soil is known as soil immobilization. It is accomplished through the leaching of nutrients by rainfall and throughfall and by the efforts of detritivores. It contributes to the cation exchange capacity of the soil and is responsible for global carbon fluxes. The most extreme variability of litterfall is seen as a function of seasonality; each individual species of plant has seasonal losses of certain parts of its body.

Surface detritus facilitates the capture and infiltration of rainwater into lower soil layers. Soil litter protects soil aggregates from raindrop impact, preventing the release of clay and silt particles from plugging soil pores. Organic matter accumulation also helps protect soils from wildfire damage. Net primary production and litterfall are intimately connected, with litterfall patterns similar to global patterns of net primary productivity. Climate also influences the depth of plant litter, with humid tropical and subtropical climates having reduced organic matter layers and horizons due to year-round decomposition.

21.7.11.5 Plant Roots

The plant root system is a community that develops beneath the surface. Its fundamental form is divided into four areas: the root cap, the meristem apical, the hair field, and the elongation region. The root hair, epidermis, epibymis, cortex, endodermal tissue, and vascular tissue are positioned at the center of the root for transfer to other parts of the plant through water absorption by the root. It absorbs and transmits water and required minerals from the soil. Roots hold the plant firmly to the ground, and some also act as storage for extra food in plants. The rhizosphere consists of dead roots, 'sloppy' epidermal root cells, and carbon (C) compounds released into the surrounding soil from living roots, both of which contribute to rhizosphere carbon. Contributions are impossible to quantify, but research that has placed a plant shoot in a carbon isotope (13C)-labeled atmosphere suggests a 5–10% release to the rhizosphere of the entire plant carbon, except C breathed as CO_2 from both the roots and the microorganisms living in the rhizosphere (Tinker and Nye, 2000). Some crops, miscanthus, form roots that contribute to nitrogen-fixing bacteria known as rhizobia. They form a symbiotic relationship with bacteria, taking carbon compounds from the plant to fuel the process. The energy needed to fix nitrogen comes from the atmosphere, and the crop, in particular, uses ammonia-producing nitrogen compounds. The root serves as the niche zone for many soil fauna.

21.7.12 Soil Fauna

Soil fauna is a major factor in the resilience of the soil as it affects carbon and nitrogen turnover and cycling, organic soils, and land build up. They conserve habitats on and below the ground depending on demographic differences and the composition of soil animals. The macrofauna (e.g., earthworms, termites, ants), through pedoturbation and soil composition, contribute to the structuring of the soil (Wright and Jones, 2004). A good soil is full of life and comprises a number of macro and microorganisms that drive principal processes of soil resistance.

The macrofauna (for example, earthworms, termites, ants) through pedoturbation mixing of soil materials helps in structuring the soil (Wright and Jones, 2004). There is an extraordinary number of macroorganisms living in healthy soil. The microfauna (<100 μm diameter), mesofauna (100 μm to 2 m diameter) and macrofauna (>2 mm diameter) classify the soil animals into three key classes (Bradford et al., 2002). They can vary in size and behavior, but their tolerance to the soil is similar.

Earthworms blend inorganic and organic particles of soil and maximize porosity and aggregation. The interconnected, heterogeneous, vertical, and large biological macropores (e.g., wormholes) are formed (e.g., wormholes). The biopores are the paths for penetration by rain and runoff, minimizing rush and length. In soil dynamics, meso and microfauna are no less significant. They influence chemical reactions (solubilization and processing) and plant root-soil exchanges. The soil restructuring, nitrogen cycling, and soil organic turnover affect the relationship of earthworms, bacteria, and plant roots.

21.7.12.1 Earthworms

Earthworms, also called "ecosystem engineers," have been the focus of specific research efforts and more general field trials for a period in excess of a century (Darwin, 1881). The invertebrate phylums annelida and oligochaeta are found predominantly in moist, rich land. The cylindrical, soft-bodied animals, along with their bodily structures, have a uniform ring. Such bodies can be divided into linear series and are externally represented by circular grooves called annuli. Rombke et al. (2005) and Tarfa (2021) present a schematic representation of the functional relationships between earthworms and their external environment. This schematic is based on their ecotypes, feeding mechanisms, and habitat. Earthworms can be divided into different ecotypes based on their habitats. These ecotypes include epigeic, anecic, and endogeic.

- **Epigeics:** These are species living above the mineral soil surface. Generally, they have no effect on soil structure because they are phytophagous, small in size, and cannot dig into the soil (Lee, 1985).
- **Anecic:** These are species living above layers of soil minerals. These species move to the surface to feed on litter and pull the material into their burrows. This process of burying surface litter is highly essential. They are geophytophagous because they feed on both plants and soil (Lee, 1985).
- **Endogenic:** These are species living in the mineral soil horizons while feeding on soil enriched with organic matter. They are geophagous, and they build horizontal branches during burrowing (Lee, 1985).

Although there are mainly three types of ecotypes based on their habitat, based on the nature of diets, earthworms can be classed as detritivorous, which feed on high-quality raw humus and geophagous, which feed on amorphous humus and mineral materials (Lee, 1985). The consistency of litter (C:N ratio of root biomass) has been found to be more extreme under grass-white clover blends, which indicates an important variable controlling earthworm abundance (C:N ratio of root biomass) (van Eekeren et al., 2010).

21.7.12.2 Earthworm Casts

The earthworm cast is a structure naturally erected on the soil by worms (Vidal et al., 2019). It is formed when earthworm ingestion of mineral soil or organic particulate matter is mixed and enriched by organic secretions in the intestines and then processed as slurry or discrete fecal pellets. It is a very fertile material, which includes digested soils, litter, and microbes, which continuously convert nutrients to bioavailable forms. Casts also contain enzymes such as protease, amylase, lipase, cellulase, and chitinase, which continue to disintegrate organic matter even after they have been excreted. Depending on the earthworm species, fecal pellets may be excreted inside or on the soil. Turnover rates vary in grassland from 40 to 70 t/ha (Bouché, 1983).

When casts are in the earthworm gut, microbes that colonize the gut start breaking up organic matter in the soil. When casts accumulate in the soil, bacterial colonization and development proceed until compounds readily decompose. Mechanisms of cast stabilization include organic bonding of particles by polymers secreted by earthworms and microbes, mechanical stabilization by plant fibers and fungal hyphae, and stabilization due to wetting and drying cycles and age-hardening effects (Tomlin et al., 1995). Mineralization of organic matter in earthworm casts and burrow linings produces zones of nutrient enrichment compared to bulk soil. Enzymatic catalyzation by enzymes such as amylase, which hydrolysis starch into sugars, is also a key process.

These zones are referred to as the "drilosphere" and are often sites of enhanced activity of plant roots and other soil biota (Lavelle et al., 1998). Plant growth-promoting substances have also been suggested as constituents of earthworm casts. Many earthworm castings from commercial vermicomposting operations are sold commercially as soil amendments to improve soil physical properties and enhance plant growth (Edwards, 1998).

21.7.12.3 NEP Budget Model Pools and Fluxes of C and N

The presence of earthworms could change dramatically the sizes of different pools of nutrients and the flows of C and N, relative to the plant tissues. To define the role of earthworms in the sustainability of the agroecosystem, it is essential to concentrate on processes that increase the storage or loss of nutrients or reduce them, and on how they affect production and nutrient intake by crops (Bohlen et al. (2004) presents a diagram showing pools and fluxes of C and N.

The key ways that earthworms can alter the preservation and loss of C and N and integrate the impact on the biological, physical, and chemical processes of the soil are emphasized by this model. Interactions between earthworms and the microbial community, and by processing OM, earthworms can increase the system flux of CO_2 (gaseous C loss). These same interactions, coupled with earthworm casts, can also lead to increased availability of C and N.

21.7.12.4 Factors Affecting Cast Production

Several factors influence the production of cast; some of the main ones are food, moisture, temperature, light, pH, and predators.

21.7.13 Soil Organic Matter

The organic matter of soil arises from the debris of green plants, animal residues, and excreta deposited on the surface and mixed to a variable extent with the mineral component. The combination of living and dead organic matter, irrespective of its source or stage of decomposition (but excluding the living parts of plants above ground), is called soil organic matter. It is mainly made up of carbon (50%), nitrogen (35%), hydrogen (5%), and oxygen (5%). It also contains small amounts of other elements, such as phosphorus, sulfur, potassium, calcium, and magnesium, contained in organic residues. It can be grouped into biotic and abiotic components and can range from very recent inputs, such as stubble, to largely decayed materials that are thousands of years old. About 10% of belowground SOM, such as roots, fauna, and microorganisms is found in particulate organic matter (POM). Griffin (2013) shows a pie chart of the forms of SOM in a report on sustainable natural resource use in agriculture.

SOM exists in four distinct fractions, which vary widely in size, turnover time, and composition in the soil. The key property that influences soil health and its biophysical and chemical functions is SOM, which is greatly influenced by management and cropping systems and potential climate change. Maintaining SOM is well-linked to the type of tillage and crop rotations or cropping systems that have been practiced. No-till and continuous tilling systems increase soil aggregate stability and resiliency over time when subjected to prolonged wet conditions, soil C stock, and water infiltration (Guzman and Al-Kaisi, 2011, 2014). Table 21.2 below shows its distribution pathways and pattern consisting of DOM, POM, humus, and resistant organic

TABLE 21.2
Soil Organic Matter Fraction

Fraction	Size (μm and mm)	Turnover Time	Composition
Dissolved Organic Matter (DOM)	<45μm (in solution)	Minutes to days	Soluble root exudates, simple sugars and decomposition by-products. It accounts for 5% of total soil organic matter.
Particulate organic matter (POM)	53μm–2mm	2–50 years	Plant and animal materials fresh or decomposing with a cell framework that can be identified. It accounts for 2–25% of total soil organic matter.
Humus	<53μm	Decadal (10s to 100s of years)	Older, decayed organic compounds that have resisted decomposition. Can make up more than 50% of total soil organic matter.
Resistant organic matter (ROM)	<53μm–2mm	100s to 1,000s of years	Relatively inert material, such as chemically resistant materials or organic remnants (e.g., charcoal). Can be up to 10% of soil organic matter.

matter (ROM). Soil health indicators are strongly influenced by climate parameters, precisely, the difference in SOM fractions. The decomposition of various SOM fractions is closely related to the decomposition of SOM or mineralization and its stabilization. Rapid mineralization of labile C components is the dominant mechanism during the first process of decomposition.

The aggregation of refractory molecules is reduced during the mineralization in the second step of decomposition (Zech et al., 1997). Regardless of the original chemical composition, the SOC pool is deposited in biologically unfavorable soil space where it is physically shielded from microbial development (Six et al., 2000). Tillage and crop rotation, as well as other management methods and cropping systems, can result in substantial losses of complete and mineralizable SOM (Schimel et al., 1985).

21.7.13.1 Soil Organic Nitrogen

The conversion of organic nitrogen in soil into mineral nitrogen is a significant source of the nitrogen required by crops. Although soil nitrogen supply is useful for estimating how much nitrogen from organic matter will become available to a crop, there is a significant difficulty with this measurement. Soil nitrogen supply estimates the quantity of nitrogen released from organic matter without giving any information about when it will be released. Most nitrogen released from organic matter occurs during the growing season, providing a steady, continuous supply of nitrogen to the crop. This is because the microorganisms responsible for releasing nitrogen from organic matter require some soil moisture, usually deposited in litter (Angus, 2001).

21.7.13.2 Soil Organic Carbon

Soil organic carbon is an important soil solid component in which all plant and animal tissues, as well as microbial biomass at different decomposition stages, are formed. The SOC sequestration refers to the "process by which plant residues and other organic materials are stored and maintained in the unit as part of the SOC with long mean residence times (MRTs) from the atmosphere to the ground matter to ensure that it is not re-emitted back to the atmosphere" (Olson et al., 2014). Sequestration of SOC could be achieved by:

- Improved plant growth within the land unit.
- Conservation of plant biomass within the land unit can be transformed into SOCs.
- Safeguarding the soil and decomposition unit in SOCs.
- Enhancing synergies between the earth, plants, and atmospheric mechanisms to produce a positive soil C budget before the soil C sinks.
- Increasing plant growth within the land unit.

21.7.14 Properties of Soil Used as Standard Sensitive Indicators in Soil Resilience

Resilience is an ecological field that encompasses a variety of characteristics that control soil decomposition responses to disruptions or stress. This is because soil

TABLE 21.3
Soil Properties as Quality and Resilience Indicators

Physical	Chemical	Biological	Biochemical	Ecological
Stable micro aggregates	Formation of organomineral complexes	Anaerobic microsites with inhibited microbial activity	Supra-molecular structure	Ecosystem characteristics (i.e., climate, growing season, belowground biodiversity)
Access in microbial processes	Absorption on clay particles	Earthworm population and activity	Formation and selective preservation of molecules	C:N ratio
Deep placement in subsoil		Rooting depth and abundance	Recalcitrant substances	
			Clay hutches	

decomposition is a biophysical process driven by political and economic factors such as land use and cropping/farming systems, which have a significant impact on soil quality and soil resilience. Although soil quality and soil resilience are interrelated, they have dissimilar attributes (Table 21.3).

Soil quality and resilience processes and mechanisms that set in motion the degradative trends include physical, chemical, and biological processes. Soil quality and resilience also differ in relation to critical limits and threshold values of key soil attributes. Soil quality, as measured by productivity, is affected by decomposition processes governed by the NPP and the maximum sustainable yield, while soil resilience is governed by NEP and the interaction within each ecosystem component.

21.7.15 Biomass

Biomass is a biological substance produced from live organisms or freshly dead organisms. It is usually plant-based, but recent studies also note that biomass can be derived from both plant and animal products. It is also a major source of alternative energy to fossil fuels. In response to the threats of climate change and the decline of fossil fuels, biomass contributes to the energy shift toward low-carbon economies (IPCC, 2011). There would be major growth in the use of dedicated bioenergy crops (Chum et al., 2011; Bentsen and Felby, 2012). New conversion technologies and biological refineries are being built to take a large array of candidate cultures into account (Ragauskas et al., 2006; Somerville et al., 2010). These crops would also have to meet a range of criteria, including high productivity, low emissions of GHGs, ecosystem conservation, and a low impact on the climate (Tilman et al., 2009; Karp and Richter, 2011).

21.7.15.1 Biomass Carbon

Biomass carbon is collected from a mixture of organic molecules containing hydrogen, usually including atoms of oxygen and nitrogen. In some cases, it also contains small quantities of other atoms, including alkali, alkaline earth, and heavy metals. It is usually derived from the mass of living organisms, including plants, animals, and microorganisms, or, from a biochemical perspective, cellulose, lignin, sugars, fats, and proteins. Plants that produce biomass to capture energy are capable of producing nearly the same quantity of CO_2 as fossil fuels through photosynthesis during growth, making biomass that can make bio-neutral energy sources.

21.7.15.2 Biomass Yield (Y)

The ratio of the amount of biomass produced to the amount of substrate consumed (g biomass/g substrate) relative to the electron donor used. Biomass yield can be determined by:

$$\text{Biomass yield Y} = \frac{\text{g biomass produced}}{\text{g substrate utilized}} \qquad \text{Equation 21.1}$$

Finding the differences between biomass produced and biomass utilized (Metcalf et al., 2003). High biomass yield is the main goal of sustainability because the cultivation of bioenergy crops on arable land has increased, with perennial crops being the most sustainable crop for energy transition, optimization, and material cycling.

21.7.15.3 Decomposition of Biomass and Soil Organic Matter

Endopedonic and exopedonic factors affect the rate of biomass decomposition (i.e., cultivation residues) because soil characteristics are related to endopedonic factors. The C:N relationship and other chemical features are related to biomass characteristics as exopedonic factors. In addition, N has variable effects on the factors that determine the SOC pool's mean residence time (Riggs et al. 2015). Biochemical plant residues can regulate soil C and MRT cycling (Martens, 2000). In addition, temperatures, the amount of precipitation, and its distribution also affect the decomposition of SOC and SOC inventory (Saiz et al., 2012). The equilibrium between the photosynthesis of CO_2 assimilation and the release of C from both dead and living material decides net exchanges between air and earth systems C (Post et al., 1992). Temperature shifts can have an important influence on the soil climate, influencing soil temperature and soil water evaporation rates, affecting C and soil nutrient cycles and soil biological activity. The OM decomposition mechanism is very complex and includes several factors, such as the heterogeneity of SOM, the abundance of C compounds, the stability of organic compounds within the plant cell, the relation to other nutrient cycles such as N, and the microorganisms' functional diversity, particularly organic decomposing (Prosser, 2007).

21.7.15.4 The Priming Effect

The priming effect is the increased or delayed decay of SOC after fresh biomass C or mineral N has been injected into the system. Microbial activity can release or immobilize large amounts of C, N, and other nutrients due to the initial effect over the short run (Jenkinson et al., 1985). The priming effect is due to interactions among various biomass characteristics and interactions between organic matter, both alive and dead.

The mechanisms and the nature of the results depend on factors such as:

- Effects of macro and microflora species.
- Centralized distribution of nutrients impacts (CDNI).

Priming effects' magnitude and course depend on particular site criteria. Biomass C supply can, in some cases, allow the SOC stock to decrease (Fontaine et al., 2004). The main mechanism that influences the soil C cycle in the different plant-soil interactions is the priming effect because it modifies SOM breakdown and labile C inputs. Incorporating the priming impact in earth system models boosts soil C inventory estimation. The broad heterogeneity in the priming effect across different ecosystem ranges can be seen in isotopic properties, from a rise in soil CO_2 emissions to a decrease of 50%, which is useful for exploring complex relationships in natural ecosystems.

21.7.16 Isotopic Properties

The term isotopes (from the Greek *iso*, same, and *topos*, place) identifies atoms of the same chemical element, that is, the same place in the periodic table of the elements, with the same atomic number but different atomic mass numbers. In other words, isotopes are atoms having the same number of protons and electrons (equal chemical properties) and a different number of neutrons (different physical properties). Isotopes of a single element possess almost identical properties. They are commonly classified as natural or artificial, stable or unstable. Physicochemical variations caused by differences usually contribute to the differences in the chemical activity of an isotope involved in a chemical reaction.

The primary reason isotopes occur in varying quantities and with different reactant and product values in each pool is the difference between the chemical activity of the isotopes involved in the reaction, which contributes to the differential representation of reactants and products. The number of electrons (e-) and their positions in a single shell, which are not variable between isotopes of the same element, largely determine the chemical properties of any element. As a result, isotopes of an element generally have similar chemical properties. Neutrons (N) that have a comparatively massive impact on the weight of an isotope result in different atomic mass (Am) and thus cause isotopes to react in different ways to chemical reactions due to their physical properties. This is valid as each isotope has the same atomic number (A). Any alteration that occurs in the relative nuclear abundances in an isotopic mixture mainly results from mass-dependent isotopic effects. This is particularly true for elements with low mass (Am), where the mass variations between the different isotopes and the molecules comprising these isotopes can be considerable. The impact is different physicochemical properties, mechanical quantum effects of isotopes, and changes in chemical bond strength, such as the weight of the molecules comprising various isotopes. For starters, molecules containing heavier isotopes have more stable chemical bonds and thus require more energy to sever.

21.7.16.1 What Do Isotopes in Agroecosystems Tell Us?

Isotopes are potentially used to separate photosynthetic and respiratory fluxes for terrestrial plants (e.g., Francey and Tans, 1987; Farquhar et al., 1993; Ciais et al., 1997). They provide key tools for better understanding global budgets of these trace gases (e.g., carbon). The isotopic distribution characterizing the sources is influenced by different natural phenomena, causing significant variations in final products. The quantification of the ratio between two isotopes allows researchers to determine if two chemically similar environmental samples have different origins, related to the differences of the original sources. Understanding global carbon biogeochemistry and the regulation of carbon deposition in soils elucidates humification processes responsible for transforming plant residues into soil organic matter. Peatlands and other organic soils are unusual because they do not have the same stabilization of their organic matter by associations with soil mineral matrix as other types of soil do. However, for decades and even generations, soil organic matter can be retained as a fragile record of past environmental conditions.

Several experiments and approaches have been suggested and used to study stable isotope formation pathways. Although most interpretations of label appearance (dynamic label) or label disappearance (pulse-chase label) are qualitative in respired CO_2, the number, size, kinetic properties (half-life, turnover rate), and contribution to pools constitute a system for interpretation as a quantitative and mechanistic tracer kinetics. It best applies to various problems of carbon assimilation, transport, and metabolism in plants using the statistical methods of compartmental research (Atkins, 1971; Jacques, 1994) (Moorby and Jarman, 1975; Prosser and Farrar, 1981; Rocher and Prioul, 1987; Bürkle et al., 1998; Lattanzi et al., 2005).

21.7.16.2 Stable Isotope Composition of Soil Organic Matter

Soil carbon stability and the deposited quantity of carbon rely primarily on both factors, the chemical composition and contact between the carbon molecules and mineral surfaces (Kaiser and Guggenberger, 2003). A stable organic matter isotope composition can be used to differentiate between the plant carbon input and the fresh carbon formed by microbial processes. The decomposition rate of plant litter, by comparison, will increase as a result of decomposition, depending on the consistency of the litter and stable plant molecules. Stable isotope composition can be measured for new insights into the input and storage of soil carbon by analyzing various rates of decomposition of particular chemical products, applying isotopic changes to bulk soils that simulate isotope effects or carbon differences in organic matter (Gleixner et al., 1993). This dilemma is solved by knowledge of the isotope composition of each molecule, and soil molecules with the same isotopic content as plant precursors suggest selective conservation (Kracht and Gleixner, 2000).

21.7.16.3 Carbon and Nitrogen Distribution and Their Stable Isotopes in Soil

In the last decade, several mathematical and statistical descriptions have been developed for C and N transformations in soil, but only a few specifically model a soil organism's behavior and mass. There are still considerable difficulties in setting specific conditions for the kinetics of microbial turnover; modern techniques are being researched. To examine this study, the effect of the C and N turnover on perennial and annual herbaceous cropping systems, earthworm casting, and other NEP constituents are reviewed and analyzed based on associated soil parameters described below.

21.7.16.4 Soil Moisture Content

The relationship between temperature, moisture, and species demonstrated by current climate change discussions states that gradually adding soil organic matter can hold soil moisture and provide nutrients for plant establishment. Studies suggest water content significantly affects litter decomposition. Litter mass loss results indicated greater mineralization activity in wet versus dry soils. This agrees with Thomsen et al. (1999), who showed that the decomposition of native SOC and labeled ryegrass was highly correlated with the volumetric water content.

21.7.16.5 Soil pH

Soil pH influences a number of factors affecting microbial activity, such as the solubility and ionization of inorganic and organic soil solution constituents, and these will in turn affect soil enzyme activity. There are a large number of both organic and inorganic acids found in soils; the majority of these acids are relatively weak (Eldor 2007). The bacterial diversity is strongly related to soil pH, with higher diversity in neutral samples and lower in acidic samples (Wu et al., 2017).

21.7.16.6 Soil Microbial Biomass

Soil microbial biomass (SMB) is an active component of the soil ecosystem, which regulates many critical functions and properties related to soil and environmental qualities. The functions and processes include source-sink in nutrient cycling, decomposition of organic residues, structural stability, and indicators of soil pollution and bioremediation (Marten et al.,1987). Microbial biomass measurement is an index for the response of soil microbiota to decomposition and microbial community distribution. Decomposition rates thus depend not only on the size of the SOC pool but also on the size and composition of the decomposer microbe pool (Wieder et al.,2015). To further determine if the isotope effect of microbial decomposition can induce a shift in the isotope composition of SOC and CO_2, selective utilization of SOC and isotope is used to examine if it is dependent on the growth of the soil microbial population. This can be derived by estimating the δ13C of microbial biomass. To calculate the $\delta\,^{13}C$ of C_{mic}, the following equation can be used:

$$\delta^{13}C_{mic} = \frac{c_{nf} \times \delta_{nf} - c_f \times \delta_f}{c_{nf} - c_f} \qquad \text{Equation 21.2}$$

where c_{nf} and c_f are the corresponding extracted organic C contents (μg C g^{-1} soil) of the nonfumigated and fumigated samples, and δ_{nf} and δ_f are the corresponding $\delta\,^{13}C$ values.

21.7.16.7 Stable Isotope Analysis (SIA)

The distribution of the isotopes characterizing the origins can be affected by various phenomena, which may lead to major changes in the final products. The word isotopes identifies atoms of the same chemical element. It refers to atoms that have the same atomic number but different nuclear mass numbers, meaning they occupy the same position within the periodic table of elements. In other words, isotopes are atoms with the same number of protons and electrons but a different number of neutrons (equal chemical properties and different physical properties). An analysis technique that measures the relative abundance of stable isotopes and provides a proportion of isotopes is used as a research tool for an increasing number of different fields of research and practical case studies. Isotopes of one molecule have almost identical characteristics. They are usually known as natural or artificial. The quantification of two isotopes enables one to determine whether there is a separate source for two chemically similar environmental specimens. Its ability to detect debris in environmental samples is based on various carbon isotopic signatures in plants used in biosequestration synthesis.

The probability of differentiating two samples based on their relative concentration of the isotope is based on the physical (e.g., evaporation or condensation) and biological (e.g., photosynthesis, assimilation, and excretion) processes. The physical mechanism of fractionation can be enacted by a broad variety of factors. Several natural (and anthropogenic) processes can change a chemical element's isotopic signature in a matrix by an unbalanced distribution of the isotope, resulting in a difference in its original isotope signature. As it has proven to be susceptible to particular processes/variables, the degree of the fractionation of several chemical elements can be used as an instrument for investigating the process/variable in question. In the thermodynamic isotopic fractionation pathway,the isotope energy in the molecules varies. This process suggests:

- Accumulation of high isotopes in oxidized products.
- Preference for isotopic splitting at lower temperatures, since variations between the isotopes are attenuated at high temperatures.

The mechanism is not applicable to the chemical reactions and biological reactions of gaseous liquids. In the kinetic mechanism, i.e.fast, irreversible, and unidirectional processes are typically observed. This applies to most biological processes, of which less energy is used, with lighter isotopes preferably being used. It also happens in systems such as evaporation, diffusion, etc., when the materials are quickly separated from reactors. These processes feature:

- The pre-emptive breaking of light isotope bonds.
- The selective distribution of light isotopes in products and heavy reagents.

This is done throughout the entire production chain. The relative mass plurality of its isotopes can be detected by the analysis of stable isotopes, depending on the chemical element. Technological advances in isotope analysis have led to experimental instruments that can calculate with high precision and accuracy minor differences in the abundance of stable isotopes (mass spectrometry). This enables stable isotope analysis of different elements to be applied, thereby allowing applications in various scientific fields today.

217.16.8 Carbon Isotope Ratio as a Tool in Soil Environment Studies

There are very minor differences in the background quantities of most isotopes in the various components of the biosphere. Carbon and nitrogen isotope analysis is used to analyze the trophic network and the matter flows within the key components of the soil ecosystem. It can be used to consider chemical and biological processes occurring at both ecosystem and organism levels. Stable isotope labeling includes the use of nonradioactive isotopes that can serve as tracers used to model many chemical and biochemical processes. The two major carbon reserves in nature are represented by organic and inorganic carbon, which are distinguished by various isotopic fingerprints due to the different processes in which they are active. The kinetic reactions, which mainly involve the organic carbon (i.e., photosynthetic process), determine a concentration of the lightest isotope in the synthesized organic material ($\delta\ ^{13}C$ equal to about –25%). Stable isotope is a promising method for metabolite detection.

The chosen isotope acts as a gas molecule that can be identified through mass spectrometry (MS). Some of the most common stable isotopes are 2H, 13C, and 15N, which can further be produced into solvents, amino acids, nucleic acids, lipids, common metabolites, and cell growth media. The mechanisms behind the 13C enrichment of organic matter with cast and litter are unclear; therefore, to determine if 13C isotopes contribute to decomposition patterns, 13C signatures of sieved soil, shoot, litter, earthworm cast, and earthworm will be measured. An estimation of the relative difference in stable isotope energy flow is important to identify the balance between C and N. Carbon studies gained increased interest due to the sensitivity of 13C and its nonradioactive nature (in contrast to 14C studies).

Tracing the fate of stable isotope enrichment from shoot and root litter in Cn can be visible in earthworm cast material (Vidal et al., 2019). Surface casts produced by epi-anecic earthworms in the presence of 13C-labeled shoot or root litter deposited onto the soil surface. The alteration in the chemical composition from initial litter to POM and mineral-associated organic matter (MOM) in cast samples was studied with isotopic ratio mass spectrometry (EA-IRMS) to identify plant tissues and microorganisms involved in plant decomposition within casts. (Vidal et al., 2019).

21.7.16.9 Measurement of Isotope Ratios by Mass Spectrometry

Stable isotope abundance is most commonly measured using mass spectrometry. The past 20 years have seen rapid growth in the development of better gas-phase stable isotope instruments, interfaces, and measurements. Automated systems for the preparation of H, C, N, O, and S have seen extensive development and, coupled with the newest continuous-flow isotope ratio mass spectrometers, provide for a growing array of applications in the fields of agriculture, natural and atmospheric sciences, forensic science, and biomedical research.

21.8 RESEARCH GUIDELINES AND CONCLUSIONS

This chapter has presented various technical and research aspects of bio-impacts on the environment. The complete research guidelines, results, discussions, and conclusions can be found in Tarfa (2021). In order to plan future agroecological systems, it is important to better understand that habitats can sustain both productivity and soil quality. The core outcome of this field study provides a relationship between neighboring cropping systems and carbon natural abundance based on decomposition pathways as it relates to carbon sequestration in the soil. The main finding of this study is that the link between cropping systems and social-ecological sustainability depends on the choice of crop type. Proper recognition of the role and impact of land-use shifts toward the potential for optimization of the current material cycles on microbial activities is important for ecological sustainability. In contrast to the traditional annual crop (maize), the novel perennial energy crops examined showed better resilience in terms of soil microbial functioning even in replacement conditions.

Findings from this study also showed the influence of plant species on soil quality. The perennial crops improved the buffering capacity of soils against material cycling conditions during land-use replacement. Though the influence of these crops was not reflected in the SOC content, microbial biomass carbon still increased. An increase in soil respiration due to high microbial biomass carbon (MBC) suggests that these plants promote a microbial community with high carbon use efficiency, thus reducing the loss of CO_2 from soil to the atmosphere and promoting soil health. The high biomass yield of perennial bioenergy crops in treatment, compared to maize, supports the importance of these crops in bioenergy cropping.

Relevant process parameters for the latter, such as pH, temperature, and carbonization time, and their influences are presented, and the exemplary phosphate extraction potential (as P_2O_5 in struvite) was modeled. Neighboring cropping systems are a sustainable agriculture means for social-ecological considerations. Clear evidence shows the distribution of carbon on the same field differs with crop type. Annual crops tend to have low ecological values, such as decreased soil quality, lower biomass yield, low resistance varieties, low C:N ratio content, and prone to soil erosion. Growing perennial crops indicates a higher C:N ratio compared to annual crops. Exploring strategies to enhance soil health by restoring SOC concentration by reducing annual cultivation with neighboring cropping systems.

The cup plant had an average biomass yield, didn't support microbial growth, and exhibited the lowest MBC. The low MBC observed in cup plants suggests that identifying plant lifetimes that enhance microbial growth and improve soil microbial activities and biomass yield is important for ecological sustainability. Among the studied plants, miscanthus outperformed the others in terms of biomass yield, microbial biomass growth, and other measured activities.

All microbial, soil, and plant biomass parameters examined indicate that perennial energy crops are more ecologically sustainable than annual crops. Hence, annual crops can be replaced with these crops to improve plant biodiversity and also utilize marginal soil fauna environments. Soil organic matter is well decomposed, chemically modified, and more stable over time relative to the original organic residues. Soil fauna govern the behavior and role of soil microorganisms and their physical-chemical interconnections with soil organic materials. The direct and indirect impacts of soil animals on nutrient supply, carbon sequestration, greenhouse gas emissions, and plant growth are critical. The study found a link between cropping system and agroecosystem NEP components, serving as indicators of the sustainability of agricultural practices as global plant biomass increases with perennial crop replacement in neighboring annual cropping systems.

Constant monitoring is necessary as MBC at a certain period cannot reveal if soil quality is improving, deteriorating, or static. Thus, connecting MBC to other soil parameters is important in evaluating overall soil health and ecological sustainability. Furthermore, more studies on the adaptation mechanisms of these plants (*Miscanthus giganteus* [miscanthus], *Triticum aestivum* [winter wheat], *Silphium perfoliatum* [cup plant], *Zea mays* [maize]) will give a clearer picture of their buffering ability in very moist soils, as little is known about each plant.

REFERENCES

Abelho M. 2001. From litterfall to breakdown in streams: A review. The Scientific World Journal 1:180292.

Aira M, Sampedro L, Monroy F, Domínguez J. 2008. Detritivorous earthworms directly modify the structure, thus altering the functioning of a microdecomposer food web. Soil Biology and Biochemistry 40(10):2511–2516.

Aira M, Domínguez J. 2011. Earthworm effects without earthworms: inoculation of raw organic matter with worm-worked substrates alters microbial community functioning. PLoS One 6(1):e16354.

Anderson, E. K., Voigt, T. B., and Bollero, G. A. 2014. Miscanthus × giganteus seedling establishment and growth across a range of field conditions in the Midwestern USA. *Global Change Biology Bioenergy* 6(5): 644–655. https://doi.org/10.1111/gcbb.12192.

Atkins CA, Pamtterso BD, Graham D. 1971. Plant carbonic anhydrases. I. Distribution of types among species. Plant Physiol 50:214-217.

Angus, J. F. 2001. Nitrogen supply and demand in Australian agriculture. *Australian Journal of Experimental Agriculture* 41: 277–288.

Badiru, A. B. 2008. *Triple C Model of Project Management: Communication, Cooperation, and Coordination*, Taylor & Francis Group/CRC Press, Boca Raton, FL.

Badiru, A. B. 2019. *Project Management: Systems, Principles, and Applications, Second Edition*, Taylor & Francis/CRC Press, Boca Raton, FL.

Bentsen NS, Felby C. 2012. Biomass for energy in the European Union - a review of bioenergy resource assessments. Biotechnol Biofuels 5:25.

Badiru, A. B. 2023. *Systems Engineering Using the DEJI Systems Model: Evaluation, Justification, and Integration with Case Studies and Applications*, Taylor & Francis Group/CRC Press, Boca Raton, FL.

Berry, W. 2009. Perennialism and stewardship. *American Society of Plant Biologists Newsletter* May/June 2009: 14–15.

Biertuempfel A, Graf T. 2013. Cultivation suitability and yield capacity of aniseed under Thurinaian site conditions. Journal of Medicinal and Spice Plants 18(4):177–179.

Bohlen, P. J., Scheu, S., Hale, C. M., McLean, M. A., Sonja, M., Groffman, P. M., and Parkinson, D. 2004. Non-native invasive earthworms as agents of change in northern temperate forests source. *Frontiers in Ecology and the Environment* 2(8): 427–435.

Bouche M. 1983. The establishment of earthworm communities. In Earthworm Ecology: From Darwin to Vermiculture. Ed.]E Satchell. pp. 431-448. Chapman and Hall, London.

Bradford MA, Tordoff GM, Eggers T, Jones TH, Newington JE. 2002. Microbiota, fauna, and mesh size interactions in litter decomposition. Oikos 99:317-323.

Bregliani MM, Ros GH, Temminghoff EJM, Van Riemsdijk WH. 2010. Nitrogen mineralization in soils related to initial extractable organic nitrogen: Effect of temperatureand time. Comm Soil Sci Plant Anal 41(11):1383–1398.

Brookes P.C., Cayuela M.L., Contin M., De Nobili M., Kemmitt S.J., and Mondini C. 2008. The mineralisation of fresh and humified soil organic matter by the soil microbial biomass. Waste Management 28(4):716–722.

Brown I, Castellazzi M. 2014. Scenario analysis for regional decision making on sustainable multifunctional land uses. Regional Environmental Change 14:1371.

Burkle L, Hibberd JM, Quick WP, Kuhn C, Hirner B, Frommer WB. 1998. The H+-sucrose cotransporter NtSUT1 is essential for sugar export from tobacco leaves. Plant Physiol 118:59–68.

Byrd KB, Flint LE, Alvarez P, Casey CF, Sleeter BM, Soulard CE, Flint AL, Sohlet TL. 2015. Integrated climate and land use change scenarios for California rangeland ecosystem services: wildlife habitat, soil carbon, and water supply. Landscape Ecol 30:729–750.

Chum H, Faaij A, Moreira J, Berndes G, Dhamija P, Dong H, Gabrielle B, Eng AG, Lucht W, Mapako M, Cerutti OM, McIntyre T, Minowa T, Pingoud K. 2011. Bioenergy. In: Edenhofer O, Pichs-Madruga R, Sokona Y, et al., eds. Renewable Energy Sources and Climate Change Mitigation: Special Report of the Intergovernmental Panel on Climate Change. Cambridge University Press; 2011:209-332.

Ciais P, Denning AS, Tans PP, Berry JA, Randall DA, Collatz GJ, Sellers PJ, White JWC, Trolier M, Meijer HAJ, Francey RJ, Monfray P, Heimann M. 1997. A three-dimensional synthesis study of δ18O in atmospheric CO2: 1. Surface fluxes, J. Geophys. Res., 102(D5):5857–5872.

CIMMYT. 1996. World wheat facts and trends 1995/96: Understanding global trends in the use of wheat diversity and international flows of wheat genetic resources. International Maize and Wheat Improvement Center (CIMMYT), Mexico, D.F.

Collinson, A. S. 1988. Introduction to world vegetation. Unwin Hyman, London.

Curtis, B. C., Rajaram, S., and Gómez Macpherson, H. (eds.). 2002. Wheat in the world. In *Bread Wheat: Improvement and Production* (FAO Plant Production and Protection Series No. 30), pp. 1–17. Food and Agriculture Organization of the United Nations (FAO), Rome.

Darwin CR. 1881. The formation of vegetable mould, through the action of worms, with observations on their habits. London: John Murray.

Dinsdale EA, Pantos O, Smriga S, Edwards RA, Angly F, et al. 2008. Microbial ecology of four coral atolls in the Northern Line Islands. PLOS ONE 3(2):e1584.

Dohleman, F. G., and Long, S. P. 2009. More productive than maize in the Midwest: How does Miscanthus do it? *Plant Physiology* 150(4): 2104–2115. https://doi.org/10.1104/pp.109.139162.

Edwards CA. 1998. The Use of Earthworms in the Breakdown and Management of Organic Wastes, In: C.A. Edwards, Ed., Earthworm Ecology, CRC Press, Boca Raton, pp. 327-354.

Eldor, A. P. 2007. *Soil Microbiology, Ecology, and Biochemistry*, 3rd ed.Elsevier, Amsterdam.

Farquhar GD, O'Leary MH, Berry JA. 1982. On the relationship between carbon isotope discrimination and the intercellular carbon dioxide concentration in leaves. Functional Plant Biology 9:121-137.

Farquhar G, Lloyd J, Taylor J, et al. 1993. Vegetation effects on the isotope composition of oxygen in atmospheric CO2. Nature 363:439–443.

Fontaine S, Bardoux G, Abbadie L, Mariotti A. 2004, Carbon input to soil may decrease soil carbon content. Ecology Letters 7:314-320.

Fraczek J, Mudryk K, Wróbel M. 2011. Cup plant Silphium perfoliatum L. Biomass Source for Biofuel Production. Inzynieria Rolnicza 131:21-27.

Francey R, Tans P. 1987. Latitudinal variation in oxygen-18 of atmospheric CO2. Nature 327:495–497.

Fuller, H. J., and Carothers, Z. B. 1963. *The Plant World*, 4th ed. Holt, Rinehart and Winston, New York.

Galinat, W. C. 1971. The origin of maize: The evolution of teosinte into maize. *Annual Review of Genetics* 5: 447–478. https://doi.org/10.1146/annurev.ge.05.120171.002311.

Gansberger M, Montgomery LFR, Liebhard P. 2015. Botanical characteristics, crop management and potential of Silphium perfoliatum L. as a renewable resource for biogas production: A review. Industrial Crops and Products 63:362-372.

Garbeva P, Veen JA, Elsas JD. 2004. Microbial diversity in soil: Selection of microbial populations by plant and soil type and implications for disease suppressiveness. Annual Review of Phytopathology 42:243-270.

Gleixner G, Danier HJ, Werner RA, Schmidt HL. 1993. Correlations between the 13C content of primary and secondary plant products in different cell compartments and that in decomposing basidiomycetes. Plant Physiology 102(4):1287–1290.

Glick BR, Patten CL, Holguin G, Penrose DM. 1999. Biochemical and Genetic Mechanism Used by Plant Growth Promoting Bacteria. ICP, Ontario.

Griffin RJ. 2013. The Sources and Impacts of Tropospheric Particulate Matter. Nature Education Knowledge 4(5):1.

Guzman JG, Al-Kaisi M. 2011. Landscape position effect on selected soil physical properties of reconstructed prairies in South Central Iowa. Journal of Soil and Water Conservation 66:183-191.

Guzman JG, Al-Kaisi M. 2014. Residue removal and management practices effects on soil environment and carbon budget. Soil Science Society of America Journal 78(2):609.

Haramoto, E. R., and Gallandt, E.R. 2004. Brassica cover cropping for weed management: A review. *Renewable Agriculture and Food Systems* 19(4): 187–198.

Herman DJ, Firestone MK, Nuccio E, Hodge A. 2012. Interactions between an arbuscular mycorrhizal fungus and a soil microbial community mediating litter decomposition. FEMS Microbiology Ecology 80(1):236–247.

Herman MA, Birnbaum MJ. 2021. Molecular aspects of fructose metabolism and metabolic disease. Cell Metab. 33(12):2329-2354.

Houghton J.T., Ding J.H., Griggs D.J., Noguer M., van der Linden P., Dai X., Maskell M.,and Johnson C.A. 2001. Climate Change 2001: The Scientific Basis. The Press Syndicate of the University of Cambridge, Cambridge.

Huy MT, Quilloy AJA, Cuc MT, Huong MT, Phuong DN, Hai TM. 2025. Adoption of conservation agriculture practices and its impacts on yields and incomes: Evidence from smallholder maize farmers in the Northwest mountainous region of Vietnam. Environmental Challenges 19:101143.

IPCC. 2011. Renewable Energy Sources and Climate Change Mitigation. Special Report of the Intergovernmental Panel on Climate Change (IPCC), Summary for Policymakers and Technical Summary, WMO, UNEP.

Jacques R, Garnier E. (eds.). 1994. A whole-plant perspective on carbon-nitrogen interactions. SPB Academic Publishing, The Hague, The Netherlands.

Jenkinson DS, Fox RH, Rayner JH. 1985. Interactions between fertilizer nitrogen and soil nitrogen—the so-called 'priming' effect. Journal of Soil Science, 36:425-444.

Kahle, P., Boelcke, B., and Zacharias, S. 2001. Cropping of Miscanthus in Central Europe: Biomass production and influence on nutrients and soil organic matter. *European Journal of Agronomy* 15(3): 171–184. https://doi.org/10.1016/S1161-0301(01)00102-2.

Kaiser K, Guggenberger G. 2003. Mineral surfaces and soil organic matter. European Journal of Soil Science 54:219-236.

Karp A, Richter GM. 2011. Meeting the challenge of food and energy security. J Exp Bot. 62(10):3263-3271.

Koch PL, Diffenbaugh NS, Hoppe KA. 2004. The effects of late Quaternary climate and pCO2 change on C4 plant abundance in the south-central United States. Palaeogeography, Palaeoclimatology, Palaeoecology 207:331–357.

Kracht O, Gleixner G. 2000. Isotope analysis of pyrolysis products from Sphagnum peat and dissolved organic matter from bog water. Organic Geochemistry 31(7–8):645-654.

Kwapinski W, Byrne CMP, Kryachko E, Wolfram P, Adley C, Leahy JJ, Novotny EH, Hayes MHB. 2010. Biochar from biomass and waste. Waste and Biomass Valorization 1(2):177-189.

Lal R. 2004. Soil carbon sequestration to mitigate climate change. Geoderma 123(1-2):1-22.

Lattanzi R, Spetea M, Schüllner F, Rief SB, Krassnig R, Negri L, Schmidhammer H. 2005. Synthesis and biological evaluation of 14-alkoxymorphinans. 22.(1) Influence of the 14-alkoxy group and the substitution in position 5 in 14-alkoxymorphinan-6-ones on in vitro and in vivo activities. J Med Chem. 48(9):3372-3378.

Lavelle P, Martin A. 1992. Small-scale and large-scale effects of endogeic earthworms on soil organic matter dynamics in soils of the humid tropics. Soil Biology and Biochemistry 24(12):1491-1498.

Lavelle P, Pashanasi B, Charpentier F, Gilot C, Rossi J-P, Derouard L, Andre J, Ponge J-F, Bernier N. 1998. Large-scale effects of earthworms on soil organic matter and nutrient dynamics. In: Edwards CA (ed) Earthworm ecology. St. Lucie Press, Boca Raton, pp 103–122.

Lee, K. E. 1985. Earthworms: Their ecology and relationships with soils and land use. Academic Press, Sydney.

Long, S. P. 1983. C4 photosynthesis at low temperatures. *Plant, Cell and Environment* 6(4): 345–363. https://doi.org/10.1111/j.1365-3040.1983.tb01802.x.

Marhan S, Philippot L, Bru D, Rudolph S, Franzaring J, Högy P, Fangmeier A, Kandeler E. 2011. Abundance and activity of nitrate reducers in an arable soil are more affected by temporal variation and soil depth than by elevated atmospheric [CO2]. FEMS Microbiology Ecology 76(2):209–219.

Martens R. 1987. Estimation of microbial biomass in soil by the respiration method: Importance of soil pH and flushing methods for the measurement of respired CO2. Soil Biology and Biochemistry 19(1):77-81.

Martens DA. 2000. Plant residue biochemistry regulates soil carbon cycling and carbon sequestration. Soil Biology and Biochemistry 32(3):361-369.

McCarthy J., Canziani OF., Leary N., Dokken, DJ, White KS. 2001. Climate Change 2001: Impacts, Adaptation, and Vulnerability. The Press Syndicate of the University of Cambridge, Cambridge.

Melligan F, Dussan K, Auccaise R, Novotny EH, Leahy JJ, Hayes MHB, Kwapinski W. 2012. Characterisation of the products from pyrolysis of residues after acid hydrolysis of Miscanthus, Bioresource Technology, 108:258-263,

Metcalf JC, Rose K, Rees M. 2003. Evolutionary demography of monocarpic perennials. Trends in Ecology and Evolution 18:471–480.

Monroy F, Aira M, Domínguez J. 2011. Epigeic earthworms increase soil arthropod populations during first steps of decomposition of organic matter. Pedobiologia 54(2):93–99.

Moorby J, Jarman PD. 1975. The use of compartmental analysis in the study of the movement of carbon through leaves. Planta 122:155–168.

Morita MT. 2010. Directional gravity sensing in gravitropism. Annu Rev Plant Biol. 61:705-20.

Moulia B, Der Loughian C, Bastien R, Martin O. 2011. Integrative Mechanobiology of Growth and Architectural Development in Changing Mechanical Environments. In: Wojtaszek, P. (eds) Mechanical Integration of Plant Cells and Plants. Signaling and Communication in Plants, vol 9. Springer, Berlin, Heidelberg

Olson K, Ebelhar SA, Lang JM. 2014. Long-term effects of cover crops on crop yields, soil organic carbon stocks and sequestration. Open Journal of Soil Science 4:284-292.

Pichard G. 2012. Management, production, and nutritional characteristics of cup-plant (Silphium perfoliatum) in temperate climates of southern Chile. Ciencia e Investigación Agraria 39(1):61-77.

Platen R, Konrad J, Glemnitz M. 2017. Novel energy crops: an opportunity to enhance the biodiversity of arthropod assemblages in biomass feedstock cultures? Ecosystems and People 13(1):162-171.

Post WM, Emanuel WR, King AW. 1992. Soil organic matter dynamics and the carbon cycle. In: World Inventory of Emission Potentials, NH Batjes and EM Bridges (eds.), Int. Soil Ref. Information Centre, Wageningen, The Netherlands.

Prosser J, Farrar JF. 1981. A compartmental model of carbon allocation in the vegetative barley plant. Plant, Cell & Environment 4:303-307.

Prosser J, Bohannan B, Curtis T, et al. 2007. The role of ecological theory in microbial ecology. Nat Rev Microbiol 5:384–392.

Ragauskas AJ, Williams CK, Davison BH, Britovsek G, Cairney J, Eckert CA, Frederick WJ Jr, Hallett JP, Leak DJ, Liotta CL, Mielenz JR, Murphy R, Templer R, Tschaplinski T. 2006. The path forward for biofuels and biomaterials. Science 311(5760):484-489.

Ranum, P., Peña-Rosas, J.P., and Garcia-Casal, M.N. 2014. Global maize production, utilization, and consumption. *Annals of the New York Academy of Sciences* 1312(1): 105–112. https://doi.org/10.1111/nyas.12396Scite+1NyaSPubs+1.

Riggs CE, Hobbie SE, Bach EM, Hofmockel KS, Kazanski CE. 2015. Nitrogen addition changes grassland soil organic matter decomposition. Biogeochemistry 125:203-219.

Ritz K, Harris J, Murray P. 2010. The role of soil biota in soil fertility and quality, and approaches to influencing soil communities to enhance delivery of these functions. Sub-Project A of Defra Project SP1601: Soil Functions, Quality and Degradation – Studies in Support of the Implementation of Soil Policy. Department for Environment, Food and Rural Affairs Research project final report. Available at: https://www.researchgate.net/profile/Anoop_Srivastava7/post/Is_there_any_bacterial_species_which_enhances_the_fertility_of_land/attachment/59d6434679197b807799ec00/AS%3A442407901765632%401482489671528/download/SP1601_9492_FRP.pdf accessed June 19, 2025.

Rocher JP, Prioul JL. 1987. Compartmental analysis of assimilate export in a mature maize leaf. Plant Physiol Biochem. 25:531–540.

Römbke J, Jänsch S, Didden W. 2005. The use of earthworms in ecological soil classification and assessment concepts. Ecotoxicology and Environmental Safety 62(2):249-65.

Russell JE. 1923. The Micro-organisms of Soil. Longmans, Green and Co. London.

Russell EW. 1973. Soil Conditions and Plant Growth. 10th Edition, Longman, London and New York.

Santru, H., Antru, C., Kova, C., Bird, M. I., and Lloyd, J. 2000. Microbial processes and carbon-isotope fractionation in tropical and temperate grassland soils.

Saiz G, Bird MI, Domingues T, Schrodt F, Schwarz M, Feldpausch TR, Veenendaal E, Djagbletey G, Hien F, Compaore H, Diallo A, Lloyd J. 2012. Variation in soil carbon stocks and their determinants across a precipitation gradient in West Africa. Glob Change Biol. 18:1670-1683.

Schimel DS, Coleman DC, Horton KH. 1985. Microbial carbon and nitrogen transformations and soil organic matter dynamics in paired rangeland and cropland catenas. Geoderma 36:201-214.

Six J, Paustian K, Elliott ET, Combrink C. 2000. Soil structure and soil organic matter: I. Distribution of aggregate size classes and aggregate associated carbon. Soil Science Society of America Journal 64:681-689.

Somerville C, Youngs H, et al. Taylor C, Davis SC. 2010. Feedstocks for lignocellulosic biofuels. Science 329:790-792.

Stanford G. 1990. Silphium perfoliatum (Cup-Plant) as a New Forage. American Journal of Plant Sciences 6(8):33-37.

Tarfa, A. 2021. Decomposition pathways in Net Ecosystem Production (NEP) components on cross neighboring cropping systems with a secondary focus on earthworm community. Master's Thesis, Faculty of Environmental Science, Soil Science Department, University of Trier, Trier, March.

Thomsen IK, Schjønning P, Jensen B, Kristensen K, Christensen BT. 1999. Turnover of organic matter in differently textured soils – II. Microbial activity as influenced by soil water regimes. Geoderma 89:199–218.

Tilman D, Socolow R, Foley JA, Hill J, Larson E, Lynd L, Pacala S, Reilly J, Searchinger T, Somerville C, Williams R. 2009. Beneficial biofuels—The food, energy, and environment trilemma. Science 325:270-271.

Tinker PBH, Nye PH. 2000 Solute Transport in the Rhizosphere. Oxford University Press, Oxford.

Tomlin AD, Shipitalo MJ, Edwards WM, Protz R. 1995. Earthworms and their influence on soilstructure and infiltration, in P.F. Hendrix, Ed., Earthworm Ecology and Biogeography in NorthAmerica, Lewis Publishing, Boca Raton, FL, pp. 159–183.

United Nations. 2017. Global opportunity report.Available at: https://unglobalcompact.org/library/5081 (accessed June 19, 2025).

Valckx J, Govers G, Hermy M, Muys B. 2011. Optimizing Earthworm Sampling in Ecosystems. In: Karaca, A. (eds) Biology of Earthworms. Soil Biology, vol 24. Springer, Berlin, Heidelberg.

Van Eekeren N, de Boer H, Hanegraaf M, Bokhorst J, Nierop D, Bloem J, Schouten T, de Goede R, Brussaard L. 2010. Ecosystem services in grassland associated with biotic and abiotic soil parameters. Soil Biology and Biochemistry 42(9):1491–1504.

Vidal A, Watteau F, Remusat L, Mueller CW, Nguyen T T-T, Buegger F, Derenne S, Quenea K. 2019. Earthworm cast formation and development: A shift from plant litter to mineral associated organic matter. Frontiers in Environmental Science 7:55.

Waksman SA. 1932. Principles of Soil Microbiology, Soil Science 33(3):239.

Wieder WR, Allison SD, Davidson EA, Georgiou K, Hararuk O, He Y, Hopkins F, Luo Y, Smith MJ, Sulman B., et al. 2015. Explicitly representing soil microbial processes in Earth system models. Global Biogeochem. Cycles 29:1782–1800.

Wilkes, H. G. 1972. Hybridization of maize and teosinte, in Mexico and Guatemala and the improvement of maize. *Economic Botany* 26(3): 245–254. https://doi.org/10.1007/BF02866877.

Wright JP, Jones CG. 2004. Predicting effects of ecosystem engineers on patch-scale species richness from primary productivity. Ecology 85(8):2071–2081.

Wu, Y., Zeng, J., Zhu, Q., Zhang, Z., and Lin, X. 2017. pH is the primary determinant of the bacterial community structure in agricultural soils impacted by polycyclic aromatic hydrocarbon pollution. *Scientific Reports* 7: 40093.

Yurova AY, Volodin EM, Ågren GI, Chertov OG, Komarov AS. 2010, Effects of variations in simulated changes in soil carbon contents and dynamics on future climate projections. Global Change Biology 16:823–835.

Zech W, Senesi N, Guggenberger G, Kaiser K, Lehmann J, Miano TM, Miltner A, Schroth G. 1997. Factors controlling humification and mineralization of soil organic matter in the tropics. Geoderma 79(1–4):117–161.

22 Climate Change Drivers for Emergency Response

Adedeji Badiru

22.1 INTRODUCTION

Not all calls for emergency response result from disasters and catastrophic singular events. Just as there are instances of weather disasters, accidents, natural events, deliberate sabotage, mischievous arson, errors of incompetence, and destructive vandalism that can necessitate an emergency response, there are also environmental-related degradations that impact the integrity of the environment to the extent that an emergency response would be needed. In other words, the need for an emergency response can arise from the gradual degradation of the environment, just as it can arise from precipitous disaster events. The emergency responses for catastrophic singular events must follow the same management principles as other events. Thus, it is essential to understand the parameters and scenarios caused by climate change that could necessitate an emergency response. If we can make a case for the existence of climate change, then it becomes easier to understand why emergency responses may be needed for climate change-induced incidents. The premise of this chapter centers around understanding the adverse environmental issues to the extent that the issues could drive an emergency response. A systems view of climate change and its broad impacts is the primary methodology of this chapter.

In *Climate Change: Evidence and Causes* (NAS & TRS, 2020), the US National Academy of Sciences and the British Royal Society provide an instructive setting for how we must respond to climate change from a systems perspective. The joint report affirms that climate change is one of the defining issues of our time. There is no doubt about this, based on recent experiences with extreme weather patterns. According to the report, it is now more obvious and certain than ever before, based on many lines of evidence, that humans are changing Earth's climate. The atmosphere and oceans have warmed, which has been accompanied by sea level rise, a noticeable decline in Arctic sea ice, and related catastrophic weather patterns. The impacts of climate change on people and nature are increasingly observed. Unprecedented flooding, heat waves, and wildfires have caused billions of dollars in damages. Human and animal habitats are undergoing rapid shifts in response to changing temperatures and precipitation patterns. It is a sorry and discouraging narrative all across the planet (see NRC, 2010 and NAS, 2018). There is only one planet, and we are all interconnected residents of it. We must all work together to protect the planet and make

 DOI: 10.1201/9781003648178-24

it livable for everyone. Whether we love our neighbors or not, we must all remain on the same planet together. What affects one affects all. If we all work together, from a systems perspective, we can build a more sustainable planet that can facilitate a healthier future for all. Let's join the journey, as enjoined by Badiru and Agustiady (2021).

Whether we see it or not, we are in a rapidly changing world. Our actions are essential and significant as impacts on the world system. Every little action can go a long way, but only if we all realize what actions can help. This book is about the what, who, when, where, how, and why of influencing our planet positively.

Men and women form the core of any system. This is in alignment with the recognition that organizations operate and thrive on the efficient interplay of people, processes, and tools. The first object of any good system is the people. Thus, developing first-class people in the workforce must be a priority of any organization or group making up a work system. From a systems perspective, every little bit contributed by a whole lot of people can amount to a monumental accomplishment.

It is a systems world. We must treat it as such in order to influence it positively. Things often start gradually. One thing leads to another and another. Before we know it, the whole system is affected. We need to reengineer our actions. The problem of climate change has been creeping on us for years. Although a potpourri of concerns, actions, and pledges has been floating around for years, everything came to a head in 2021 when we suddenly realized the immense changes in the climate, manifested in more frequent and more extreme weather patterns. A recent US national weather warning says:

> Temperatures across the country will hit record highs and lows as a huge winter storm sweeps across much of the country. In D.C., temperatures will reach nearly 80 degrees before plummeting to below freezing. The National Weather Service says the storm will be disruptive to travel, infrastructure, livestock, and recreation in affected areas.

Ouch!

The premise of this chapter is that there is something each one of us can do at our own personal level to influence our planet positively, thereby mitigating the need for emergency responses. Unfortunately, we, as individuals, do not always realize the extent that our actions can go in impacting the planet, either positively or negatively. As a case example, I once witnessed a simple action that caused a huge impact, but to the nonchalance of the actor. I was stopped at a red light. A pickup truck in the adjacent lane sped up furiously across the intersection in an attempt to beat the red light. He made it. But at what expense? A huge black smoke spewed out from the pickup's exhaust and drifted into the atmosphere. The driver jubilated happily for beating the light. He was happy. But the environment was sad because of yet another human assault. It is my belief, as an author, that the more we know what is expected of us and the more we know the implications, and the more likely we are to join the global efforts to save our planet. Badiru (2016) raised an alarm about climate change from a systems engineering framework. Some of his arguments center on several factors, including the following:

- Water, land, and air all interface rhythmically to create the environment in which humans live and work.
- Climate is the precursor to all human activities.
- We must take a systems view of the world to respond to climate change issues.

22.2 EVOLUTION AND REVOLUTION OF EMERGENCY RESPONSE

There is no shortage of papers, journal articles, seminars, presentations, statements, communiques, conventions, conferences, and press releases on the urgency of taking action on the prevailing environmental issues on our planet. The problem has not been neglected, yet it doesn't appear that we are making progress in remediating the damage already done and stemming future damages. Jones (2014) presents a warning that the energy landscape of the future won't be a sudden break from the past. Organizations will have to evolve their portfolios and actions along the paths of the energy revolution. He provides the following heads-up on what the world needs to do:

- Seek out alternatives.
- Leverage the local advantage.
- Find the way that works.
- Make smart investments.
- Expect the unexpected.
- Adapt to the environment.
- Learn from the past.

It is the position of this book that doing what we need to do can best be approached from a global systems framework. In a related case study, Gamble (2014), presents how Australia is taking the lead in many environmental strategies. His conclusion highlights how an Australian project proved that renewable energies can play more than a supporting role in addressing global climate change dilemmas.

22.3 THE ROLE OF RENEWABLES

Sambo (2023) emphasizes that a reasonable standard of living and economic growth both require adequate, reliable, and affordable energy supplies for households, business services, commercial enterprises, transportation systems, and industrial sectors of all national economies. Fossil-type energy resources, like oil, natural gas, and coal, which have been the dominant sources of energy for electrification, transport, and industrial production, are highly polluting and exhaustible. 87% of CO_2 emissions from human sources arise from the combustion of fossil fuels, and it has four major components:

- Electricity generation: 41%
- Transportation: 23%

- Industry: 20%
- Others: 16%

Renewable energy (RE) sources, like solar, wind, hydro, geothermal, biomass, and so on, are, however, in principle, non-exhaustible, as they are always available on a cyclic or periodic basis, and they emit negligible greenhouse gases. There is an urgent need to significantly minimize carbon dioxide (CO_2) emissions in the power and transportation sectors. Sustainable pathways should be adopted for environmental stability and remediating impacts of climate change. It is noted that in 2015, the United Nations adopted the 17 Sustainable Development Goals (SDGs) to, among other things, by 2030, curtail the catastrophe that will befall the world from the increasing menace of global warming and climate change. The 17 SDGs are:

Goal 1: End poverty in all its forms everywhere.
Goal 2: End hunger, achieve food security and improved nutrition, and promote sustainable agriculture.
Goal 3: Ensure healthy lives and promote well-being for all at all ages.
Goal 4: Ensure inclusive and equitable quality education and promote lifelong learning opportunities for all.
Goal 5: Achieve gender equality and empower all women and girls.
Goal 6: Ensure availability and sustainable management of water and sanitation for all.
Goal 7: Ensure access to affordable, reliable, sustainable, and modern energy for all.
Goal 8: Promote sustained, inclusive, and sustainable economic growth, full and productive employment, and decent work for all.
Goal 9: Build resilient infrastructure, promote inclusive and sustainable industrialization, and foster innovation.
Goal 10: Reduce inequality within and among countries.
Goal 11: Make cities and human settlements inclusive, safe, resilient, and sustainable.
Goal 12: Ensure sustainable consumption and production patterns.
Goal 13: Take urgent action to combat climate change and its impacts.
Goal 14: Conserve and sustainably use the oceans, seas, and marine resources for sustainable development.
Goal 15: Protect, restore, and promote sustainable use of terrestrial ecosystems, sustainably manage forests, combat desertification, halt and reverse land degradation, and halt biodiversity loss.
Goal 16: Promote peaceful and inclusive societies for sustainable development, provide access to justice for all, and build effective, accountable, and inclusive institutions at all levels.
Goal 17: Strengthen the means of implementation and revitalize the global partnership for sustainable development.

The best way to achieve most or all the above goals is to use a comprehensive systems-based approach, specifically, leveraging the efficacy of systems engineering. This is where, why, and when individual contributions are essential, primarily through our energy consumption practices. Badiru and Osisanya (2013) present the systems-based interrelationships of energy generation, transmission, distribution, and consumption as summarized below:

- Exploration: Drilling, fracking, dissolution removal technology.
- Generation: Fossil, fission, fusion, fusion.
- Distribution: Transmission technology, wireless transfer, storage movement.
- Consumption: Households, industry, transportation, business, construction.

In tackling the climate change problems, both qualitative and quantitative approaches must be pursued. This allows us to bring in technological approaches (Lathan, 2022) as well as human-centered social considerations. Again, the premise of this book is that a systems engineering approach is key to making the desired progress. As such, this book contains a mix of technical, social, economic, engineering, and political considerations.

22.4 IMPLICATION OF THE HYDROGEN ANGLE

One of the emerging, exciting technical approaches to the future of energy on Earth is hydrogen-based technologies. A 2023 article (Mines Staff 2023) on the ongoing research at the Colorado School of Mines is captioned, "Green Hydrogen: Empowering the Future of Energy – A Closer look at hydrogen's roles in the energy transition." The article advises that hydrogen has emerged as a key player in the energy transition, identified by the International Energy Agency as a "versatile energy carrier" with a diverse range of applications that can be deployed in a variety of sectors. But is hydrogen a moonshot? Or does it really have the potential to change the energy game? At Colorado School of Mines, teams of researchers are working on the hydrogen problem, from developing electrolyzers to separate hydrogen from other energy sources to developing and testing the ceramic materials in fuel cells and making them commercially viable and cost-effective. The research team confirms that hydrogen truly has the potential to supplement the world's energy profile in meaningful ways and help society successfully navigate the energy transition. The article highlights the researchers working on projects across the scope of the hydrogen approach for a deeper dive into hydrogen technology, the challenges they are facing today, and how they are overcoming these challenges, as well as what the future looks like when powered by hydrogen. Colorado School of Mines faculty across multiple disciplines actively perform collaborative research and bring diverse perspectives to the field. Close ties with industry partners enable the researchers to meet today's technological development needs. The research scope of the Colorado School of Mines includes the following:

- Proton-conducting ceramic fuel cells and electrolyzers
- Solid-oxide fuel cell (SOFC) development and testing

- Fuel processing
- Modeling and simulation
- Advanced materials processing and evaluation
- Manufacturing technology development
- Systems integration

It is of particular interest that "systems integration" is included in the scope of research at the Colorado School of Mines. Systems integration happens to be a cornerstone of the approach recommended in this book through the application of the trademarked DEJI Systems Model, which is covered in Chapter 3.

The Colorado example is just one of the multitude of efforts going on around the world, either small or large. For example, the lomi.com website has a "trash-to-treasure" program that aims to address environmental issues by solving daily food waste problems, thus making ordinary families a part of the global teams of planet-conscious citizens. Lomi's participative approach suggests a role for everyone, both children and adults, in reducing food waste footprint, converting household waste to useful garden energy, using technology to divert organic waste from undesirable landfills, and so on. That is the essence of a systems approach to solving complex problems. Hendrickson et al. (2006) present a systems assessment framework for the environmental life cycle of goods and services. Their presentation aligns with the theme of this book on using systems engineering to reengineer our actions and impacts on the environment.

22.5 SYSTEMS APPROACH TO EMERGENCY RESPONSE

Systems engineering involves the recognition, appreciation, and integration of all aspects of an organization or facility. A system is defined as a collection of interrelated elements working together in synergy to produce a composite output that is greater than the sum of the individual outputs of the components. A systems view of a process facilitates a comprehensive inclusion of all the factors involved in the process. Blanchard and Fabrycky (2006) emphasize that systems are as pervasive as the universe in which they exist. Basically, systems engineering inculcates systems science and engineering into the problem-solving domain. The systems engineering approach (Badiru, 2014) facilitates the inclusion of all pertinent elements from a technical linkage perspective. It leverages the conventional engineering problem-solving methodology, as summarized here. The typical eight-step process for engineering problem-solving approach consists of the following:

Step 1: Gather data and information pertinent to the problem.
Step 2: Develop an explicit problem statement.
Step 3: Identify what is known and unknown.
Step 4: Specify assumptions and circumstances.
Step 5: Develop schematic representations and drawings of inputs and outputs.
Step 6: Perform engineering analysis using equations and models as applicable.
Step 7: Compose a cogent articulation of the results.
Step 8: Perform verification, presentation, and "selling" of the result.

The steps may be tweaked, condensed, or expanded depending on the specific problem being tackled. Regardless, the steps in the framework facilitate the application of a systems-integration model. The good thing about the engineering process is that technical, social, political, economic, and managerial considerations can be factored into the solution process. The end justifies the details at hand. Systems engineering embodies the following elements:

- Economics and evaluations of the components of the system.
- Quantitative probabilistic and statistical assessment of the system components.
- Scientific and mathematical realities governing the system.
- Hard system characteristics, dealing with technical aspects.
- Soft system characteristics, dealing with human elements.

In the above context, a system is a set of interrelated components working together toward some common objective or purpose, which fits the goal of our climate change response. Systems are composed of components, attributes, and relationships as summarized below:

System components: Components are the operating parts of a system, consisting of input, process, and output. Each system component may assume a variety of values to describe a system state, as determined by some control action and one or more restrictions. The technique of state-space modeling can be applicable in this regard. Technical systems, such as electronic gadgets, consist of several intricate operating components.

System attributes: Attributes are the properties or identifiable manifestations of the components or a system. The collection of these attributes helps to characterize and describe the system. So, the system can be clearly distinguished from other systems. In some cases, similar systems may look identical on the surface, until the defining components and attributes are examined. A good example is distinguishing a male human from a female human, even though many of the defining elements are similar. The flavoring of culinary products is what can distinguish one meal item from another.

System relationships: Relationships are the links between components and attributes. Some system elements may have one-to-one correspondence. It is an understanding of the relationships between system elements that makes systems integration possible. The following considerations set the foundation for a systems approach to operational challenges:

The properties and behavior of each component of the set have an effect on the properties and behavior of the set as a whole.

The properties and behavior of each component of the set depend on the properties and behavior of at least one other component in the set.
Each possible subset of components satisfies the two considerations listed above, and the components cannot be divided into independent subsets.

As a complement to the above discussions, systems are embedded in the principles and practice of industrial engineering, as illustrated in the definition of *industrial engineering* below:

> *Industrial engineering is concerned with the design, installation, and improvement of integrated systems of people, materials, information, equipment, and energy by drawing upon specialized knowledge and skills in the mathematical, physical, and social sciences, together with the principles and methods of engineering analysis and design to specify, predict, and evaluate the results to be obtained from such systems.*

The integrative process of industrial and systems engineering creates a sort of "topping out" of a project. Topping out is the term used in construction to indicate the final piece of steel being hoisted into place on a building, bridge, or other large structure. At the topping-out point, the project is not complete, but it has reached its maximum height and peripheral construction still has to continue. In this context of climate change, it means that we are instituting a systems engineering approach that tops out, forming the platform for continuing the other related efforts. A systems engineering approach provides workable intersections of engineering, technology, science, mathematical modeling, ethics, socio-economic considerations, and legal implications.

The industrial and systems engineering (Badiru 2014) approaches use a variety of tools, techniques, models, principles, and methodologies, many of which are covered in this book. Nasr (2023) highlights the importance of taking urgent action regarding responses to climate change. Despite several attempts by COPs (Conference of the Parties), including COP27 in Egypt (November 2022), many key agreements are still languishing in implementation. Industrial and systems engineering approaches can help in this regard. As an upfront summary, Table 22.1 presents selected tools and techniques from industrial and systems engineering that can be brought to bear on environmental sustainability and climate change challenges. Obviously, users can add to the list as opportunities develop and new tools emerge.

22.5.1 System of Systems

In the context of applying systems engineering to climate change response, the definition of a system is not complete unless we consider its position within the hierarchical structure of the overall systems that make up the environment. Every system is made up of components, and any component can be broken down into smaller components. If two hierarchical levels are involved in a given system, the lower-level hierarchy is referred to as a subsystem. In any environmental sustainability or

TABLE 22.1
Selected Tools and Techniques of Industrial and Systems Engineering

Process Management Tools	
• Affinity Diagram	• DEJI Systems Model
• Benchmarking	• Flowchart
• Block Diagram	• Graph
• Brainstorming	• Interview
• Cause and Effect Diagram	• Multivoting
• Cause and Effect	• Nominal Group Technique
• Force Field Analysis	• Pareto Diagram
• Control Chart	• Q-MAP
• Customer Needs Analysis	• Survey
• Customer/Supplier Questionnaire	• Tree Diagram
Process Improvement Tools	
• Action Plan	• Flowchart
• Block Diagram	• Graphs
• Brainstorming	• Histogram
• Cause and Effect Diagram	• Interview
• Cause and Effect Analysis	• Multivoting
• Control Chart	• Nominal Group Technique
• Customer Needs Analysis	• Pareto Diagram
• Customer/Supplier Modeling	• Problem Definition Checklist
• Customer/Supplier Questionnaire	• Process Map
• Data Collection Form	• Survey
• Decision Matrix	• Theory of Constraints
• DMAIC, SIPOC, PDCA, etc.	• Triple C Model

climate change scenario, it is important to define the system under consideration by specifying its limits, boundaries, constraints, and scope. Everything located outside the system is considered the external environment of the system. We should, however, note that no system is completely closed and isolated from its environment. Material, energy, information, and/or influence (soft or hard) must often pass back and forth through the system boundaries. The level of granularity defined for a system will determine the level of control that can be exercised on the system from external or internal sources. The term SoS (system of systems) has emerged as an effective way of managing complex systems. For the purpose of this book, climate change consists of a multitude of systems, subsystems, and systems of systems. NASA (2007) presents several examples of system of systems related to research and development in space exploration. In exploring system of systems characteristics, some of the attributes of interest include security, reliability, accessibility, safety, agility, and adaptability.

22.5.2 Preemption Is Better than Correction

Systems engineering provides an opportunity to practice the concept of "preemption is better than correction" in a manner similar to the proverbial saying that prevention is better than a cure. If we can preempt an adverse impact on the environment in the first place, we can contribute positively to preserving our planet. Every little damage adds up to decimating the overall environment. A case example is the hazardous train derailment in East Palestine, Ohio, February 3, 2023. The train derailment and subsequent spill of thousands of gallons of chemicals into the land and water near East Palestine led to fears among its residents that the crash may affect their health. The Norfolk Southern train had about 150 cars, of which 20 were carrying hazardous materials. The crash resulted in a fire that burned chemicals in derailed the train cars. Initial assessment was that the accident could have been prevented. Only time will tell the extent and duration of the adverse environmental impact of the train accident. Typical fallouts from such scenarios include political insinuations and accusations. Disastrous impacts on the environment can happen due to a variety of causes, including the following:

- Catastrophic weather event
- Incompetence
- Mismanagement
- Sabotage
- Mischief
- Terrorism
- Deliberate act
- Negligence
- Distraction
- Natural accident

A priori systems engineering approaches can help with preemptive processes and actions to prevent disasters or mitigate the adverse impacts.

22.6 DYNAMICS OF CLIMATE CHANGE

No matter what we believe and conjecture about climate change, the reality is that something feels different in the human experience over the preceding centuries in the history of our Earth. From a personal perspective, growing up in Lagos, Nigeria, in the 1950s, 1960s, and 1970s, I can tell the difference in environmental temperature, as I can feel it. To put things in a general perspective, I recall a narrative analogy presented by the "Ask Marilyn" column in *Parade* magazine some years ago. The question addressed was about the importance of human history. The columnist's response was that the chronicle of historical events teaches us, bit by bit by bit, about civilization, human nature, human actions, and their implications and consequences. We were told to imagine two men after a centuries-long journey in time: One was asleep all the way; the other was awake throughout the journey. The one who stayed awake witnessed and experienced every catastrophe that occurred and every success that happened. He learned where triumphs occurred and how to leverage them. He saw where and how evil developed and how to avoid it. He learned the differences between good and evil. He knew what to avoid and what to embrace. By comparison, the somnolent man has no idea what has transpired and has no basis for a comparative analysis of before and after. Which of these two men should we select as our leader? Only historical accounts can guide us toward the better decision. Do we want the man who saw everything or the man who saw nothing? Thus, the physics of climate change can embody both the physical aspects of change and the sociological aspects of our experiences and reactions.

The consensus is that human activities are responsible for climate change. For billions of years, the elements of the world had co-existed in a mutual balance, precarious as it might have been. With more and more human activities generating more and more carbon into the atmosphere, the precarious world atmospheric balance is being assaulted and disrupted. Unfortunately, the reality of life is that humans burn fossil fuels, which generates environmentally adverse increases of carbon in the atmosphere. Global warming is one immediate notice of a changing climate around us. We are all experiencing more extreme and more frequent weather patterns, manifested in harsh winds, massive flooding, extreme temperatures, unusual cold spells, uncontrollable raging fires, and so on. The delicate balance of our environment is being disrupted before our eyes, above our heads, and below our feet. Figure 22.1

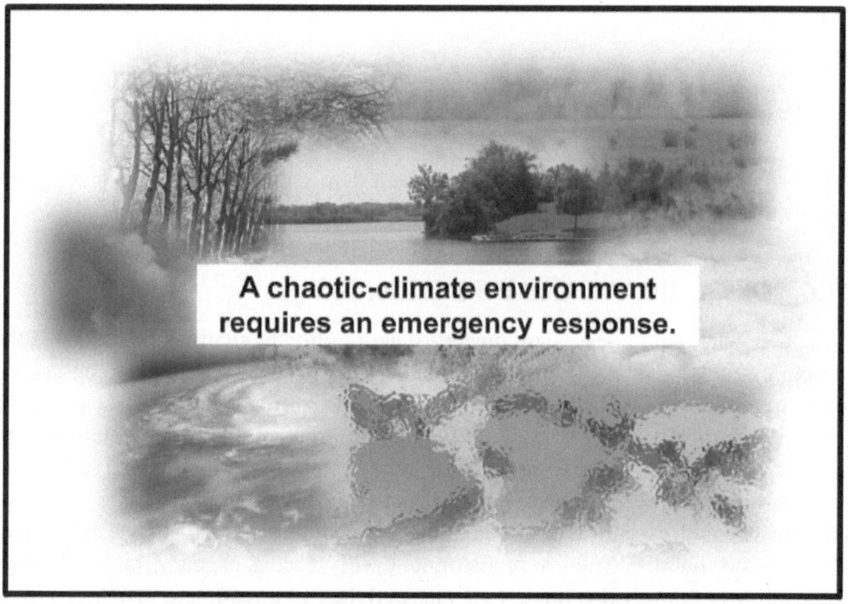

FIGURE 22.1 A turbulent mix of land, sea, and air disasters necessitating emergency response

illustrates the precarious enmeshment of components of environmental components leading to the need for emergency responses.

22.6.1 Beyond Rhetoric

As a young climate activist said (Thunberg 2021), it seems that the world leaders are engaging in more blah, blah, blah, and more blah, blah, blah, all over again, with no real actions. Sustainable world actions have been few and far between, prompting the activist to characterize world actions as just more blah, blah, blah. What do we need to do collectively to remediate the recurrence of blah, blah, blah? The approach of this book is to bring the tools and techniques of industrial and systems engineering to bear on the problems of climate change. We often tend to limit our understanding and actions to the scientific frameworks of addressing climate change. However, this book suggests a broader, systems-based approach that encompasses humans, processes, tools, technologies, and science.

In the context of systems engineering coverage, Figure 22.2 suggests a comprehensive systems-based framework of research, policy, and education as the launch pad for the diverse actions needed to address climate change. A climate resolution will not happen in one fell swoop. We must continue to chip away at the problem gradually, with each action feeding into additional complementary actions. Education is

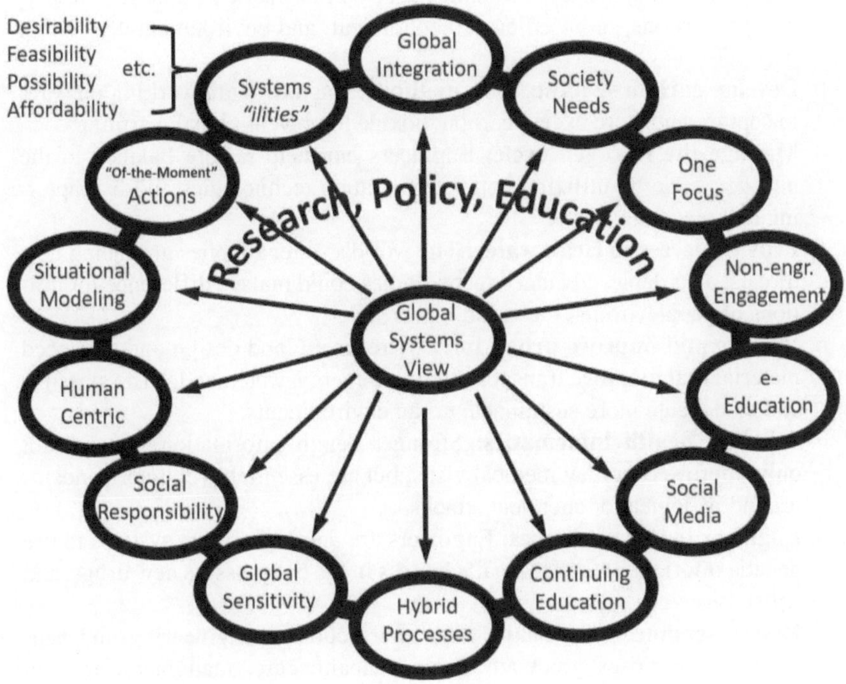

FIGURE 22.2 Systems view of climate change impacts

a strong element of the systems engineering approach because it can foster a better understanding of what is going on and what individual actions are required.

22.6.2 Our Climate as a System

A system is a collection of interrelated subsystems whose collective output is greater than the sum of the outputs of the subsystems. In the context of the theme of this book, that output is the climate. A world system affects all of us in all corners of the world, which points to the need for systems engineering. We must address climate change from a world-systems perspective.

22.7 PLATFORM FOR EMERGENCY ACTION

In 2008, the US National Academy of Engineering released the 14 Grand Challenges for Engineering (NAE, 2008). Several of the topics covered by the challenges have environmental and climate implications. The list provided below paves the way for considering several broad aspects that affect us, our environment, and our planet.

1. **Make solar energy economical:** Solar energy provides less than 1% of the world's total energy, but it has the potential to provide much, much more.
2. **Provide energy from fusion:** Human-engineered fusion has been demonstrated on a small scale. The challenge is to scale up the process to commercial proportions, in an efficient, economical, and environmentally benign way.
3. **Develop carbon sequestration methods:** Engineers are working on ways to capture and store excess carbon dioxide to prevent global warming.
4. **Manage the nitrogen cycle:** Engineers can help restore balance to the nitrogen cycle by utilizing better fertilization technologies and by capturing and recycling waste.
5. **Provide access to clean water:** The world's water supplies are facing new threats; affordable, advanced technologies could make a difference for millions of people around the world.
6. **Restore and improve urban infrastructure:** Good design and advanced materials can improve transportation and energy, water, and waste systems, and also create more sustainable urban environments.
7. **Advance health informatics:** Stronger health information systems not only improve everyday medical visits, but are essential to counter pandemics and biological or chemical attacks.
8. **Engineer better medicines:** Engineers are developing new systems to use genetic information, sense small changes in the body, assess new drugs, and deliver vaccines.
9. **Reverse-engineer the brain:** The intersection of engineering and neuroscience promises great advances in health care, manufacturing, and communication.

10. **Prevent nuclear terror:** The need for technologies to prevent and respond to a nuclear attack is growing.
11. **Secure cyberspace:** It's more than preventing identity theft. Critical systems in banking, national security, and physical infrastructure may be at risk.
12. **Enhance virtual reality:** True virtual reality creates the illusion of actually being in a different space. It can be used for training, treatment, and communication.
13. **Advance personalized learning:** Instruction can be individualized based on learning styles, speeds, and interests to make learning more reliable.
14. **Engineer the tools of scientific discovery:** In the century ahead, engineers will continue to partner with scientists in the great quest to understand many unanswered questions of nature.

Many of the topics are intertwined. If we make solar energy economical, we can lessen the need to use fossil fuels, thereby lessening the pressure on the environment. Ditto if we make energy available through fusion. If we succeed in developing carbon sequestration methods, we can contribute to the remediation of global warming. If we can manage the nitrogen cycle effectively, we can move toward restoring the balance of critical environmental ingredients. If we provide clean water to more of our population, we can impede environmentally damaging acts to obtain drinking water. If we improve urban infrastructure, we can slow down the decaying impacts of building materials that decimate the environment with respect to transportation movements, energy consumption, waste generation, and waste disposal. If we advance health informatics, we create opportunities for cleaner living for humans, thus reducing the chances for the occurrence and spread of pandemics. If we can engineer better medicines, we can facilitate a healthier society that is less susceptible to adverse genetics. If we can reverse-engineer the brain, we can strengthen the intersection of human existence and the advancement of society. If we can prevent nuclear terror, we lessen the risk of environmental disaster from nuclear war. If we can secure cyberspace, we can create a more responsible society that is less subject to damaging acts on critical infrastructure. If we can enhance virtual reality, we can better simulate what the future portends for the purpose of creating preventive actions. If we can advance personalized learning, we can expand knowledge and belief in how the environment is impacted by human actions. If we can engineer dependable tools of scientific discovery, we can dig deeper into the interplay of social, economic, scientific, and technological assets affecting the environment. The efficacy of using a systems approach to positively influence our planet is that, if we all work together, each of us will have less work to do. That is, little contributions from many people translate to a large contribution by all. If we want to go far, we must go together, from a systems engineering perspective.

As NAE (2008) reminds us, throughout human history, engineering has driven the advance of civilization. From the metallurgists who ended the Stone Age to the shipbuilders who united the world's peoples through travel and trade, the past has witnessed many marvels of engineering prowess. As civilization grew, it was nourished and enhanced with the help of increasingly sophisticated tools for agriculture, technologies for producing textiles, and inventions transforming human interaction and communication. Inventions such as the mechanical clock and the printing press irrevocably changed civilization (NAE, 2008). In the modern era, the Industrial Revolution brought engineering's influence to many parts of human endeavors (Badiru and Omitaomu, 2023). Machines supplemented and replaced human labor for many production activities. Improved systems for sanitation enhanced human health. The steam engine facilitated transportation and supply chains. New energy-generating techniques provided benefits for factories to increase manufacturing yield and improve product quality.

Under the purview of NAE's 14 grand challenges, topics of urgent interest include research, policy, education, communication, cooperation, collaboration, and coordination, from a systems viewpoint. Figure 22.3 presents the comprehensive span of strategic and multi-faceted actions needed to address climate change problems.

There is potential for collaborative actions in every topic covered by the possible roles of engineers and the methodology of systems engineering in addressing the requirements of NAE's grand challenges, as listed below.

1. **Advance Personalized Learning**

A growing appreciation of individual preferences and aptitudes has led toward more "personalized learning," in which instruction is tailored to a student's individual needs. Given the diversity of individual preferences and the complexity of each

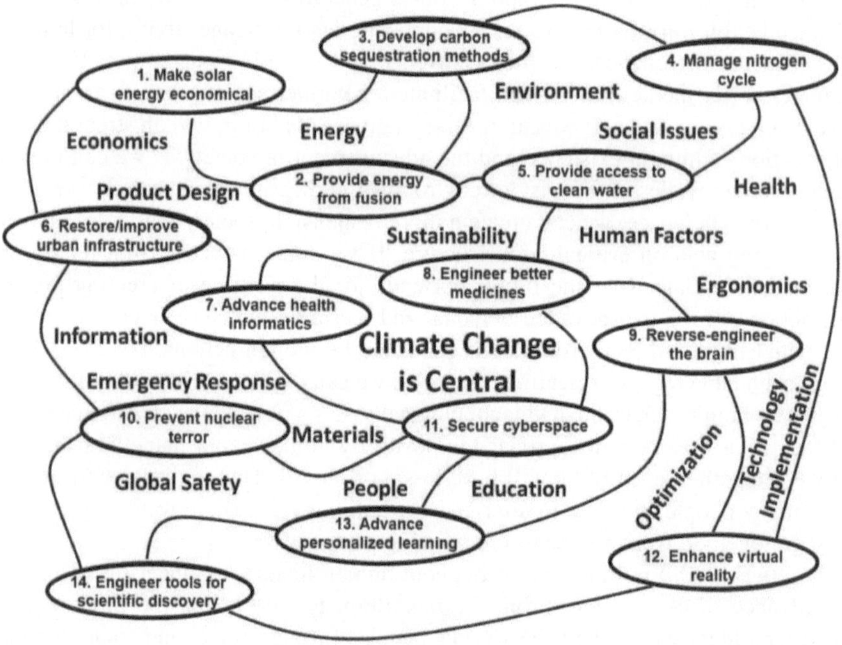

FIGURE 22.3 Environmental systems integration for emergency response

human brain, developing teaching methods that optimize learning will require engineering solutions of the future. The emergence of COVID-19 has made this topic even more relevant and urgent due to the need to embrace remote learning.

2. **Make Solar Energy Economical**

As of 2008, when the list was first published, solar energy provided less than 1% of the world's total energy, but it has the potential to provide much, much more. There has been some increase in the percentage of solar usage, but there is room for more. We need to continue our systems-driven efforts in this endeavor.

3. **Enhance Virtual Reality**

Within many specialized fields, from psychiatry to education, virtual reality is becoming a powerful new tool for training practitioners and treating patients, in addition to its growing use in various forms of entertainment. Mixed-mode simulation of production systems has been practiced by industrial engineers for decades. The same operational wherewithal can be applied to enhancing virtual reality in the context of the new world order in business, industry, academia, and government.

4. **Reverse-Engineer the Brain**

A lot of research has been focused on creating thinking machines – computers capable of emulating human intelligence; however, reverse-engineering the brain could have multiple impacts that go far beyond artificial intelligence and will promise great advances in health care, manufacturing, and communication. The same technical principles of reverse engineering, which business and industry already use, can be applied to human anatomy and physiological challenges.

5. **Engineer Better Medicines**

Engineering can enable the development of new systems to use genetic information, sense small changes in the body, assess new drugs, and deliver vaccines to provide health care directly tailored to each person. The furious worldwide search for a vaccine for COVID-19 comes to mind in this regard. We need ways to engineer and develop better medicines quickly, effectively, and efficiently. Such a process is the bastion of industrial engineers, who can work with a diverse collection of scientists to expedite and secure production processes. Industrial engineering tools, such as lean production and Six Sigma, are very much needed for engineering better medicines.

6. **Advance Health Informatics**

As computers have become available for all aspects of human endeavors, there is now a consensus that a systematic approach to health informatics – the acquisition, management, and use of information in health – can greatly enhance the quality and efficiency of medical care and the response to widespread public health emergencies.

The rapid emergence of new disciplines in data analytics and data science is in line with this stated area of need included in the 14 grand challenges.

7. **Restore and Improve Urban Infrastructure**

Infrastructure is the combination of fundamental systems that support a community, region, or country. Society faces the formidable challenge of modernizing the fundamental structures that will support our civilization in the centuries ahead. Industrial engineers have facility design and urban infrastructure planning in their skill set. Thus, there is an alignment between this area of urgent need and the ready capabilities of industrial engineers.

8. **Secure Cyberspace**

Computer systems are involved in the management of almost all areas of our lives, from electronic communications and data systems to controlling traffic lights to routing airplanes. It is clear that engineering needs to develop innovations to address a long list of cybersecurity priorities. The increasing threat to cyberspace and the risk of unexpected hacking and unauthorized data incursion have made it imperative to expedite research and development in cyberspace security.

9. **Provide Access to Clean Water**

The world's water supplies are facing new threats; affordable, advanced technologies could make a difference for millions of people around the world. Efficient management of resources is an area of interest and expertise for industrial engineers. Water is a resource that we often take for granted. With a systems-oriented view of all resources, industrial engineers can be instrumental in the global efforts to provide access to clean water.

10. **Provide Energy from Fusion**

Human-engineered fusion has been demonstrated on a small scale. The challenge is to scale up the process to commercial proportions, in an efficient, economical, and environmentally benign way. This is a highly technical area of pursuit. But it is still an area that can benefit from better managerial policies and procedures from the perspectives of industrial and systems engineering. No matter how technically astute a system might be, it will still need good policies and collaborative governance. This is something that industrial engineers can contribute to in the pursuit of providing energy from alternate sources.

11. **Prevent Nuclear Terror**

The need for technologies to prevent and respond to a nuclear attack is growing. The threat of a nuclear attack is always human-driven. The more we can understand how the other side thinks and operates, the better our handle on how to prevent nuclear terror. The human-focused practice of industrial engineering may have something to offer with respect to understanding human behavior, reactions, and tendencies. Both preparation and prevention are essential in the endeavor to better leverage nuclear capabilities while limiting the chances for terror.

12. **Manage the Nitrogen Cycle**

Engineers can help restore balance to the nitrogen cycle with better fertilization technologies and by capturing and recycling waste. Managing the nitrogen cycle requires management from the standpoint of technical requirements and human sensitivities. The reuse, recover, and recycle programs that industrial engineers often participate in can be applied to this topic.

13. **Develop Carbon Sequestration Methods**

Engineers are working on ways to capture and store excess carbon dioxide to prevent global warming. Industrial engineers already work within the domain of designing efficient storage systems, whether for physical industrial assets or non-physical resources. It is all about the strategic placement of things, while considering the systems influences coming from other things.

14. **Engineer the Tools of Scientific Discovery**

In the century ahead, engineers will continue to partner with scientists in the great quest to understand many unanswered questions of nature. The toolbox of industrial engineers contains what it takes to advance and leverage the tools and processes for scientific discovery.

Our society will be tackling these grand challenges for the foreseeable future. Project management is one avenue through which we can ensure that the desired products, services, and results can be achieved. With the positive outcomes of these projects achieved, we can improve the quality of life for everyone, and our entire world can benefit positively. In the context of tackling the grand challenges as system-based projects, some of the critical issues to address are:

- Strategic implementation plans
- Strategic communication
- Knowledge management
- Evolution of virtual operating environment
- Structural analysis of projects
- Analysis of integrative functional areas
- Project concept mapping
- Prudent application of technology
- Scientific control
- Engineering research and development

TABLE 22.2
Climate Change Research Needs and Opportunities for 2022–2031

Areas of Focus	Systems Studies
Systems	**Natural Systems:** physical climate system and ecosystems; dynamics governed by biophysical and/or physical processes. **Human Systems:** systems managed by people to meet specific needs of society; dynamics governed by human actions. **Coupled Human-Natural Systems:** systems with interconnected, interdependent, and complex interactions among human systems, the physical climate system, and ecosystems.
Risks	**Risks:** the potential for adverse consequences for human or natural systems from exposure to hazards. **Integrated Risks:** risks to coupled human-natural systems.
Risk Management Approaches	**Management Approaches:** strategies to minimize risks to systems; include mitigation, adaptation, and strategies that combine them. **Integrated Risk Management Approaches:** address risks to human and natural systems, as well as synergies and tradeoffs, to increase the security of the integrated system.

Much research remains to be done. Research must be followed by sustainable development. A recent NAS (2021) report presents a summary of the climate change research needs and opportunities for 2022 to 2031. A systems view of energy security is a focused item on the research agenda highlighted in the consensus report. The other key items addressed in the report are summarized in Table 22.2.

22.8 THE ESSENCE OF SYSTEMS INTEGRATION

We must integrate all the elements of a project on the basis of alignment of functional goals. Systems overlap for integration purposes can conceptually be represented as projection integrals by considering areas bounded by the common elements of subsystems. Multi-disciplinary education is essential in grasping the integrated concepts and principles that exist among the elements of the 14 grand challenges for engineering.

In response to a need to actualize NAE's 14 grand challenges in the context of engineering education, Badiru (2013) and Badiru (2015) present Badiru's 15 grand strategies for global engineering education on climate change. The elements of his strategies are summarized below:

1. Systems view of the world in educational delivery modes and methods in order to leverage unique learning opportunities around the world.
2. Pursuit of integration and symbiosis of global academic programs. Through global educational system integration, we can move toward a mutually

assured advancement of engineering education. Think global, but educate locally to fit domestic needs. Language diversity, for example, can expand thought and understanding to facilitate global communication, cooperation, and coordination.

3. Linking engineering education to the present and future needs of society rather than just a means to better employment.
4. Commitment to embracing all engineering disciplines in a collaborative, one-focus alliance to address societal challenges.
5. Engagement of non-engineering disciplines, such as management and the humanities, in addressing high-value societal problems collectively. There are now medical humanities programs. Consider incorporating humanities programs into engineering to put a human face on engineering solutions.
6. Adoption and adaptation of e-education to facilitate blended learning modes, flexibility of learning, and diversity of thought in a fast-paced society. Of interest in this regard is the evolution of measurement scales for pedagogy and andragogy.
7. Leveraging of social media tools and techniques to facilitate serious and rigorous transmission of knowledge.
8. Extension of formal engineering education to encompass continuing engineering education and sustainability of learning.
9. Creation of hybrid method of teaching what is researched and researching what is taught.
10. Inculcation of global sensitivity into engineering education programs.
11. Inclusion of social responsibility in engineering education, research, and practice.
12. Making engineering solutions more human-centric solutions. Use engineering to solve real human problems. Keep engineering education relevant to the needs of society.
13. Teaching representational modeling in engineering education. Modeling can provide historical connectivity to recognize the present as an output of the past and a pathway for the future.
14. Teaching "of-the-moment creativity" to spur innovation for the current, prevailing, and attendant problem.
15. Introduction of engineering solution "ilities" covering feasibility, sustainability, viability, and desirability of engineering solution approaches.

Badiru (2014, 2019a, 2019b, 2020, 2023) presents the various tools and techniques of industrial and systems engineering for accomplishing the strategic elements outlined above. Some of these are addressed fully in subsequent chapters of this book. Education is the avenue through which the goals and objectives of the 14 grand challenges can be realized. It could be education in terms of preparing future engineers or education in the form of raising the awareness of members of society. Table 22.3 presents a taxonomy of education implications of the 14 grand challenges.

Energy, in its various forms, appears to be a common theme in many of the 14 grand challenges. In addition to teaching the technical and analytical topics related

TABLE 22.3
Taxonomical Analysis of Research, Education, and Practice Alignment in NAE's Grand Challenges

NAE's 14 Grand Challenges	Research Topics	Education Topics	Practice Topics
2. Make solar energy economical	Strategic investments	Engineering economics	Portfolio management
3. Provide energy from fusion	Design safety	Energy management	Energy strategies
4. Develop carbon sequestration methods	Natural science analytics	Storage systems design	Global systems interfaces
5. Manage the nitrogen cycle	System planning	Systems optimization	Environmental science
6. Provide access to clean water	Environmental science	Water resource engineering	Water management and remediation
7. Restore and improve urban infrastructure	Resilience engineering	Construction management	Infrastructure design
8. Advance health informatics	Health systems engineering	Computer science and bioinformatics	Health informatics
9. Engineer better medicines	Personalized pharmaceuticals	Biomedical engineering	Health systems engineering in medicine
10. Reverse-engineer the brain	Human factors	Cognitive psychology	Behavioral science
11. Prevent nuclear terror	Deterrent strategies	Emergency response	Social responsibility and negotiation
12. Secure cyberspace	Information resources research	Enterprise design and management	Information security
13. Enhance virtual reality	Software engineering	Software design and programming	Game design
14. Advance personalized learning	Active learner systems	Blended hybrid learning	Distance learning systems
15. Engineer the tools of scientific discovery	Product design	Scientific inquiry	Ergonomics

to energy, energy-requirement analysis must consider the social and cultural aspects involving the three primary focus areas listed below.

- **Energy Generation:** Fossil, fission, fusion, renewable, non-renewable, safety, security, energy independence.
- **Energy Distribution:** Transmission technology, hydrogen, distributed energy sources, market.
- **Energy Consumption:** Transportation, storage, product requirements, conservation, recovery, recycling.

These focus areas give us, as individuals and groups, multiple opportunities to reengineer our actions in ways that positively influence our planet, which is the premise of this book.

Climate-centric education must be delivered within the context of the proper systems. Education misapplied is education missed. A systems model that can help ensure effective design, evaluation, justification, and integration is the DEJI model (Badiru, 2019b, 2023). The model has been applied to product quality management as well as aerospace product development (Badiru, 2013) to effect the cycle of desig n-evaluation-justification-integration in the operating environment. Education is the ultimate operating environment where several subsystems must interact to bring about a successful outcome. Some unique education environments require specialized views and practices. For example, in military education systems, a hybrid credit assessment process leverages military service for advancing science, technology, engineering, and mathematics (STEM) career development. In general, every aspect of engineering education, from curriculum development to educational outcome assessment, can benefit from a structured application of a systems model. Using climate-focused curriculum development as an illustrative example, consider the following stages:

Design of curriculum: An educational curriculum must be designed to fit the current technological tools and the prevailing needs in the job market.

Evaluation of curriculum: The curriculum must be evaluated periodically to ensure that it continues to meet the identified needs of the education process.

Justification of curriculum: There should not be a de facto curriculum. Every curriculum should be evaluated and justified to ensure a continuity alignment with educational objectives.

Integration of curriculum: Each educational outcome must be integrated into the prevailing needs of the society. What is desirable and practical in one system may not be realistic in other systems. To minimize disconnect, the local environment of education must be considered when designing, evaluating, and justifying new or existing curricula. For example, the social environment, economic scenario, cultural needs, and political requirements are all essential within the systems view of global engineering education. Some of the critical issues to be brought to the forefront as a result of applying a structural model to engineering education include the following:

- Focus on learner-centered curriculum design.
- Pursuit of transformational engineering education that is aligned with the prevailing times.
- Recognition of active and passive learning modes.
- A holistic view of engineering education input and output processes.
- Essentials of teaching with the latest technology.
- Appreciation of the cultural, social, political, and economic limitations affecting engineering education in some nations.

- Governmental competence in initiating and/or supporting engineering education programs.
- Appreciation of hybrid education resources, including distance learning and online resources.
- Emergence of new engineering education standards as a result of structural design, evaluation, justification, and integration of engineering education processes.
- Encouragement of engineering education outcomes through diversity of backgrounds and views.
- Facilitation of self-motivational and self-regulated student learning.

22.9 CITIZEN ACCOUNTABILITY FOR ACTION

Demonstrating personal accountability for actions related to climate change is essential for achieving global success in positively influencing our planet. A personal commitment to sustainability is a ready approach to making a contribution. Sustainability is not just for the environment. Although environmental concern is what immediately comes to mind whenever the word "sustainability" is mentioned, there are many languages (i.e., modes) of sustainability, depending on whatever perspective is under consideration. The context determines the interpretation. Each point of reference determines how we, as individuals or groups, respond to the need for sustainability. Pursuits in green building, green engineering, clean water, climate research, energy conservation, eco-manufacturing, clean product design, lean production, and so on remind us of the foundational importance of sustainability in all we do.

Commitment to sustainability is in vogue these days, be it in the corporate world or personal pursuits. But what exactly is sustainability? Definitions of the word contain verbs, nouns, and adjectives such as "green," "clean," "maintain," "retain," "stability," "ecological balance," "natural resources," and "environment." The definition of sustainability implies the ability to sustain (and maintain) a process or object at a desirable level of utility. The concept of sustainability applies to all aspects of functional and operational requirements, embracing both technical and managerial needs. Sustainability requires methodological, scientific, and analytical rigor to make it effective for managing human activities and resources.

In the above context, sustainability is nothing more than prudent resource utilization. The profession of industrial engineering is uniquely positioned to facilitate sustainability, especially as it relates to the environment, technical resources, management processes, human interfaces, product development, and facility utilization. Industrial engineers have creative and simple solutions to complex problems. Sustainability is a complex undertaking that warrants the attention and involvement of industrial engineers. A good example of the practice of sustainability is how a marathon runner strategically expends stored energy to cover a long-distance race. Burning up energy too soon means that the marathon race will not be completed. Erratic expenditure of energy would prevent the body from reaching its peak performance during the race. Steady-state execution is a foundation for achieving sustainability in all undertakings where the decline of an asset is a concern. An example is an analysis of how much water or energy it takes to raise cattle for human consumption. Do we ever wonder about this as we delve into our favorite steaks? Probably not. Yet, this is, indeed, an issue of sustainability. For this reason, we present the following succinct definition of the role of industrial engineers in sustainability:

> *Industrial engineers make systems function better together with less waste, better quality, fewer resources, and on target with goals, objectives, and requirements.*

22.10 RESOURCE-BASED CONSCIOUSNESS

This section aligns with the theme of dedicating this book to "Aina," the Hawaiian word for "land," and its value to human existence. The often-heard debate about what constitutes sustainability can be alleviated if we adopt the context of "resource consciousness," which, in simple terms, conveys the pursuit of conservation in managing our resources. All the resources that support our objectives and goals are amenable to sustainability efforts. For example, the expansion of a manufacturing plant should consider sustainability, not only in terms of increased energy consumption but also in terms of market sustainability, intellectual property sustainability, manpower sustainability, product sustainability, and so on. The limited resources may be spread too thin to cover the increased requirements for a larger production facility. Even a local community center should consider sustainability when contemplating expansion projects, just as the local government should consider tax base sustainability when embarking on new programs. The mortgage practices that led to the housing industry bust in the US were due to financial expectations that were unsustainable. In the context of energy consumption, buying a bigger house implies a higher level of energy consumption, which ultimately undermines the goal of environmental sustainability. Similarly, a sports league that chooses to expand haphazardly will eventually face a non-sustainability dilemma. Every decision is tied back to the conservation of some resource (whether a natural or a manufactured resource), which directly links to the conventional understanding of sustainability.

22.11 SUSTAINING EMERGENCY RESPONSE

There are several moving parts in sustainability. Only a systems view can ensure that all components are factored into the overall pursuit of sustainability. A systems view of the world allows an integrated design, analysis, and execution of sustainability projects. It would not work to have one segment of the world embarking on sustainability efforts while another segment embraces practices that impede the overall achievement of sustainability. In the context of production for the global market, whether a process is repeatable or not, in a statistical sense, is an issue of sustainability. A systems-based framework allows us to plan for prudent utilization of scarce resources across all operations. Some specific areas of sustainability include the following:

- Environmental sustainability
- Operational sustainability
- Energy sustainability
- Health and welfare sustainability
- Safety and security sustainability
- Market sustainability
- Financial sustainability
- Economic sustainability
- Health sustainability
- Family sustainability
- Social sustainability

The long list of possible areas means that sustainability goes beyond environmental concerns. Every human endeavor should be planned and managed with a view toward sustainability.

Sustainability imparts value to any organizational process and product. Even though the initial investment and commitment to sustainability might appear discouraging, it is a fact that sustainability can reduce long-term costs, increase productivity, and promote the achievement of global standards. Sample questions for value sustainability are provided below:

- What is the organizational mission in relation to the desired value stream?
- Are personnel aware of where value resides in the organization?
- Will value assignment be on a team, individual, or organizational basis?
- Is the work process stable enough to support the acquisition of value?
- Can value be sustained?

22.12 HUMAN HIERARCHY OF NEEDS IN EMERGENCY RESPONSE

Sustainability is often tied to the basic needs of humans. The psychology theory of "Hierarchy of Needs" postulated by Abraham Maslow in his 1943 paper, "A Theory of Human Motivation," still governs how we respond along the dimensions of sustainability, particularly where group dynamics and organizational needs are involved. An environmentally induced disparity in the hierarchy of needs implies that we may not be able to fulfill personal and organizational responsibilities along the spectrum of sustainability. In a diverse workforce, the specific levels and structure of needs may be altered from the typical steps suggested by Maslow's Hierarchy of Needs. This calls for evaluating the needs from a multi-dimensional perspective. For example, a three-dimensional view of the hierarchy of needs can be used to coordinate personal needs with organizational needs with the objective of facilitating sustainability. People's hierarchy of basic needs will often dictate how they respond to calls for sustainability initiatives. Maslow's hierarchy of needs consists of five stages:

1. **Physiological needs:** These are the fundamental necessities of life, including food, water, housing, and clothing (i.e., survival needs). This is the level where access to money is most critical. *Sustainability applies here.*
2. **Safety needs:** These are the needs for security, stability, and freedom from physical harm (i.e., desire for a safe environment). *Sustainability applies here.*
3. **Social needs:** These are the needs for social approval, friends, love, affection, and association (i.e., desire to belong). For example, social belonging may bring about a better economic outlook, enabling each individual to be in a better position to meet his or her social needs. *Sustainability applies here.*
4. **Esteem needs:** These are the needs for accomplishment, respect, recognition, attention, and appreciation (i.e., desire to be known). *Sustainability applies here.*
5. **Self-actualization needs:** These are the needs for self-fulfillment and self-improvement (i.e., desire to arrive). This represents the stage of opportunity to grow professionally and be in a position to selflessly help others. *Sustainability applies here.*

Ultimately, the need for and commitment to sustainability boils down to each person's perception based on his or her location on the hierarchy of needs and level of awareness of sustainability. How do we explain to a hungry, poor family in an economically depressed part of the world the need to conserve forestry? Or, how do we dissuade an old-fashioned professor from the practice of making volumes of hardcopy handouts instead of using electronic distribution? Cutting down on printed materials is an issue of advancing sustainability. In each wasteful eye, "the *need* erroneously justifies the *means*" (author's variation of the common phrase). This runs counter to the principle of sustainability. We can expand the hierarchy of needs to generate a multi-dimensional view that incorporates an organizational hierarchy of needs. The location of each organization along its hierarchy of needs will determine how the organization perceives and embraces sustainability programs. Likewise, the hierarchical position of each individual will determine how he or she practices commitment to sustainability.

In an economically underserved culture, most workers will be at the basic level of physiological needs, and there may be constraints on moving from one level to the next higher level. This fact has implications for how human interfaces impact sustainability practices. In terms of the organizational hierarchy of needs, the levels are characterized as follows:

Level 1 of Organizational Needs: This refers to the organizational need for the essentials of economic vitality to support the provision of value to stockholders and employees. Can the organization fund projects from cash reserves? *Sustainability applies here.*

Level 2 of Organizational Needs: This refers to the need for organizational defense. Can the organization feel safe from external attacks? Can the organization protect itself from cyber attacks or brutal take-over attempts? *Sustainability applies here.*

Level 3 of Organizational Needs: This refers to an organization's need to belong to market alliances. Can the organization be invited to join trade groups? Does the organization have a presence on some World stage? *Sustainability applies here.*

Level 4 of Organizational Needs: This is the level of having market respect and credibility. Is the organization esteemed in some aspect of the market, economic, or technology movement? What positive thing is the organization known for? *Sustainability applies here.*

Level 5 of Organizational Needs: This is the level of being classified as a "power" in the industry of reference. Does the nation have a recognized niche in the market? *Sustainability applies here.*

Obviously, where the organization stands in its hierarchy of sustainability goals will determine how it influences its employees, as individuals, to embrace, support, and practice sustainability. How each individual responds to organizational requirements depends on that individual's own level in the hierarchy of needs. We must all recognize the factors that influence sustainability in our strategic planning programs. In order for an organization to succeed, sustainability must be expressed explicitly as a goal across organizational functions.

22.13 THE SUSTAINABILITY MATRIX

The coupling of technical assets and managerial tools is essential for realizing sustainability. This section presents an example of the *sustainability matrix* introduced by Badiru (2013). The matrix is a simple tool for organizing the relevant factors associated with sustainability. It overlays sustainability awareness factors, technical assets, and managerial tools. The sample elements illustrate the nature and span of factors associated with sustainability projects. Each organization must assess its environment, including relevant factors and issues, within the context of prevailing sustainability programs. Without a rigorous analytical framework, sustainability will merely be a matter of talk rather than action. One viable strategy is to build collaborative STEM alliances for sustainability projects. The analytical framework of systems engineering provides a tool for this purpose from an interdisciplinary perspective. With this, environmental systems, industrial systems, and societal systems can be sustainably tied together to provide win-win benefits for all. An effective collaborative structure would include researchers and practitioners from a wide variety of disciplines (civil and environmental engineering, industrial engineering, mechanical engineering, public health, business, etc.).

Project sustainability is as much a need as the traditional components of project management, spanning planning, organizing, scheduling, and control. The proactive pursuit of best sustainability practices can pave the way for project success on a global scale. In addition to people, technology, and process issues, there are project implementation issues. In terms of performance, if we need a better policy, we can develop it. If we need technological advancements, we have the capabilities to achieve them. The items that are often beyond reach relate to project lifecycle management issues. Project sustainability implies that sustainability exists in all aspects related to the project. Thus, we should always focus on project sustainability.

The vertical dimension of the matrix consists of the following *technical factors*:

- Physical infrastructure
- Work design
- Analytical modeling
- Scientific limitation
- Technology constraints

The horizontal dimension of the matrix consists of the following *managerial environmental factors*:

- Organizational behavior
- Personnel culture
- Resource base
- Market influence
- Share capital

The cells within the matrix consist of a variety of attributes, factors, and indicators, including the following: communication modes, cooperation incentives, coordination techniques, building performance, energy economics, technical acquisitions, work measurement, project design, financial implications, project control, resource combinations, qualitative risk, engineering analysis, value assessment, forecast models, fuel efficiency, technical workforce, contingency planning, contract administration, green purchases, energy conservation, training programs, quantitative risk, public acceptance, and technology risks.

Think "sustainability" in all you do, and you are bound to reap the rewards of better resource utilization, operational efficiency, and process effectiveness. Both management and technical issues must be considered in the pursuit of sustainability. People issues must be placed at the nexus of all sustainability considerations. Otherwise, sustainability itself cannot be sustained. Many organizations are adept at implementing rapid improvement events (RIE). This chapter recommends a shift from mere RIE to sustainable improvement events (SIE).

Change is the root of advancement. Sustainability requires change. Our society must be prepared for change in order to achieve sustainability. Efforts that support sustainability must be integrated into every aspect of society's activities. If society is better prepared for change, then positive changes can be achieved. The "pain but no gain" aspects of sustainability can be avoided if proper preparations have been made for societal changes. Sustainability requires an increasingly larger domestic market to preserve precious limited natural resources. The social systems that make up such markets must be carefully coordinated. The socio-economic impact on sustainability cannot be overlooked.

Social changes are necessary to support sustainability efforts. Social discipline and dedication must be instilled in society to make sustainability changes possible. The roles of the members of a society in terms of being responsible consumers and producers of consumer products must be outlined. People must be convinced of the importance of the contribution of each individual, whether that individual is acting as a consumer or as a producer. Consumers have become so choosy that they no longer will simply accept whatever is offered in the marketplace. In cases where social norms dictate that consumers behave in ways that are not conducive to sustainability, gradual changes must be facilitated. If necessary, an acquired taste must be developed to like and accept the products of local industry. To facilitate consumer acceptance, the quality of industrial products must be improved to competitive standards. In the past, consumers were expected to make do with the inherent characteristics of products, regardless of potential quality and functional limitations. This has changed drastically in recent years. For a product to satisfy the sophisticated tastes of the modern consumer, it must exhibit a high level of quality and responsiveness to the consumer's needs with respect to global expectations. Only high-quality products and services can survive the prevailing market competition and, thus, fuel the enthusiasm for further sustainability efforts. Some of the approaches for preparing a society for sustainability changes are listed below:

- Make changes in small increments.
- Highlight the benefits of sustainability development.
- Keep citizens informed of the impending changes.
- Get citizen groups involved in the decision process.
- Promote sustainability change as a transition to a better society.
- Allay fears about potential job losses due to new sustainability programs.
- Emphasize the job opportunities that can be created through sustainability investments.

Addressing the above issues means using a systems view to tackle the various challenges of executing sustainability. As has been discussed in the preceding sections, the concept of sustainability is a complex one. However, with a systems approach, it is possible to delineate some of its most basic and general characteristics. For our sustainability purposes, a system is simply defined as a set of interrelated elements (or subsystems). The elements can be molecules, organisms, machines, machine components, social groups, or even intangible abstract concepts. The relations, interlinks, or "couplings" between the elements may also have very different manifestations (e.g., economic transactions, energy flows, material exchanges, causal linkages, control pathways, etc.). All physical systems are *open* in the sense that they exchange energy, matter, and information with their environment, which is significant for their functioning. Therefore, what the system "does," in its behavior depends not only on the system itself but also on the factors, elements, or variables coming from the system's environment. The environment impacts "inputs" on the system, while the system impacts "outputs" on the environment. This, in essence, is the systems view of sustainability.

REFERENCES

Badiru, A. B. (2013), "NAE's 14 grand challenges and 2020 skills for engineers," Distinguished Keynote Address, World Congress on Engineering Education (WCEE2013), Doha, Qatar, January 7–9.

Badiru, A. B., ed. (2014), *Handbook of Industrial & Systems Engineering*, 2nd edition, Taylor & Francis/CRC Press, Boca Raton, FL.

Badiru, A. B. (2015), "A systems model for global engineering education: The 15 grand challenges," *Engineering Education Letters*, vol. 1, no. 1, p. 3, 1–14, http://dx.doi.org/10.5339/eel.2015.3.

Badiru, A. B. (2016), "A global systems view of climate change: Research, policy, and education," Presentation at the London Climate Change Conference, Westminster, London, October 25.

Badiru, A. B. (2019a), *Project Management: Systems, Principles, and Applications*, Second Edition, Taylor & Francis/CRC Press, Boca Raton, FL.

Badiru, A. B. (2019b), *Systems Engineering Models: Theory, Methods, and Applications*, Taylor & Francis/CRC Press, Boca Raton, FL.

Badiru, A. B. (2020), *Innovation: A Systems Approach*, Taylor & Francis/CRC Press, Boca Raton, FL.

Badiru, A. B. (2023), *Systems Engineering Using DEJI Systems Model: Design, Evaluation, Justification, and Integration with Case Studies and Applications*, Taylor & Francis/CRC Press, Boca Raton, FL.

Badiru, A. B., & Agustiady, T. (2021), *Sustainability: A Systems Engineering Approach to the Global Grand Challenge*, Taylor & Francis/CRC Press, Boca Raton, FL.

Badiru, A. B., & Omitaomu, O. A. (2023), *Systems 4.0: Systems Foundation for Industry 4.0*, Taylor & Francis/CRC Press, Boca Raton, FL.

Badiru, A. B., & Osisanya, S. O. (2013), *Project Management for the Oil & Gas Industry*, Taylor & Francis/CRC Press, Boca Raton, FL.

Blanchard, B. S., & Fabrycky, W. J. (2006), *Systems Engineering and Analysis*, Prentice-Hall, Upper Saddle River, NJ.

Gamble, S. (2014), "Taking the lead," *PM Network*, vol. 28, no. 10, pp. 36–37.

Hendrickson, C. T., Lave, L. B., & Matthews, H. S. (2006), *Environmental Life Cycle Assessment of Goods and Services: An Input-Output Approach*, RFF (Resources for the Future), Washington, DC.

Jones, T. (2014), The energy revolution," *PM Network*, vol. 28, no. 10, pp. 30–35.

Lathan, C. (2022), *Inventing the Future: Stories from a Techno-Optimist*, Lioncrest Publishing, Carson City, NV.

Mines Staff (2023), "Green hydrogen: Empowering the future of energy – A closer look at hydrogen's roles in the energy transition," Colorado School of Mines Research Report, Golden, CO, pp. 18–25.

NAE (2008), *NAE Grand Challenges for Engineering*, US National Academy of Engineering, The National Academies Press, Washington, DC.

NAS (2018), *Review of the Draft Fourth National Climate Assessment: Consensus Study Report*, US National Academy of Science, The National Academies Press, Washington, DC.

NAS (2021), *Global Change Research Needs and Opportunities for 2022-2031: Consensus Study Report*, US National Academy of Science, The National Academies Press, Washington, DC.

NAS & TRS (2020), *Climate Change Evidence and Causes: Update 2020 – An Overview from the Royal Society and the US National Academy of Sciences*, US National Academy of Sciences and the British Royal Society, The National Academies Press, Washington, DC.

NASA (2007), *NASA Systems Engineering Handbook*, National Aeronautical and Space Administration, NASA Headquarters, Washington, DC, December.

Nasr, N. (2023), "Another step toward climate action," *ISE Magazine*, vol. 55, no. 2, p. 24.

NRC (2010), *Verifying Greenhouse Gas Emissions: Methods to Support International Climate Agreements*, National Research Council, The National Academies Press, Washington, DC.

Sambo, A. S. (2023), "The increasing global uptake of renewable energy and the way forward for Nigeria," Presentation of the Renewable Energy Committee of the Nigerian Academy of Engineering, Abuja, Nigeria, February 21.

Thunberg, G. (2021), "Blah, blah, blah: Greta Thunberg lambasts world leaders over climate crisis," https://www.theguardian.com/environment/2021/sep/28/blah-greta-thunberg-leaders-climate-crisis-co2-emissions (accessed February 20, 2023).

23 Qualitative Impact of Climate Change, Infrastructure Integrity, Sustainability, and Environmental Degradation on Emergency Response Programs

Adedeji B. Badiru, Khalilat Usman Naibi, and Ahmed Usman Naibi

23.1 INTRODUCTION

Wagenknecht et al. (2022) presents the backdrop for this chapter. Emergency response is effective only to the extent that the affected critical infrastructure has proper integrity. Climate change agreements provide the platform over which organizations and individuals can develop effective and sustainable emergency response programs. The chapter addresses the qualitative issues related to the legal and business aspects of executing climate change agreements. The original report was specifically on COP26 (Conference of the Parties, 26th edition) (United Nations/United Kingdom government 2021), but the discussions are relevant for all future COP conventions with respect to environmental emergency response programs.

23.2 LEGAL AND REGULATORY ASPECTS OF CLIMATE CHANGE

Within the framework of international climate diplomacy, nations have committed themselves to achieving certain goals. The current US administration has pledged to cut greenhouse gas emissions by 50–52% below 2005 levels by 2030, aiming to

DOI: 10.1201/9781003648178-25

reach a 100% carbon pollution-free power sector by 2035 and achieve a net-zero economy by no later than 2050. The European Union (EU) announced its intention to cut greenhouse gas emissions by 55% below 1990 levels in 2030 and achieve a net-zero economy by no later than 2050 (European Commission 2019).

Every nation and supranational organization, such as the EU, is free to decide whether to cut greenhouse gas emissions, to what extent, and how to deliver on these goals. This is in line with the aforementioned conclusion that there are operational differences among nations, and goals need to be adapted and integrated into the prevailing local practices of the target system. Hence, it is also important to note that from a regulatory point of view, the commitments from each nation are implemented by the respective nation at its sole/own discretion.

23.3 LEGAL PROBLEM-SOLVING METHODOLOGY

Similar to the typical eight-step process for engineering problem-solving, it is common in the legislative process to also consider potential consequences prior to passing a certain regulation. In principle, there is a prerogative in favor of the legislative branch. That means the legislative power is, in principle, free to decide which measures it wants to apply in order to serve a certain matter in the public interest. Hence, measures enacted by the legislative are only subject to a limited review by the judiciary power. According to European law, for example, every measure attributed to member states and the EU itself must comply with the principle of proportionality. The principle of proportionality is used, among other things, as a logical method to balance the restrictions imposed by a certain measure with its intended aim.

The stages of the proportionality test are as follows:

- There must be a legitimate aim for a measure.
- The measure must be suitable to achieve the aim (potentially with a requirement to provide evidence that it will have that effect).
- The measure must be necessary to achieve the aim, meaning there cannot be any less onerous way of doing it.
- The measure must be reasonable, considering the competing interests of different groups at hand.

It is not just good practice to foresee any adverse effects, as the case may be, by way of applying the proportionality test. It has also become mandatory to conduct a so-called "regulatory impact analysis" in advance of a planned regulation. Such an approach aims to make measures by the State more efficient, reduce harmful effects to the absolute minimum, and consider potential alternatives. In this regard, aimed effects and unwanted disadvantages are analyzed. In the US, regulatory impact analyses are governed by guidance issued by the Office of Management and Budget (OMB) Circular A-4. Circular A-4 requires agencies to clearly identify the need for regulation and its impacts. Within the OMB, the Office of Information and Regulatory Affairs (OIRA) reviews regulatory impact analyses for transparency, utility, and objectivity. According to the aforementioned guideline, the regulatory impact analysis comprises the following assessment steps:

- Why regulation is needed.
- Consider a reasonable number of alternative regulatory approaches.
- Conduct a rigorous and objective cost-benefit analysis for each alternative.

The EU applies a similar scheme according to the so-called "integrated impact assessment." Details to such an approach are contained in different guidelines by the European Commission.

23.4 IMPLEMENTATION OF POLICIES THROUGH REGULATION

States that have pledged to decarbonize usually issue policies on how to reach their self-defined goals. In particular, the following policy tools are available in the context of decarbonization:

- Tax credits and promotion/funding of investments in new technologies, e.g.:
  - Carbon capture and storage.
  - Carbon dioxide removal.
  - Geoengineering the oceans.
  - Solar radiation management.
  - Electrification or the use of hydrogen made with renewable electricity.
  - Fusion energy.
  - Enhanced rock weathering.
- Spending on climate-smart programs and infrastructure.
- Sector-specific performance standards such as a clean electricity standard and zero emissions vehicle standard, e.g., clean car rules.
- Carbon pricing.
- Make the federal government lead by example by way of slashing government's greenhouse gas emissions faster and/or earlier.
- Impose tariff on imports from countries that contribute to climate change.
- Mandate for companies to disclose climate-related risks and opportunities.

Once the policies have been agreed upon, they need to be implemented. Usually, the implementation of policies is conducted by specific regulations. Without a sufficient legal framework (and government funding or tax incentives), there would be no investments in new technologies or actions intended to support decarbonization.

23.5 CARBON CAPTURE AND REMOVAL

The carbon budget set by nations will likely be exceeded. As a consequence, according to the United Nations Intergovernmental Panel on Climate Change (IPCC) the world cannot only rely on slashing emissions to lower the excess carbon dioxide. However, IPCC's April 2022 report also mentions that there are strategies existing according to which excess carbon can be removed from the atmosphere. Some forest-based methods refer to planting more trees. Others deal with new technologies (e.g., carbon capture and storage). According to the IPCC, such solutions are required to decarbonize and mitigate climate change. Carbon capture with carbon storage is the process in which carbon is caught from industrial emissions at their source, thus preventing them from entering the atmosphere at all. The carbon is then pumped underground for long-term storage.

Another similar technology is also being developed and called carbon dioxide (CO_2) removal. This approach aims to build large machines to extract CO_2 out of the atmosphere and store it underground. It is also referred to as vacuuming CO_2 from the sky. From a legal point of view, it is required to establish a legal framework for direct air capture and CO_2 removal in advance. Such a framework needs to address the conditions for respective activities, e.g., liability of operators for certain events and a scheme to transport and store CO_2. Otherwise, there would be no certainty as regards to the specific conditions, and as a consequence, no respective investments in new technologies.

Since carbon capture and storage, as well as CO_2 removal, are relatively expensive technologies, substantial government funding and tax incentives are required to help demonstrate them at a commercial scale in different applications in the first place. Furthermore, capturing carbon adds cost, and companies would understandably demand subsidies to cover the expenses. Besides, proposals to build a network of CO_2 pipelines might only be prepared if tax credits provide companies with a certain amount of money per metric ton for capturing and storing CO_2. Hence, it appears that entrepreneurial activity and corporate investment in carbon removal are, at least for the time being, exclusively driven by government funding and tax incentives. Another legal issue relates to the pipelines that are required to transport the captured CO_2. There is a risk that unwilling property owners do not agree that pipelines are laid out on their property. It might be disputed whether property rights and other concerns outweigh the potential benefits of the pipelines to local industry and the climate.

Usually, companies conclude agreements with landowners, entitling them to install and maintain pipelines that are designed to transport carbon captured for underground injection. If this is not feasible, a seizure of land might be conducted provided that such approach is in the public interest and a compensation is paid to the affected land owner. This has been practiced in the past for pipelines that were used for transporting oil and gas. The decisive question in this case would be whether pipelines which are supposed to transport captured CO_2 also serve a public purpose. It would then need to be assessed whether carbon capture and storage as a means to meet the nation's climate targets qualifies as "public purpose." This question might be subject to a potential future litigation case in which a landowner challenges the seizure of his or her land.

23.6 GEOENGINEERING THE OCEANS

Carbon removal is not limited to the above-described carbon capture technologies. Carbon removal can also take place by way of making use of the oceans. In 2021, the

US National Academy of Sciences released a report (NASM 2021) which describes six different approaches to how the oceans could be used to pull even more carbon dioxide out of the atmosphere:

- Nutrient fertilization
- Artificial upwelling and downwelling
- Seaweed cultivation
- Ecosystem recovery
- Ocean alkalinity enhancement
- Electrochemical processes

However, the identified techniques are still subject to further research and are far from being implemented in the near future. The rationale for this is that any harmful (side) effects on marine life needs to be excluded. This applies for any of the aforementioned measures. Another reason why none of the measures can be implemented directly is the absence of a legal framework. Similar to carbon capture and storage or CO_2 removal technologies, a legal framework is required in advance of any implementation. Even if some existing regulations on the national or international level might cover aspects of geoengineering the oceans, there is no specific regulation regarding CO_2 removal by way of using the oceans.

Regulations on carbon capture and removal technologies are likely to be set up soon, in large measure because these technologies are generally considered to have no harmful effects on the environment. However, regulations that govern the conditions of ocean-geoengineering technologies will most likely not be set up any time soon. It first needs to be assessed whether the specific technology in question is truly effective and has no harmful effects on marine life. Accordingly, it has been acknowledged in the context of the report by the National Academy of Sciences that "all techniques have multiple hurdles to overcome, ranging from feasibility to regulatory," and moving forward will require "a deeper dive on research and regulations in tandem."

23.7 SOLAR RADIATION MANAGEMENT

The term "solar radiation management" encompasses different options that aim to reduce the intensity of solar radiation so that global warming will decline accordingly. One highly disputed way of solar radiation provides for the injection of sulfur into the stratosphere. The sulfur is supposed to reflect solar radiation into space, thus cooling down the Earth. A similar effect occurs following a major volcanic eruption. This technique is also referred to as "global dimming."

Global dimming is controversial because some fear that it might create droughts in the Amazon region as well as in regions of South Asia and West Africa. Further, this approach would not remove any CO_2 at all. At present it cannot be completely ruled out that a State or a private party nonetheless starts to apply solar radiation management as it is not explicitly prohibited. Hence, some call for such explicit prohibition of any respective measures on the international level and even demand that any patent application in the context of solar radiation management shall be rejected. It can be expected that this issue will be further discussed on the international level in the framework of the United Nations.

23.8 LEGAL IMPLEMENTATION OF POLICIES

23.8.1 Reduction of the Government's Greenhouse Gas Emissions

As previously described, the US administration pledged to reach a 100% carbon pollution-free power sector by 2035 and achieve a net-zero economy by no later than 2050. It has to be noted that according to a presidential executive order (White House 2021), a special scheme applies in order to slash the US government's greenhouse gas emissions:

- By 2023: Cut greenhouse gas emissions by 65%.
- By 2027: All "light duty" government vehicles to be electric.
- By 2032: Half of all US facilities and properties to have net-zero emissions.
- By 2030: Slash government's greenhouse gas emissions by 65%; 100% carbon pollution-free electricity.
- By 2035: 100% of federally owned vehicles to be electric; Entire US electricity sector to be carbon-free.
- By 2045: All 300,000 leased or owned federal properties to have net-zero emissions.
- By 2050: Net-zero emissions from all federal operations, including contracts for goods and services.

The changes outlined in the executive order are designed to make the federal government lead by example. It has to be noted that there are no rules governing the implementation of the directive yet. However, such rules are necessary to ensure transparent and competitive procurement processes. For example, with regard to the future procurement of federally owned vehicles to be electric, the detailed conditions for this approach need to be further stipulated. Furthermore, following the completion of the rulemaking process, government staff has to be trained accordingly with regard to the application of the new procurement rules.

23.8.2 Mandate for Companies to Disclose Climate-Related Risks and Opportunities

The US Securities and Exchange Commission (SEC) recently proposed mandatory climate risk disclosure rules for certain US companies, while in the EU, companies are addressed by the proposal for a Corporate Sustainability Reporting Directive. According to the aforementioned rules by the SEC, such companies are obliged to disclose information to investors about their emissions and how they are managing risks related to climate change and future climate regulations through annual reports. The draft rules are subject to public comment, and thereafter, the final rules will be issued by the SEC.

There are critics of climate disclosures that provide that the SEC has no authority to require disclosures that are not financially material. As a consequence, the disclosure requirements might be legally challenged. The Administrative Procedure Act allows courts to vacate SEC rules that are deemed arbitrary or capricious because the agency failed to offer sufficient justification for choosing the proposal over alternatives.

However, according to the SEC, the information is financially material for shareholders, noting that "physical and transition risks from climate change can materialize in financial markets in the form of credit risk, market risk, insurance or hedging risk, operational risk, supply chain risk, reputational risk and liquidity risk." If the SEC eventually enacts the mandatory climate risk disclosure rules, companies may become targets of litigation. This is at least true for companies that are relevant contributors to climate change, are failing to manage the risks posed by climate change to their businesses, or are providing inadequate or incomplete disclosure.

23.8.3 Impose Tariffs on Imports from States that Contribute to Climate Change

Another policy is to impose tariffs on imports from states that contribute to climate change or on the imports of major energy-intensive goods (e.g., iron, steel, aluminum, cement, fossil fuels, and petrochemicals). Such a policy does not remove or reduce any CO_2 at all. However, it (indirectly) induces other countries to make more efforts in this regard. In general, tariffs are considered trade barriers and are, as such, not in line with the General Agreement on Tariffs and Trade (GATT). However, GATT Article XX contains a catalog of general exceptions to its obligations. According to GATT Article XX(b), measures "necessary to protect human, animal or plant life or health" are justified. GATT Article XX(g) covers measures "relating to the conservation of exhaustible natural resources." If a State imposes tariffs on imports from another State that contributes to climate change, it might be the case that this measure will be challenged by the exporting State. It will then be decisive whether the tariffs can be regarded as justified according to GATT Article XX(b) or (g).

23.9 ECONOMIC IMPLICATIONS OF CLIMATE CHANGE

The general economic perspective of climate change-related reflections implies two main spheres. Both can be directly derived from the COP26 achievement segments as well as from the Sixth IPCC Assessment report. The two relevant spheres of economic impacts from climate change are outlined as:

- Adoption and Protection
- Response and Mitigation

23.9.1 Adoption and Protection Sphere of Economic Impacts

On the one hand, states, their governments, societies, and private organizations across the globe have to cope with the weather and climate extremes caused by global warming. The changes in extremes, which are strengthened in their development and partially irreversible, have been observed and also physically confirmed (IPCC 2021), directly related to human influence on climate change. Since the magnitude and worldwide experience with climatic changes are expected to increase as global temperatures continue to rise, adaption, protection, and risk reduction measures are being introduced to mitigate the impact. Following the IPCC Working Group II report contribution (IPCC 2022), the vulnerability to the fall-outs of climate change is substantially dependent on the region and is reinforced by several factors such as socio-economic development, governance, and inequity, among others. Consequently, the adaption sphere is influenced by the region and its particularities.

Supporting efforts to tackle climate impacts is also an important part of the COP26 pledges, which include a surge in funding for protection measures, especially in developing countries, and adaption plans to strengthen preparedness for climatic risks. According to the World Economic Forum's Global Risks Report (2022), the results of the recent Global Risks Perception Survey reveal broad concern about environmental risks. They are among the perceived short-term risks as well as – in the long-term perspective – the perceived predominant threats and those considered the most severe and damaging to humans and ecosystems, with "climate action failure" or "extreme weather" as exemplary named forms.

Adaption to and protection from the risks of climate change have economic relevance, revealed in aspects of a wide variety of fields and sectors. Examples of economic fall-outs related to the scope of adaption to climate risks are presented below, with respect to possible economic impacts.

- A trade-off between a fast, disordered transition to green economies and decelerated, or respectively insufficient measures can be observed. With the intensification of the physical risks of climate change, the corresponding consequences for societies and economic systems gain urgency. The challenges of a divisive, disordered, and inequality-creating accelerated transition to carbon net-zero emissions within states and among states worldwide on the one hand, and the risk of slow and superficial measures to achieve substantial emissions reductions with devastating outcomes for prosperity and economic development on the other hand, illustrate the extent of the threat to global and national economies.
- Strengthening domestic preparedness for climate change risks competes with other future-focused, topical domains, as well as with the allocation of public and private investment. Government and business financial aid to boost, adapt, and protect domestic societies and economies from climate change impacts compete with measures, for example, to address pandemics, digitalization, and other future-relevant issues, alongside regular domestic government and private investment programs. The long-term perspective

of climate change adaption aggravates the political and actual feasibility of measures, especially when compared to other short- and mid-term domains of critical dimension and high public significance.

- Supply-side as well as demand-side economic shocks related to climate change impacts endanger economic growth, productivity, work force availability, and private consumption. Physical climate change threats like severe weather events and climate disasters can cause economic shocks, which can be driven by both supply and demand factors. Agricultural products and raw materials shortfalls as well as damage to production plants can heavily disrupt global and national supply chains and affect the production capabilities of economies. Property damage, business disruptions, and productivity losses represent serious threats to businesses and the broad economy. Losses of work force can be a further adverse implication in this context.
- Ruined homes and livelihoods, and the resulting monetary losses impair demand from affected households; poor income prospects as well as uncertainty, may lead to less private investments and consumption. A worsening aspect in strongly affected regions consists of potential risk surcharges on loans and insurance or reduced coverage.
- High recovery and adaption costs and substantial global gross domestic product (GDP), as well as human welfare losses with varying degrees of regional impacts, are to be expected in case of minor progress toward climate goals or absent climate action ("business-as-usual"). From the scientific perspective of the United Nations Framework Convention on Climate Change (UNFCCC) Sixth Assessment Report, limiting global warming requires curbing CO_2 emissions, reaching at least net-zero emissions (IPCC 2021). Hence, the severity of future impacts of climate change depends on global greenhouse gas emissions, and even ambitious achievements in mitigating the progress of climate change cannot prevent, but at least limit it. Global GDP impacts of climate change appear to be permanent, long-term, and worse with climate action inactivity. Accordingly, economic impacts related to adaption and protection are strongly dependent on current and future commitments to climate goals, particularly those focused on limiting global warming. The projected global GDP losses and the particular vulnerability within certain world regions, therefore, hinge on the scope of collective fulfillment to achieve carbon net-zero emissions. The COP26 Glasgow Climate Pact asks the global community to move forward with Nationally Determined Contributions (NDCs) containing ambitious emissions-reduction goals committed to reaching net-zero emissions by 2050. Examples of rising costs include dropping outputs and economic losses in adversely affected regions, such as falling productivity in the agricultural sector, infrastructure destruction, decreasing tourism activity, health hazards, and global warming with adverse effects on labor productivity. Besides lower productivity and reduced work capacity, another channel of amplifying output losses is reduced investment activity, for example due to pessimistic future expectations for ongoing operations or due to damages

to capital stock like infrastructure or equipment. Consumer spending is affected adversely in a similar way, for example, as far as worsening future expectations or damages to home infrastructure are concerned. Overall, adverse economic impacts arise through increased volatility, pressure on production, output declines, price hikes, and reduced future economic growth potential.

- The disproportionate vulnerability to and the distribution of the consequences of climate change are likely to lead to a redistribution of wealth and economic development worldwide. Adverse impacts of climate change, damages, and losses are observed to affect highly vulnerable people and systems throughout sectors and regions disproportionally (e.g., tropical or low-lying regions). Examples are climate change-related impacts like droughts or rising sea levels. Movements of benefits and losses related to climate change among countries and regions, causing a turn in comparative (dis)advantages, are supposed to be one of the consequences, potentially benefiting polar regions and disadvantaging (sub)tropical regions. This trend does not necessarily depend on the respective region's role as the main harmful emission producer; it rather depends on its particular exposure and susceptibility to the adverse physical impacts of global warming. Supply chain disruptions might economically impact trade-dependent sectors; countries and regions might be economically affected by severe weather events, natural disasters, and other events related to climate change. Import, export, world markets, global supply chains, product streams, and trade resilience, in general, will probably be affected by changes in climate-sensitive sectors and the corresponding contributing factors, attributes, and indicators. Examples can be seen in commodities or agricultural goods, but also manufactured products. The economic impact potentially rises with the level of dependence of a country, region, corporation, or organization on trade. Conversely, the severity of climate change impacts on vulnerable systems – including the national government's and domestic private sector's capacity, as well as the cost-intensity of adaption and protection measures – also play a part. In this context, the success of COP26 commitments, especially in the "Adaption," "Finance," and "Collaboration" dimensions, is particularly relevant.

23.9.2 Response and Mitigation Platform

This platform is characterized by worldwide plans, measures, and actions taken to deliver climate goals, reduce carbon dioxide emissions, and achieve net-zero emissions by 2050. The response and mitigation sphere is linked to the major commitment to keep the increase in global average temperature well below 2°C and the pledge to undertake further efforts to limit global warming to 1.5°C. The path towards climate goal achievements has been updated at the COP26 Conference in Glasgow by setting more ambitious 2030 interim goals and an elaborated global system of accordingly adjusted NDCs.

The "Mitigation" segment of the COP26 arrangements, for instance, includes decarbonization and defossilization objectives in the shape of phasing down coal power or phasing out of fossil fuel subsidies. Not only national governments are addressed by the Glasgow Pact, but, due to its importance in delivering global net-zero emissions – in the "Finance" and "Collaboration" segments of the Climate Pact – the private sector (e.g., financial institutions and businesses) is also addressed.

A recent McKinsey report classifies sectors primarily responsible for carbon dioxide and methane emissions that contribute to climate warming into seven systems: power, industry, mobility, buildings, agriculture, forestry and waste (McKinsey 2022). Presumably, most economic changes in the relevant sphere are to be expected to be directly or indirectly related to these systems. Thus, they bear particular importance in the mitigation and response sphere underway in a climate-resilient transformation. The following section outlines possible economic impacts with reference to mitigation and response measures for climate change, especially "green" transitions to limit and to reduce greenhouse gas emissions.

- The transformation process to carbon net-zero emissions is marked enormous complexity and widespread economic impacts on both global and domestic economies. According to UN experts, an immediate, rapid, extensive, decisive, and sustained approach is necessary to mitigate global warming and climate change – an assessment that formed the basis for the COP26 Glasgow Pact. Enormous investment activities are required to enable a broad transition, from both the public and the private sector, which means immense expenditure. The shift to net-zero emissions implies a historic global transformation and structural change of both global and national economies. Substantial risks include, for instance, job losses in emission-intensive industries and the fossil fuel-producing sector, stranded assets, climbing energy prices or generally shifting prices, and energy supply volatility. However, significant opportunities and promising perspectives can also be expected from a green transformation and climate-resistant development. Such opportunities could be newly created jobs, efficient defossilization processes, low-emission products, or new, sustainable technologies, such as in power generation, transport, and agriculture. The extraordinary transformation requires extensive capital spending on assets, processes, and supply chain adaptions of greenhouse gas emitting systems, an outlook that underlines the important role of the private sector in the mitigation sphere. This aspect is aligned with the systems-thinking perspective where different nuances can be factored in and become a substantial part of a process, integrating technical, social, political, economic, cultural, and managerial considerations. A certain disorder in the execution of climate transition despite common goals is to be expected: rising costs and job losses in carbon-intensive economic sectors, missed technological developments, or increasing inequality could become unintended consequences, reinforcing frictions and undermining acceptance. The economic risks of complexity may become manageable through intensive and broad cooperation. The

Working Group II contribution to the IPCC Sixth Assessment report points out that climate-resilient development is effectively promoted by inclusive governance, decisions, and actions, involving national governments, civil societies, and the private sector as well as international cooperation and partnerships with traditionally marginalized groups.

- Carbon trading and pricing are likely to become key instruments for managing climate change mitigation – they affect governments, businesses, and consumers economically. CO_2 pricing, such as taxes, transparently fixes prices typically for a certain level of CO_2. Hence, it raises prices and reduces the profitability of carbon-footprinted products and services, thereby incentivizing both CO_2-emitting systems and private consumers to shift to climate-friendly products and services. Examples include heating systems, high-emission foods, or vehicles. COP26 achievements denounce coal as the most polluting of the existing fossil fuels. Moving away from coal power, though, could reinforce certain global economic imbalances. Acknowledging that industrialized nations are by far more responsible for the climate problem could force developed economies to suspend their use of cheap fossil fuels, while encouraging continued use of inefficient fossil fuel systems in coal-dependent, developing nations. In a globalized world, this trend could lead to competitive disadvantages and distortions, especially if occurring in combination with financial burdens companies already face, such as carbon emissions trading. Carbon emissions trading corresponds to a carbon cap system, which allows transferring carbon dioxide emission "credits" to other market participants, charging over-polluters, and rewarding those who can reduce emissions below the permitted limit. Economic opportunities potentially arise from the relatively low costs to societies as a whole as well as the political feasibility, and the incentive-basing approach to stimulate market-driven climate transformation efforts. Carbon trading charges certain market participants and disadvantages, for instance, financially weak, less climate innovative, emission-intensive, or fossil fuel-dependent businesses, industries, and sectors.
- Economic shocks and dislocations can also accompany mitigation efforts. Economic shocks can not only be caused by physical impacts such as severe weather events or natural disasters. They can also be triggered by stringent low-carbon climate policies, causing disruptions and dislocations in certain carbon-intensive sectors. Fossil fuel subsidies elimination or carbon taxes are examples of response policies to mitigate climate change that could have adverse impacts on the competitiveness, economic contribution, and workforce of highly carbon-emitting sectors.
- Cross-border trade aspects linked to climate change mitigation could also include economic impacts. Implemented climate standards or requirements on products and for production, similar to safety standards for labor protection in manufacturing, have the potential to affect cross-border trade. Examples include introduced climate standards on certain products or border CO_2 taxes. Impacts of response policies to climate change on trade and

economic development in this context are complex to estimate, in general, and depend on several connected factors such as transportation costs or competitive advantages of certain sectors. Nevertheless, trade-related mitigation measures could also lead to incentives, and a "drive" in moving forward to meet emission limiting requirements. On the other hand, they carry economic risks for regions, companies and the work force facing impacts from rising costs or shrinking revenues.

- Public investments compete with private investments in a low-carbon transition. In this context, COP26 achievements are expected to have a boost effect on the efforts by the private business sector to achieve net-zero emissions. Adapted NDCs, a major part of COP26 results, tend to strengthen national ambitions to align strategies, initiatives, endeavors, and policies with the net-zero goal. In general, not only political negotiations but also impulses and pushes from the private sector towards a climate-resistant transition were an important part of the COP26 agreements (Collaboration segment). Decarbonization could be based on different, potentially imbalanced, investments – a primary government investment could crowd out private sector investments. However, reassessed business and government strategies taking into account carbon balances, increasing pressure on emitting sectors, and policies to realign with more ambitious climate action, including climate-related investments, could become significantly more important. This is why political endeavors, organizations, or businesses without an affiliated low-carbon plan could be affected adversely, for example, in terms of credit ratings, risk and insurance assessments, or attractiveness to talent. Examples are waiver of air traffic, rail, or public transport promotion measures, usage of renewable energy sources, and zero-emission duty vehicle fleets.

23.10 BASIS FOR SYSTEMS INTEGRATION

In the final analysis, all organizations are interested in the bottom line (i.e., the economic basis) of their operations. In this regard, we provide additional perspectives in this section. Evaluation is an essential part of the DEJI Systems Model, beyond the "design" phase. This stage has an engineering and technical focus, allowing the DEJI Systems Model to provide an economic evaluation of the overall system, with particular emphasis on the systems-integration requirement. The evaluation stage mainly includes the economic feasibility of the considered system within a system-of-systems approach. This stage may be supplemented or expanded by a cost-benefit analysis, adding a **utility dimension**. The so-called **cost-benefit analysis** can be used as a supplement to conventional monetary profitability calculations, especially when two or more options have almost the same characteristics and evaluation variables.

23.10.1 Cost-Benefit Analysis

Benefit can be understood as utility. For example, suppose a corporation in a critical infrastructure sector (see Figure 23.1) plans to invest in a production line connected

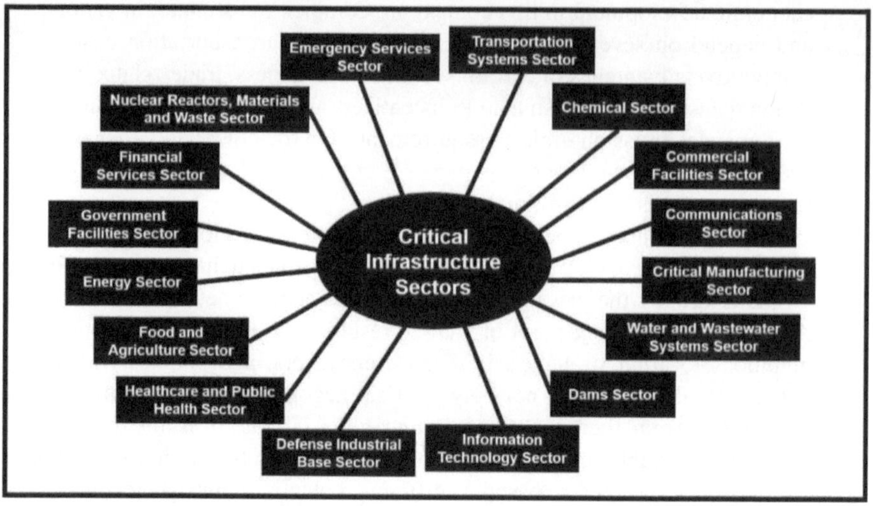

FIGURE 23.1 The 16 critical infrastructure sectors in the US (adapted from CISA 2022)

to an autonomous energy-generating and energy-providing system. The company has calculated the investment costs for three different system options, including their residual values at the end of the evaluation period. We assume that "classic" investment accounting, based on the capital-value method (Vanek et al. 2016), yields preliminary results but does not provide a clear decision, as net present values and internal rates of return are only marginally different. After carrying out the first part of the economic analysis – the investment cost perspective – the available production line systems are analyzed for their utility contributions and benefits from avoided costs. Utility modeling techniques can be used to assess the relative utilities of sub-elements in the system (Badiru and Foote 1992). Below are examples of benefits considered in our hypothetical economic assessment.

- Reduction of lead/turnaround/processing times.
- Reduction of scrap and error rate.
- Strengthening of strategic cooperations and partnerships with associated organizations.
- Improvement of delivery readiness.
- Improvement of work processes and working conditions.
- Amplification of employee skills, knowledge, and capabilities.
- Improvement of service or product quality and reduction of penalty costs related to quality.
- Enhancement of customer satisfaction and reduction of customer complaints.
- Avoidance of fossil fuels and enhancement of the use of renewable energy sources.
- Improvement of employee motivation and increasing attractiveness to talents.

- Improvements in communication and information flow.
- Improvement of the company image and reputation.
- Reduction of overtime and avoidance of extra work.
- Increased autonomy and independence from suppliers.
- Reduction of energy consumption, saving energy costs, increasing energy efficiency.
- Improvement of adherence to delivery dates.
- Reduction of internal transport routes and times.

An example of a beneficial outcome within this microeconomic perspective is the potentially positive reputation effect of an emissions-neutral and climate-conscious investment option, connected with an autonomous energy system that is based on renewable energy sources. With the aid of the cost-benefit analysis, the climate-related perspective can thus be easily integrated and evaluated within the micro-economic sphere of an organization. The expected "green" impacts can even be pertinently isolated and measured (Williams and Phillips 2011). In the hypothetical study, reinforcement of energy efficiency, raising attractiveness to the potential workforce, and greater independence are further exemplary beneficial factors regarding climate change. As outlined earlier, climate change mitigation takes hold in the microsphere of a company, among others. Hence, reassessed business strategies taking into account carbon emission balances, as well as climate-related action and investments have the potential to gain significance in this economic dimension.

In the case example, the utility of the new energy system, quantitatively measured in benefits, can be related to the investment costs of the respective production line with its connected energy system and incorporated into an extended profitability analysis – extended by the sum of total annual benefits over the period of consideration of the investment case. A major prerequisite is the requirement to convert identified benefits into a monetary value, based on comparable units (Williams and Phillips 2011). The result of the cost-benefit analysis should be, in the above-mentioned example, the deciding factor due to the similar net present values and the significant differences in benefit factors. Additionally, this approach provides a "bottom-up" microeconomic perspective on climate change mitigation, as discussed above. In the case example, we suppose Option A has the highest overall efficiency due to the leading cost-benefit relation in comparison to the competing options, hypothetically foremost regarding climate-related benefits.

Such a cost-benefit analysis can, in general, be performed for various areas of application. There are, however, several challenges to address, such as differing expectations regarding the specific benefits of measures. One further characteristic of the cost-benefit analysis is the necessity for comparable utility units among different options, requiring the most objectification and precise monetarization of the respective benefit aspects.

In almost every investment project, there are non-monetary factors that are not considered or only marginally considered in classic profitability analyses. Among other things, this approach enables us to assess an investment, system, or project more comprehensively and thoroughly. This is one of the beneficial features of the

DEJI Systems Model. It may turn out after the evaluation that a project that has the greatest advantage from a monetary point of view is not the most beneficial. A weighting, for example, which considers 80% of the results of the monetary profitability analysis and 20% of the results of the cost-benefit analysis, helps to objectify the results. This is an example of the classic Pareto distribution analysis of investment projects.

23.10.2 Macroeconomic Perspective

Due to its comprehensive character, the cost-benefit analysis serves as an appropriate procedure for the assessment of macroeconomic efficiency, for example, in evaluating government policies or law initiatives. Concerning the COP26 pledges, adapted NDCs are the means to express national contributions and actions to reduce emissions, deliver on goals, and mitigate climate change. On this macroeconomic level, the cost-benefit analysis also enables the incorporation of the beneficial outcomes of climate-related measures. Benefits are part of an extensive approach to efficiency assessment. They can be directly related to the monetary perspective on legislation and public investments and therefore supplement the wide-ranging evaluation of the impacts of measures. In contrast to the microeconomic approach described above, in this case, a macroeconomic view on measures is adopted, i.e., all positive and negative effects of the measure are taken into account, irrespective of the reason for their occurrence. Depending on the degree of detectability and the possibility of monetization, the effects which can be considered in the analysis involve:

- *Direct costs*, for example, *revenues* that can be directly determined based on available market prices. For example, investment costs of a railroad and railway station construction and permanent revenues from the use by railroad companies.
- *Indirect costs*, for example, *benefits* that can be monetarized through comparative estimates. For instance, the increased noise pollution caused by the station and the railroad traffic; the strengthening effect on the city's attractiveness to new residents and purchasing power, or the climate-related impact of emission avoidance.
- *Non-monetizable costs*, for example, *benefits* that can be evaluated through an advantage and disadvantage-illustration or a pure utility value analysis. Examples include changes to the landscape by the railroad station, or a modern construction design.

An important prerequisite for the use of cost-benefit analysis, especially to ensure comparability, is a set of specifications including the respective objectives, measure effects to be captured, the evaluation scale, etc. Monetizable costs and benefits occurring at different times have to be taken into account with their net present values (see methodology of the microeconomic perspective).

A challenge with particular regard to the involvement of climate change mitigation in the conduct of macroeconomic cost-benefit analyses is to quantify the impacts of climate-related policies. As these impacts have a temporal aspect, and furthermore, often no reliable market prices exist to evaluate them, it is necessary to connect them with the physical impact as well as the mitigation impact perspective of the relevant world region and nation. Thus, the described spheres (adaption and protection, mitigation and response) with the corresponding expected economic and environmental impacts inclusively trade-offs and side effects, are relevant for the macroeconomic cost-benefit assessment of measures. The methodology is similar to the microeconomic perspective – measurable, comparable units form the basis for a calculation of monetary climate-related factors. In addition, non-monetizable factors are also assessed on a utility value basis.

The dimension of a macroeconomic perspective on cost-benefit analyses is probably more complex than the microeconomic one. Such analyses require fundamental data sources and a clear set of specifications, as mentioned above. On the other hand, this instrument is, for instance, well suited to supporting assessments of national contributions to climate change adaption and mitigation. Its methodology enables the incorporation of change aspects in national legislation, initiatives, and policies, as well as sharpening political arguments. Examples of measurable and evaluable impacts in this context are outlined below.

- Quantified environmental damages and adverse economic impacts saved by certain protection policies and investments.
- Influence on crop yield security by measures implemented to curb physical threats from climate change.
- Corresponding avoidance of carbon dioxide emissions through a cut of fossil fuel subsidies in relation to the loss of workforce in the fossil fuel sector.
- New labor opportunities related to a carbon net-zero transition of the energy generation sector.
- Technological progress emerging through shifting to emission-reducing means of transport, waste processing and recycling, or manufacturing technologies.
- Consideration of threat-minimizing, emissions-reducing and renewable energy-producing effects in infrastructure construction and restructuring projects.
- Public profits from reinvestments of carbon revenues in return for impacts from carbon pricing and energy costs on demand and growth (Andersson et al. 2020).
- Fossil fuel energy savings from power line investments in renewable energies.

All in all, the macroeconomic cost-benefit approach allows the consideration of quantified avoided costs, prevented environmental damages, and other benefits attributable to policies, and relates economic impacts to climate change mitigation strategies. Without a pervasive quantification of benefits of domestic policy endeavors, it will become more difficult to perform a successful climate change adaption and transition to achieve climate goals, as well as to convince stakeholders and the public.

23.10.3 Life Cycle Cost Management

Life cycle cost management is a further methodology that allows incorporating economic impacts of climate change, the adaption as well as the mitigation dimension. In general, the **life cycle costing** approach is a means to estimate the entire costs of products, services or work processes. It includes and takes into account the whole life cycle of products from "cradle to grave." In the domain of business decisions, it is conducive to evaluate and to consider the total product prices comprehensively, for example, when investing in new assets for manufacturing. In this domain, many economic impacts of climate change, which directly affect the cost consideration of the respective company for the particular investment project, can be integrated. Examples are summarized below (aligned with NGFS 2021).

- Impacts of supply shocks such as raw materials, agricultural goods shortfalls, and energy prices risings.
- Investments in sustainability, defossilization, climate resilience, technological progress, emission mitigating transition as additional expenditures/further apportionment costs on products/services.
- Climate risk (physical as well as transition risks) and venture cost reconsideration.
- Additional disposal costs for environmentally harmful waste and carbon emission-intensive product removals.
- Finance costs/interest rates reconsideration: e.g., risk surcharges on insurance fees and credit costs.
- Consideration of underinsurance and lack of coverage in case of significant physical climate risks.
- Losses, damage, and depreciation in capital stock/assets according to climate change threats.
- Carbon pricing and carbon trading.
- Affecting changes in public subsidies (e.g., for fossil fuels) and government priority adaption.
- Prolonged stock holding due to supply chain disruptions.
- Cross-border trade impacts related to climate change, such as product climate standards.
- Impacts on labor force productivity and outages caused by severe weather events like heat waves.

23.10.4 ROI and EVA Dimensions

Climate change measures are, to a certain extent, comparable to regular business investments: they require financial efforts and provide benefits, mostly long-term, due to the strengthening of preparedness to tackle physical threats of climate change and the transition towards emission reduction goals. This is why climate-related investments help to avoid future economic losses on the one hand, and to develop climate-resistant economic progress, profiting from opportunities of decarbonization. Climate action measures require investments, which ideally "pay off" in a lifecycle approach by providing substantial benefits. The mathematical equation for the **return on investment** (ROI), useful in this context, is described as follows:

$$\boldsymbol{ROI} = \frac{Net\ investment\ gain\ /\ loss}{Cost\ of\ investment} \times 100$$

$$= \frac{\left(Current\ value\ of\ investment - Initial\ costs\ of\ investment\right)}{\left(Initial\ costs\ of\ investment\right)} \times 100$$

Equation 23.1

To measure, track, and compare efficiency of "green" investments, a **climate-related ROI** can be derived from the above principle to assess climate-related investment benefits:

$$\boldsymbol{Climate\text{ - }related\ ROI} = \frac{\left(Net\ Benefits\ from\ climate\ investments\ \right)}{\left(Costs\ of\ climate\ investments\right)} \times 100$$

Equation 23.2

Even though certain aspects, such as the time dimension of the investment or different types of costs, are excluded from this approach, it nevertheless provides a feasible option to assess climate investment initiatives from an economic perspective. As with the other introduced instruments, the supplementary ROI dimension also requires measurable units of gained benefits, which help translate climate change contributions into value.

A possible alternative, with a generally similar implication, methodological principle, and meaning to evaluate and compare the efficiency of climate action spending and measures, is the **economic value added** (EVA) approach. The equation for EVA can be described as follows:

$$\boldsymbol{EVA} = Net\ Operating\ Profit(After\ Taxes) - \left(Weighted\ Average\ Cost\ of\ Capital \times Capital\ Invested\right)$$

Equation 23.3

A supplementary view of the above instrument could involve net benefits gained from climate-related investments and relate them to the costs of the invested capital:

$$\boldsymbol{Climate\text{ - }related\ EVA} = Net\ benefits\ from\ climate\ investments$$
$$- \left[Cost\ of\ Capital\ Invested\ \text{´}\ Capital\ Invested\right]$$

Equation 23.4

In simple terms, climate-related EVA describes whether the value of generated benefits exceeds the cost of invested capital. This approach contributes to the comparability of climate-relevant expenses and gains across different organizations and periods. Thus, it allows, in particular, the measurement of the efficiency of investments meant to protect from and to respond to climate change. Furthermore, the EVA instrument draws on its economic origin to measure the capability to generate additional value beyond the costs of invested capital, but it is not limited to a financial view of businesses. The principle applies to a variety of cases, domains, and organizations facing and operating climate action investment cases.

23.10.5 Target Agreements

From an economic perspective, another potentially appropriate tool to deliver, manage, and break down climate goals is worth considering. COP26 agreements, pledges, commitments, and the derived NDCs could be operationalized by embedding them into target agreements and sub-targets in politics, business, financial institutions, private organizations, and administration according to the SMART principle of operations management (Specific actions, Measurable metrics, Achievable goals, Relevant plans, and Time action plan). As previously mentioned, a systems approach facilitates endeavors following the SMART principle of operations management, which is shown in Figure 23.2.

Applying the SMART principle of operations for target operationalization and tracking management within different target spheres, measured top-down, is a possible vehicle to strengthen domestic efforts toward national climate ambitions. Without an appropriate operationalization and tracking system, the most ambitious global climate goal is worthless – the "drive" created by national impulses from governments, the private sector, and societies can only accelerate if COP26 pledges

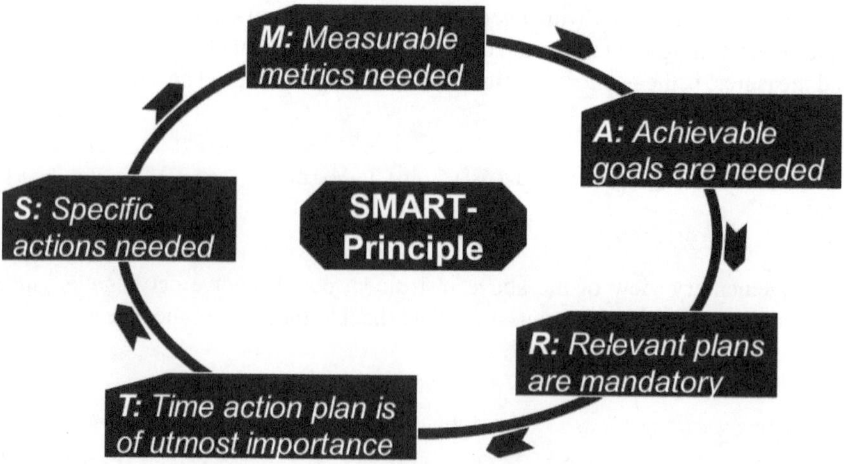

FIGURE 23.2 SMART principle of operations management

are brought to life by global stakeholders. The systems modeling view is highly relevant in this context: divergent national platforms of political, cultural, legal, financial, educational, media, and trade systems require these dissimilarities and disconnections to be appropriately addressed. Hence, the integration stage of systems modeling, considering cultural and operational differences and accompanied by accordingly operationalized climate goals, allows an effective and efficient move forward in climate change action.

Target agreements based on the SMART principle of operations can be implemented in almost every hierarchical sphere. Examples include politics (e.g., chiefs of government, secretaries, and parliamentary state secretaries), business (e.g., CEOs, COOs, heads of departments, and subsidiaries), and administration (e.g., state secretaries, heads of directorates, and heads of subordinate agencies). A highly relevant part of target agreements is an effective tracking and controlling system, embedding itself into the operations of different organizations. Moreover, incentives and consequences in cases of achievement, underfulfillment, and failure to reach goals complete a pertinent establishment of target agreement systems. The following table illustrates examples of the content of operationalized national target agreements.

- Targets on zero-emission duty vehicle fleets.
- Zero-carbon-oriented procurement goals.
- Defossilization cooperation goals (e.g., joint ventures, supplier alliances).
- Guidelines and standards for the use of renewable energy sources in manufacturing processes.
- Emission reduction goals for duty transportation and traveling (e.g., waiver of air traffic and promotion of rail and public transport).
- Training and education goals to enhance acceptance and consciousness.
- Goals on system-thinking, comprehensive cooperation with civil society, educational bodies, and scientific institutions in climate-related aspects, including marginalized groups.
- Prescriptive consideration of climate aspects in negotiations, contracting, and trade.
- Goals on emission-reducing public construction measures and government investments.
- Installed representatives or persons in charge of climate change issues within organizations.
- Prescriptive implementation into decision-making processes and consideration in guidelines.

23.10.6 Systems Efficacy

Without a systems view, we cannot be sure we are pursuing the right outputs that can be integrated into the prevailing operating environment. Thus, the DEJI Systems Model allows for a multi-dimensional analysis of climate matters, considering many of the typical "ilities" attributes related to a system-of-systems view. It focuses on specific goals of a system, considering the specifications, prevailing constraints, possible behaviors, and structure of the system, and involves a consideration of the activities required to ensure that the system's performance matches specified goals. Concretely, this means the measures and activities to fulfill global climate objectives, reaffirmed at COP26, passed through a system engineering perspective and its particular integrative process methodology on a stage-by-stage approach. The methodology contains an interdisciplinary assessment of the legal, economic, and technical nuances impinging on the viability of implementing the pledges and premises that emanated from COP26 in Glasgow, Scotland, in 2021, particularly related to the thematic dimension of critical infrastructure.

The implementation of policies regarding decarbonization is conducted through specific regulations. This is especially true for the promotion of new technologies, such as carbon capture and storage/removal and geoengineering. In addition, different aspects of administrative, civil, constitutional, and (international) trade law need to be considered when implementing further policies like adjustments of public procurement procedures, adoption of a mandate to disclose climate-related risks, and imposition of tariffs on imports. Some of the identified open questions have not yet been subject to any legal proceedings. Hence, no relevant precedent exists. This might lead to new litigation cases but also creates an opportunity to conduct further research on specific issues from a legal point of view.

All in all, there are economic risks and threats related to the transformation to carbon net-zero emissions, especially for jobs, industries, and sectors with particular emission intensity and reliance to fossil fuel. The global economic structure will certainly change significantly. However, costs and GDP losses in a business-as-usual or delayed transition scenario in which the global community fails to undertake necessary efforts to respond to climate change and deliver climate goals have the very likely potential to cause extensive adverse economic fallout and irreversible damages to human life. The COP26 Climate Pact, with its various segments, involves a promising toolbox to deal with both the adaption and mitigation spheres so that the states and their decision-makers in governments, private organizations, financial institutions, industries, and companies have been provided with an effective perspective on an ambitious pathway to curb climate change-related threats to their societies and economies. The effectiveness of decisive climate change policies is essentially supported by strong international cooperation as well as a comprehensive, collaborative approach between societies, governments, and the private sector, consistently including traditionally marginalized population groups. In addition, there are also economic opportunities with regard to climate transitions, awaiting those who respond to climate change in the framework of a "green" transformation.

In this context, the methodology of various economic techniques and tools is strongly applicable to the systems view on climate change agendas, initiatives, and policies presented in this paper. The supplementary consideration of these business aspects allows for measuring the efficiency of climate action measures and therefore involves the capability to accompany the development of protection against climatic threats and mitigation, as well as "green" transition towards carbon net-zero.

In correspondence with the systems-thinking perspective of systems engineering, different nuances consisting of technical, social, political, economic, cultural, and managerial considerations, among others, are factored into and form a substantial part of a system-of-systems view on a complex process, such as climate change adaptation and mitigation based on COP26 is.

23.11 CONCLUSIONS

Outputs of system-of-systems follow an integrative process that must be evaluated in a stage-by-stage approach. This requires research, application, and implementation strategies that consider several pertinent factors. This collaborative paper suggests the DEJI Systems Model, which has been used successfully for product development applications, as a viable methodology for system design, system evaluation, system justification, and system integration. The integrative approach of the DEJI Systems Model can facilitate the intricate and complex interrelation between climate change, COP26 Glasgow Climate Pact agreements, and critical infrastructure by application of a systems view and consideration of existing analytical tools and techniques. The systematic involvement of additional technical-engineering, legal, and economic perspectives as parts of the systems approach represents the main focus and output. The paper reveals that the climate change resilience endeavor is coherently combinable with the structured framework of systems modeling. It also stresses the alignment to the scope of practical systems implementations in business, industry, government, financial institutions, and private organizations, among others.

It is anticipated that this chapter will spark the interest of researchers in the DEJI Systems Model and emphasizes its polyvalent problem-solving applicability to multifaceted problem domains like climate change and critical infrastructure, so that collaborative research can help advance the mathematical and graphical representation of the model elements, with a special focus on the metrics of complex systems integration. It is also hoped that it will provide a pertinent platform to contribute to the climate change debate in a global context.

Such an application will expand the applicability of the DEJI Systems Model to platforms of national debates related to climate change mitigation initiatives. Hence, it can also be applied to evaluate and justify a designed politically driven national proposal, with a specific template for integration into the expectations and peculiarities of the local or regional environment.

REFERENCES

Andersson, M., Baccianti, C., & Morgan, J. (2020), *Climate Change and the Macro Economy*, Occasional Paper Series, European Central Bank, No. 243, June.

Badiru, A. B., & Foote, B. L. (1992), Utility based justification of advanced manufacturing technology. *Manufacturing Research and Technology, 14*, 189–207.

Cybersecurity & Infrastructure Security Agency (CISA) (2022), *Infrastructure security: Critical infrastructure sectors,* https://www.cisa.gov/critical-infrastructure-sectors (accessed April 14, 2022).

European Commission (2019), *A European Green Deal*, https://ec.europa.eu/info/strategy/priorities-2019-2024/european-green-deal_en (accessed May 12, 2022).

IPCC (2021), *Sixth Assessment Report, Working Group I: The Physical Science Basis; Headline Statements from the Summary for Policymakers*, August 9.

IPCC (2022), *Working Group II Contribution to the Sixth Assessment Report of the IPCC: Climate Change 2022, Impacts, Adaption and Vulnerability; Headline Statements from the Summary for Policymakers*, February 28.

McKinsey (2022), The net-zero transition: What it would cost, what it could bring, https://www.mckinsey.com/business-functions/sustainability/our-insights/the-net-zero-transition-what-it-would-cost-what-it-could-bring (accessed April 26, 2022).

National Academies of Sciences, Engineering, and Medicine (2021), *A Research Strategy for Ocean-based Carbon Dioxide Removal and Sequestration*, Washington, DC: The National Academies Press, https://doi.org/10.17226/26278.

Network for Greening the Financial System (NGFS) (2021), *Climate Scenarios for Central Banks and Supervisors*, June.

United Nations/United Kingdom Government (2021), *UN Climate Change Conference UK 2021, COP26 – The Glasgow Climate Pact,* https://ukcop26.org (accessed April 19, 2022).

Vanek, F. M., Albright, L. D., & Angenent, L. T. (2016), *Energy System Engineering: Evaluation and Implementation*, 3rd ed., New York: McGraw-Hill Education.

Wagenknecht, N., Mertens, A., Omitaomu, O., & Badiru, A. (2022), Legal and business aspects of COP26 agreements, Research Exchange Research Report, Graduate School of Engineering and Management, Air Force Institute of Technology, Wright-Patterson Air Force Base, Dayton, OH.

White House (2021), Fact sheet: Executive order catalyzing America's clean energy economy through federal sustainability, December 8, https://www.whitehouse.gov/briefing-room/statements-releases/2021/12/08/fact-sheet-president-biden-signs-executive-order-catalyzing-americas-clean-energy-economy-through-federal-sustainability/ (accessed December 8, 2022).

Williams, P. P., & Phillips, J. J. (2011), *The Green Scorecard: Measuring the Return on Investment in Sustainability Initiatives*, Boston, MA and London: Nicholas Brealey Publishing.

World Economic Forum (2022), *The Global Risks Report 2022, 17th Edition*, https://www.weforum.org/reports/global-risks-report-2022.

Index